EFFECTIVE TREATMENTS
FOR PTSD

Effective
Treatments
for PTSD

Practice Guidelines
from the International Society
for Traumatic Stress Studies

SECOND EDITION

edited by
Edna B. Foa
Terence M. Keane
Matthew J. Friedman
Judith A. Cohen

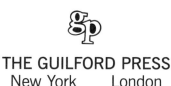

THE GUILFORD PRESS
New York   London

© 2009 The Guilford Press
A Division of Guilford Publications, Inc.
72 Spring Street, New York, NY 10012
www.guilford.com

Part IV, Treatment Guidelines, © 2009 International Society
for Traumatic Stress Studies

Printed in the United States of America

This book is printed on acid-free paper.

Last digit is print number: 9 8 7 6 5 4 3

The authors have checked with sources believed to be reliable in their efforts to provide information that is complete and generally in accord with the standards of practice that are accepted at the time of publication. However, in view of the possibility of human error or changes in medical sciences, neither the authors, nor the editors and publisher, nor any other party who has been involved in the preparation or publication of this work warrants that the information contained herein is in every respect accurate or complete, and they are not responsible for any errors or omissions or the results obtained from the use of such information. Readers are encouraged to confirm the information contained in this book with other sources.

Library of Congress Cataloging-in-Publication Data
Effective treatments for PTSD : practice guidelines from the International Society for Traumatic Stress Studies / edited by Edna B. Foa . . . [et al.].—2nd ed.
     p. ; cm.
  Includes bibliographical references and index.
  ISBN 978-1-60623-001-5 (hardcover : alk. paper)
   1. Post-traumatic stress disorder—Treatment—Standards.   2. Psychic trauma—Treatment—Standards.   3. Psychotherapy—Standards.   I. Foa, Edna B.   II. International Society for Traumatic Stress Studies.
   [DNLM: 1. Stress Disorders, Post-Traumatic—therapy—Practice Guideline.
2. Psychotherapy—methods—Practice Guideline. WM 170 E275 2009]
  RC552.P67E35 2009
  616.85′21—dc22
                                                                                    2008022316

About the Editors

Edna B. Foa, PhD, is Professor of Clinical Psychology in Psychiatry at the University of Pennsylvania, where she is also Director of the Center for the Study and Treatment of Anxiety.

Terence M. Keane, PhD, is Director of the National Center for PTSD, Behavioral Sciences Division, VA Boston Healthcare System, where he is also Associate Chief of Staff for Research and Development, and Professor and Vice Chairman of Psychiatry at Boston University School of Medicine.

Matthew J. Friedman, MD, PhD, is Executive Director of the National Center for PTSD, White River Junction VA Medical Center, and Professor of Psychiatry and Pharmacology at Dartmouth Medical School.

Judith A. Cohen, MD, is a board-certified child and adolescent psychiatrist and Medical Director of the Center for Traumatic Stress in Children and Adolescents, Department of Psychiatry, Allegheny General Hospital, Pittsburgh, Pennsylvania.

Contributors

Lisa Amaya-Jackson, MD, MPH, UCLA–Duke National Center for Child Traumatic Stress, Duke University, Durham, North Carolina

Sudie E. Back, PhD, Department of Psychiatry, Clinical Neuroscience Division, Medical University of South Carolina, Charleston, South Carolina

Victor Balaban, PhD, Travelers Health and Animal Importation Branch, Division of Global Migration and Quarantine, Centers for Disease Control and Prevention, Atlanta, Georgia

Lucy Berliner, MSW, Harborview Center for Sexual Assault and Traumatic Stress, Seattle, Washington

Jonathan I. Bisson, DM, Department of Psychological Medicine, Cardiff University, Cardiff, United Kingdom

Arthur S. Blank Jr., MD, Washington Center for Psychoanalysis, Washington, DC; Department of Psychiatry, George Washington University, Washington, DC; Department of Psychiatry, Uniformed Services University of Health Sciences, Bethesda, Maryland

Elisa Bolton, PhD, VA Medical Center, Manchester, New Hampshire

Kathleen T. Brady, MD, PhD, Department of Psychiatry, Clinical Neuroscience Division, Medical University of South Carolina, Charleston, South Carolina

Richard A. Bryant, PhD, School of Psychology, University of New South Wales, Sydney, Australia

Melissa J. Brymer, PhD, PsyD, Department of Psychiatry and Biobehavioral Sciences and UCLA/Duke University National Center for Child Traumatic Stress, University of California, Los Angeles, California

Shawn P. Cahill, PhD, Center for the Study and Treatment of Anxiety, Department of Psychiatry, University of Pennsylvania, Philadelphia, Pennsylvania

John Canterino, BA, Center for the Study and Treatment of Anxiety, Department of Psychiatry, University of Pennsylvania, Philadelphia, Pennsylvania

Etzel Cardeña, PhD, Department of Psychology, Lund University, Lund, Sweden

Linda M. Chapman, MA, San Francisco Injury Center for Research and Prevention, University of California, San Francisco, California

Judith A. Cohen, MD, Center for Traumatic Stress in Children and Adolescents, Department of Psychiatry, Allegheny General Hospital, Pittsburgh, Pennsylvania

Karen Cusack, PhD, Department of Psychiatry, University of North Carolina, Chapel Hill, North Carolina

Jonathan R. T. Davidson, MD, Department of Psychiatry and Behavioral Sciences, Duke University Medical Center, Durham, North Carolina

Esther Deblinger, PhD, Department of Psychiatry, School of Osteopathic Medicine, University of Medicine and Dentistry of New Jersey, Stratford, New Jersey

Craig L. Donnelly, MD, Department of Psychiatry, Dartmouth–Hitchcock Medical Center, Lebanon, New Hampshire

Charles Drebing, PhD, Bedford VA Medical Center, Bedford, Massachusetts

Edna B. Foa, PhD, Center for the Study and Treatment of Anxiety, Department of Psychiatry, University of Pennsylvania, Philadelphia, Pennsylvania

Victoria M. Follette, PhD, Department of Psychology, University of Nevada, Reno, Nevada

Matthew J. Friedman, MD, PhD, National Center for PTSD, Veterans Affairs Medical Center, White River Junction, Vermont, and Departments of Psychiatry and Pharmacology, Dartmouth Medical School, Hanover, New Hampshire

Linda Gantt, PhD, Intensive Trauma Therapy, Inc., Morgantown, West Virginia

Shirley M. Glynn, PhD, Greater Los Angeles Healthcare System at West Los Angeles, Los Angeles, California, and Semel Institute for Neuroscience and Human Behavior, University of California, Los Angeles, California

Robin F. Goodman, PhD, A Caring Hand, The Billy Esposito Foundation Bereavement Center, New York, New York

Amber Gray, MPH, Restorative Resources Training and Consulting, Santa Fe, New Mexico

Judith L. Herman, MD, Department of Psychiatry, Harvard Medical School, Cambridge, Massachusetts

Mardi J. Horowitz, MD, Department of Psychiatry, University of California, San Francisco, California

Chandra Ghosh Ippen, PhD, Child Trauma Research Project, University of California, San Francisco, California

Anne K. Jacobs, PhD, Clinical Child Psychology Program, University of Kansas, Lawrence, Kansas

Lisa H. Jaycox, PhD, RAND Corporation, Arlington, Virginia

David Read Johnson, PhD, Post Traumatic Stress Center, New Haven, Connecticut

Terence M. Keane, PhD, National Center for PTSD, VA Boston Healthcare System, Boston, Massachusetts, and Department of Psychiatry, Boston University, Boston, Massachusetts

Ellen Koch, PhD, Department of Psychology, Eastern Michigan University, Ypsilanti, Michigan

Janice L. Krupnick, PhD, Department of Psychiatry, Georgetown University School of Medicine, Washington, DC

Harold S. Kudler, MD, Department of Psychiatry and Behavioral Sciences, Duke University Medical Center, Durham, North Carolina, and Mental Illness, Education, and Clinical Center, Durham Veterans Affairs Medical Center, Durham, North Carolina

Mooli Lahad, PhD, Departments of Psychology and Dramatherapy, Tel Hai Academic College, Upper Galilee, Israel

Christopher M. Layne, PhD, Department of Psychiatry and Biobehavioral Sciences and UCLA/Duke University National Center for Child Traumatic Stress, University of California, Los Angeles, California

Alicia F. Lieberman, PhD, Child Trauma Research Project, University of California, San Francisco, and San Francisco General Hospital, San Francisco, California

Brett T. Litz, PhD, VA Boston Healthcare System, Boston, Massachusetts, and Department of Psychiatry, Boston University, Boston, Massachusetts

José R. Maldonado, MD, Department of Psychiatry and Behavioral Sciences, Stanford University School of Medicine, Stanford, California

Anthony P. Mannarino, PhD, Center for Traumatic Stress in Children and Adolescents and Department of Psychiatry, Allegheny General Hospital, Pittsburgh, Pennsylvania

Steven Marans, MSW, PhD, Yale Child Study Center and Department of Psychiatry, Yale University, New Haven, Connecticut

Meghan McDevitt-Murphy, PhD, Department of Psychology, University of Memphis, Memphis, Tennessee

Alexander C. McFarlane, MD, Department of Psychiatry, University of Adelaide, Woodville, Australia

Candice M. Monson, PhD, National Center for PTSD, VA Boston Healthcare System, Boston, Massachusetts, and Department of Psychiatry, Boston University, Boston, Massachusetts

Kim T. Mueser, PhD, Department of Psychiatry, New Hampshire–Dartmouth Psychiatric Research Center, Dartmouth Medical School, Concord, New Hampshire

Lisa M. Najavits, PhD, National Center for PTSD, VA Boston Healthcare System, Boston, Massachusetts, and Department of Psychiatry, Boston University, Boston, Massachusetts

Sherry Pagoto, PhD, Division of Preventive and Behavioral Medicine, Department of Medicine, University of Massachusetts Medical School, Worcester, Massachusetts

Walter Penk, PhD, ABPP, Department of Psychiatry and Behavioral Sciences, Texas A&M College of Medicine, College Station, Texas, and Central Texas VA Health Care System, College Station, Texas

Robert S. Pynoos, MD, MPH, Department of Psychiatry and Biobehavioral Sciences and UCLA/Duke University National Center for Child Traumatic Stress, University of California, Los Angeles, California

David J. Ready, PhD, Atlanta Veterans Affairs Medical Center, Decatur, Georgia, and Department of Psychiatry and Behavioral Sciences, Emory University School of Medicine, Atlanta, Georgia

Patricia A. Resick, PhD, National Center for PTSD, VA Boston Healthcare System, Boston, Massachusetts, and Department of Psychiatry, Boston University, Boston, Massachusetts

David S. Riggs, PhD, Center for Deployment Psychology, Department of Medical and Clinical Psychology, Uniformed Services University of the Health Sciences, Bethesda, Maryland

Suzanna Rose, PhD, Berkshire Healthcare NHS Foundation Trust, Berkshire, United Kingdom

Barbara Olasov Rothbaum, PhD, Trauma and Anxiety Recovery Program and Department of Psychiatry, Emory University School of Medicine, Atlanta, Georgia

Josef I. Ruzek, PhD, National Center for PTSD, VA Palo Alto Health Care System, Menlo Park, California

Donna Ryngala, PhD, Department of Psychology, University of Montana, Missoula, Montana

Paula P. Schnurr, PhD, National Center for PTSD, Veterans Affairs Medical Center, White River Junction, Vermont, and Department of Psychiatry, Dartmouth Medical School, Hanover, New Hampshire

M. Tracie Shea, PhD, VA Medical Center and Department of Psychiatry and Human Behavior, Alpert Medical School, Brown University, Providence, Rhode Island

C. Richard Spates, PhD, Anxiety Disorders Laboratory, Department of Psychology, Western Michigan University, Kalamazoo, Michigan

David Spiegel, MD, Department of Psychiatry and Behavioral Sciences, Stanford University School of Medicine, Stanford, California

Bradley D. Stein, MD, MPH, Department of Psychiatry, University of Pittsburgh School of Medicine, Pittsburgh, Pennsylvania, and RAND Corporation, Pittsburgh, Pennsylvania

Dan J. Stein, MD, Department of Psychiatry, Groote Schuur Hospital, University of Cape Town, Cape Town, South Africa

Alan M. Steinberg, PhD, Department of Psychiatry and Biobehavioral Sciences and UCLA/Duke University National Center for Child Traumatic Stress, University of California, Los Angeles, California

Onno van der Hart, PhD, Department of Clinical and Health Psychology, Utrecht University, Utrecht, The Netherlands

Eric M. Vernberg, PhD, Clinical Child Psychology Program, University of Kansas, Lawrence, Kansas

Stacey Waller, PhD, Department of Behavioral Medicine and Psychiatry, West Virginia University School of Medicine, Morgantown, West Virginia

Patricia J. Watson, PhD, National Center for PTSD, Veterans Affairs Medical Center, White River Junction, Vermont, and Department of Psychiatry, Dartmouth Medical School, Hanover, New Hampshire

Frank W. Weathers, PhD, Department of Psychology, Auburn University, Auburn, Alabama

Contents

Contents

PART IV. Treatment Guidelines

PART V. Conclusion

CHAPTER 1

Introduction

Edna B. Foa, Terence M. Keane, Matthew J. Friedman, and Judith A. Cohen

The revised treatment guidelines presented in this book were developed under the auspices of the Posttraumatic Stress Disorder (PTSD) Treatment Guidelines Task Force established by the Board of Directors of the International Society for Traumatic Stress Studies (ISTSS) in 2005. The goal was to update the first set of treatment guidelines published in 2000. As was the case in the first set of guidelines, the revised guidelines are based on an extensive review of the clinical and research literature prepared by experts in each field. The book comprises two major parts. The first comprises position papers that describe the salient literature; the second, the much briefer treatment guidelines themselves. These guidelines are intended to inform the clinician on what experts have determined to be the best practices in the treatment of individuals with a diagnosis of PTSD. PTSD is a serious psychological condition that occurs following exposure to a traumatic event. The symptoms that characterize PTSD are reliving the traumatic event or frightening elements of it; avoiding thoughts, memories, people, and places associated with the event; emotional numbing; and elevated arousal. Often accompanied by other psychological disorders, PTSD is a complex condition that can be associated with significant morbidity, disability, and impairment of life functions.

In the development of these practice guidelines, the Task Force acknowledged that traumatic experiences in some individuals can lead to the development of several different disorders, including major depression; specific phobias; disorders of extreme stress not otherwise specified (DESNOS); and personality disorders (e.g., borderline personality disorder and panic disor-

1

der), other individuals are resilient and recover after experiencing trauma. Yet the focus of these guidelines is specifically on the treatment of PTSD and its symptoms as defined in the text revision of the fourth edition of the *Diagnostic and Statistical Manual of Mental Disorders* (DSM-IV-TR; American Psychiatric Association, 2000).

It is also recognized that the PTSD diagnostic framework is inherently limiting, and these limitations may be particularly salient for survivors of early childhood sexual and physical abuse or domestic violence. Individuals with these histories display a wide range of relational and interpersonal problems that contribute to distressed lives and disability. Yet relatively little is known about the successful treatment of patients with these trauma histories. There is a growing clinical consensus, with a degree of empirical support, that some patients with these histories require multimodal interventions, applied consistently over a longer time period.

The Task Force also recognized that PTSD is often accompanied by other psychological conditions, and that such comorbidity requires clinical sensitivity, attention, and evaluation at the point of diagnosis and throughout the process of treatment. Disorders of particular concern are substance abuse and major depression, the most frequently co-occurring conditions. In recognition of the common comorbidity of PTSD with other disorders, the revised version includes a new chapter that focuses specifically on the treatment of PTSD in the presence of comorbid psychiatric conditions.

These guidelines are intended to assist clinicians who provide treatment for adults, adolescents, and children with PTSD. Because clinicians with diverse professional backgrounds provide mental health treatment for PTSD, the guidelines were developed with interdisciplinary input. Psychologists, psychiatrists, social workers, creative arts therapists, marital therapists, and others actively contributed to, and participated in, the developmental process. Accordingly, the guidelines are suitable for the diversity of clinicians who treat PTSD.

The original Task Force explicitly excluded from consideration individuals who are currently living in violent or abusive relationships because their treatment, and the related forensic and ethical issues that arise, differ fundamentally from those individuals whose traumatic events are over. Individuals in the midst of a traumatic situation require special considerations from the clinician. However, the revised guidelines recognize that children in particular may be living in ongoing traumatic circumstances, such as violent neighborhoods or homes in which domestic violence is occurring intermittently, if not repeatedly; testing of treatment modalities for these populations are also expressly noted in the literature review. In recognition of the real-life circumstances of many individuals treated by clinicians reading these guidelines, these treatments are also included.

Little is known about the treatment of PTSD in nonindustrialized countries. Research and scholarly treatises on the topic come largely from the Western industrialized nations. The Task Force acknowledges this cultural limitation explicitly. There is growing recognition that PTSD is a universal response to exposure to traumatic events observed in many different cultures and societies. Yet there is a need for systematic research to determine the extent to which the treatments, both psychological and psychopharmacological, that have proven efficacy in Western societies are indeed effective in non-Western cultures. When available, the revised guidelines include enhanced cultural considerations and adaptations of Western treatments for additional cultural groups.

Finally, clinicians following these guidelines should not limit themselves only to these approaches and techniques. All current treatments have limitations; either not all patients respond to them, patients drop out of treatment, or, for various reasons, therapists are not comfortable using a particular intervention. To promote the development of improved treatments, creative integration of new approaches driven by sound theoretical principles is most welcome in the field. Promoting new treatments ultimately enhances and optimizes treatment outcome, thus contributing to optimal public health across national boundaries.

The Process of Developing the Guidelines

The process of developing these guidelines was as follows. A decision was made by the original Task Force co-chairs to expand the Task Force to include a greater emphasis on children and adolescents for the revised edition. This decision was based on both the growing empirical literature about effective treatments for children and increasing information about the critical risk that childhood trauma contributes to the later development of PTSD in diverse groups of trauma-exposed individuals, including combat veterans. The co-chairs identified an additional co-chair with child and adolescent expertise, and these co-chairs then assembled a new Task Force by identifying experts in the major fields of therapy and treatment modalities currently used for patients with PTSD. The new Task Force included expanded child and adolescent experts who wrote summary chapters that generally corresponded with adult therapies. These chapters included early interventions, cognitive-behavioral therapy (CBT), pharmacotherapy, psychodynamic therapy, school-based treatment, and creative arts therapies. Other chapters that focused primarily on adults but included information on children are eye movement desentization and reprocessing (EMDR), group therapy, psychosocial rehabilitation, hypnosis, couple and family therapy, and treatment of PTSD with comorbid disorders. Thus, the Task Force addressed treatment across the developmental spectrum, with experts who represented diverse clinical approaches, theoretical orientations, schools of therapy, and professional training. The focus of the guidelines and their format was determined by the co-chairs based on the previous guidelines and recent developments in the field.

The Task Force co-chairs commissioned summary papers on the major treatment areas or modalities from Task Force members. Each paper was to be written by a designated member, with assistance from other members or clinicians of their choosing as deemed necessary by that member. The summary papers included literature reviews of research and clinical practice.

The literature reviews on each of the topics involved the use of online literature searches, such as Published International Literature on Traumatic Stress (PILOTS), MEDLINE, PsycLIT, the National Child Traumatic Stress Network (NCTSN), and other relevant literature searches. The resulting papers adhered to a standard format and were generally restricted in length. Authors reviewed the literature in their assigned area, presented the clinical findings, reviewed critically the scientific support for the approach, and presented the papers to the co-chairs. Completed papers were then distributed to all co-chairs for comments and active discussion. These reviews resulted in further revisions to the papers, which eventually became the chapters in this book.

Because of concerns voiced by some ISTSS members about this process with respect to the EMDR chapter, an additional step was taken for that chapter only. Dr. Bonnie Green served as a guest editor, and the position paper was sent out for blind review. Upon satisfactory completion of this process, the EMDR chapter was accepted for inclusion in the book (Chapter 11 by Spates, Koch, Cusack, Pagoto, & Waller).

On the basis of the position papers and careful attention to the literature review, a draft of the practice guidelines for each treatment approach was developed. These appear in Part II of this text. In these guidelines, each treatment approach or modality was assigned ratings with respect to strength of evidence regarding its efficacy. These ratings were standardized with a coding system adapted from the Agency for Health Care Policy and Research (AHCPR; U.S. Department of Health and Human Services, Public Health Service), which is now called the Agency for Healthcare Research and Quality (AHRQ). This rating system, presented below, represents an effort to formulate recommendations for practitioners based on the available scientific evidence. The guidelines were reviewed by the co-chairs for concurrence and then presented to the Board of Directors of the ISTSS, and placed on the ISTSS website for comments from the membership. Feedback obtained from this iterative process was incorporated into the guidelines. The revised guidelines were then deliberated by the ISTSS Board of Directors and approved after some further revisions.

As with all psychological disorders, limitations exist in the scientific treatment outcome literature for PTSD. Specifically, most studies use inclusion and exclusion criteria to define participants appropriately; accordingly, each study may not fully represent the complete spectrum of patients seeking treatment. It is customary, for example, in studies of PTSD treatment to exclude patients with active substance dependence, acute suicidal ideation, neuropsychological deficits, retardation, and/or cardiovascular disease. Therefore, generalization of the findings, and the resulting guidelines, to these populations may not extend to patients with these concurrent conditions.

Clinical Issues

Type of Trauma

Most, but not all, randomized clinical trials (RCTs) with combat (mostly Vietnam War) veterans showed less treatment efficacty than RCTs with nonveterans whose PTSD was related to other traumatic experiences (e.g., sexual assaults, accidents, natural disasters). Therefore, some experts believe that combat veterans with PTSD are less responsive than survivors of other traumas to treatment. Such a conclusion is premature. For example, recent studies of Gulf War veterans suggest a link between previous child sexual abuse and development of combat-related PTSD. The difference between veterans and other patients with PTSD may be related to the greater severity and chronicity of veterans' PTSD rather than to differences inherent to combat traumas. Furthermore, the poor treatment response in veterans may be a sampling artifact because Vietnam veterans currently receiving treatment at Department of Veteran Affairs (VA) facilities may constitute a self-selected group of chronic patients with multiple impairments. Furthermore, clinical trials conducted in non-VA settings have shown that veterans do at least as well as civilian participants. Finally, veterans treated for noncombat traumatic events appear to respond as well as nonveterans to these same traumatic events. Importantly, veterans in Israel respond as well to CBT (i.e., prolonged exposure) as do samples of civilians; in Europe, veterans appear to respond to medication as well as or better than civilians. In short, there is no conclusive evidence at this time that PTSD following certain traumas is especially resistant to treatment. More clinical trials with combat veterans would be important and welcome additions to this literature.

Much of the child treatment research has been conducted with children who have experienced sexual abuse, domestic violence, and community violence (these often co-occur). Although these problems are sometimes associated with severe problems, such as DESNOS in adulthood, when treated in childhood they are responsive to a broad range of trauma-focused treatments, as described in these guidelines. Notably, in studies of adult survivors of sexual assault, those whose PTSD was related to child sexual abuse responded as well to exposure therapy as those whose PTSD was related to adult sexual or physical abuse.

Single versus Multiple Traumas

No clinical studies have been designed to address the question of whether the number of previous traumas predicts treatment response among adult patients with PTSD. Because most treatment studies have been conducted with either military veterans or female adult survivors of sexual assault, many of whom have a history of multiple assaults, it appears that much of the current knowledge about treatment efficacy applies to people who have been traumatized more than once. It would be of great interest to conduct studies comparing individuals with single versus multiple traumas to find out whether, as expected, the former would be more responsive to treatment. Recruitment for such studies might be very difficult, however, because the research design would have to control for PTSD severity and chronicity, as well as for comorbid diagnoses—each of which may be more predictive of treatment response than the precise number of traumatic events experienced.

One study of children has evaluated the relative efficacy of two treatments for single versus multiple traumas, and the relative contribution of coexisting depressive symptoms. This multisite study showed the greater benefit of trauma-focused CBT over child-centered therapy for children who had experienced multiple traumas, as well as for those with higher initial depressive symptoms. More studies of this type will not only help to explicate superior treatments but also better match treatments to specific children.

Chronicity of PTSD

There is growing interest in clinical approaches that emphasize prevention, identification of risk factors, early detection of PTSD, and acute intervention. This is based on the idea that, as with many medical and mental disorders, PTSD has a better prognosis if clinical intervention is implemented early. One study in Israel suggests that early treatment (within the first month) leads to better outcomes than does treatment provided later. There is abundant evidence that many people who develop PTSD continue to have the disorder indefinitely. Although it is unclear whether chronic PTSD is inherently (e.g., psychobiologically) different than more acute clinical presentations, it is generally believed that chronic PTSD is more difficult to treat. However, in several studies, chronicity was unrelated to treatment outcome. Some patients with chronic PTSD develop a persistent, incapacitating psychiatric condition marked by severe and intractible symptoms; marital, social, and vocational disability; as well as extensive use of psychiatric and community services. Such patients may benefit more from case management and psychosocial rehabilitation than from psychotherapy or pharmacotherapy (see Glynn, Drebing, & Penk, Chapter 16, this volume).

Gender

Although lifetime prevalence rates of PTSD are twice as high in women as in men (10.4 vs. 5%) and women are four times more likely to develop PTSD when exposed to the same trauma, gender differences in response to treatment have not been studied systematically. Therefore, we do not know whether gender is predictive of treatment outcome. It is important to emphasize this point because a superficial review of the treatment literature suggests that women are more responsive than men to treatment. On further inspection, however, several differences between treatment studies with men and women can be noted, making direct comparisons difficult. First, the PTSD studies of women to date largely involve (childhood or adult) sexual trauma and motor vehicle accidents (MVAs), whereas studies with men have usually involved war veterans. Second, in some large, multisite medication trials, men responded as well as women to treatment. Finally, other factors, such as treatment modality, PTSD severity/chronicity, or the presence of comorbid disorders, need to be systematically controlled in future studies before differences in treatment outcome can be attributed to gender. In short, it is impossible to conclude that gender is predictive of treatment response at this time.

Age

Two questions are relevant concerning the effects of age on treatment outcome:

1. Does the age at which the trauma occurred influence response to treatment?
2. Does the age at which treatment begins affect treatment outcome?

Neither question has been studied systematically; hence, there are no conclusive data on either question. Adults and children have responded to some treatments and not to others. Age of trauma exposure has not predicted treatment outcome in studies published to date.

Children

Perhaps due to the creation of the NCTSN there has been a proliferation of empirical studies of trauma and PTSD in children since the publication of the last Guidelines. In addition, children present so many distinct challenges for assessment and treatment that seven chapters in this volume are devoted to treatment of children with PTSD. Developmental level is particularly important because it may influence the clinical phenomenology of PTSD in children, as well as the choice of treatment. In addition, parental factors must be carefully considered when treating children. Developmental biological factors may also influence choice of drug, if pharmacotherapy is indicated. In addition, cognitive-developmental factors may influence the choice of assessment and treatment strategies.

Elder Adults

PTSD may have its onset or reoccurrence at any point in the life cycle. It may persist for decades and even intensify in old age. Developmental factors unique to older adults may influence susceptibility to PTSD among older adults, including a sense of helplessness produced by illness, diminished functional capacity and cognitive capacity, or social marginalization. Death of loved ones can trigger intrusive recollections of traumatic losses, thereby precipitating a relapse of PTSD symptoms that may have been in remission for decades. Retirement and the life review process of old age can also increase vulnerability to the development of PTSD for the first time, exacerbation of an existing condition, or relapse. Developmental biological factors may influence both the choice and recommended dosage of any drug selected for pharmacotherapy, while cognitive status may influence the approach to both assessment and psychotherapy for older patients with PTSD. Recent studies on elders with PTSD suggest that CBT may be helpful with this population.

Factors Affecting Treatment Decisions

At present, few empirical data exist to guide us in the question of how to decide the course of treatment for PTSD. However, some clinical considerations are discussed below.

Treatment Goals

All treatments presented in these guidelines have proponents who claim that they are clinically useful for patients with PTSD. The therapeutic goals for each treatment, however, are not necessarily the same. Some treatments (e.g., CBT, pharmacotherapy, and EMDR) target PTSD symptom reduction as the major clinical outcome by which efficacy should be judged. Other treatments (e.g., hypnosis, art therapy, and possibly psychodynamic therapy) emphasize the capacity to enrich the therapeutic process rather than the ability to improve directly PTSD symptoms. Still other treatments (e.g., psychosocial rehabilitation) emphasize functional improvement, with or without reduction of PTSD symptoms. Finally, some interventions (e.g., hospitalization, substance abuse treatment) focus primarily on severe disruptive behaviors or comorbid disorders that must be addressed before PTSD treatment per se can be initiated. More recently, there is an increased awareness among clinical researchers that the goals of treatment should include reduction of not only PTSD symptom severity but also associated symptoms, such as depression, general anxiety, anger, shame, and guilt, as well as improved quality of life. Ultimately, this recognition will yield a broader range of assessment within clinical trials and perhaps the development of additional targets for treatment.

Treatment of PTSD

"Successful treatment" of PTSD is the major criterion by which all clinical practice is evaluated in these guidelines. Our definition for this is based in a reduction of symptom frequency, intensity, or severity as a function of the intervention. Some treatments appear to reduce all clusters of PTSD symptoms, whereas others seem to be effective in attenuating one symptom cluster (e.g., intrusion [Criterion B], avoidant/numbing [Criterion C], or arousal [Criterion D] symptoms) but not others. In this volume, Weathers, Keane, and Foa (Chapter 2) and Balaban (Chapter 3) discuss state-of-the-art methods for assessing and monitoring PTSD symptom severity during treatment trials for adults and children, respectively. Some experts have challenged the focus on specific symptoms when evaluating various therapeutic approaches, arguing that the best gauge of clinical efficacy is the capacity of a given treatment to produce global improvement in PTSD rather than specific symptom reduction. In these guidelines, however, the major criterion for treatment efficacy is reduction of PTSD symptoms, although clinical global improvement is indicated when available.

Comorbidity

As do persons with other mental disorders, patients with PTSD usually have at least one other psychiatric disorder. Indeed, U.S. epidemiological findings indicate that 80% of patients with lifetime PTSD have lifetime depression, another anxiety disorder, or chemical abuse/dependency. Good clinical practice dictates that the best treatment is one that might be expected to ameliorate both PTSD and comorbid symptoms. Therefore, the presence of a specific comorbid disorder may prompt a clinician to choose one particular treatment rather than another. In recognition of this principle, the revised guidelines have added a chapter focused on the treatment of PTSD with comorbid psychiatric conditions. Again, it must be emphasized, however, that treatment of PTSD is the major criterion by which all the clinical practices have been evaluated. It is notable that some treatments aimed at reduction of PTSD symptoms, such as CBT, were found concomitantly to reduce associated symptoms, such as depression, general anxiety, guilt, and anger.

Suicidality

Self-destructive and impulsive behaviors, although not part of the core PTSD symptom complex, are recognized as associated features of this disorder that may profoundly affect clinical management. Therefore, the routine assessment of all patients presenting with PTSD should include a careful evaluation of current suicidal ideation and past history of suicidal attempts. Risk factors for suicide should also be assessed, such as current depression and substance abuse. If significant suicidality is present, it must be addressed before any other treatment is initiated. If the patient cannot be safely managed as an outpatient, hospitalization should be the immediate clinical focus. If suicidality is secondary to depression and/or substance abuse, clinical attention must focus on either or both of these conditions before initiating treatment for PTSD.

Chemical Abuse/Dependence

Lifetime prevalence rates of alcohol abuse/dependence among men and women with PTSD are approximately 52 and 28%, respectively, whereas lifetime prevalence rates for drug abuse/dependence are 35 and 27%, respectively. Such comorbid disorders not only complicate treatment but in some cases may also exacerbate PTSD itself. In addition, a number of legal substances, such as nicotine, caffeine, and sympathomimetics (e.g., nasal decongestants) may interfere with treatment and should therefore be carefully assessed in all patients with PTSD. In many cases, if significant chemical abuse/dependency is present, it should be treated until it is under control, and before treatment for PTSD is initiated. As noted by Najavits, Ryngala, Back, and Bolton (Chapter 21, this volume, regarding comorbid disorders), clinical trials are underway and researchers have recently examined approaches designed for concurrent treatment of PTSD and comorbid alcohol/substance misuse. One of these studies shows that patients with comorbid alcohol dependence and PTSD show excellent outcome when treated simultaneously for both disorders by exposure therapy, yielding reductions in both drinking and PTSD symptoms. These results suggest that, whenever possible, a concurrent approach may be better than treating each disorder sequentially.

Concurrent General Medical Conditions

There is mounting evidence that traumatized individuals appear to be at greater risk of developing medical illnesses. Compared to nontraumatized individuals, trauma survivors report more medical symptoms, use more medical services, have more medical illnesses detected during a physical examination, and display higher mortality. A few studies suggest that such adverse medical consequences may be mediated by PTSD. This has generated considerable interest in screening primary and specialty medical patients for both trauma histories and symptoms of PTSD. This work is in its infancy, however, and there are no studies examining the effects of treatment of PTSD among medical patients.

Disability and Functional Impairment

People with PTSD differ greatly from one another with respect to symptom severity, chronicity, complexity, comorbidity, associated symptoms, and functional impairment. These differences may affect both choice of treatment and clinical goals. For some patients with chronic PTSD, functional improvement may be much more important than reduction of PTSD symptoms. In others (especially those who have been subjected to protracted child sexual abuse or politically motivated torture), clinical interventions often need to focus primarily on symptoms of dissociation, impulsivity, affect liability, somatization, interpersonal difficulties, or pathological changes in identity. Therefore, although the major emphasis in these guidelines is on reduction of core PTSD symptoms, clinicians may find that functional improvement is the most important or appropriate clinical priority for some patients.

Indications for Hospitalization

Inpatient treatment should be considered when the individual is in imminent danger of harming self or others, has experienced functional or psychological destabilization, exhibits a significant loss of functioning, is in the throes of major psychosocial stressors, and/or is in need of specialized observation/ evaluation in a secure environment. The general recommendation is that such a hospitalization must occur in collaboration with outpatient providers and be integrated into the overall long-term treatment plan that has been developed. We have not included a separate chapter on inpatient treatment, as we did in the first edition, because many different types of treatment reviewed in these chapters may be provided during hospitalization.

What Treatments Are Included in the Guidelines?

For more than 100 years, the treatment for trauma-related disturbances has appeared in professional literature. This rich literature has provided us with much clinical wisdom. In the last two decades, researchers have studied several treatments for PTSD studied using experimental and statistical methods. Thus, at the present time, we have both clinical and scientific knowledge about what treatment modalities may help patients with posttrauma problems. Accordingly, the guidelines contain a variety of psychotherapies and pharmacotherapies developed for trauma survivors. The scientific and clinical evidence for the efficacy of these therapies in reducing PTSD and related symptoms varies greatly. In this volume we have decided to present the various treatments that are being applied to PTSD rather than focusing only on evidence-based treatments, which at this point comprise exclusively psychopharmacological and direct therapeutic methods (i.e., CBT and EMDR).

Clinical Research Issues

What Are Well-Controlled Studies?

The use of rigorous scientific methods in PTSD clinical trials has increased dramatically in the last 25 years of clinical research. Well-controlled studies should have the following features:

1. *Clearly defined target symptoms.* Merely experiencing a trauma in and of itself is not an indication for treatment. Significant trauma-related symptoms, such as PTSD or depression, should be present to justify treatment. Whatever the target symptom or syndrome, it should be defined clearly, so that appropriate measures can be employed to assess improvement. Ascertaining the diagnosis is important, as is specification of a precise threshold for symptom severity as an inclusion criterion for entering treatment (see Weathers et al., Chapter 2, and Balaban, Chapter 3, this volume).

Clear articulation of inclusion and exclusion criteria is a key feature of scientific rigor. Delineation of inclusion–exclusion criteria can assist both in examining predictors of outcome and in evaluating the efficacy of the treatment and its generalizability beyond the studied sample. A treatment that is effective regardless of sample differences is a more robust and more useful treatment.

2. *Reliable and valid measures.* Once target symptoms have been identified and the population defined, measures with good psychometric properties should be employed (see earlier discussion on measures). For studies targeting a particular diagnosis, assessment should include instruments designed to yield diagnoses and symptom severity. Measures must be developmentally appropriate for young children because current DSM-IV-TR criteria do not adequately capture how PTSD symptoms are developmentally manifested.

3. *Use of blind evaluators.* Early studies of treatment of traumatized individuals relied primarily on therapist and patient reports to evaluate treatment efficacy, and introduced expectancy and demand biases into the evaluation. The use of blind evaluators is a current requirement for a credible treatment outcome study. Two procedures are involved in keeping an evaluator blind. First, the evaluator should not be the same person conducting the treatment. Second, patients should be trained not to reveal their treatment condition during the evaluation, so as not to bias the blind evaluator's ratings.

4. *Assessor training.* The reliability and validity of an assessment depends largely on the skill of the evaluator; thus, training of assessors is critical, and a minimum criterion should be specified. This includes demonstrating interrater reliability and calibrating assessment procedures over the course of the study to prevent evaluator drift.

5. *Manualized, replicable, specific treatment programs.* It is also important that the chosen treatment is designed to address the target problem defined by inclusion criteria. Thus, if PTSD is the disorder targeted for treatment, employing a treatment specifically developed for PTSD would be most appropriate. Use of a detailed treatment manual is of utmost importance in evaluating treatment efficacy because it helps to ensure consistent treatment delivery across patients and across therapists, and affords replicability of the treatment to determine generalizability.

6. *Equipoise with regard to treatment conditions.* To eliminate the potential for bias, if more than one active treatment is being provided, therapists must

have equivalent backgrounds, experience, allegiance, and training in each treatment provided by an equivalently experienced trainer in that treatment model, with equivalent amounts of ongoing supervision in each model.

7. *Unbiased assignment to treatment.* To eliminate one potential source of bias, neither patient nor therapist should be allowed to choose the patient's treatment condition. Instead, a patient should be assigned randomly to a treatment condition, or assigned via a stratified sampling approach. This helps to ensure that observed differences or similarities among treatments are due to the techniques employed rather than to extraneous factors. To separate the effects of treatment from those of the therapist, each treatment should be delivered by at least two therapists, and patients should be randomly assigned to therapists within each condition.

8. *Treatment adherence.* Another component of a well-controlled study is the use of treatment adherence ratings. These ratings indicate whether the treatments were carried out as planned, and whether components of one treatment condition drifted into another.

9. *Data analysis conducted according to accepted procedures.* The final component of a well-controlled study is the use of accepted data-analytic procedures. All participants who are randomized and who receive treatment should be included in all data analyses. Selective administration of instruments to only a portion of participants, or data analyses of only some instruments, can potentially bias outcomes. There is surely value in calculating "competer" analyses, but a comprehensive view of the effectiveness of a treatment comes only from "intent-to-treat" analyses.

Limitations of Well-Controlled Studies

Although controlled studies are essential for evaluating the efficacy of a given treatment approach, the data emerging from such studies are by no means without problems. The stringent requirements of such studies can render unrepresentative samples; therefore, the generalizablity of the results may be limited. For example, the requirement of random assignment to studies that include placebo may be acceptable to some patients but not to others, and the factors that lead someone to enroll in such studies may be germane to how well he or she responds to treatment. Differential rates of dropout also need to be considered when evaluating completed studies. Some treatments by their very nature are powerful and/or may not be consistent with the patient's expectations of treatment, leading to dropout. This can and should influence conclusions.

Another source of bias in knowledge derived from controlled studies is that certain treatment approaches are more amenable than others for scientific study. For example, short-term and structured treatments, such as CBT and medication, are more suitable for controlled trials than longer, less structured treatments. As a result, there is more knowledge about the efficacy of the former than of the latter.

What Is Effect Size?

There are many ways to calculate the effectiveness of a given treatment in ameliorating a clinical condition. One way is to examine how many treated people lose their diagnosis. Another way is to calculate reduction in symptom severity from pre- to posttreatment or to follow-up. "Effect size" is a statistical method developed to evaluate in a standardized manner how much, on average, a given treatment program reduces the severity of target symptoms. Using an effect size method enables us to compare efficacy of different types of treatments across studies. We applied effect size analyses to all empirical studies discussed in this volume. To enhance comparability among the position papers, procedures for calculating and presenting effect sizes were standardized in two ways. First, a single effect size statistic was adopted: a member of Cohen's *d* family of effect size estimators known as Hedges's unbiased *g*. Like Cohen's *d*, Hedges's unbiased *g* is easy to conceptualize. It is based on the standardized difference between two means, typically the mean of a treatment sample minus the mean of a comparison sample divided by pooled standard deviations of the two samples. Therefore, each whole number represents one standard deviation away from the comparison sample mean. For example, if *g* = 0.5, the mean of the treatment sample would be estimated to be 0.5 standard deviation above the comparison sample. Unlike Cohen's *d*, which systematically overestimates when used with small samples, Hedges's unbiased *g* includes a mathematical adjustment for small-sample bias. To further ease comparability, the signs of all effect sizes were then adjusted such that positive effect sizes always represent better outcome than the comparison group.

Second, a hierarchical procedure was adopted for selecting the studies to be included in each position paper. This was done because studies with different kinds of comparison groups produce effect sizes that are not directly comparable, even when utilizing the same effect size statistic. If enough studies that utilized comparison groups, such as a waiting list or a nonspecific control treatment, were available for inclusion in a position paper, studies utilizing other comparison group types were not included. If the number of "no-treatment" comparison studies was inadequate for drawing conclusions, studies utilizing "placebo" comparison groups were included, with the caution that the effect sizes calculated from these studies would tend to be smaller by comparison, even if the treatments were equally effective.

Only if enough studies of either type were not available would purely within-subjects experimental designs with no comparison group be included. In these designs, the only way to calculate a standardized difference effect size is to estimate a comparison group's scores by using the pretreatment scores of the treatment group. Because these estimated scores are not independent, effect sizes resulting from these calculations are inflated compared to effect sizes from the other two comparison group types and should not be compared directly with them.

The State of Current Knowledge about Treatment of PTSD

Research on treatment efficacy for PTSD began in the early 1980s, with the introduction of the disorder into DSM-III. Since then, many case reports and studies have been published. These studies vary with respect to their methodological rigor; therefore, the strength of conclusions that can be drawn from them is different for different treatments. Since the initial guidelines were published in 2000, several new studies have been added to the guidelines, and a number of treatments have advanced in their level of evidence. However, the absence of evidence for a technique or approach does not imply that it does not work, only that it has not yet been subjected to rigorous scientific scrutiny.

Controlled research on additional approaches to treating PTSD is needed; many international projects are ongoing as of the writing of these guidelines. Most conclusions on the treatment of PTSD are based on efficacy trials and should be viewed cautiously as a result. The field awaits the completion of effectiveness trials to determine the extent to which findings in controlled treatment trials generalize to other clinical environments. As with all disorders, periodic updates of these guidelines are needed to track progress in the field.

Combined Treatments

Few studies systematically examined the value of combining psychotherapy with medication, or combinations of medications. Research on other disorders (e.g., depression) has shown benefits from combination approaches. One small study of combined trauma-focused CBT (TF-CBT) and sertraline showed no added benefit to TF-CBT alone for sexually abused children. Furthermore, one study with adults has shown that the average partial responders to medication (e.g., sertraline) benefited from the addition of prolonged exposure therapy. Only a few studies examined whether programs that include a wide variety of cognitive-behavioral techniques yield better outcome than programs that include fewer techniques. On the whole, these studies do not support the administration of more complex programs. Despite the scarcity of knowledge, clinical wisdom dictates the use of combined treatments for some patients. Many patients with PTSD also have depression. If depression is severe, a combination of psychotherapy and medication is often desired.

The Coding System

To help clinicians appropriately evaluate the treatment approaches presented in the guidelines, the following coding system was devised to denote the strength of the evidence for each approach. Each recommendation is identified as falling into one of six categories of endorsements, each indicated by a letter. The six categories represent varying levels of evidence for the use of a specific treatment procedure, or for a specific recommendation. This system was adopted from the AHCPR classification of Level of Evidence.

> *Level A:* Evidence is based on randomized, well-controlled clinical trials for individuals with PTSD.
> *Level B:* Evidence is based on well-designed clinical studies, without randomization or placebo comparison for individuals with PTSD.
> *Level C:* Evidence is based on service and naturalistic clinical studies, combined with clinical observations that are sufficiently compelling to warrant use of the treatment technique or follow the specific recommendation.
> *Level D:* Evidence is based on long-standing and widespread clinical practice that has not been subjected to empirical tests in PTSD.
> *Level E:* Evidence is based on long-standing practice by circumscribed groups of clinicians that has not been subjected to empirical tests in PTSD.
> *Level F:* Evidence is based on recently developed treatment that has not been subjected to clinical or empirical tests in PTSD.

Treatment Considerations

Therapist Training

To utilize most appropriately the information contained in these guidelines, individuals should be professionally trained and licensed in their state or country. Typical training would include a graduate-level degree, a clinical internship or its equivalent, and past supervision in the specific technique or approach employed.

Choice of Treatment Setting

Most treatments for PTSD take place in an outpatient setting, such as psychiatric or psychological clinics and counseling centers. For children, treatment may occur in schools, homes, community settings, or residential treatment facilities. However, an inpatient setting may be required when the patient manifests a significant tendency for suicidality or severe comorbid disorders (e.g., psychotic episode, severe borderline personality). The treatment setting should be determined during the initial diagnostic evaluation. Careful monitoring of the patient's mental status throughout treatment may indicate the appropriateness of changes in the treatment setting.

Treatment Management

A comprehensive diagnostic evaluation should precede treatment to determine the presence of PTSD and whether PTSD symptoms constitute the predominant problem of the patient. Once the diagnosis is ascertained, irrespective of the treatment chosen, the clinician should establish a professional milieu. First, the clinician must form and maintain a therapeutic alliance. Special attention should be given to trust and safety issues. Many individuals with PTSD have difficulties trusting others, especially if the trauma had interpersonal aspects (e.g., assault, rape). Other patients have related problems in recognizing and respecting personal boundaries when they enter a therapeutic relationship. Therefore, during the first stage of therapy, attention should be directed to these sensitive issues and to providing reassurance that the patient's welfare is the priority of the therapeutic relationship. Second, the therapist should demonstrate concern with the patient's physical safety when planning the treatment, such as appraising the safety of places selected for exposure exercises, or monitoring the safety of the woman who has just left an abusive relationship. Third, the clinician should provide education and reassurance with regard to the PTSD symptoms and related problems. Fourth, the patient's PTSD symptoms and general functioning should be monitored over time. Fifth, comorbid conditions should be identified and addressed. When necessary, it is important to work with other health professionals and with the patient's family members and significant others.

Many patients with PTSD require dependable and steady therapeutic relationships because their symptoms do not remit completely and can exacerbate with anniversary reactions and trauma reminders. For these reasons, it is important to assure the patient of the continued availability of his or her therapist. Finally, many patients with PTSD have ongoing crises in their lives and may need to rely intermittently upon a supportive therapist. Crises that arise during the course of therapy have clear implications for the sequencing of treatments for some patients. Starts and pauses in treatment may characterize the only way that they can engage the process of change. Acknowledging this, and accounting for this in designing a treatment plan may avert problems during the intensive therapeutic phase. Additional treatment considerations are presented by Friedman, Cohen, Foa, and Keane in Chapter 22, this volume.

When working with traumatized children and adolescents it is usually optimal to include parents or other caregivers in treatment, and it is crucial to form a therapeutic alliance with these caregivers as well. When treating children, therapists often interact with school, child protection, child advocacy, juvenile justice, and a variety of other child and family child welfare agencies. It is crucial that therapists working with traumatized children become familiar with these systems. At the same time, therapists need to be sensitive to the complex relationship between adolescents and their parent or guardians, and allow flexible relationships with them depending on the individual circumstances.

Treatment Resistance

Despite the progress that has been achieved in the treatment of PTSD, many patients do not benefit from the first line of treatment. The phenomenon of treatment resistance has been particularly noted among Vietnam War veterans receiving VA treatment in the United States, but other trauma populations have their share of treatment failures. It seems that patients with chronicity, pervasive dysfunction, and/or high comorbidity are especially resistant to first-line therapy. These patients may be especially good candidates for programs that include multiple treatment modalities such as meditation, psychotherapy, family therapy, and rehabilitation therapy.

Readiness for Treatment

Several factors deter many traumatized individuals with acute PTSD from seeking treatment for the disorder: They assume that the symptoms will dissipate with time; they feel that nothing can help them, or that there is an element of shame surrounding their traumatic experiences. In addition, PTSD is characterized by avoidance of reminders of the traumatic event (Criterion C for the diagnosis). If the patient views therapy as a forum for discussing or approaching the topic of the trauma, it is understandable that many people with PTSD delay or refuse treatment. Accordingly, attempts to offer treatment in this initial stage often fail. Even when PTSD becomes chronic, many either do not seek treatment or they present to treatment with related symptoms, such as depression. Therefore, after diagnosing the disorder, a crucial first step to prepare the patient for treatment of PTSD is educating him or her about the disorder and its high rates among trauma survivors. Many are reluctant to enter treatment because they view their PTSD symptoms as a personal failure. For many patients, normalization of their symptoms results in immediate relief and reduces their reluctance to continue treatment.

Some patients are reluctant to enter treatment because it often entails discussing the traumatic event either during the assessment or in therapy. The clinician should encourage patients to express their misgivings and be sensitive to the distress they experience when discussing or recounting their traumatic experiences, so that their concerns can be addressed in the first stage of therapy.

Validity of Memories of Traumatic Events

To receive the diagnosis of PTSD, one must first be exposed to a traumatic event. Treatment of PTSD typically involves the processing of this event, its meaning, and its consequences. All the methods in the guidelines presuppose the existence of a verifiable and valid traumatic event. The guidelines do not address the use of any of these treatment approaches in an effort to recover unconscious memories of past traumatic events.

The Task Force does acknowledge that memories for traumatic events are sometimes not reported, or are forgotten by individuals who seek mental health treatment. But because of lack of scientific evidence, the Task Force does *not* support the position that the presence of some of the symptoms of PTSD (emotional numbing, concentration problems, etc.) is clear evidence that the patient experienced a traumatic event. To be clear, this Task Force does not support the use of these guidelines to assist in the recovery of forgotten traumatic memories.

How to Use the Guidelines

These guidelines summarize the state of the art in the treatment of PTSD to inform mental health professionals about the care of patients with PTSD. They begin when the patient has been diagnosed as having PTSD, according to the DSM-IV criteria. The guidelines also assume that the patient has been evaluated for comorbid disorders and include treatments with various degrees of evidence for efficacy, indicated by the coding system described earlier and the conclusions section for each treatment approach.

The clinician is encouraged to adopt treatments that have been proven effective. However, it is important to remember that several treatments with proven efficacy are available. Also, many treatments that have not been evaluated in well-controlled studies have been practiced extensively and have accumulated clinical evidence for their efficacy. The distinction between clinical wisdom and scientific knowledge is emphasized here. Not all of the art of psychotherapy has been examined in RCTs. Experienced and sensitive clinicians are often in the best position to determine the nature and the timing of specific psychological and psychopharmacological interventions.

We also recognize that not all treatments are universally effective. Even the best treatments we have to offer fail in certain circumstances. Clinicians are encouraged to assess systematically those patients who do not respond to interventions to determine the presence of undisclosed or undetected conditions that might be responsible for a nonresponse. Detection of factors related to a lack of full participation in a treatment plan may also assist the clinician in understanding a poor outcome. Given that several treatments for PTSD have empirical support, the clinician can apply these treatments sequentially to optimize treatment success.

Finally, the choice of treatment approach should depend on the clinical circumstances presented by the specific patient (e.g., the presence of comorbid disorders and the patient's preferences), as well as the efficacy of the treatment modality. Although clinicians have learned much about the treatment of PTSD in the past 28 years, they still need to learn much more. Clinicians are encouraged to incorporate into their clinical practice the approaches that have proven efficacy. In this way, the public health of society will be enhanced. This is the goal of the ISTSS and its production of these treatment guidelines.

Reference

American Psychiatric Association. (2000). *Diagnostic and statistical manual of mental disorders* (4th ed., text revision). Washington, DC: Author.

PART I

ASSESSMENT AND DIAGNOSIS OF PTSD

CHAPTER 2

Assessment and Diagnosis of Adults

Frank W. Weathers, Terence M. Keane, and Edna B. Foa

Posttraumatic stress disorder (PTSD) is a complex, often chronic and debilitating mental disorder that develops in response to catastrophic life events such as combat, sexual assault, natural disasters, and other extreme stressors. As currently conceptualized in DSM-IV-TR (American Psychiatric Association, 2000) the core PTSD syndrome involves 17 symptoms in three symptom clusters: reexperiencing the trauma, avoidance and numbing, and hyperarousal. In addition, the clinical picture for trauma survivors is often complicated by associated features, such as guilt, dissociation, alterations in personality, affect dysregulation, and marked impairment in intimacy and attachment (Herman, 1992; Wilson, 2004); comorbid disorders, such as depression, substance abuse, and other anxiety disorders (Brown, Campbell, Lehman, Grisham, & Mancill, 2001; Kessler, Sonnega, Bromet, Hughes, & Nelson, 1995; Orsillo et al., 1996); and a variety of physical health complaints (Kimerling, Clum, McQuery, & Schnurr, 2002; Schnurr, Green, & Kaltman, 2007). Thus, PTSD is a multifaceted disorder that manifests in cognitive, affective, behavioral, and physiological response channels. In its most severe form, PTSD can disrupt virtually every aspect of normal functioning and presents multiple targets for assessment and intervention.

The effects of psychological trauma have been noted throughout history and intermittently have been a focus for mental health professionals (Herman, 1992; Trimble, 1985; van der Kolk, 2007). However, the introduction of PTSD as a formal diagnosis in DSM-III (American Psychiatric Association, 1980) prompted a remarkably active and sustained period of investigation, resulting in a voluminous and ever-expanding empirical literature on trauma and trauma-related syndromes. On the one hand, PTSD has been the focus of much of this resurgence of interest in trauma and has had substantial utility and heuristic value as the central construct in the field of traumatic stress.

On the other hand, PTSD also has been the subject of considerable controversy, and critics have challenged many of its underlying assumptions (e.g., Rosen, 2004b). Some of the most salient issues include long-standing debate regarding the nature of trauma and its unique effects; extensive revision of the diagnostic criteria; poorly defined and overlapping symptom criteria; high rates of comorbidity and concerns regarding differential diagnosis; lack of an objective, definitive test or biological marker; overreliance on retrospective self-report; and concerns about response bias, especially the potential for symptom exaggeration or malingering.

Although many of these issues are general and constitute important concerns in almost all areas of psychopathology, some are specific to PTSD. Together, they challenge the field of traumatic stress to clarify the conceptual underpinnings of PTSD and provide empirically based answers to the following questions: What is the nature of psychological trauma, and how is it best defined? What is the link between trauma and PTSD? What are the defining features of the PTSD syndrome? How is PTSD different from other disorders? Although much work clearly remains, substantial progress has been made thus far in addressing these and other important questions. The various criticisms notwithstanding, the fact remains that PTSD is an extensively investigated and well-validated disorder, with more than 25 years of rigorous and programmatic research into its phenomenology, etiology, and treatment (for a recent summary, see Friedman, Resick, & Keane, 2007). From a construct validation perspective (Cronbach & Meehl, 1955), PTSD is defined by an extensive and increasingly well-articulated nomological network, based on empirical validity evidence from a wide variety of sources.

Moreover, these research achievements would not have been possible without the development of a psychometrically sound measurement technology. As with any mental disorder, advances in the scientific understanding of PTSD depend on the availability and appropriate use of reliable and valid assessment instruments and procedures. Fortunately, assessment has been one of the most active, productive areas of investigation in the field of traumatic stress. Over the last 20 years considerable progress has been made in the development and empirical evaluation of assessment instruments for measuring trauma exposure and PTSD, as well as related syndromes, such as acute stress disorder and complex PTSD. In the years immediately following the introduction of PTSD in DSM-III, few measures were available. Since the mid-1980s, however, dozens of measures have been developed, including questionnaires, structured interviews, and psychophysiological procedures, and more continue to appear every year. Some interview and self-report measures, such as the Impact of Events Scale (IES; Horowitz, Wilner, & Alvarez, 1979), the Mississippi Scale for Combat-Related PTSD (Mississippi Scale; Keane, Caddell, & Taylor, 1988), the PTSD Checklist (PCL; Weathers, Litz, Herman, Huska, & Keane, 1993), the Interview and Self-Report versions of the PTSD Symptom Scale (PSS; Foa, Riggs, Dancu, & Rothbaum, 1993), and the Clinician-Administered PTSD Scale (CAPS; Blake et al., 1995), have been extensively validated and widely adopted. In addition, a broad array of assessment protocols have been developed, ranging from single-measure surveys to comprehensive multimeasure approaches (Schlenger, Jordan, Caddell, Ebert, & Fairbank, 2004). Furthermore, assessment of trauma and PTSD has been the focus of several books, some of which have now appeared in revised editions (Briere, 2004; Carlson, 1997; Wilson & Keane, 2004).

Thus, ample resources are now available to conduct psychometrically sound assessments of trauma survivors in any context, and it is no longer defensible for clinicians to do otherwise. When we summarized the state of PTSD assessment in the mid-1990s (Weathers & Keane, 1999), we noted that although the use of standardized measures was becoming the norm, it was lacking even in some published studies, and almost certainly absent in many clinical settings because of the lag time in disseminating empirically based procedures. Ten years later, however, the use of standardized measures is a requirement for research and is strongly encouraged as part of best practice for clinical work. This welcome progress has been facilitated by several factors. First, there have been continued advances in the measurement of trauma and PTSD. New measures have been developed and existing measures have been extensively validated. Many of these measures are in the public domain and are disseminated widely through outlets such as the National Center for PTSD (*www.ncptsd.va.gov*). Second, a new generation of clinicians and investigators has been trained in settings where such measures are used and, consequently, has incorporated evidence-based measures into routine assessment and treatment activities.

Third, there is a growing emphasis in the mental health field more broadly on evidence-based assessment (EBA; Hunsley & Mash, 2005). EBA complements the long-standing emphasis on evidence-based treatment and is a key component of a comprehensive and integrative evidence-based approach to mental health services. From the outset, research and practice in PTSD assessment have been firmly grounded in empirical methods, drawing on both classic psychometric and behavioral assessment traditions (Fairbank, Keane, & Malloy, 1983; Malloy, Fairbank, & Keane, 1983). Over time, PTSD assessment has continued to exhibit many of the hallmarks of EBA, including (1) the development of psychometrically sound individual instruments; (2) a focus on multimethod assessment across multiple response channels, as well as empirical methods for combining information from multiple sources (Keane, Wolfe, & Taylor, 1987; Kulka et al., 1991); and (3) investigations of the generalizability of measures across different trauma populations and settings, including consideration of the impact of gender, ethnicity, and culture

(Kimerling, Ouimette, & Wolfe, 2002; Marsella, Friedman, Gerrity, & Scurfield, 1996). PTSD assessment clearly exemplifies the principles of EBA and is in many respects a model for the evidence-based approach to assessment of mental disorders.

In this chapter we provide an overview of the conceptual and practical considerations involved in designing and implementing an assessment protocol for trauma and PTSD. We outline the basic tasks and issues in the assessment of trauma survivors. Next, we provide an overview of some of the most commonly used measures. Last, we offer recommendations for tailoring a protocol for a given clinical or research application. Due to the enormous scope of the literature, our coverage is selective. We focus on the PTSD syndrome rather than trauma exposure per se or other trauma-related syndromes, such as acute stress disorder or complex PTSD. We also focus on self-report and interview measures rather than on physiological procedures or other assessment modalities. Furthermore, we focus primarily on diagnosis. Although diagnosis is an essential goal in most assessments, there are other important goals and activities in a comprehensive assessment of trauma survivors, including clinical management, history taking, functional analysis of problem behaviors, case formulation, and treatment planning (see Briere, 2004; Carlson, 1997; Litz & Weathers, 1994; Wilson & Keane, 2004). Finally, we limit our discussion to the assessment of adults.

Tasks and Issues

PTSD is a multifaceted disorder that poses a number of significant conceptual and practical challenges with regard to accurate assessment and diagnosis. In this section we outline the main tasks involved in a comprehensive evaluation of trauma exposure and trauma-related symptoms, and discuss some of the most salient issues associated with each task. In contemporary clinical practice, establishing a diagnosis involves adherence to DSM-IV-TR guidelines and diagnostic criteria. Although there are limitations of the DSM approach in general (e.g., the issue of categorical vs. dimensional approaches to classification), and limitations of the PTSD criteria specifically, DSM-IV-TR represents the current official conceptualization of PTSD and should be followed closely to maintain a consistent operational definition of the construct throughout the field of traumatic stress. In clinical settings a PTSD diagnosis is part of a DSM-IV-TR multiaxial diagnosis; thus, it should always conform to the official diagnostic criteria. In research settings it may be useful in some cases to investigate alternative operational definitions of trauma and PTSD. However, even then, it would be essential also to provide a standard DSM-IV diagnosis to serve as a reference point for evaluating the impact of adopting a different definition.

Current diagnostic criteria for PTSD include exposure to a traumatic stressor (Criterion A); development of a characteristic syndrome involving reexperiencing, avoidance and numbing, and hyperarousal symptoms (Criteria B–D); duration of at least 1 month (Criterion E); and clinically significant distress or impairment in social or occupational functioning (Criterion F). Unlike most other anxiety disorders, or even acute stress disorder, PTSD criteria do not include the usual exclusion criteria that the syndrome is not due to the physiological effects of a substance or a general medical condition, and is not better accounted for by another disorder.

A comprehensive PTSD assessment would evaluate all of the diagnostic criteria, and would also evaluate associated features and comorbid disorders, establish differential diagnosis, and measure and identify the effects of response bias. Although some of these tasks can be accomplished satisfactorily with the use of self-report measures, most are best accomplished with a structured interview, and much of the discussion in this section of the various issues associated with diagnosing PTSD is most directly relevant for an interview format. Self-report measures are limited by their fixed item content and rating scale format, and their effectiveness is dependent on respondents' ability to interpret items accurately and make appropriate ratings. In contrast, interviews provide ample opportunity to ask follow-up questions, clarify items and responses, and use clinical judgment in making the final ratings. Although a putative diagnosis can be made on the basis of a self-report measure, a formal diagnosis is not ordinarily made on the basis of self-report measures alone. It may be appropriate in some research settings to derive a putative diagnosis based only on a self-report measure, but in clinical settings this is rarely an adequate substitute for a diagnosis made by a qualified clinician using a well-validated structured interview.

Assess Criterion A

The first step in assessing PTSD is to establish that an individual has been exposed to an extreme stressor that satisfies the DSM-IV-TR definition of a trauma described in Criterion A. "Trauma" has proven to be remarkably difficult to define, and Criterion A has evolved considerably since PTSD was introduced in DSM-III. Criterion A in DSM-IV-TR comprises a two-part definition of a traumatic event and incorporates three distinct elements. Criterion A1 presents the first two elements. The first element involves the type of exposure (i.e., whether an individual directly experienced the event, witnessed, or learned about it indirectly). The second element, which is the basis for distinguishing traumatic stressors from ordinary stressors, requires that the event entail life threat, serious injury, or threat to physical integrity. Criterion A2 presents the third element, which requires that the event trigger an intense emotional response of fear, horror, or helplessness.

Criterion A has been the subject of considerable controversy. Critics have questioned whether trauma can be adequately defined and distinguished from ordinary stressors, and some have called for eliminating Criterion A altogether and defining PTSD only in terms of the characteristic symptoms (e.g., Maier, 2006; Solomon & Canino, 1990; for a full discussion of the Criterion A problem, see Weathers & Keane, 2007). One of the most important criticisms of Criterion A in DSM-IV-TR is that it represents an overly broad definition of trauma that allows too many stressors to be categorized as traumas, a situation that McNally (2004) has labeled "conceptual bracket creep." Several aspects of DSM-IV-TR Criterion A potentially contribute to bracket creep, including the ambiguous phrases "confronted with" and "threat to physical integrity," both of which could be interpreted in ways that represent a marked departure from the original intent of Criterion A. However, as we have argued elsewhere (Weathers & Keane, 2007), these aspects are essential to provide sufficient coverage for the wide range of stressors that could be traumatic. Any risk for bracket creep that they create can be mitigated by considering the accompanying text, which clearly emphasizes direct personal involvement with extreme stressors, where "extreme" refers primarily to life-threatening.

Despite its limitations, Criterion A plays an important role in the current conceptualization of PTSD; thus, its assessment requires careful attention. In practical terms, Criterion A serves a gatekeeping function by establishing a threshold of stressor severity that must be met before a diagnosis of PTSD can be made. Unless exposure to an unequivocal traumatic stressor can be established, a diagnosis of PTSD cannot be made, even if the rest of the criteria are met. According to DSM-IV-TR, in those cases in which the syndrome is present but the stressor does not meet Criterion A, the appropriate diagnosis is adjustment disorder. Thus, Criterion A is a crucial consideration in differential diagnosis. Although it provides flexibility to allow for clinical judgment in determining whether a stressor constitutes a trauma, it is important to maintain a threshold of stressor severity to guard against bracket creep. For example, when assessing events that involve indirect exposure (i.e., that happened to someone else), it is essential to establish that the respondent had a very close relationship with the individual directly exposed to the trauma.

The primary goal for assessing Criterion A is to identify at least one event that satisfies Criteria A1 and A2, and can be used as the index event for symptom inquiry. This can be accomplished in a variety of ways. In some cases the index event will be the main reason for a clinical referral (or for recruitment into a research study); thus, it may have been identified prior to the assessment. In addition, some interviews and self-report measures provide a means of screening for possible traumas and identifying an index event for symptom inquiry. Another alternative is to administer a dedicated trauma exposure measure. These range from broad-spectrum measures that evaluate exposure to a broad range of stressors, to focal measures that evaluate exposure to a single type of trauma, such as combat (for recent reviews of trauma exposure measures, see Keane, Street, & Stafford, 2004; Norris & Hamblen, 2004). In addition to identifying an index event for symptom inquiry, whenever possible it also important to assess for exposure to other traumatic events across the lifespan. Exposure to multiple lifetime traumas is typical (e.g., Breslau et al., 1998; Kessler et al., 1995), and previous traumas may influence reactions to the index event.

The assessment of Criterion A becomes more challenging when the stressor cannot readily be conceptualized as a unitary event. DSM-IV-TR refers to "a stressor," "an event," or "the traumatic event," thus implying that the stressor is a single, well-delineated event. Some traumas, such as a sexual or physical assault, a motor vehicle accident (MVA), or an earthquake or tornado are relatively circumscribed and provide a reasonable fit for the single-event model. However, this does not reflect the reality of many types of trauma, such as combat, childhood sexual abuse, community violence, domestic violence, or a life-threatening illness, which may comprise multiple traumatic stressors or multiple occurrences of the same stressor over months or even years. In such cases, a reasonable approach would be to ensure that at least one aspect of the stressor meets Criterion A, then ask the respondent to consider the stressor as a whole and link symptoms to the most traumatic aspects. Therefore, for some trauma types, the index "event" may actually be a summary label for multiple Criterion A events (e.g., "the most difficult parts of your combat experiences"). Another possible approach is to ask the respondent to identify one of the multiple traumatic events as the most distressing at present in terms of causing the most frequent and severe symptoms, then use that event as the basis for symptom inquiry.

Assess Symptom Criteria

The next step is to assess the 17 symptoms of PTSD and determine whether the respondent has the requisite number of symptoms in each of the three symptom clusters (i.e., at least one of five reexperiencing symptoms, at least three of seven avoidance and numbing symptoms, and at least two of five hyperarousal symptoms). There are a number of potential difficulties in accomplishing this task. First, PTSD is a multifaceted disorder with a large number of symptoms, representing a broad array of overt and covert behaviors in multiple response channels. Second, some of the symptoms, particularly flashbacks, amnesia, and sense of foreshortened future, are poorly conceptualized and vaguely defined in the diagnostic criteria. They are not well understood by many experienced clinicians, much less by respondents, which makes them subject to idiosyncratic interpretation leading to substantial error variance in inquiry, response, and rating.

Third, some of the symptoms overlap substantially, both within a cluster (e.g., overlap within the reexperiencing symptoms among intrusive thoughts, cued distress, cued physiological reactivity) and across clusters (e.g., nightmares and sleep disturbance), and are difficult to assess and to rate independently. This can lead to "double-coding," whereby respondents are credited with two or more symptoms for essentially the same problem, which can result in inflation of the overall PTSD severity score. Fourth, many of the symptoms, such as the emotional numbing, are negative symptoms or behavioral deficits. These are particularly difficult to assess because to respondents they may not be as evident as are the positive symptoms, such as the reexperiencing and hyperarousal symptoms (Keane, 1989). Furthermore, inquiring about negative symptoms is difficult because it often amounts to asking the awkward question of how often something does *not* occur.

Determine Presence or Absence of Individual Symptoms

Assessing individual symptoms involves two objectives. The first objective is to evaluate whether the respondent's description of a symptom fits the diagnostic criterion phenomenologically. For example, for the symptom *reacting or feeling as if the traumatic event were recurring*, commonly referred to as a "flashback," it is essential to determine that the respondent's experience involves a true dissociative quality, with a distinct alteration in mental status. Without the dissociative quality, this symptom would be difficult to distinguish from other reexperiencing symptoms, such as intrusive recollections. Similarly, for the symptom *inability to recall an important aspect of the trauma*, it is essential to determine that the "amnesia" is functioning as a type of avoidance of a feared part of the trauma memory. Other reasons for amnesia, such as having been unconscious during part of the traumatic event, or even ordinary forgetting with the passage of time, would not count for this symptom. Elsewhere we have provided a full description of all 17 symptoms and guidelines for their assessment (Weathers et al., 2004).

The second objective is to evaluate whether the respondent's description of a symptom represents a clinically significant problem and not simply an expectable, normative reaction that is not indicative of mental disorder and does not require treatment. As Spitzer, First, and Wakefield (2007) recently noted, PTSD symptoms may be worded so broadly that some respondents may make false-positive endorsements because they interpret them as referring to normal rather than pathological reactions to stress. Spitzer et al. suggested that one solution for the DSM-V revision of PTSD criteria might be to raise the threshold of symptom severity by adding qualifiers, such as "excessively intense, frequent, or enduring," to the symptom descriptors. This approach would make the threshold between normal and pathological reaction more explicit. However, this distinction is already evident in several DSM-IV-TR symptoms (e.g., *intense psychological distress, markedly diminished interest, exaggerated startle response*) and in Criterion F (*clinically significant distress*), and should be routinely factored into clinical judgment on structured interviews. On self-report measures, an appropriately stringent threshold can be achieved by identifying appropriate cutoffs for item severity ratings.

Link Symptoms to the Index Event

Once the presence of individual symptoms is established, the next step is to establish an explicit link between the symptoms and the index event. For the symptoms to count toward a diagnosis of PTSD, they must have developed following exposure to the trauma and must be attributable to it, at least in the sense of it being the immediate precipitant. For respondents with previous trauma exposure or previous PTSD symptoms, it must be clear that the current syndrome was exacerbated by the index event. In any case, it must be clear that the symptoms represent a distinct change from a previous level of functioning prior to the index event.

This is a relatively straightforward task for the five reexperiencing symptoms (B1–B5), the two effortful avoidance symptoms (C1–C2), and amnesia (C3) because all are inherently linked to the trauma in that they explicitly refer to the index event. The remaining nine symptoms, the rest of the Cluster C symptoms (C4–C7) and the hyperarousal symptoms (D1–D5), are not inherently linked to the trauma, so specific inquiry is required to establish that these symptoms are functionally related to the index event. This is a much more difficult task, especially in a self-report format. It is more feasible in a structured interview, but in many cases, especially when the index trauma occurred many years prior to the diagnostic interview, as with childhood sexual abuse, the link to the symptoms is still ambiguous and requires clinical judgment. To make this task explicit and to assist interviewers in making the appropriate determination, the CAPS, for example, includes a trauma-related inquiry and rating for each of the last nine symptoms. Interviewers ask about the onset of the symptom and rate the link between the symptom and the index event as *definite, probably,* or *unlikely*. Symptoms rated as *definite* or *probably* are counted toward a PTSD diagnosis. Symptoms rated as *unlikely* because they are explicitly attributable to some other cause, are not counted toward a diagnosis.

Quantify Symptom Severity

Although it is not essential for diagnosis, quantifying PTSD symptom severity is very useful for a variety of clinical and research applications. Having a continuous measure of severity for the syndrome, for symptom clusters, or even for individual items, provides a more flexible, sensitive metric than dichotomous present–absent ratings. Among their most important functions, continuous measures of PTSD (1) dimensionalize PTSD severity and allow for more precise statements about current clinical status; (2) permit the evaluation of group differences in mean PTSD severity; (3) provide PTSD variables for use in correlational and regression analyses (e.g., to evaluate convergent and discriminant validity, employ PTSD severity as a predictor or criterion in multiple regression, or include individual symptom scores in factor analysis); and (4) permit the assessment of changes in symptom severity over time, especially in treatment outcome studies.

Clarify Chronology

DSM-IV-TR requires that the PTSD symptoms have lasted at least 1 month to distinguish short-term, normative reactions to stress from a more chronic syndrome indicative of a mental disorder. The syndrome is specified as "acute" if symptoms have lasted at least 1 month but less than 3 months, and as "chronic" if symptoms have lasted longer than 3 months. In addition, if the symptoms began 6 months or more after the index event, the syndrome is specified as "with delayed onset."

Evaluate Subjective Distress and Functional Impairment

Following the assessment of symptom criteria, the next task is to evaluate Criterion F, which requires that the syndrome cause clinically significant subjective distress or functional impairment. The degree of subjective distress is typically evident from assessment of the individual symptoms. Distress is included explicitly as part of the criterion language for several of the reexperiencing symptoms and is implicit for a number of other symptoms in all three symptom clusters. With structured interviews, clinicians consider subjective distress as they determine the presence or absence of individual symptoms; thus, the global evaluation of distress for Criterion F is essentially redundant with symptom inquiry. Self-report measures typically do not include a separate, overall rating of subjective distress, so this aspect of Criterion F is inferred from the total severity score. In contrast, although functional impairment can be inferred from symptom-level inquiry, it is often better evaluated globally, at the syndrome level, to understand how the combined impact of all symptoms in the clinical presentation are affecting current social and occupational functioning. Several structured interview and self-report measures include separate ratings to assess the impact of the syndrome on key domains of functioning.

It notable that in DSM-IV-TR, Criterion F is satisfied by the presence of either clinically significant distress or functional impairment. Individuals may experience substantial distress but still manage to get through their daily lives, although perhaps with diminished productivity and interpersonal connectedness; thus, they may report only moderate or even mild impairment. In such cases, on the one hand, a diagnosis of PTSD would still be appropriate, at least according to the current conceptualization of the disorder. On the other hand, it is somewhat implausible that an individual would have clinically significant distress but not have at least some degree of impaired functioning, so subjective distress and functional impairment typically are both involved in the clinical presentation.

Establish Differential Diagnosis

As with any mental disorder, differential diagnosis is a crucial task in assessing PTSD. An important discrimination that must be made is between PTSD and adjustment disorder. According to DSM-IV-TR, a diagnosis of adjustment disorder is warranted when either the symptoms that develop following a Criterion A stressor do not meet full PTSD criteria or the symptoms develop following a stressor that does not meet Criterion A. The latter distinction is crucial because it provides diagnostic coverage for individuals who develop symptoms in response to low-magnitude stressors, yet maintains a relatively stringent threshold of stressor severity, thereby addressing the problem of bracket creep and excessive diagnosis of PTSD.

Apart from the distinction between PTSD and adjustment disorder, the differential diagnosis of PTSD and other disorders is generally unambiguous and typically much less difficult than the differential diagnosis between, say, a mood disorder with psychotic features and schizophrenia. PTSD is easily distinguished from acute stress disorder in that PTSD involves symptoms that persist beyond 1 month following the index event. Beyond that, although there is some symptom overlap with other disorders, such as major depression and other anxiety disorders, no other disorder could plausibly account for the characteristic syndrome of PTSD, particularly the defining features of reexperiencing and effortful avoidance. Furthermore, the usual exclusion criteria regarding the physiological effects of a substance or a general medical condition are not directly relevant because there is no evidence that any substance use syndrome or medical condition could account for the PTSD syndrome.

Assess Comorbid Disorders

Although PTSD can usually be readily distinguished from other disorders, it often co-occurs with other disorders, especially major depression, substance use disorders, and other anxiety disorders (Keane & Kaloupek, 1997; Kessler et al., 1995). The presence of additional disorders indicates a more complicated and severe clinical presentation, with multiple targets for assessment and intervention. Therefore, a comprehensive assessment of PTSD must include a thorough evaluation of comorbidity, with the goals of determining what other disorders may be present, prioritizing targets for intervention, and developing an appropriate treatment plan. As discussed below, multiscale inventories can play a valuable role in alerting the clinician to the presence of comorbid problems, but the best approach is to administer a structured diagnostic interview, such as the Structured Clinical Interview for DSM-IV (SCID; First, Spitzer, Gibbon, & Williams, 1996).

Assess Associated Features

In addition to comorbid disorders, the clinical presentation of PTSD often involves other clinically significant clinical problems, most notably guilt (i.e., survivor guilt, guilt over acts of commission or omission), as well as a group of symptoms referred to as "complex PTSD," which may result from chronic interpersonal trauma such as physical and sexual abuse or marital violence (Herman, 1992). The main symptoms of complex PTSD include affect dysregulation, dissociation, alterations in perceptions of self and perpetrator, markedly impaired interpersonal relationships, and alterations of meaning, including a loss of faith accompanied by feelings of hopelessness and despair. Although not currently part of the diagnostic criteria for PTSD, these symptoms are listed as associated features to alert those who work with victims of chronic interpersonal trauma to give special attention to these problem areas. It is important to note that problems such as guilt, shame, and alterations in perceptions of self and other are also often seen in individuals whose PTSD stems from events other than interpersonal traumas (Foa, Ehlers, Clark, Tolin, & Orsillo, 1999).

Assess Response Bias

A crucial task in the assessment of PTSD is a thorough evaluation of response bias, particularly symptom exaggeration or malingering (Guriel & Fremouw, 2003; Rosen & Taylor, 2007). More than other mental disorders, PTSD is particularly susceptible to malingering because it is a highly compensable disorder, both within the Veterans Department of Affairs (VA) for combat veterans seeking service-connected disability compensation and in the context of civil litigation. Malingering poses a threat not only to the validity of clinical assessment but also to the integrity of the research database in the field of traumatic stress (Rosen, 2004a). In the differential diagnosis section of the PTSD text, DSM-IV-TR includes the instruction to rule out malingering when there is the possibility of secondary gain.

In practice, though, this can be difficult to accomplish. On most PTSD measures, including self-report measures and structured interviews, the items are transparent, the pathological response is easily discerned, and there is no means of detecting response bias, all of which make it relatively easy to invent or exaggerate a pathological presentation. Nevertheless, several different approaches to clinical assessment can potentially detect malingering and other types of response bias, and one or more of these should be used whenever possible. One approach is to draw on multiple sources of information, such as public records, medical records, and collateral reports from friends, family members, or others who know the respondent well, to corroborate the trauma exposure, as well as the presence and impact of any PTSD symptoms. A second approach is to administer a multiscale inventory, such as the Minnesota Multiphasic Personality Inventory—2nd edition (MMPI-2) and Personality Assessment Inventory (described below), which include psychometrically sound scales to detect response bias. A third approach is to administer a dedicated malingering instrument, such as the Structured Interview of Reported Symptoms (SIRS; Rogers, Bagby, & Dickens, 1992). Each of these strategies will require additional time and resources, but will increase confidence in the validity of responses and the final outcome of the assessment process.

Integrate Information across Measures

The use of multiple measures has long been advocated in the assessment of PTSD (Keane, Fairbank, Caddell, Zimering, & Bender, 1985; Keane et al.,

1987; Kulka et al., 1991), and a typical comprehensive protocol may include a trauma exposure measure, a structured interview for PTSD, one or more self-report measures of PTSD, a multiscale inventory, and possibly even a psychophysiological assessment. From a construct validity perspective, each PTSD measure is seen as a fallible indicator of the underlying construct, and the limitations of any single measure are offset by the strengths of another measure. However, combining information across measures can be difficult, and currently few empirical guidelines are available. Sequential decision rules can be developed, and scores from different measures can be combined with regression techniques (Kraemer, 1992; Kulka et al., 1991), but these approaches require very large samples and may be impractical in many settings. A second approach is to use clinical judgment. When all indicators are positive or negative, the decision would be considered settled. When indicators are discordant, however, there are several options. One is to give priority to the best measures (e.g., structured interviews). A second option is to debrief the respondent and inquire about attributions for the discordance. A third option is to administer additional measures, or gather other, additional information that might help to account for the discordance.

Measures

In this section we describe some of the most widely used measures of PTSD, including structured interviews and self-report measures (for a comprehensive list of measures of trauma and PTSD, and an estimate of frequency of their use, see Elhai, Gray, Kashdan, & Franklin, 2005). These measures vary in the extent to which they correspond to DSM diagnostic criteria for PTSD. All of the interviews correspond directly to DSM criteria. However, the self-report measures can be divided into those that correspond directly to DSM and those that assess trauma-relevant symptoms but do not correspond directly to DSM. PTSD measures also vary in format, especially in terms of the wording of items, the number of response options, the type of response dimension (e.g., symptom frequency, level of subjective distress), and time frame (e.g., past week, past month). Therefore, when selecting a measure, it is important to review it carefully to ensure that it is appropriate for the intended purpose. We conclude this section with a discussion of the use of multiscale personality inventories in the assessment of PTSD. This review is selective and focuses on instruments that are likely to be useful in a wide variety of settings. In addition to the resources already cited, further information and access to specific instruments is available from the International Society for Traumatic Stress Studies (ISTSS; *www.istss.org/resources/browse.cfm*) and the National Center for PTSD (NCPTSD; *www.ncptsd.va.gov*), which also provides a link for accessing and searching the Published International Literature on Traumatic Stress (PILOTS) database.

Structured Interviews

Structured interviews are considered the "gold standard" in the diagnosis of mental disorders. Thus, whenever possible, a structured interview should be included in the assessment of PTSD. Several well-validated interviews exist for PTSD and meet a variety of clinical and research needs. In this section we describe four interviews that vary in their features, and in their potential utility, for different applications. In considering the relative merits of these interviews, it is important to recognize that an interview is more than just the words on the page. The standard administration and scoring of a structured interview for PTSD requires expertise in diagnostic interviewing and differential diagnosis, a thorough conceptual understanding of trauma and the clinical presentation of PTSD, and extensive experience with that particular interview. Therefore, it is not appropriate to compare interviews simply by examining written features, such as the content of the prompts and the nature of the rating scale. An adequate description of an interview must include information about how it is to be administered and by whom. This description should specify how follow-up inquiry after an initial prompt is handled, and how much clinical judgment is involved in translating responses into ratings. It should also specify the appropriate qualifications for interviewers, including training in diagnostic interviewing, experience in assessing trauma survivors, and documented reliability for the specific interview. This is particularly relevant for interviews that provide relatively less structure and guidance in terms of prompts and rating scale anchors, and that rely more heavily on the clinical skill and judgment of the interviewer.

Structured Clinical Interview for DSM-IV

The SCID (First et al., 1996) is a comprehensive structured interview designed to diagnose all the major DSM-IV disorders. There are a number of versions of the SCID, including three research versions and a clinical version for Axis I disorders, and a version to diagnose personality disorders (for extensive information on the various versions, see the SCID website at *www.scid4.org*). The PTSD module of the SCID can be administered in the context of the full SCID but often is administered alone or with a few additional modules to assess the disorders most highly comorbid with PTSD (e.g., depression, other anxiety disorders). As with all SCID modules, the PTSD module maps directly on to DSM-IV diagnostic criteria. It begins with a brief screening for potentially traumatic events, followed by two questions to identify the worst event for symptom inquiry and to determine whether that event satisfies Criterion A. The symptom inquiry section is next and comprises a single prompt for each of the 17 PTSD symptoms, although interviewers may ask additional questions as needed to clarify responses. The module concludes with several questions regarding the onset and course of symptoms. All criteria are rated as ? = *inadequate information*, 1 = *absent*, 2 = *subthreshold*, or 3 = *threshold*. A respondent is diagnosed with PTSD if all diagnostic criteria are met (i.e., are rated as 3 = *threshold*).

The SCID PTSD module appears to have good reliability and convergent validity. Kulka and colleagues (1991) found a kappa of .93 for interrater reliability. Similarly, Keane and colleagues (1998) found good interrater reliability for PTSD ratings of current, never, and lifetime, with 77% agreement and a weighted kappa of .68. They also found good test–retest reliability, with 78% agreement and a weighted kappa of .66. Both of these reports involved a large sample of male veterans in a PTSD-focused study. Other investigators have found strong reliability in other samples and settings. Skre, Onstad, Torgersen, and Kringlen (1991) found a kappa of .77 for interrater reliability. Zanarini and colleagues (2000) found kappas of .88 for interrater reliability and .78 for test–retest reliability. In a second study, Zanarini and Frankenburg (2001) found kappas of 1.0 for both interrater and test–retest, indicating perfect reliability. With respect to validity, Schlenger and colleagues (1992) found that the SCID PTSD module was positively associated with self-report measures of PTSD, including the Mississippi Scale (kappa = .53) and the Keane PTSD Scale (PK) of the MMPI (kappa = .48), and had excellent diagnostic utility against a composite PTSD diagnosis (e.g., sensitivity = .81, specificity = .98).

The SCID PTSD module has several advantages. It is relatively brief, it corresponds to DSM criteria for PTSD, and it incorporates the other well-established features of the SCID. However, it also has some disadvantages. One limitation is that the trauma screening section is cursory and may not provide a sufficient context for eliciting reports of traumatic events. The primary limitation, however, is that it yields essentially present–absent ratings for individual symptoms and for the diagnosis. Because it does not provide continuous severity scores, it cannot be used as a dimensional measure of PTSD, nor can it be used to detect changes in symptom severity.

PTSD Symptom Scale—Interview

The PTSD Symptom Scale—Interview (PSS-I; Foa et al., 1993), a structured interview originally developed to assess DSM-III-R criteria for PTSD, comprises 17 questions that correspond to the 17 symptom criteria for PTSD. The severity of each symptom over the past 2 weeks is rated on a 4-point scale. In the original version, the rating scale anchors were 0 = *not at all*, 1 = *a little bit*, 2 = *somewhat*, or 3 = *very much*. These were modified in the current version for DSM-IV, so they now include combined frequency and intensity ratings (e.g., 1 = *once per week or less/a little* and 3 = *five or more times per week/very much*) (Foa & Tolin, 2000). The rationale for combining severity and frequency ratings on the PSS-I is that for some symptoms, such as nightmares, frequency is the most relevant dimension because nightmares are by definition severe. For other symptoms, such as hypervigilance and sense of foreshortened future, which typically are experienced continuously, severity is the only relevant dimension. The PSS-I yields a severity/frequency score for each of the three

PTSD symptom clusters, as well as a total PTSD severity score. It also yields a PTSD diagnosis, which is obtained by following a rationally derived scoring rule, whereby an item is counted as a symptom toward a diagnosis if it is rated as 1 = *once per week or less/a little.*

The PSS-I has excellent psychometric properties. In its original report (Foa et al., 1993), the PSS-I demonstrated strong internal consistency, with an alpha coefficient of .85 for all 17 items. It also demonstrated good test–retest reliability (r = .80 for total severity) and very high interrater reliability (kappa = .91) for a PTSD diagnosis, and an intraclass correlation of .97 for total severity. Validity is also excellent. The PSS-I had a sensitivity of .88, a specificity of .96, and an efficiency of .94 for predicting a diagnosis of PTSD based on the SCID. Furthermore, it correlated strongly with several self-report measures of PTSD, depression, and anxiety.

More recently, Foa and Tolin (2000) also reported excellent psychometric properties and concluded that, in general, the PSS-I compares favorably with the CAPS. In this study, the PSS-I again demonstrated strong internal consistency, with an alpha of .86 for total severity, and excellent interrater reliability, with correlations ranging from .91 to .93 for the three symptom clusters, and .93 for total severity. The PSS-I also showed good correspondence with the SCID PTSD module and the CAPS. PSS-I total severity score correlated .73 with the SCID PTSD module and .87 with CAPS total severity score. At the diagnostic level, the PSS-I had a kappa of .65, with the CAPS scored with the original Frequency (F) = 1/Intensity (I) = 2 rule, and a kappa of .56 with the SCID PTSD module. Foa and Tolin also found that the PSS-I took significantly less time to administer than did the CAPS (22 vs. 33 minutes for the full sample; 29 vs. 43 minutes for those with PTSD based on the PSS-I).

Advantages of the PSS-I are that it is relatively brief and easy to administer; it yields a PTSD diagnosis, as well as continuous severity scores for the three symptom clusters and the full syndrome; and it has strong reliability and validity. One disadvantage is that it includes only a single question for each symptom. However, the PSS-I manual (Hembree, Foa, & Feeny, 2002) provides instructions and additional questions to guide interviewers in following up on ambiguous responses. Another disadvantage is that the diagnostic scoring rule was rationally derived, and alternative rules have not been proposed or evaluated. This scoring rule may be relatively liberal in that it yields PTSD prevalence rates substantially higher than the original F1/I2 scoring rule for the CAPS (Foa & Tolin, 2000), which is the most lenient CAPS rule recommended for routine use.

Structured Interview for PTSD

The Structured Interview for PTSD (Davidson, Smith, & Kudler, 1989) was developed to assess DSM-III and DSM-III-R criteria for PTSD. Originally referred to as the SI-PTSD, it was modified in 1997 to correspond to DSM-IV criteria and relabeled as the SIP (Davidson, Malik, & Travers, 1997). The SIP comprises 19 items, including 17 items that correspond to DSM-IV diagnostic criteria for PTSD and two items measuring trauma-related guilt. Items are rated on a 5-point scale (0–4), and those that are rated as 2 = *moderate* or higher are considered symptom endorsements. The SIP yields a continuous measure of PTSD symptom severity, as well as a dichotomous DSM-IV PTSD diagnosis.

The SIP appears to have good psychometric properties. In the original report, Davidson and colleagues (1989) reported a full-scale alpha of .94, test–retest reliability of .71, and excellent interrater reliability, with intraclass correlations ranging from .97 to .99, and perfect diagnostic agreement. They also reported good diagnostic utility against the SCID PTSD module, with a sensitivity of .96, a specificity of .80, and a kappa of .79. For the revised version, Davidson and colleagues (1997) reported a full-scale alpha of .80, test–retest reliability of .89, and interrater reliability of .90. They also reported moderate to strong correlations with self-report measures of PTSD, and moderate correlations with measures of depression and anxiety. Diagnostic utility against the SCID PTSD module varied by cutoff of the Total Severity score, but at a cutoff of 20 the SIP achieved perfect agreement with the SCID. Finally, the SIP demonstrated good sensitivity to clinical change as a treatment outcome measure.

As with the PSS-I, the advantages of the SIP are that it is relatively brief and easy to administer; it yields a continuous measure of PTSD symptom severity, as well as a dichotomous PTSD diagnosis; and it appears to be psychometrically sound. In addition the SIP provides follow-up prompts and rating scale descriptors to help clarify symptom inquiry and ratings. One disadvantage is that the SIP relies on a single, rationally derived scoring rule for obtaining a diagnosis. Furthermore, the psychometric findings, although promising, are somewhat limited and have not been independently confirmed by other investigators.

Clinician-Administered PTSD Scale

Developed in 1989 at the NCPTSD, the CAPS (Blake et al., 1990, 1995) is a comprehensive structured interview for PTSD. The CAPS comprises 30 items, including 17 items that assess the DSM-IV symptoms of PTSD; 5 items that assess onset, duration, subjective distress, and functional impairment; 3 items that assess overall response validity, symptom severity, and symptom improvement; and 5 items that assess associated symptoms, including trauma-related guilt and dissociation. In addition, the CAPS assesses Criterion A by means of the Life Events Checklist, which screens for possible trauma exposure, and a trauma inquiry section that evaluates both parts of Criterion A and identifies an index event for symptom inquiry. At the symptom level, the CAPS yields continuous and dichotomous scores for each item, and at the syndrome level, it yields a continuous measure of overall PTSD symptom severity, in addition to a dichotomous PTSD diagnosis.

The CAPS has several distinctive features. First, it assesses the frequency and intensity of each symptom on separate 5-point (0–4) rating scales. Second, CAPS items include initial prompt questions, as well as a number of follow-up questions to help clarify ambiguous responses. Third, CAPS prompt questions and rating scale anchors contain clear behavioral referents to increase the uniformity of inquiry and the accuracy of ratings. Fourth, the CAPS includes a "trauma-related" inquiry and rating scale for the numbing and hyperarousal symptoms to assess explicitly the link between these symptoms and the index event. Fifth, the CAPS provides a procedure for determining lifetime diagnostic status. Finally, a variety of scoring rules are available for converting CAPS scores into a PTSD diagnosis, which allows the CAPS diagnosis to be adjusted for different assessment tasks (Weathers, Ruscio, & Keane, 1999).

As we have discussed in detail elsewhere (Weathers, Keane, & Davidson, 2001), the CAPS has been studied extensively and has excellent psychometric properties. It is the most widely used structured interview for PTSD and has proven useful for a variety of clinical and research assessment needs. The CAPS is available in a published version, which includes the interview booklet, an interviewer's guide, and a technical manual (Weathers et al., 2004). It is also available in many languages with information accumulating about its psychometric characteristics in these different languages (e.g., Charney & Keane, 2007). Qualified investigators may obtain a research version of the CAPS and an abbreviated manual from the NCPTSD website. The main disadvantages of the CAPS are that it takes longer than other interviews to administer and requires more extensive training to become proficient in its administration and scoring.

Self-Report Measures

DSM-Correspondent Measures

PTSD CHECKLIST

The PCL (Weathers et al., 1993) is a self-report measure of PTSD developed at the National Center for PTSD in 1990. The 17 PCL items correspond to the 17 DSM-IV symptoms of PTSD. Respondents rate how much they were bothered by each symptom over the past month using a 5-point scale, ranging from 1 = *not at all* to 5 = *extremely*. The three versions of the PCL are identical except for the description of the target event in the first eight items (i.e., items tapping reexperiencing, effortful avoidance, and amnesia). The Civilian Version (PCL-C), which refers to "a stressful experience from the past," and the Military Version (PCL-M), which refers to "a stressful military experience," are appropriate when a specific stressor has not been identified. In contrast, the Specific Version (PCL-S) refers to a specific stressor identified by either the participant or, in some research applications, the investigator. The PCL yields a continuous measure of PTSD symptom severity for each of the three symptom clusters and for the whole syndrome. It may also be scored to yield a dichotomous PTSD diagnosis, by counting items rated 3 = *moderately* or higher as a symptom toward a diagnosis, then following the DSM-IV diagnostic rule of at least one reexperiencing symptom, at least three avoidance and numbing symptoms, and at least two hyperarousal symptoms.

The PCL has been widely adopted and extensively evaluated, and has excellent psychometric properties across a variety of trauma populations. In the original work with male combat veterans (Weathers et al., 1993) the PCL demonstrated high internal consistency for the full scale, with an alpha of .97, and excellent test–retest reliability, with a correlation of .96 between separate administrations 2–3 days apart. The PCL also correlated strongly with other measures of PTSD and combat exposure, and demonstrated good diagnostic utility against the SCID PTSD module, with a sensitivity of .82, a specificity of .83, and a kappa of .64. Also, in a sample of victims of MVAs or sexual assault, Blanchard, Jones-Alexander, Buckley, and Forneris (1996) reported excellent internal consistency, with a full-scale alpha of .94, and strong correspondence with the CAPS. Using a slightly lower PCL cutoff of 44, they found a sensitivity of .94, a specificity of .86, and an efficiency of .94 against a CAPS diagnosis of PTSD. They also found that each PCL item correlated significantly with its counterpart on the CAPS, with seven correlations higher than .70, and all but three higher than .60. Furthermore, in a sample of college students with mixed civilian trauma, Ruggiero, Del Ben, Scotti, and Rabalais (2003) reported excellent internal consistency, with a full-scale alpha of .94; test–retest reliability ranging from .68 to .92, depending on the retest interval; and strong correlations with self-report measures of PTSD, depression, and anxiety.

In addition to its ability to predict an interview-based diagnosis of PTSD, the PCL is useful for a range of other assessment tasks, including screening for possible PTSD (e.g., Andrykowski, Cordova, Studts, & Miller, 1998; Dobie et al., 2002), detecting clinical change (e.g., Forbes, Creamer, & Biddle, 2001), and estimating PTSD prevalence in large-scale epidemiological surveys (e.g., Kang, Natelson, Mahan, Lee, & Murphy, 2003). The PCL was also used extensively in factor-analytic studies of PTSD (e.g., Asmundson et al., 2000; DuHamel et al., 2004; Palmieri, Weathers, Difede, & King, 2007; Simms, Watson, & Doebbeling, 2002), the cumulative findings of which have challenged the DSM-IV three-cluster approach to PTSD symptoms.

One concern about the PCL literature is that different studies have used different versions, and the version used is not always clearly specified. Therefore, it cannot be assumed that the psychometric findings for one version generalize to the others. Another question that needs further investigation involves the choice of specific cutoff scores on the PCL. The optimal cutoff score has varied across trauma type, setting, and task (e.g., screening vs. differential diagnosis), and clearly no single cutoff is appropriate for all applications. The best approach in selecting a PCL cutoff for a trauma type in a given setting is to use cutoffs identified in studies of similar samples.

DAVIDSON TRAUMA SCALE

The Davidson Trauma Scale (DTS; Davidson, 1996) is another 17-item, self-report measure that assesses the DSM-IV diagnostic criteria for PTSD. The item format is similar that of the CAPS, in that the frequency and severity of each symptom is rated on separate 4-point scales. The Frequency scale ranges from 0 = *not at all* to 4 = *every day*, and the Severity scale ranges from 0 = *not at all distressing* to 4 = *extremely distressing*. The time frame for ratings is the past week. This allows for frequent administrations, which is valuable in treatment outcome studies, but limits the use of the DTS as a diagnostic measure because it does cover the required duration for PTSD symptoms of at least 1 month. Although the main purpose of the DTS is to provide a continuous measure of PTSD symptom severity, the manual provides a table for converting DTS total scores into a probability of having a PTSD diagnosis.

The DTS appears to have good psychometric properties. Davidson (1996) found high internal consistency, with alphas for frequency, severity, and total scores all above .90, and strong test–retest reliability with a correlation of .86 between administrations over a 1-week interval. The DTS also demonstrated good convergent and discriminant validity, correlating strongly with several other PTSD measures, and not correlating with a measure of extraversion. In addition, the DTS distinguished between groups that varied in PTSD severity and was sensitive to changes in PTSD severity as a function of treatment. Finally, the DTS demonstrated good diagnostic utility against the SCID PTSD module. A cutoff of 40, which was described as the most accurate, had a sensitivity of .69, a specificity of .95, and an efficiency of .83.

The DTS appears to be a useful measure of PTSD. It is well suited for tracking changes in symptom severity in treatment outcome studies and has been widely adopted for this purpose (Davidson, Tharwani, & Connor, 2002). One limitation is that little additional psychometric work has been conducted, so it is not clear how well the original findings generalize to other samples and settings.

POSTTRAUMATIC STRESS DIAGNOSTIC SCALE

The Posttraumatic Stress Diagnostic Scale (PDS; Foa, 1995; Foa, Cashman, Jaycox, & Perry, 1997), a 49-item self-report measure of PTSD, is designed to assess all of the DSM-IV diagnostic criteria for PTSD. The PDS, which is based on the self-report counterpart (PSS-SR) of the PSS-I described earlier (Foa et al., 1993), is one of only two self-report instruments that assess all DSM-IV PTSD criteria and was designed as a screening instrument for identifying a diagnosis of PTSD in the general population or in a population of trauma survivors. Accordingly, the PDS include four sections. The first two sections assess Criterion A. The first comprises a list of common potential traumatic events and asks respondents to indicate whether they have experienced one or more of those events. The second section establishes which event that they endorsed in the first section is the most distressing to them at present, how long ago this most distressing event occurred, and whether they were horrified, terrified, or feeling helpless during the event. The third section asks respondents to rate the frequency/severity of the 17 PTSD symptoms, linking them to the traumatic event identified in the second section. The fourth section assesses functional impairment. Symptoms are rated on a 4-point frequency scale with respect to the past month, with 0 = *not at all or only one time*, 1 = *once a week or less/once in a while*, 2 = *two to four times a week/half the time*, and 3 = *five or more times a week/almost always*. Symptom scores are summed to yield a total symptom severity score, which ranges from 0 to 51 and is classified into one of four severity categories: *mild* (10 or lower), *moderate* (11–20), *moderate to severe* (21–35), and *severe* (36 or higher). The PDS also yields a dichotomous PTSD diagnosis.

The PDS is psychometrically sound. In terms of reliability, Foa and colleagues (1997) reported strong internal consistency, with an alpha of .92 across the 17 symptom items, and good test–retest reliability, with a correlation of .83 for total severity and a kappa of .74 for a PTSD diagnosis. In terms of validity, Foa et al. found that the PDS strongly correlated with self-report measures of PTSD, depression, and anxiety. Furthermore, the PDS total severity score and the total number of symptoms endorsed significantly discriminated individuals with and without a PTSD diagnosis based on the SCID PTSD module. Finally, the PDS demonstrated adequate diagnostic utility against the SCID, with a sensitivity of .89, a specificity of .75, an efficiency of .82, and a kappa of .65.

Advantages of the PDS are that it assesses all the PTSD diagnostic criteria, it was developed with careful attention to content validity, it yields both a continuous measure of symptom severity and a PTSD diagnosis, and it appears to have good psychometric properties in an initial sample of trauma survivors. Because of its ability to assess all the PTSD diagnostic criteria, it has been widely used in studies examining the rate of PTSD in populations that experienced a traumatic event (e.g., earthquakes, war). The PDS have been translated into numerous languages (e.g., Croatian, Hebrew, Spanish, Chinese, Japanese, German, French, Persian, Arabic, Dutch, and Lughara). The psychometric properties of the PDS have been examined in several cultures, replicating those found in the original study. For example, Powell and Rosner (2005) administered the Croatian version of the PDS and other measures of trauma-related psychopathology (IES and Beck Depression Inventory [BDI]) to 812 people living in Sarajevo or Benja Luka in Bosnia and Herzegovina, of whom the majority had experienced a high number of traumatic war events. The correlations between the total scale and the subscales were all quite high at .89, .93, and .87 for reexperiencing, avoidance, and hyperarousal, respectively. Convergent and discriminant validity were also adequate. The correlation between the PDS and the IES was .75, whereas the correlation between the PDS and the BDI was .60. Similar results were reported by Griesel, Wessa, and Flor (2006), who used the German version of the PDS with 143 trauma survivors. One possible disadvantage is that because the PDS relies on a single, rationally derived diagnostic scoring rule, alternative rules have not been proposed or evaluated.

DETAILED ASSESSMENT OF POSTTRAUMATIC STRESS

The Detailed Assessment of Posttraumatic Stress (DAPS; Briere, 2001) is a 104-item, comprehensive, self-report measure of trauma and PTSD. Similar to the PDS, the DAPS evaluates all DSM-IV diagnostic criteria for PTSD, including trauma exposure, the 17 PTSD symptoms, and the degree of functional impairment. Beyond that, though, the DAPS includes scales assessing peritraumatic distress and dissociation, trauma-specific dissociation, substance abuse, and suicidality. Furthermore, the DAPS includes scales to assess positive and negative response bias, and is the only dedicated PTSD measure, self-report or interview, to do so. T-scores based on a normative sample of approximately 400 trauma-exposed adults are used to generate a dimensional profile incorporating the two response validity scales and 11 clinical scales. For the clinical scales, T-score elevations of 65 and above are considered clinically significant. In addition, decision rules are provided for generating a probable diagnosis of PTSD or acute stress disorder.

As reported in the professional manual, the DAPS initial psychometric analyses are promising. Internal consistency was excellent, with high alpha coefficients for all scales except for Negative Bias (NB) and Relative Trauma Exposure (RTE), which are not expected to be internally consistent, because they do not tap a coherent construct. In addition, the response bias scales demonstrated good convergent and discriminant validity with other self-report measures of response validity, and the clinical scales demonstrated good convergent and discriminant validity with other self-report measures of PTSD and other types of psychopathology. Finally, a PTSD diagnosis based on the DAPS had good diagnostic utility against the CAPS, with a good balance between sensitivity (.88) and specificity (.86), a high level of efficiency (.87), and a good kappa coefficient (.73).

The DAPS appears to be a valuable addition to the PTSD assessment toolkit and would be useful for a range of research and clinical applications. Its main advantages are the inclusion of response validity scales, complete coverage of all PTSD diagnostic criteria, thorough assessment of peritraumatic responses and various associated features of PTSD, and the availability of normative data. A potential disadvantage is that it is longer than other self-report PTSD measures. Also, the DAPS is a relatively new instrument, and little additional psychometric work has appeared in the literature. However, Elhai et al. (2005) found that the DAPS is in reasonably widespread use in clinical and research settings, so more empirical reports are likely to emerge soon.

Other PTSD-Focused Measures

IMPACT OF EVENT SCALE

Developed prior to the formal recognition of PTSD as a mental disorder in DSM-III, the IES (Horowitz et al., 1979) is the oldest standardized measure of posttraumatic symptoms. The IES is the most widely used self-report measure in the field of traumatic stress and has played an invaluable role by providing a common metric across studies with diverse assessment batteries. Based on Horowitz's biphasic model of stress response, the IES comprises 15 items, 7 of which assess intrusive symptoms, and 8 of which assess avoidance. The frequency of each symptom's occurrence over the past week is rated on a 4-point scale, ranging from 0 = *not at all*, 1 = *rarely*, 3 = *sometimes*, and 5 = *often*. The psychometric properties of the IES have been extensively evaluated and, as Sundin and Horowitz (2002) concluded in a recent review, it has proven to be a consistently reliable and valid measure of trauma-related symptoms.

However, the IES does not assess hyperarousal symptoms; therefore, it does not provide complete coverage of the PTSD symptom criteria. To address this limitation Weiss and Marmar (1997) developed a 22-item revised version (IES-R) by adding six hyperarousal items and one dissociative item. They also made several important modifications to the rating scale, which include changing the response dimension from symptom frequency to degree of subjective distress, expanding the number of response options from four to five, and relabeling the anchors so that 0 = *not at all*, 1 = *a little bit*, 2 = *moderately*, 3 = *quite a bit*, and 4 = *extremely*. Although the addition of the new items brought the IES-R more in line with DSM-IV criteria, it still does not directly correspond to the diagnostic criteria, unlike the measures discussed in the previous section. Some DSM-IV PTSD symptoms are not assessed at all (diminished interest, estrangement, sense of foreshortened future), and others are assessed somewhat ambiguously (amnesia, restricted range of affect). Nonetheless, the various modifications make the IES-R an attractive measure for many applications. Its use has steadily increased since its introduction, and accumulating psychometric evidence indicates that the revised version demonstrates the same high level of reliability and validity as the original IES (Weiss, 2004). It should be emphasized that introduction of the IES-R does not mean that the IES is now considered obsolete (Sundin & Horowitz, 2002). Both measures are currently in use and can be used effectively to assess trauma-related symptomatology.

MISSISSIPPI SCALE FOR COMBAT-RELATED PTSD

The Mississippi Scale (Keane et al., 1988) is a 35-item self-report measure of PTSD symptoms and associated features. Items are rated on a 5-point scale, with anchors that vary according to item content (e.g., 1 = *never* to 5 = *very frequently*, 1 = *never true* to 5 = *always true*). The Mississippi Scale is the most widely used measure of combat-related PTSD. It has excellent psychometric properties (e.g., Keane et al., 1988; King & King, 1994; King, King, Fairbank, Schlenger, & Surface, 1993; McFall, Smith, Mackay, & Tarver, 1990) and was selected as the primary PTSD measure in the National Vietnam Veterans Readjustment Study (NVVRS; Kulka et al., 1991).

A Civilian Version of the Mississippi Scale (CMS) was developed for assessing nonmilitary PTSD in the NVVRS. The most significant change involved revision of items containing references to the military, either by deleting the reference or by rephrasing items so that they referred instead to events "in the past." Four items were subsequently added to provide better coverage of the DSM-III-R PTSD criteria, creating a 39-item version, as well as a 35-item version of the CMS. Vreven, Gudanowski, King, and King (1995) evaluated the 35-item version and concluded that it performed reasonably well but warranted some revisions. However, Lauterbach, Vrana, and King (1997), after evaluating both the 35-item and 39-item versions, concluded that the CMS performed more like a general measure of distress, and cautioned against interpreting it as a specific measure of PTSD. In an effort to enhance the utility of the CMS for specific applications, investigators have revised the it by deleting, adding, and modifying items, and by using uniform response options for all items (e.g., Inkelas, Loux, Bourque, Widawski, & Nguyen, 2000; Norris & Perilla, 1996). Despite these efforts, generally the CMS has not performed as well as the original combat version, although it is difficult to reach firm conclusions because of variability across studies in the format, method of administration, and nature of the sample. One consistent concern has focused on the reverse-scored items, which have proven to be particularly problematic and may need to be revised or dropped (Conrad, Wright, & McKnight, 2004; Inkelas et al., 2000).

Multiscale Personality Inventories

The two measures discussed in this section, the Minnesota Multiphasic Personality Inventory—2nd edition (MMPI-2; Butcher et al., 2001) and the Personality Assessment Inventory (PAI; Morey, 2007) are broad spectrum instruments that assess a wide variety of aspects of personality and psychopathology. They have several advantages for the assessment of PTSD. First, they include specialized PTSD scales. Second, they permit the assessment of comorbid disorders and associated clinical features. Third, they allow an estimate of overall severity of disturbance. Fourth, they allow the evaluation of response bias.

MINNESOTA MULTIPHASIC PERSONALITY INVENTORY

The Minnesota Multiphasic Personality Inventory (MMPI; Hathaway & McKinley, 1951) is one of the oldest and most widely used psychological assessment instruments. The MMPI was revised in 1989, and the MMPI-2 (Butcher et al., 2001), which incorporated a number of innovative new features, has continued the tradition of the MMPI as a preeminent multiscale personality inventory. The MMPI-2 permits a broad, psychometrically sound assessment of personality, psychopathology, and various forms of response bias.

The MMPI/MMPI-2 has been used extensively in the assessment of PTSD, particularly in combat veterans. The earliest studies that employed the MMPI led to the identification of a mean F-2-8 PTSD profile, as well as the construction of a specialized PTSD scale, the Keane PTSD Scale (PK; Fairbank et al., 1983; Keane, Malloy, & Fairbank, 1984). Subsequent researchers have found that although scales F, 2, and 8 typically figure prominently in mean PTSD profiles, other scales are often elevated, and in general there is substantial heterogeneity in profiles both within and across studies (e.g., Glenn, Beckham, & Sampson, 2002; Wise, 1996). This has led some investigators to supplement the mean profile approach with an individualized approach based on the frequency of code types for individual respondents (e.g., Glenn et al., 2002).

More directly relevant for PTSD diagnosis is the PK. The original PK comprised 49 MMPI items that discriminated between Vietnam War combat veterans with PTSD and Vietnam veterans with other psychiatric disorders. For the MMPI-2, three redundant items were dropped and one item was reworded (Lyons & Keane, 1992). Keane and colleagues (1984) found that a cutoff of 30 (27 in the MMPI-2) provided the best discrimination, with 82% correct classification in both a derivation and a cross-validation sample. Subsequent research has generally confirmed the diagnostic utility of the PK, although performance has varied, possibly as a function of sample characteristics and diagnostic procedures, and the cutoff scores have tended to be lower (e.g., Cannon, Bell, Andrews, & Finkelstein, 1987; Watson, Kucala, & Manifold, 1986).

The PK has also been used successfully in civilian trauma samples (e.g., Koretzky & Peck, 1990). However, some investigators have cautioned that it may be more a measure of general distress than a specific measure of PTSD. For example, Scheibe, Bagby, Miller, and Dorian (2001) found that several standard MMPI-2 clinical and content scales, especially Scales 7 and 8 and the Anxiety and Anger content scales, were more effective than the PK for predicting PTSD in workplace accident victims. Finally, the PK has been evaluated for use as a stand-alone measure, with a performance in this format that appears comparable to its performance when administered in the context of the full MMPI/MMPI-2 (Herman, Weathers, Litz, & Keane, 1996; Lyons & Scotti, 1994).

One of the most valuable features of the MMPI-2 is the availability of an array of response validity indicators. Given the concerns about malingering in PTSD, the MMPI-2 scales that detect a fake-bad response style, especially Infrequency (F), Infrequency-Back (Fp), and Gough's Dissimulation scales (Ds) (Rogers, Sewell, Martin, & Vitaco, 2003), are particularly useful in the assessment of PTSD. In addition, a new scale, the Infrequency-PTSD (Fptsd), was developed to improve discrimination of genuine and feigned PTSD

(Elhai, Ruggiero, Frueh, Beckham, & Gold, 2002). In the original study Elhai and colleagues (2002) found that Fptsd outperformed existing MMPI-2 scales in detecting feigned PTSD. However, a follow-up study revealed that Fptsd improved detection of feigned PTSD over F but not Fp. Furthermore, Marshall and Bagby (2006) recently found that Fptsd did not improve detection over the existing family of F scales, possibly because Fptsd shares a substantial proportion of items with Fp. Clearly, more research is needed to determine the clinical usefulness of this scale.

In summary, the MMPI-2 is a valuable addition to a PTSD assessment battery. It assesses the wide range of problems typically seen in the clinical presentation of PTSD and provides sophisticated methods for detecting malingering and other types of response bias. Penk, Rierdan, Losardo, and Robinowitz (2006) provide a thorough overview of the various clinical applications of the MMPI-2, and describe in some detail how information from the MMPI-2 can be integrated effectively with information from other sources.

PERSONALITY ASSESSMENT INVENTORY

Developed in 1991, the PAI (Morey, 2007) has grown rapidly in popularity in clinical, research, and forensic settings. The PAI comprises 344 items that make up 22 nonoverlapping scales, including 4 response validity scales, 11 clinical scales, 5 treatment scales, and 2 interpersonal scales. In addition, 9 of the clinical scales and 1 of the treatment scales have subscales reflecting key aspects of the construct assessed by the parent scale (e.g., the Cognitive, Affective, and Physiological subscales of the Depression scale). The validity scales detect random or careless responding and the tendency to present in an overly positive or negative manner, and include Inconsistency (ICN), Infrequency (INF), Negative Impression (NIM), and Positive Impression (PIM). The clinical scales assess well-established clinical syndromes, and include Somatic Complaints (SOM), Anxiety (ANX), Anxiety-Related Disorders (ARD), Depression (DEP), Mania (MAN), Paranoia (PAR), Schizophrenia (SCZ), Borderline Features (BOR), Antisocial Features (ANT), Alcohol Problems (ALC), and Drug Problems (DRG). The treatment scales assess several key areas relevant to clinical management, and include Aggression (AGG), Suicidal Ideation (SUI), Stress (STR), Nonsupport (NON), and Treatment Rejection (RXR). Finally, the interpersonal scales assess two aspects of normal personality, and include Dominance (DOM) and Warmth (WRM).

In contrast to the MMPI/MMPI-2, which was developed using an empirical criterion keying method, the PAI was developed using a construct validation approach that emphasized explication of the constructs to be assessed and content validity of the items for assessing the constructs. In addition, rather than a true–false response format, PAI items are rated on a 4-point scale, with anchors of *false, not at all true*; *slightly true; mainly true;* and *very true*. PAI profiles are presented in *T*-scores, based on a census-matched normative sample. *T*-scores of 70 and higher are considered clinically significant.

Another reference point for scale interpretation is the "skyline," which represents scores that are two standard deviations above the mean of a clinical normative sample.

Because the PAI is a relatively new instrument, only a limited number of studies have investigated its use in the assessment of PTSD. However, studies that have emerged indicate that the PAI has considerable promise and may be very useful as a research and clinical tool with trauma survivors. A focal point for PTSD assessment with the PAI is the Traumatic Stress subscale of the Anxiety-Related Disorders scale (ARD-T), which comprises eight items: Five items primarily assess reexperiencing, one assesses effortful avoidance, one assesses loss of interest in usual activities, and one assesses guilt. Each *ARD-T* item is linked to a previous experience, sometimes referred to broadly and not necessarily as a stressor ("about my past") and other times more specifically as a trauma ("something horrible" or "since I had a very bad experience"). Although it does not explicitly assess Criterion A and covers only about half of DSM-IV PTSD symptom criteria, ARD-T does assess some of the most distinctive aspects of PTSD and typically is the most elevated PAI scale in individuals with PTSD. In addition, several other conceptually relevant PAI scales and subscales appear to be elevated in PTSD. For example, Mozley, Miller, Weathers, Beckham, and Feldman (2005) administered the PAI to 176 male combat veterans with PTSD. They found significant elevations on NIM, SOM, ANX, ARD, DEP, and SCZ, with the highest elevations on ARD-T and DEP. They also found that ARD-T correlated strongly with the Mississippi Scale (.67) and moderately with the PK scale of the MMPI-2 (.58) and the DTS (.44).

Furthermore, McDevitt-Murphy, Weathers, Adkins, and Daniels (2005) compared PAI profiles in a community sample of 55 women with and without PTSD. The PTSD group scored significantly higher than the non-PTSD group on a number of scales, including ANX, DEP, ARD, SOM, PAR, BOR, and SCZ, as well as NON and RXR. The largest group differences were for ARD-T and the Physiological subscale of Depression (DEP-P). ARD-T and DEP-P also had the highest correlations with CAPS total severity ($r = .72$ for ARD-T, $r = .66$ for DEP-P). Finally, ARD-T and DEP-P demonstrated strong diagnostic utility against the CAPS at levels comparable to that of the PCL, which had the highest quality of efficiency of all the measures in the study.

In a subsequent study, McDevitt-Murphy, Weathers, Flood, Eakin, and Benson (2007) compared the discriminant validity of the PAI and MMPI-2 for distinguishing PTSD, depression, and social phobia in college students. The PAI and MMPI-2 differentiated the PTSD and well-adjusted control groups, with substantially higher elevations for the PTSD group on a number of scales on both measures. For the PAI, the largest group difference was for ARD-T, with other large differences on PIM, ANX, ARD, DEP, BOR, and RXR. The PAI and MMPI-2 also differentiated the PTSD and social phobia groups, although the pattern of group differences varied somewhat and the effect sizes were smaller. However, the PAI was more effective than the MMPI-2 in differentiating the PTSD and depression groups. For the PAI, significant group differences between PTSD and depression were found for PIM, ARD-T, the Grandiosity subscale of the Mania scale (MAN-G), and the Antisocial Behaviors (ANT-A) and Egocentricity (ANT-E) subscales of the Antisocial Features scale. In contrast, for the MMPI-2, a significant group difference was found only for the Low Self-Esteem content scale (LSE).

Based on the relatively small literature thus far, the PAI appears to have considerable merit for the assessment of PTSD. As with the MMPI-2, the PAI rigorously evaluates various forms of response bias, assesses a wide range of comorbid syndromes, and contains a specialized PTSD scale. Because it was developed with a construct validation approach, the PAI provides a straightforward assessment of contemporary constructs related to diagnosis and clinical management. In addition, preliminary evidence suggests that it has better discriminant validity for distinguishing PTSD from other commonly comorbid disorders, such as depression.

Recommendations for Designing a PTSD Assessment

In this section we offer some recommendations and guidelines to assist in selection of PTSD assessment instruments and creation of an appropriate assessment battery protocol for a given setting, target population, and intended application. These guidelines are not necessarily relevant to all situations, but they are generally applicable to most PTSD assessments.

1. *Establish explicit goals.* All decisions regarding the selection of assessment measures should grow out of a clear statement of what the assessment is intended to accomplish. What are the goals for the assessment, and what end products are desired (i.e., inferences, conclusions, and decisions made based on the assessment)? The most common goals for PTSD assessment include screening for possible trauma exposure and PTSD, establishing a diagnosis of PTSD, and quantifying PTSD symptom severity. These goals have direct implications for instrument selection. For example, self-report measures are useful for screening and quantifying symptom severity but should not be used as the sole basis for diagnosis. Structured interviews are useful for diagnosis and, in some cases, for quantifying symptom severity, but are too inefficient for large-scale screening. When resources are available, it may be tempting to use a shotgun approach and administer as many measures as possible. However, this raises the question of incremental validity and creates the problem of respondent burden and possible noncompliance with the assessment tasks.

2. *Consider the target population and assessment context.* Taking into account the nature of the target population and the context will help to guide selection of appropriate measures. Key variables include sex, age, type of trauma (e.g., combat, sexual assault, mixed civilian trauma; also, relatively circum-

scribed vs. chronic, repeated trauma), and the setting (clinic vs. community; inpatient vs. outpatient; trauma-focused vs. general psychiatric or medical). It is important to select measures that have been well-validated for the specific population. The nature of the population may also help to determine what domains other than the core syndrome of PTSD to emphasize, such as lifetime trauma history, comorbidity, associated features of PTSD, malingering, and other types of response bias.

3. *Consider the available resources.* The types of measures that can be administered and the scope of the assessment will depend on personnel and the amount of time available. What assessment personnel are available, what training and qualifications do they have, and how much time are they able to devote to the assessment protocol? Questionnaires may be administered and scored by clerical staff, and trained lay interviewers may administer highly structured research interviews, but appropriately trained and credentialed clinicians are required for conducting clinical interviews and making a clinical diagnosis. Furthermore, how much time is available for the assessment? Key considerations include the time commitment and cost of assessment personnel, as well as respondent burden and any logistical constraints in the assessment context. Regarding respondent burden, are respondents able to tolerate the assessment procedure and provide valid information? Will the assessment need to be abbreviated or divided into multiple sessions? Time considerations will also determine the emphasis given to the various assessment domains. Most assessment protocols involve trade-offs and compromises, with more time and resources given to the primary targets of PTSD diagnostic status and symptom severity, and relatively less time to other targets, such as comorbidity and response bias.

4. *Enhance compliance with the assessment.* To obtain the most valid information, it is important for respondents to be invested in the assessment process. Trauma is associated with a sense of powerlessness and helplessness, and extensive avoidance and lack of trust are often central issues. An effort should be made to engage and to empower respondents by offering encouragement and support to confront feared material, and by increasing predictability and controllability. Predictability can be enhanced by being transparent and explaining clearly all aspects of the assessment process, including specific assessment activities, specific questions, and the rationale for each. Controllability can be enhanced by promoting respondents' autonomy and choice throughout the assessment, emphasizing informed consent and the right to withdraw at any point or take a break if the process becomes too emotionally taxing, and reassuring respondents about confidentiality.

5. *Use an interview whenever possible.* As discussed earlier, interviews have several advantages over self-report measures. When time is limited, either the SCID or PSS-I is appropriate. The SCID evaluates all DSM-IV-TR criteria and yields a diagnosis of PTSD. The PSS-I yields both a diagnosis and a continuous measure of PTSD symptom severity, although the index trauma must be identified by some other measure, and it is necessary to ensure that

the symptoms have lasted at least a month. When there is sufficient time, the CAPS is a good choice. It too yields a diagnosis and a continuous measure of severity, and also provides more detailed information that may be useful for functional analysis and treatment planning.

6. *Use a DSM-correspondent self-report measure whenever possible.* Apart from interviews, DSM-correspondent self-report measures are the most important component of a multimeasure PTSD assessment and for some applications may serve as the primary or even sole measure. Many of the non-DSM-correspondent measures make useful supplements but provide only an indirect evaluation of DSM-IV-TR PTSD criteria. If an interview is not administered, and only one DSM-correspondent measure is used, then the PDS or DAPS is a good choice because each measure covers all the criteria and provides a diagnosis and continuous measure of severity.

7. *Use the most appropriate scoring rule for a given application.* Although indispensable in the assessment of PTSD, continuous measures introduce an additional layer of complexity when there is a need to convert them to dichotomous scores (i.e., by selecting a cutoff score to define caseness, or by dichotomizing item scores and following DSM-IV-TR criteria to derive a diagnosis). Whenever possible it is crucial to select the appropriate scoring rule for a given population, context, and assessment task (e.g., screening, differential diagnosis). The available empirical evidence indicates that the performance of cutoffs and scoring rules varies widely across samples. Unfortunately, for many measures, there is not sufficient research to guide the selection of an optimal rule because either alternative rules have not been proposed or the rules have not been adequately validated.

8. *Use multiple measures whenever possible.* As noted earlier, the use of multiple measures has long been advocated in the assessment of PTSD. A battery that would meet most clinical and research needs would include a PTSD interview; a DSM-correspondent measure; a supplemental measure, such as the IES or the Mississippi Scale; and either the MMPI-2 or the PAI. If time permits, an interview covering other disorders, such as the non-PTSD portions of the SCID, would be very helpful. In choosing between the MMPI-2 and PAI, the advantages of the MMPI-2 are that it has a much more extensive research base and has been used to assess PTSD for more than 25 years. The advantages of the PAI are that it is shorter (344 vs. 567 items), the scales correspond to familiar concepts in contemporary diagnosis and clinical management, and the specialized PTSD scale appears to have greater discriminant validity than do any of the MMPI-2 scales.

9. *Evaluate response bias.* Response bias, particularly malingering, should be assessed routinely in all clinical and research assessments of PTSD. The MMPI-2 and PAI are excellent resources in this regard because of their rigorous, well-validated procedures for evaluating under- and overreporting. In settings with a very high potential for malingering, it might be necessary to include a dedicated malingering instrument, such as the SIRS. This crucial assessment domain has been given insufficient attention in the field of trau-

matic stress in particular, and in the assessment of mental health disorders more broadly (Rosen, 2004; Rosen & Taylor, 2007).

Summary and Future Directions

Considerable progress has been made in the development and evaluation of standardized measures for assessing trauma exposure and PTSD. Clinicians and investigators now have available a wide variety of instruments and protocols that provide psychometrically sound and practicable measurement of PTSD for almost any application across settings. As noted earlier, the use of such instruments is now *de rigueur* for empirical studies, and is increasingly expected in clinical settings as well. The increasing focus on the use of EBA procedures will foster the continued dissemination of such measures, until they become part of routine clinical practice.

Although progress has been made, much remains to be done. First, as we noted nearly a decade ago (Weathers & Keane, 1999), there are actually too many measures of trauma and PTSD, and more new measures appear every year. Although progress in instrument development is always welcome, rarely do new measures represent an improvement over existing ones. Most are largely redundant and represent minor variations on previous measures. However, they do differ in at least some respects, thus hindering progress in PTSD research by reducing comparability of findings across studies. A more productive approach would be to expand the empirical foundation for the best existing measures, thereby moving toward a consensus battery for the field of traumatic stress. This would involve the accumulation of validity evidence from multiple sources, including evidence of convergent and discriminant validity, diagnostic utility, sensitivity to clinical change, and structural evidence from factor-analytic studies. At this point, discriminant validity is arguably the most important source of evidence and, unfortunately, the one that to date is the most underdeveloped. Given the high rates of comorbidity in PTSD, particularly the overlap with depression and other anxiety disorders, it is crucial to demonstrate that PTSD assessment instruments measure symptomatology uniquely attributable to PTSD rather than simply reflecting nonspecific distress.

Second, more research is needed to evaluate the generalizability of standardized measures across trauma types (e.g., combat vs. sexual assault), settings (e.g., inpatient vs. outpatient, clinical vs. research, trauma clinic vs. primary care), key demographic characteristics (age, gender, ethnicity), and cultures, including the comparability and psychometric performance of translations of measures into other languages. It is essential to document empirically, rather than to assume, that a measure developed and evaluated primarily in one population will perform similarly in a different context. Closely related to this is the need to evaluate different scoring rules and cutoff scores for standardized measures to identify the optimal scoring method for a given assessment task in a given population. Third, much more work is needed to develop methods for combining the information from multiple measures. Although the use of multiple measures is recommended, currently there is little empirical guidance as to how to integrate findings across measures.

Fourth, PTSD diagnostic criteria have evolved considerably since DSM-III and likely will continue to evolve, so PTSD assessment measures need to be updated accordingly. Apropos of this issue, Spitzer and colleagues (2007), responding to a series of articles criticizing the PTSD construct, recently proposed several revisions of the PTSD criteria for DSM-V. For example, to address the apparent nonspecificity of the PTSD syndrome, they suggested eliminating PTSD symptom criteria that are also criteria for other disorders—specifically, irritability, insomnia, difficulty concentrating, and diminished interest—then combining the remaining symptoms in Criteria C and D into a single cluster. Spitzer and colleagues emphasized that they were not being prescriptive, and that experts in the field of traumatic stress would be in the best position to generate the most appropriate revisions.

Such changes in the diagnostic criteria are largely speculative at this point. What is clear, however, is that scientific knowledge regarding the phenomenology, etiology, and treatment of PTSD will continue to broaden and deepen, and that sound measurement will play a vital role. The construct of PTSD has fostered a sustained and systematic investigation of the human response to trauma, and EBA will continue to provide the foundation for the study and care of those individuals who suffer the psychological toll of catastrophe.

References

American Psychiatric Association. (1980). *Diagnostic and statistical manual of mental disorders* (3rd ed.). Washington, DC: Author.

American Psychiatric Association. (2000). *Diagnostic and statistical manual of mental disorders* (4th ed., text revision). Washington, DC: Author.

Andrykowski, M. A., Cordova, M. J., Studts, J. L., & Miller, T. W. (1998). Posttraumatic stress disorder after treatment for breast cancer: Prevalence of diagnosis and use of the PTSD Checklist—Civilian version (PCL-C) as a screening instrument. *Journal of Consulting and Clinical Psychology, 66*, 586–590.

Asmundson, G. J. G., Frombach, I., McQuaid, J., Pedrelli, P., Lenox, R., & Stein, M. B. (2000). Dimensionality of posttraumatic stress symptoms: A confirmatory factor analysis of DSM-IV symptom clusters and other symptom models. *Behaviour Research and Therapy, 38*, 203–214.

Blake, D. D., Weathers, F. W., Nagy, L. M., Kaloupek, D. G., Gusman, F. D., Charney, D. S., et al. (1995). The development of a clinician-administered PTSD scale. *Journal of Traumatic Stress, 8*, 75–90.

Blake, D. D., Weathers, F. W., Nagy, L. M., Kaloupek, D. G., Klauminzer, G., Charney, D. S., et al. (1990). A clinician rating scale for assessing current and lifetime PTSD: The CAPS-1. *Behavior Therapist, 13*, 187–188.

Blanchard, E. B., Jones-Alexander, J., Buckley, T. C., & Forneris, C. A. (1996). Psychometric properties of the PTSD Checklist (PCL). *Behaviour Research and Therapy, 34*, 669–673.

Breslau, N., Kessler, R. C., Chilcoat, H. D., Schultz, L. R., Davis, G. C., & Andreski, P. (1998). Trauma and posttraumatic stress disorder in the community: The 1996 Detroit Area Survey of Trauma. *Archives of General Psychiatry, 55*, 626–631.

Briere, J. (2001). *Detailed Assessment of Posttraumatic Stress (DAPS)*. Odessa, FL: Psychological Assessment Resources.

Briere, J. (2004). *Psychological assessment of adult posttraumatic states: Phenomenology, diagnosis, and measurement* (2nd ed.). Washington, DC: American Psychological Association.

Brown, T. A., Campbell, L. A., Lehman, C. L., Grisham, J. R., & Mancill, R. B. (2001). Current and lifetime comorbidity of the DSM-IV anxiety and mood disorders in a large clinical sample. *Journal of Abnormal Psychology, 110*, 585–599.

Butcher, J. N., Graham, J. R., Ben-Porath, Y. S., Tellegen, A. M., Dahlstrom, W. G., & Kaemmer, B. (2001). *Minnesota Multiphasic Personality Inventory–2: Manual for administration, scoring, and interpretation* (rev. ed.). Minneapolis: University of Minnesota Press.

Cannon, D. S., Bell, W. E., Andrews, R. H., & Finkelstein, A. S. (1987). Correspondence between MMPI PTSD measures and clinical diagnosis. *Journal of Personality Assessment, 51*, 517–521.

Carlson, E. B. (1997). *Trauma assessments: A clinician's guide*. New York: Guilford Press.

Charney, M. E., & Keane, T. M. (2007). Psychometric analysis of the Clinician-Administered PTSD Scale (CAPS)—Bosnian translation. *Cultural and Ethnic Minority Psychology, 13*, 161–168.

Conrad, K. J., Wright, B. D., & McKnight, P. (2004). Comparing traditional and Rasch analyses of the Mississippi PTSD Scale: Revealing limitations of reverse-scored items. *Journal of Applied Measurement, 5*, 15–30.

Cronbach, L. J., & Meehl, P. E. (1955). Construct validity in psychological tests. *Psychological Bulletin, 52*, 281–302.

Davidson, J. (1996). *Davidson Trauma Scale* [Manual]. Toronto, Ontario, Canada: Multi-Health Systems.

Davidson, J. R. T., Malik, M. A., & Travers, J. (1997). The Structured Interview for PTSD (SIP): Psychometric validation for DSM-IV criteria. *Depression and Anxiety, 5*, 127–129.

Davidson, J. R. T., Smith, R. D., & Kudler, H. S. (1989). Validity and reliability of the DSM-III criteria for post-traumatic stress disorder: Experience with a structured interview. *Journal of Nervous and Mental Disease, 177*, 336–341.

Davidson, J. R. T., Tharwani, H. M., & Connor, K. M. (2002). Davidson Trauma Scale (DTS): Normative scores in the general population and effect sizes in placebo-controlled SSRI trials. *Depression and Anxiety, 15*, 75–78.

Dobie, D. J., Kivlahan, D. R., Maynard, C., Bush, K. R., McFall, M. E., Epler, A. J., et al. (2002). Screening for post-traumatic stress disorder in female Veteran's Affairs patients: Validation of the PTSD Checklist. *General Hospital Psychiatry, 24*, 367–374.

DuHamel, K. N., Ostroff, J. S., Ashman, T., Winkel, G., Mundy, E. A., Keane, T. M., et al. (2004). Construct validity of the Posttraumatic Stress Disorder Checklist in cancer survivors: Analyses based on two samples. *Psychological Assessment, 16,* 255–266.

Elhai, J. D., Gray, M. J., Kashdan, T. B., & Franklin, C. L. (2005). Which instruments are most commonly used to assess traumatic event exposure and posttraumatic effects?: A survey of traumatic stress professionals. *Journal of Traumatic Stress, 18,* 541–545.

Elhai, J. D., Ruggiero, K. J., Frueh, B. C., Beckham, J. C., & Gold, P. B. (2002). The Infrequency-Posttraumatic Stress Disorder Scale (Fptsd) for the MMPI-2: Development and initial validation with veterans presenting with combat-related PTSD. *Journal of Personality Assessment, 79,* 531–549.

Fairbank, J. A., Keane, T. M., & Malloy, P. F. (1983). Some preliminary data on the psychological characteristics of Vietnam veterans with posttraumatic stress disorders. *Journal of Consulting and Clinical Psychology, 51,* 912–919.

First, M. B., Spitzer, R. L., Gibbon, M., & Williams, J. B. W. (1996). *Structured Clinical Interview for DSM-IV Axis I Disorders, Clinician Version (SCID-CV).* Washington, DC: American Psychiatric Press.

Foa, E. B. (1995). *Posttraumatic Stress Diagnostic Scale* [Manual]. Minneapolis, MN: National Computer Systems.

Foa, E. B., Cashman, L., Jaycox, L., & Perry, K. (1997). The validation of a self-report measure of posttraumatic stress disorder: The Posttraumatic Diagnostic Scale. *Psychological Assessment, 9,* 445–451.

Foa, E. B., Ehlers, A., Clark, D. M., Tolin, D. F., & Orsillo, S. M. (1999). The Post-Traumatic Cognition Inventory (PTCI): Development and validation. *Psychological Assessment, 11,* 303–314.

Foa, E. B., Riggs, D. S., Dancu, C. V., & Rothbaum, B. O. (1993). Reliability and validity of a brief instrument for assessing post-traumatic stress disorder. *Journal of Traumatic Stress, 6,* 459–473.

Foa, E. B., & Tolin, D. F. (2000). Comparison of the PTSD Symptom Scale—Interview version and the Clinician-Administered PTSD Scale. *Journal of Traumatic Stress, 13,* 181–191.

Forbes, D., Creamer, M. C., & Biddle, D. (2001). The validity of the PTSD Checklist as a measure of symptomatic change in combat-related PTSD. *Behaviour Research and Therapy, 39,* 977–986.

Friedman, M. J., Keane, T. M., & Resick P. A. (Eds.). (2007). *Handbook of PTSD: Science and practice.* New York: Guilford Press.

Glenn, D. M., Beckham, J. C., & Sampson, W. S. (2002). MMPI-2 profiles of Gulf and Vietnam combat veterans with chronic posttraumatic stress disorder. *Journal of Clinical Psychology, 58,* 371–381.

Griesel, D., Wessa, M., & Flor, H. (2006). Psychometric qualities of the German version of the Posttraumatic Diagnostic Scale (PTDS). *Psychological Assessment, 18,* 262–268.

Guriel, J. L., & Fremouw, W. (2003). Assessing malingered posttraumatic stress disorder: A critical review. *Clinical Psychology Review, 23,* 881–904.

Hathaway, S. R., & McKinley, J. C. (1951). *Minnesota Multiphasic Personality Inventory: Manual for administration and scoring.* New York: Psychological Corporation.

Hembree, E. A., Foa, E. B., & Feeny, N. C. (2002). *Manual for the administration and scoring of the PTSD Symptom Scale—Interview (PSS-I).* Unpublished manuscript available online at *www.istss.org/resources/browse.cfm*

Herman, D. S., Weathers, F. W., Litz, B. T., & Keane, T. M. (1996). Psychometric properties of the embedded and stand-alone versions of the MMPI-2 Keane PTSD Scale. *Assessment, 3,* 437–442.

Herman, J. L. (1992). *Trauma and recovery.* New York: Basic Books.

Horowitz, M. J., Wilner, N., & Alvarez, W. (1979). Impact of Event Scale: A measure of subjective stress. *Psychosomatic Medicine, 41,* 209–218.

Hunsley, J., & Mash, E. J. (2005). Introduction to the special section on developing guidelines for the evidence-based assessment (EBA) of adult disorders. *Psychological Assessment, 17,* 251–255.

Inkelas, M., Loux, L. A., Bourque, L. B., Widawski, M., & Nguyen, L. H. (2000). Dimensionality and reliability of the Civilian Mississippi Scale for PTSD in a postearthquake community. *Journal of Traumatic Stress, 13,* 149–167.

Kang, H. K., Natelson, B. H., Mahan, C. M., Lee, K. Y., & Murphy, F. M. (2003). Posttraumatic stress disorder and chronic fatigue syndrome-like illness among Gulf War veterans: A population-based survey of 30,000 veterans. *American Journal of Epidemiology, 157,* 141–148.

Keane, T. M. (1989). Post-traumatic stress disorder: Current status and future directions. *Behavior Therapy, 20,* 149–153.

Keane, T. M., Caddell, J. M., & Taylor, K. L. (1988). Mississippi Scale for Combat-Related Posttraumatic Stress Disorder: Three studies in reliability and validity. *Journal of Consulting and Clinical Psychology, 56,* 85–90.

Keane, T. M., Fairbank, J. A., Caddell, J. M., Zimering, R. T., & Bender, M. E. (1985). A behavioral approach to the assessment and treatment of post-traumatic stress disorder in Vietnam veterans. In C. R. Figley (Ed.), *Trauma and its wake: Vol. I. The study and treatment of post-traumatic stress disorder* (pp. 257–294). New York: Brunner/Mazel.

Keane, T. M., & Kaloupek, D. G. (1997). Comorbid psychiatric disorders in PTSD: Implications for research. *Annals of the New York Academy of Sciences, 821,* 24–34.

Keane, T. M., Kolb, L. C., Kaloupek, D. G., Orr, S. P., Blanchard, E. B., Thomas, R. G., et al. (1998). Utility of psychophysiological measurement in the diagnosis of posttraumatic stress disorder: Results from a Department of Veterans Affairs Cooperative Study. *Journal of Consulting and Clinical Psychology, 66,* 914–923.

Keane, T. M., Malloy, P. F., & Fairbank, J. A. (1984). Empirical development of an MMPI subscale for the assessment of combat-related posttraumatic stress disorder. *Journal of Consulting and Clinical Psychology, 52,* 888–891.

Keane, T. M., Street, A. E., & Stafford, J. A. (2004). The assessment of military-related PTSD. In J. P. Wilson & T. M. Keane (Eds.), *Assessing psychological trauma and PTSD* (2nd ed., pp. 262–285). New York: Guilford Press.

Keane, T. M., Wolfe, J., & Taylor, K. L. (1987). Post-traumatic stress disorder: Evidence for diagnostic validity and methods of psychological assessment. *Journal of Clinical Psychology, 43,* 32–43.

Kessler, R. C., Sonnega, A., Bromet, E., Hughes, M., & Nelson, C. B. (1995). Posttraumatic stress disorder in the National Comorbidity Survey. *Archives of General Psychiatry, 52,* 1048–1060.

Kimerling, R., Clum, G. A., McQuery, J., & Schnurr, P. P. (2002). PTSD and medical comorbidity. In R. Kimerling, P. C. Ouimette, & J. Wolfe (Eds.), *Gender and PTSD* (pp. 271–302). New York: Guilford Press.

Kimerling, R., Ouimette, P. C., & Wolfe, J. (Eds.). (2002). *Gender and PTSD.* New York: Guilford Press.

King, D. W., King, L. A., Fairbank, J. A., Schlenger, W. E., & Surface, C. R. (1993).

Enhancing the precision of the Mississippi Scale for Combat-Related Posttraumatic Stress Disorder: An application of item response theory. *Psychological Assessment, 5*, 457–471.

King, L. A., & King, D. W. (1994). Latent structure of the Mississippi Scale for Combat-Related Posttraumatic Stress Disorder: Exploratory and higher-order confirmatory factor analyses. *Assessment, 1*, 275–291.

Koretzky, M. B., & Peck, A. H. (1990). Validation and cross-validation of the PTSD subscale of the MMPI with civilian trauma victims. *Journal of Clinical Psychology, 46*, 296–300.

Kraemer, H. C. (1992). *Evaluating medical tests: Objective and quantitative guidelines.* Newbury Park, CA: Sage.

Kulka, R. A., Schlenger, W. E., Fairbank, J. A., Hough, R. L., Jordan, B. K., Marmar, C. R., et al. (1991). Assessment of posttraumatic stress disorder in the community: Prospects and pitfalls from recent studies of Vietnam veterans. *Psychological Assessment, 3*, 547–560.

Lauterbach, D., Vrana, S., & King, D. W. (1997). Psychometric properties of the Civilian Version of the Mississippi PTSD Scale. *Journal of Traumatic Stress, 10*, 499–513.

Litz, B. T., & Weathers, F. W. (1994). The diagnosis and assessment of post-traumatic stress disorder in adults. In M. B. Williams & J. F. Sommer, Jr. (Eds.), *Handbook of post-traumatic therapy* (pp. 9–22). Westport, CT: Greenwood Press.

Lyons, J. A., & Keane, T. M. (1992). Keane PTSD Scale: MMPI and MMPI-2 update. *Journal of Traumatic Stress, 5*, 111–117.

Lyons, J. A., & Scotti, J. R. (1994). Comparability of two administration formats of the Keane Posttraumatic Stress Disorder Scale. *Psychological Assessment, 6*, 209–211.

Maier, T. (2006). Posttraumatic stress disorder revisited: Deconstructing the A-Criterion. *Medical Hypotheses, 66*, 103–106.

Malloy, P. F., Fairbank, J. A., & Keane, T. M. (1983). Validation of a multimethod assessment of posttraumatic stress disorders in Vietnam veterans. *Journal of Consulting and Clinical Psychology, 51*, 488–494.

Marsella, A. J., Friedman, M. J., Gerrity, E. T., & Scurfield, R. M. (Eds.). (1996). *Ethnocultural aspects of posttraumatic stress disorder: Issues, research, and clinical applications.* Washington, DC: American Psychological Association.

Marshall, M. B., & Bagby, R. M. (2006). The incremental validity and clinical utility of the MMPI-2 Infrequency Posttraumatic Stress Disorder Scale. *Assessment, 13*, 417–429.

McDevitt-Murphy, M. E., Weathers, F. W., Adkins, J. W., & Daniels, J. B. (2005). Use of the Personality Assessment Inventory in assessment of posttraumatic stress disorder in women. *Journal of Psychopathology and Behavioral Assessment, 27*, 57–65.

McDevitt-Murphy, M. E., Weathers, F. W., Flood, A. M., Benson, T., & Eakin, D. E. (2007). A comparison of the MMPI-2 and PAI for discriminating PTSD from depression and social phobia. *Assessment, 14*, 181–195.

McFall, M. E., Smith, D. E., Mackay, P. W., & Tarver, D. J. (1990). Reliability and validity of the Mississippi Scale for Combat-Related Posttraumatic Stress Disorder. *Psychological Assessment, 2*, 114–121.

McNally, R. J. (2004). Conceptual problems with the DSM-IV criteria for posttraumatic stress disorder. In G. M. Rosen (Ed.), *Posttraumatic stress disorder: Issues and controversies* (pp. 1–14). New York: Wiley.

Morey, L. C. (2007). *Personality Assessment Inventory: Professional manual* (2nd ed.). Lutz, FL: Psychological Assessment Resources.

Mozley, S. L., Miller, M. W., Weathers, F. W., Beckham, J. C., & Feldman, M. E. (2005). Personality Assessment Inventory (PAI) profiles of male veterans with combat-related posttraumatic stress disorder. *Journal of Psychopathology and Behavioral Assessment, 27,* 179–189.

Norris, F. H., & Hamblen, J. L. (2004). Standardized self-report measures of civilian trauma and PTSD. In J. P. Wilson & T. M. Keane (Eds.), *Assessing psychological trauma and PTSD* (2nd ed., pp. 63–102). New York: Guilford Press.

Norris, F. H., & Perilla, J. L. (1996). The revised Civilian Mississippi Scale for PTSD: Reliability, validity, and cross-language stability. *Journal of Traumatic Stress, 9,* 285–298.

Orsillo, S., Weathers, F. W., Litz, B. T., Steinberg, H. R., Huska, J. A., & Keane, T. M. (1996). Current and lifetime psychiatric disorders among veterans with war-zone-related post-traumatic stress disorder. *Journal of Nervous and Mental Disease, 184,* 307–313.

Palmieri, P. A., Weathers, F. W., Difede, J., & King, D. W. (2007). Confirmatory factor analysis of the PTSD Checklist and the Clinician-Administered PTSD Scale in disaster workers exposed to the World Trade Center Ground Zero. *Journal of Abnormal Psychology, 116,* 329–341.

Penk, W. E., Rierdan, J., Losardo, M., & Robinowitz, R. (2006). The MMPI-2 and assessment of posttraumatic stress disorder (PTSD). In J. N. Butcher (Ed.), *MMPI-2: A practitioner's guide* (pp. 121–141). Washington, DC: American Psychological Association.

Powell, S., & Rosner, R. (2005). The Bosnian version of the international self-report measure of posttraumatic stress disorder, the Posttraumatic Stress Diagnostic Scale, is reliable and valid in a variety of different adult samples affected by war. *BMC Psychiatry, 5,* 11.

Rogers, R., Bagby, R. M., & Dickens, S. E. (1992). *Structured Interview of Reported Symptoms (SIRS) and professional manual.* Odessa, FL: Psychological Assessment Resources.

Rogers, R., Sewell, K. W., Martin, M. A., & Vitacco, M. J. (2003). Detection of feigned mental disorders: A meta-analysis of the MMPI-2 and malingering. *Assessment, 10,* 160–177.

Rosen, G. M. (2004a). Malingering and the PTSD data base. In G. M. Rosen (Ed.), *Posttraumatic stress disorder: Issues and controversies* (pp. 85–99). New York: Wiley.

Rosen, G. M. (Ed.). (2004b). *Posttraumatic stress disorder: Issues and controversies.* Chichester, UK: Wiley.

Rosen, G. M., & Taylor, S. F. (2007). Pseudo-PTSD. *Journal of Anxiety Disorders, 21,* 201–210.

Ruggiero, K. J., Del Ben, K. S., Scotti, J. R., & Rabalais, A. E. (2003). Psychometric properties of the PTSD Checklist—Civilian version. *Journal of Traumatic Stress, 16,* 495–502.

Scheibe, S., Bagby, R. M., Miller, L. S., & Dorian, B. J. (2001). Assessing posttraumatic stress disorder with the MMPI-2 in a sample of workplace accident victims. *Psychological Assessment, 13,* 369–374.

Schlenger, W. E., Jordan, B. K., Caddell, J. M., Ebert, L., & Fairbank, J. A. (2004). Epidemiological methods for assessing trauma and PTSD. In J. P. Wilson & T.

M. Keane (Eds.), *Assessing psychological trauma and PTSD* (2nd ed., pp. 226–261). New York: Guilford Press.

Schlenger, W. E., Kulka, R. A., Fairbank, J. A., Hough, R. L., Jordan, B. K., Marmar, C. R., et al. (1992). The prevalence of post-traumatic stress disorder in the Vietnam generation: A multimethod, multisource assessment of psychiatric disorder. *Journal of Traumatic Stress, 5*, 333–363.

Schnurr, P. P., Green, B. L., & Kaltman, S. (2007). Trauma exposure and physical health. In M. J. Friedman, T. M. Keane, & P. A. Resick (Eds.), *Handbook of PTSD: Science and practice* (pp. 406–424). New York: Guilford Press.

Simms, L. J., Watson, D., & Doebbeling, B. N. (2002). Confirmatory factor analyses of posttraumatic stress symptoms in deployed and nondeployed veterans of the Gulf War. *Journal of Abnormal Psychology, 111*, 637–647.

Skre, I., Onstad, S., Torgersen, S., & Kringlen, E. (1991). High interrater reliability for the Structured Clinical Interview for DSM-III-R Axis I (SCID-I). *Acta Psychiatrica Scandinavica, 84*, 167–173.

Solomon, S. D., & Canino, G. J. (1990). Appropriateness of DSM-III-R criteria for posttraumatic stress disorder. *Comprehensive Psychiatry, 31*, 227–237.

Spitzer, R. L., First, M. B., & Wakefield, J. C. (2007). Saving PTSD from itself in DSM-V. *Journal of Anxiety Disorders, 21*, 233–241.

Sundin, E. C., & Horowitz, M. J. (2002). Impact of Event Scale: Psychometric properties. *British Journal of Psychiatry, 180*, 205–209.

Trimble, M. R. (1985). Post-traumatic stress disorder: History of a concept. In C. R. Figley (Ed.), *Trauma and its wake: Vol. I. The study and treatment of post-traumatic stress disorder* (pp. 5–14). New York: Brunner/Mazel.

van der Kolk, B. A. (2007). The history of trauma in psychiatry. In M. J. Friedman, T. M. Keane, & P. A. Resick (Eds.), *Handbook of PTSD: Science and practice* (pp. 19–36). New York: Guilford Press.

Vreven, D. L., Gudanowski, D. M., King, L. A., & King, D. W. (1995). The civilian version of the Mississippi PTSD Scale: A psychometric evaluation. *Journal of Traumatic Stress, 8*, 91–109.

Watson, C. G., Kucala, T., & Manifold, V. (1986). A cross-validation of the Keane and Penk MMPI Scales as measures of post-traumatic stress disorder. *Journal of Clinical Psychology, 42*, 727–732.

Weathers, F. W., & Keane, T. M. (1999). Psychological assessment of traumatized adults. In P. A. Saigh & J. D. Bremner (Eds.), *Posttraumatic stress disorder: A comprehensive approach to research and treatment* (pp. 219–247). Boston: Allyn & Bacon.

Weathers, F. W., & Keane, T. M. (2007). The Criterion A problem revisited: Controversies and challenges in defining and measuring psychological trauma. *Journal of Traumatic Stress, 20*, 107–121.

Weathers, F. W., Keane, T. M., & Davidson, J. R. T. (2001). The Clinician-Administered PTSD Scale: A review of the first ten years of research. *Depression and Anxiety, 13*, 132–156.

Weathers, F. W., Litz, B. T., Herman, D. S., Huska, J. A., & Keane, T. M. (1993, October). *The PTSD Checklist (PCL): Reliability, validity, and diagnostic utility.* Paper presented at the annual meeting of the International Society for Traumatic Stress Studies, San Antonio, TX.

Weathers, F. W., Newman, E., Blake, D. D., Nagy, L. M., Schnurr, P. P., Kaloupek, D. G., et al. (2004). *Clinician-Administered PTSD Scale (CAPS)—Interviewer's guide.* Los Angeles: Western Psychological Services.

Weathers, F. W., Ruscio, A. M., & Keane, T. M. (1999). Psychometric properties of nine scoring rules for the Clinician-Administered Posttraumatic Stress Disorder Scale. *Psychological Assessment, 11,* 124–133.

Weiss, D. S. (2004). The Impact of Event Scale—Revised. In J. P. Wilson & T. M. Keane (Eds.), *Assessing psychological trauma and PTSD* (2nd ed., pp. 168–189). New York: Guilford Press.

Weiss, D. S., & Marmar, C. R. (1997). The Impact of Event Scale—Revised. In J. P. Wilson & T. M. Keane (Eds.), *Assessing psychological trauma and PTSD* (pp. 399–411). New York: Guilford Press.

Wilson, J. P. (2004). PTSD and complex PTSD: Symptoms, syndromes, and diagnoses. In J. P. Wilson & T. M. Keane (Eds.), *Assessing psychological trauma and PTSD* (2nd ed., pp. 7–44). New York: Guilford Press.

Wilson, J. P., & Keane, T. M. (Eds.). (2004). *Assessing psychological trauma and PTSD* (2nd ed.). New York: Guilford Press.

Wise, E. A. (1996). Diagnosing posttraumatic stress disorder with the MMPI clinical scales: A review of the literature. *Journal of Psychopathology and Behavioral Assessment, 18,* 71–82.

Zanarini, M. C., & Frankenburg, F. R. (2001). Attainment and maintenance of reliability of Axis I and Axis II disorders over the course of a longitudinal study. *Comprehensive Psychiatry, 42,* 369–374.

Zanarini, M. C., Skodol, A. E., Bender, D., Dolan, R., Sanislow, C., Schaefer, E., et al. (2000). The Collaborative Longitudinal Personality Disorders Study: Reliability of Axis I and II diagnoses. *Journal of Personality Disorders, 14,* 291–299.

CHAPTER 3

Assessment of Children

Victor Balaban

As recently as the 1980s, children's psychological responses to many types of traumatic events were widely assumed to be transient and not overly important (Rigamer, 1986). It is now accepted that a wide variety of traumas can have devastating effects on children. The study of children's psychological responses to trauma is still at an early stage; many published studies on children's psychological responses to trauma are contradictory, and even basic questions such as age and gender differences have not yet been resolved (Yule, 2001). Children and adolescents have been found to experience posttraumatic stress symptoms from many types of events, including war (Allwood, Bell-Dolan, & Husain, 2002; Balaban, 2006), illness (Brown, Madan-Swain, & Lambert, 2003), community violence (Cooley-Quille, Boyd, Frantz, & Walsh, 2001), family violence (Grych, Jouriles, Swank, McDonald, & Norwood, 2000), and natural disasters (McFarlane, Policansky, & Irwin, 1987).

Accurate and timely assessment of posttraumatic stress disorder (PTSD) symptoms in children is extremely important because poor developmental outcomes are associated with untreated trauma symptoms (Grych et al., 2000; Yates, Dodds, Sroufe, & Egeland, 2003). Posttraumatic stress can impact cognitive functioning, initiative, personality style, self-esteem, outlook, and impulse control (Pynoos & Nader, 1991). Personality changes have been reported in very young children (Gislason & Call, 1982; Terr, 1988). Childhood trauma studies have also consistently found regressive behavior and a marked change in attitude toward the future, with negative expectations and a sense of foreshortened future (Pynoos & Eth, 1986; Pynoos & Nader, 1991).

One reason for the lack of definitive knowledge about the epidemiology of traumatic responses in children is that researchers have carried out assessments with a variety of instruments of differing levels of reliability. As a result, there is a tremendous need for systematic psychological assessment of children after trauma to better establish the prevalence and etiology of children's posttraumatic symptomatology, and to be able to design interventions more effectively.

Diagnostic Criteria for PTSD

PTSD is an anxiety disorder that can occur after exposure to traumatic stress, and symptoms of PTSD are among the most common types of psychological distress observed in children after trauma. PTSD is characterized by (1) persistent reexperiencing of the traumatic event, such as recurring or intrusive thoughts; (2) avoidance of cues associated with the trauma, or emotional numbing; and (3) persistent physiological hyperreactivity or arousal. Signs and symptoms must be present for more than 1 month following the traumatic event and cause clinically significant disturbance in functioning. A child is considered to have acute stress disorder (ASD) when these criteria are met during the month following a traumatic event. PTSD is further characterized as acute when present for less than 3 months, chronic when present for more than 3 months, or delayed onset when symptoms develop initially 6 months or more after the trauma (American Psychiatric Association, 1994 [DSM-IV]; Pfefferbaum, 1997; Yule, 1999).

DSM-IV diagnostic criteria for PTSD are designed for adults, not for children. Instruments used in postemergency assessment of young children must take into account their limited verbal skills and different ways of reacting to stress. For example, children who are too young to verbalize their symptoms may not be able to express signs of numbing and withdrawal, and they may show reexperiencing symptoms in the form of play reenactment rather than flashbacks or intrusive thoughts (Eth, Silverstein, & Pynoos, 1985; Scheeringa, Zeanah, Drell, & Larrieu, 1995).

Choosing the Appropriate Assessment Instrument

"Psychological assessment" is the area of psychology devoted to examination and analysis of behaviors and/or psychological characteristics by means of construction, administration, scoring, and interpretation of tests and other measurement devices (Anastasi & Urbino, 1996). When conducting posttrauma assessments, there is generally not a single "best" instrument. Different instruments are appropriate for different contexts, and even psychometrically sound instruments may have other characteristics that could limit their usefulness in different types of populations or emergencies. A good psychological instrument should be both reliable and valid, although validity is generally considered to be the measure of the usefulness of a test (Anastasi & Urbino, 1996).[1]

Thousands of assessment interviews, instruments, and rating scales have been developed to assess hundreds of different constructs, and simply using a well-known instrument, without taking into consideration its specific characteristics and the context in which it will be used, can result in wasted opportunities and effort. For example, because the majority of psychological instruments were not developed for assessing traumatized populations, they do not assess symptoms that are known empirically to be associated with child and adolescent trauma (Balaban, 2006; Saylor & DeRoma, 2002). In addition, many older scales that may have impressive bodies of psychometric data behind them were not developed explicitly for children, or may have been based on older or unclear definitions of underlying constructs. Newer scales often have been designed to overcome these problems, but they may not yet have been in use long enough to establish definitive conclusions on their validity or reliability. Until recently, one of the factors which hampered the assessment of trauma-related mental health effects in children and adolescents was a lack of reliable, validated instruments, but there is now a range of acceptable instruments available for assessing child and adolescent psychopathology (Myers & Winters, 2002).

This chapter is intended to help bring methodological consistency to future assessments by providing a review of instruments appropriate for assessing PTSD in children and adolescents. Two categories of instruments are reviewed: questionnaires and self-report instruments, and structured and semistructured interviews. The instruments for assessing PTSD in children discussed in this chapter, and information on obtaining and administering them, are summarized in Table 3.1.

Questionnaires and Self-Report Instruments

Child PTSD Reaction Index

The Child PTSD Reaction Index (CPTSD-RI), one of the mostly widely used measures in childhood PTSD research, is a scale for assessing posttrauma symptoms and PTSD in children ages 6–17 after exposure to a broad range of traumatic events. It contains 20 items that are scored 0 to 4 points according to presence of symptoms, and takes 15–20 minutes to administer. CPTSD-RI items are written in age-appropriate language. It has been translated into several different languages and used with children and adolescents in the aftermath of many different types of traumas. The CPTSD-RI has more psychometric research behind it than most other assessment scales for juvenile trauma, and it has shown good reliability and validity. A shorter, seven-question version of the CPTSD-RI has also been developed (Ohan, Myers, & Collett, 2002; Pynoos et al., 1987, 1993).

The CPTSD-RI is most likely to be appropriate for assessing children after disasters and emergencies. Explicitly designed for children and adolescents, it has been used in a variety of emergency contexts. In addition, it is

TABLE 3.1. Instruments for Assessing PTSD in Children

Instrument	Description	Availability	Length/administration time	Ages	Reliability
Questionnaires and self-report measures					
UCLA PTSD Reaction Index for DSM-IV (Pynoos et al., 1998)	Assessing posttrauma symptoms and PTSD in children	No cost. Available at *rpynoos@mednet.ucla.edu.*	22 items; 20–30 minutes	6–17	Internal consistency .69–8; interrater reliability 0.88, test–retest reliability .93 over 1 week; convergent validity .91 with measures of PTSD
Impact of Event Scale—Revised (IES-R; Weiss & Marmar, 1997)	Measuring symptoms of PTSD after a traumatic event	No cost. Available at many sites online (e.g., *www.swin.edu.au/victims/resources/assessment/ptsd/ies-r.html*). A 13-item version of IES-R (IES-13) developed for children affected by war is available at *www.childrenandwar.org/cries-13.doc.*	22 items; 10–15 minutes	Used with children as young as 7 (not designed for children)	(validation data only available for adults) Internal consistency .79–.90 for subscales, .60–.90 total; interrater reliability not reported; test–retest reliability .79–.89 over 1 week; convergent validity .41–.78 with measures of PTSD
Posttraumatic Stress Symptoms in Children (PTSS-C; Ahmad et al., 2000)	Identifying pediatric posttraumatic symptoms in chaotic disaster contexts	No cost. Available at *abdulbaghi.ahmad@bupinst.uu.se.*	30 items; 30 minutes	6–18	Internal consistency .78–88; interrater reliability .94; test–retest reliability not reported; convergent validity .64–.95 with measures of PTSD
Child PTSD Symptom Scale (CPSS; Foa et al., 2001)	Assessing symptoms and functional impairment related to PTSD	No cost. Available at *foa@mail.med.upenn.edu.*	24 items; 15 minutes	8–18	Internal consistency .70–80 for subscales, .89 total; test–retest .63–.85 for subscales, .84 total; interrater reliability not reported; convergent validity .80 with measures of PTSD

(continued)

65

TABLE 3.1. (continued)

Instrument	Description	Availability	Length/administration time	Ages	Reliability
Questionnaires and self-report measures (cont.)					
Trauma Symptom Checklist for Children (TSCC; Briere, 1996)	Assessing PTSD symptoms after trauma, particularly sexual abuse	Licensed through *www.parinc.com*	54 items; 20 minutes	7–16	Internal consistency .70–.90 for subscales, .89 total; interrater reliability not reported; test–retest reliability not reported; convergent validity .75–.82 with measures of PTSD
Trauma Symptom Checklist for Young Children (TSCYC; Briere et al., 2001)	Caretaker report measure for trauma symptoms	Licensed through *www.parinc.com*	90 items	3–12	Internal consistency (clinical scales) .73–.93, convergent validity .52–.82 with CBCL, CSBI, CD
PTSD Symptoms in Preschool-Age Children (PTSDPAC; Levendosky et al., 2002)	Caregiver-completed measure for PTSD	No cost. Available online at *levendo1@msu.edu*	18 items	3–5	Internal consistency .79
Child Behavior Checklist—PTSD subscale (CBCL; Achenbach & Rescorla, 2000)	Caregiver-completed behavior checklist	Licensed through *www.aseba.org*	13 items	1.5–5, 4–18 depending on version	Internal consistency .80–.89; convergent validity .66 with structured interview

Structured and semistructured interviews

Diagnostic Interview for Children and Adolescents (DICA; Reich, Leacock, & Shanfield, 1994)	Semistructured interview designed to assess present and lifetime diagnoses of PTSD	Multi-Health Symptoms (MHS) Publishers (*www.mhs.com*)	1–2 hours	6–17	N/A
Kiddie Schedule for Affective Disorders and Schizophrenia for School-Age Children (K-SADS-PL; Kaufman et al., 1997)	Semistructured interview to assess present and lifetime diagnosis of PTSD	Available online at *www.wpic.pitt.edu/ksads/default.htm*	45 minutes	7–17	Internal consistency N/A; interrater reliability 98% agreement on current/lifetime diagnoses; interrater reliability .63 (Freeman & Beck, 2000); test–retest reliability present PTSD .67; lifetime PTSD .60 N/A; convergent validity .71 agreement with CBCL PTSD subscale (McLeer et al., 1998)
Clinician-Administered PTSD Scale for Children and Adolescents (CAPS-CA; Newman et al., 2004)	Semistructured clinical interview designed to assess PTSD symptoms and associated symptoms in children and adolescents	Western Psychological Services (*help@wpspublish.com*)	45 minutes	8–15	Internal consistency for total score .89; interrater reliability .80–1.0; convergent validity .51 correlation with CPTSD-RI
Posttraumatic Stress Disorder Semistructured Interview (Scheeringa & Zeanah, 1994)	Semistructured interview of primary caretaker with the child present in the room	Contact author at *mscheer@tulane.edu*	8 violence exposure symptoms; 29 PTSD symptoms	0–6	Interrater reliability .74–.79

inexpensive, simple, fast to administer and to score, and has a body of psychometric research to support it.

Impact of Event Scale—Revised

The Impact of Event Scale (IES), one of the first self-report measures of posttraumatic disturbance designed to measure current subjective distress related to a specific event, is a widely used instrument in adult PTSD research (Horowitz, Wilner, & Alvarez, 1979). It was developed prior to the adoption of PTSD as a legitimate diagnosis in 1980; as result, an updated version, the Impact of Event Scale—Revised (IES-R) was developed to accommodate the new DSM-IV criteria for PTSD. The IES-R comprises 22 items that measure symptoms of intrusion, avoidance, and arousal. It takes approximately 10–15 minutes to administer. It has been translated into several different languages.

It is important to note that the IES-R does not cover all the symptoms of PTSD. In addition, the instrument has not been modified to assess specific manifestation of child and adolescent trauma, and the psychometric properties of the IES-R have not yet been studied in younger children (Briere, 1997; Jones & Kafetsios, 2002; Ohan et al., 2002; Weiss & Marmar, 1997).

The IES-R is appropriate for screening children who have been exposed to a specific, discrete trauma, but its focus on effects of a specific event may limit its applicability in contexts where children have been exposed to multiple or ongoing traumas. In addition, although it has been used with children and adolescents, the IES-R was designed for adults, so it may not be the best instrument for child assessments. A shorter, 13-item version of the IES-R has been developed to assess children in postconflict settings, but psychometric data are still limited (Smith, Perrin, Dyregrov, & Yule, 2002).

Posttraumatic Stress Symptoms in Children

The Posttraumatic Stress Symptoms in Children (PTSS-C) measure was developed to be an easy-to-administer instrument for identifying posttraumatic symptoms and diagnosing PTSD in children in chaotic disaster contexts. It takes approximately 30 minutes to administer and comprises 30 yes–no items. The first 17 items are based on DSM criteria for PTSD; the rest are designed to assess child-specific posttraumatic symptoms, such as feelings of guilt, hyperactivity, and so forth. The limited available data have shown that the PTSS-C has good validity (Ahmad, Sundelin-Wahlsten, Sofi, Qahar, & von Knorring, 2000).

The PTSS-C is easy to administer and is designed specifically for assessing younger children exposed to chaotic war environment and trauma contexts. However, it is a relatively new instrument with little validation data available, which can make comparisons of its results and those of measures using other postemergency assessment scales difficult.

Trauma Symptom Checklist for Children

The Trauma Symptom Checklist for Children (TSCC), a self-report scale that assesses distress and posttraumatic symptoms after acute or chronic trauma, has been used primarily to assess children's responses to sexual abuse. It comprises 54 items divided into six subscales: Anxiety, Depression, Anger, Posttraumatic Stress, Dissociation, and Sexual Concerns. Shorter, 44- and 40-item versions of the TSCC that do not contain items relating to sexual concerns are also available.

The TSCC has been shown to have good validity, and extensive psychometric data have been collected on both clinical and nonclinical populations. It does not assess all symptoms of PTSD, though, so it may be more useful for screening than for diagnosis (Briere, 1996).

Trauma Symptom Checklist for Young Children

The Trauma Symptom Checklist for Young Children (TSCYC; Briere et al., 2001) is a caretaker report measure for children ages 3–12. Caretakers rate each symptom on a 4-point scale based on how frequently it has occurred in the last month. The TSCYC contains eight clinical scales: Posttraumatic Stress–Intrusion (PTSI), Posttraumatic Stress–Avoidance (PTS-AV), Posttraumatic Stress–Arousal (PTS-AR), Sexual Concerns (SC), Dissociation (DIS), Anxiety (ANX), Depression (DEP), and Anger/Aggression (ANG). It also contains a summary posttraumatic stress scale, Posttraumatic Stress–Total (PTS-TOT), and several scales to ascertain the validity of response level (RL) and atypical response (ATR) in caretaker reports.

The TSCYC is easy to administer and requires minimal training. However, the scale does not ask questions related to trauma-specific child symptoms (i.e., repetitive play or regression of previously learned skills).

Child PTSD Symptom Scale

The Child PTSD Symptom Scale (CPSS), a self-report scale, assesses DSM-IV symptoms and functional impairment related to PTSD in a developmentally appropriate format and language for children and adolescents ages 8–18. It comprises 17 questions that assess the frequency of symptoms of PTSD in the previous month, and seven additional questions that assess daily functioning (i.e., school performance, relationships with friends). Only preliminary validation data are available for the CPSS, but the early data are good. Sensitivity and cutoff scores for diagnosing PTSD are still being developed (Foa, Johnson, Feeny, & Treadwell, 2001; Ohan et al., 2002).

Although the CPSS is rapidly administered and designed for children, it is a relatively new instrument with little validation data available, which may make comparing its results with those from other posttrauma scales more difficult.

PTSD Symptoms in Preschool-Age Children

PTSD Symptoms in Preschool-Age Children (PTSDPAC; Levendosky et al., 2002) is a caregiver-completed measure based on DSM-IV criteria for PTSD, with additional items related to young children. Parents report the presence or absence of symptoms, and the number of endorsed items is summed to create a total score. Parents are asked to endorse the presence of symptoms, including those relevant to reexperiencing (playing out the event with toys, having dreams about the event, having flashbacks, avoidance, hyperarousal, and loss of previously attained skills). Parents are asked to answer each item in relation to their child's behavior since the traumatic event. The PTSDPAC relies solely on parent report and asks no questions about frequency or onset of symptoms.

Child Behavior Checklist

The Child Behavior Checklist (CBCL; Achenbach & Rescorla, 2000) was not specifically designed to measure PTSD in children; however, researchers have created a post hoc PTSD scale from items in previous versions of the CBCL (Levendosky, Huth-Bocks, Semel, & Shapiro, 2002). The PTSD items on the CBCL include argues, difficulty concentrating, obsessive thoughts, clinging, irrational fears, feels persecuted, nervous, nightmares, fearful/anxious, guilty, headaches, nausea, stomachaches, vomiting, secretive, sullen/irritable, labile mood, difficulty sleeping, sad, and withdrawn; parents rate each item as *not true, somewhat or sometimes true,* or *very true/often true* within the last 2 months. Levendosky and colleagues (2002) found no correlation between the CBCL PTSD scale and a measure created to assess PTSD symptoms. However, Dehon and Scheeringa (2005), using a modified version of the CBCL PTSD scale to screen for PTSD in a sample of children ages 2–6 compared to a structured clinical interview, have reported promising sensitivity and specificity.

Structured and Semistructured Interviews

Posttraumatic Stress Disorder Semistructured Interview and Observation Record

The Posttraumatic Stress Disorder Semistructured Interview and Observation Record (Scheeringa & Zeanah, 1994) is an examinee-based interview of the primary caretaker, with the child present in the room. The interviewer first asks the child's parent about a series of traumas the child may have experienced. If a parent endorses a trauma, she is then asked when it occurred and whether she considered the event traumatic for the child. Next, the interviewer reads a series of stem questions about each PTSD symptom. If a respondent endorses a symptom, then the interviewer asks for specific examples, until he or she is convinced of the presence of the symptom and some level of dysfunction as a result, for example, "Has your child had flashbacks, where it looks like he's reliving the event and reacting to it?" The interviewer asks for specific examples observed by the parent, then requests information about the onset, frequency, and duration of the symptom. Symptoms measured by the interview include those from the list of DSM-IV criteria and other developmentally based young child symptoms, such as loss of previous skills, new separation anxiety, or aggression.

This measure requires a high level of clinical skill to administer. The interviewer must observe symptoms of the child, while directing questions to the parent and making decisions about the symptoms described by the parent. The scale does come with a coding manual to help users identify signs and symptoms, and with high-quality interviewers, this measure can give an accurate diagnostic picture. Although the measure does include direct observation of the child during the course of the parent interview, it does not include any direct interviewing of the child either verbally or in play form.

Diagnostic Interview for Children and Adolescents—Revised

The Diagnostic Interview for Children and Adolescents (DICA; Reich, Leacock, & Shanfield, 1994) was developed in 1969 primarily for clinical and epidemiological research and has since undergone many revisions. The revised DICA (DICA-R), the most recent version, is a semistructured interview designed to assess present and lifetime diagnoses. The DICA-R PTSD module comprises 17 questions and is one of 18 diagnostic scales. The PTSD portion of the interview is based on an event the child identifies as traumatic. Lay interviewers who receive 2–4 weeks of training can administer the DICA-R. A diagnosis can be based on either parent or child/adolescent interview, but a thorough assessment should consider information from both sources.

Kiddie Schedule for Affective Disorders and Schizophrenia for School-Age Children—Present and Lifetime Version

The original Kiddie Schedule for Affective Disorders and Schizophrenia for School-Age Children (K-SADS; Kaufman et al., 1997) was designed as a comprehensive instrument to assess psychopathology in children. This semistructured interview assesses full and partial diagnosis, including present and lifetime diagnosis of PTSD (K-SADS-PL). The PTSD module is one of 32 scales and varies in length depending on the number of endorsed items. Intensive training is needed to administer the instrument because of the importance of diagnostic classification and differential diagnosis. The clinician integrates parent report of observable behavior and child self-report when formulating a diagnosis. In the PTSD module, the scale initially assesses whether any of a variety of traumatic events have occurred recently or in the past, then assesses PTSD diagnostic criteria for one specific event.

Clinician-Administered PTSD Scale for Children and Adolescents

The Clinician-Administered PTSD Scale for Children and Adolescents (CAPS-CA; Newman et al., 2004) is a semistructured clinical interview designed to assess PTSD symptoms and associated symptoms in children and adolescents. The CAPS-CA comprises 36 questions based on a specific event the child identifies as most distressing. The CAPS-CA evaluates current and lifetime diagnosis, frequency and intensity of symptoms, as well as social, developmental, and scholastic functioning. A diagnosis also incorporates the interviewer's clinical judgment regarding the type of trauma and impact on functioning.

Factors in Designing
Posttrauma Child Psychological Assessments

In addition to selecting the correct instrument, recent research suggests that several important factors be taken into consideration when planning post-trauma assessments of children.

Necessity of Assessing Severity and Type of Trauma

It is essential that the type, nature, and duration of trauma be assessed in children. Severity of posttraumatic symptoms in children has been found to be related to the level of exposure (Cooley-Quille et al., 2001) and number of exposures (Allwood et al., 2002). A variety of questionnaires have been designed to assess levels of exposure to various types of traumas. These questionnaires are not mental health assessment tools themselves, but they can provide an important way to identify at-risk children and adolescents and should be used whenever possible as part of posttrauma mental health assessments (for a review, see Saylor & DeRoma, 2002).

Necessity of Assessing Multiple Disorders

Youth with PTSD often carry dual diagnoses, which makes it difficult for clinicians to distinguish between overlapping symptoms. High rates of comorbidity have been documented in youth exposed to a variety of traumas (Kilpatrick et al., 2003; Sack, Seeley, Him, & Clarke, 1998). Although a great deal of the current knowledge of children's psychological responses to trauma is based on PTSD research, PTSD is only one of a range of possible responses to trauma. Traumatized children can exhibit a range of trauma-based symptoms, including anxiety, depression, somatic disturbances, learning problems, oppositional behaviors, and conduct disorder (Goenjian et al., 1995; Sack et al., 1995; Yule, 2001). Although the wide range of symptoms displayed can make diagnosis more difficult, accurate diagnosis of PTSD remains essential.

Independent Assessment of Children's Behavior

Assessing child mental health often requires input from several informants. Children have generally been found to be able to report their own internal states accurately, but often they are not reliable observers of their own behaviors. Adults, in contrast, are generally reliable observers of children's behaviors, but have a tendency to underestimate children's internal distress (Jensen, Salzberg, Richters, & Watanabe, 1993; Loeber, Green, Lahey, & Stouthamer-Loeber, 1991). Whenever possible, assessments of children should include an adult's assessment of their behavior. However, this should not be a substitute for an assessment of the children themselves.

Assessment of Family Members, Especially Mothers

If possible, the mental health status of primary caretakers should be assessed at the same time as children are assessed. A variety of studies have indicated that parental adjustment is an important predictor of children's mental health outcomes, particularly maternal reactions (Laor, Wolmer, & Cohen, 2001; McFarlane et al., 1987; Pynoos, Goenjian, & Steinberg, 1988; Smith, Perrin, Yule, & Rabe-Hesketh, 2001).

Functional Status

Whenever possible, instruments that include questions of social and behavioral functioning should be used in assessment of children after exposure to trauma. Appropriate and adaptive behaviors may be very different in the aftermath of emergencies, so the presence of symptoms does not always indicate functional disability, nor does the absence of reported symptoms indicate lack of distress (e.g., Bolton et al., 2000; Sack et al., 1995; Shalev, Tuval-Mashiach, & Hadar, 2004; Terr, 1988).

Age and Developmental Differences

Although the impact of age on children's posttraumatic behavior and psychopathology are not yet well understood, it is critically important that any assessment instruments be age- and developmentally appropriate (i.e., postemergency assessments of young children must take into account their limited verbal skills and different ways of reacting to stress). For example, children too young to verbalize their symptoms may not be able to express signs of numbing and withdrawal, and they may show reexperiencing symptoms in the form of play reenactment rather than flashbacks or intrusive thoughts (Eth et al., 1985; Scheeringa et al., 1995). In general, screening instruments for children under age 5 should only be given to adult caretakers because children this young are developmentally unable to report psychiatric symptoms of this type accurately.

Not all pediatric instruments are equally applicable for all children. Instruments for younger children must be carefully constructed with age-appropriate language and concepts; it is very important that an instrument be used with children the age for whom it was developed. In addition, there is evidence that children's reporting of physical symptoms is strongly influenced both by the level of cognitive development, and by family, parents, peers, and school and community environments (Rhee, 2003). It is likely that similar factors may influence children's reporting of psychological symptoms as well. There is a need for further studies that address these complicated developmental issues.

Risk and Resilience Factors

A variety of studies have identified risk factors that influence response to trauma and affect recovery, including exposure to previous traumas, preexisting psychopathology, and lack of social support (Caffo & Belaise, 2003; Pfefferbaum, 1997). Other studies of traumatized child populations have also indicated that family displacement and parental loss can add to the effects of the original trauma itself (Norris et al., 2002). Ideally, posttrauma assessment and screening would include questions to assess these and other potential risk factors, as a way to identify populations of children and adolescents who may be at higher risk for developing trauma-related psychopathology. One promising area for further research is the PsySTART studies, particularly the assessment of Thai children after the Asian tsunami, in which researchers accurately identified risk factors for future development of PTSD, inquiring about trauma-related experiences rather than current symptoms (Thienkrua et al., 2006).

Although most research on the effects of trauma has focused on negative impacts, recent research has also begun to evaluate positive changes (often referred to as "posttraumatic growth" or "adversarial growth") that may also occur following trauma (e.g., Linley & Joseph, 2004; Tedeschi, Park, & Calhoun, 1998). In general, it has been found that the majority of adults exposed to disasters and emergencies show resilience and do not develop trauma-related psychopathology (Shalev et al., 2004), but comparable data on children and adolescents are not yet available. Future work should include the identification and testing of measures of resilience and adversarial growth in children and adolescents.

Cross-Cultural Differences

Any scale must be used with caution when the population being assessed is different from the one on which the test was validated. Many assessment instruments may not be appropriately sensitive to cultural and ethnic variability, and simply translating an instrument into another language does not necessarily mean that the same symptoms or the same disorders are being assessed across cultures. Even when language is not an issue, original validation studies of an instrument may not be sufficient to establish cutoff scores in a new setting or population. For example, a test validated in a middle-class clinical population may need to be revalidated for use in a non-Western context or in an inner-city population exposed to chronic violence (Kleinman & Good, 1986; Mollica, Cui, McInnes, & Massagli, 2002).

If time and resources allow, there are several strategies that maximize cross-cultural validity of existing scales in settings in which they have not been validated or of new scales being developed in cross-cultural settings. The first step would be to use ethnographic methods (key informant interviewing, focus groups, free listing, pile sorts, etc.) to determine what symptoms people may be experiencing as a result of trauma, and to learn the names and symptoms of comparable, locally recognized responses to trauma. The next step would be to translate the scale into the local language(s). Accurate translation and back-translation is particularly important when assessing mental health because even minor mistranslations of expressions for mental and emotional states can often alter substantially the meaning of questions. Finally, a pilot study should be conducted to determine the validity of the instrument. At a minimum, an instrument should be shown to have adequate internal reliability, as well as adequate convergent validity with other measures of the same disorder (for more detailed explanations of the process of instrument development and validation, e.g., see Anastasi & Urbino, 1996; Bolton, 2001; Mollica et al., 1992).

Even with instruments used in cross-cultural settings, it is not always clear from published articles whether or how an instrument has actually been validated for all the various cultures. Therefore, it is always best to contact the author and/or the publisher of an instrument to be certain how much validity an instrument is known to have in any particular culture.

The fact that very few instruments have been validated in non-Western populations does not mean that psychological assessment with existing instruments cannot be carried out. Guarnaccia's (1993) comparison of anxiety and depression disorders with a local disorder, *ataques de nervios*, in the aftermath of floods in Puerto Rico, and Bolton's (2001) comparison of depression and a locally recognized grief syndrome, *agahinda gakabije* in postgenocide Rwanda, are examples of how this can be accomplished. Few current studies directly compare the psychological responses to trauma of children in one culture to those in another, although at least one ongoing study addresses these issues by evaluating HIV-affected, sexually abused children in Zambia for the presence of PTSD and depressive symptoms, assessing how these are manifested cross-culturally, validating instruments among these children, then adapting evidence-based treatment approaches using local providers (Murray, 2006). Future research should focus on understanding the impact of cultural factors on pediatric responses to trauma (Hinshaw & Nigg, 1999; Yule, 2001).

Discussion

Effective intervention for children and families following trauma can be facilitated by careful screening and assessments with valid and reliable instruments. Questionnaires and interviews are important tools that serve different functions in posttrauma child assessments. Self-report symptom checklists and questionnaires are important public health tools for mental health, and are extremely useful for screening and for epidemiological research, but they should not be the sole criteria for making clinical diagnoses. No checklist can replace the role of a mental health professional. However, diagnostic interviews are time-consuming to conduct and generally require training to administer, which can limit their use in large populations. Questionnaires and symptom checklists can be used in conjunction with structured and semistructured interviews as part of a process that includes initial screening to identify at-risk children for more thorough examination by clinicians.

This discussion has focused on instruments for the assessment of children, but it is also important to consider the interpersonal, social, and cultural contexts in which child assessments take place. Assessments should ideally be conducted in environments where children feel safe to express themselves and in ways that will not cause any additional anxiety. The design of posttrauma assessments requires careful consideration on a case-by-case basis. For example, younger children may be afraid of being separated from their parents, or in some cultures parents may not consent to children being assessed by themselves, so it may be appropriate in some settings to conduct child assessments and adult and family assessments simultaneously.

When designing posttrauma assessments it is also important to consider the role of resilience and the goal of promoting mental health, and not to focus exclusively on illness and psychopathology. Ideally, future research will identify patterns of child resilience, coping, and recovery in the aftermath of trauma.

Note

1. When choosing instruments for psychological assessment, it is important to note that whereas some instruments are in the public domain, others must be licensed to be used. In general, it is useful first to contact the author about the availability of an instrument because there are often different ways in which instruments can be used (i.e., some licensed instruments can be used at no charge, if the author of the test is involved). Further information on rating scales can generally be located in reference resources such as *Tests in Print* (Murphy, Plake, Impara, & Spies, 2002), the *Mental Measurements Yearbook* (Plake, Impara, & Spies, 2003), and electronic databases such as Health and Psychosocial Instruments (HAPI).

References

Achenbach, T. M., & Rescorla, L. (2000). *Child Behavior Checklist for Ages 1½–5*. Burlington: University of Vermont.

Ahmad, A., Sundelin-Wahlsten, V., Sofi, M. A., Qahar, J. A., & von Knorring, A. L. (2000). Reliability and validity of a child-specific cross-cultural instrument for assessing posttraumatic stress disorder. *European Child and Adolescent Psychiatry, 9*(4), 285–294.

Allwood, M. A., Bell-Dolan, D., & Husain, S. A. (2002). Children's trauma and adjustment reactions to violent and nonviolent war experiences. *Journal of the American Academy of Child and Adolescent Psychiatry, 41*, 450–457.

American Psychiatric Association. (1994). *Diagnostic and statistical manual of mental disorders* (4th ed.). Washington, DC: Author.

Anastasi, A., & Urbino, S. (1996). *Psychological testing*. New York: Prentice-Hall.

Balaban, V. (2006). Psychological assessment of children in disasters and emergencies. *Disasters, 30*(2), 178–198.

Bolton, D., O'Ryan, D., Udwin, O., Boyle, S., & Yule, W. (2000). The long-term psychological effects of a disaster experienced in adolescence: II. General psychopathology. *Journal of Child Psychology and Psychiatry, and Allied Disciplines, 41*(4), 513–523.

Bolton, P. (2001). Cross-cultural validity and reliability testing of a standard psychiatric assessment instrument without a gold standard. *Journal of Nervous and Mental Disease, 189*(4), 238–242.

Briere, J. (1996) *Trauma Symptom Checklist for Children: Professional manual*. Lutz, FL: Psychological Assessment Resources.

Briere, J. (1997) *Psychological assessment of adult posttraumatic states*. Washington, DC: American Psychological Association.

Briere, J., Johnson, K., Bissada, A., Damon, L., Crouch, J., Gil, E., et al. (2001). Trauma Symptom Checklist for Young Children (TSCYC): Reliability and association with abuse exposure in a multi-site study. *Child Abuse and Neglect, 25*, 1001–1014.

Brown, R. T., Madan-Swain, A., & Lambert, R. (2003). Posttraumatic stress symptoms in adolescent survivors of childhood cancer and their mothers. *Journal of Traumatic Stress, 16*, 309–318.

Caffo, E., & Belaise, C. (2003). Psychological aspects of traumatic injury in children and adolescents. *Child and Adolescent Psychiatric Clinics of North America, 12*, 493–535.

Cooley-Quille, M., Boyd, R. C., Frantz, E., & Walsh, J. (2001). Emotional and behavioral impact of exposure to community violence in inner-city adolescents. *Journal of Clinical Child Psychology, 30*, 199–206.

Dehon, C., & Scheeringa, M. (2005). Screening for preschool posttraumatic stress disorder with the Child Behavior Checklist. *Journal of Pediatric Psychology, 31*, 431–435.

Eth, S., Silverstein, S., & Pynoos, R. S. (1985). Mental health consultation to a preschool following the murder of a mother and child. *Hospital and Community Psychiatry, 36*(1), 73–76.

Foa, E. B., Johnson, K. M., Feeny, N. C., & Treadwell, K. R. (2001). The Child PTSD Symptom Scale: A preliminary examination of its psychometric properties. *Journal of Clinical Child Psychology, 30*(3), 376–384.

Freeman, J. B., & Beck, J. G. (2000). Cognitive interference for trauma cues in sexually abused adolescent girls with posttraumatic stress disorder. *Journal of Clinical Child Psychology, 29*, 245–256.

Gislason, I. L., & Call, J. D. (1982). Dog bite in infancy: Trauma and personality development. *Journal of the American Academy of Child Psychiatry, 21,* 203–207.

Goenjian, A. K., Pynoos, R. S., Steinberg, A. M., Najarian, L. M., Asarnow, J. R., Karayan, I., et al. (1995). Psychiatric comorbidity in children after the 1988 earthquake in Armenia. *Journal of the American Academy of Child and Adolescent Psychiatry, 34*(9), 1174–1184.

Grych, J. H., Jouriles, E. N., Swank, P. R., McDonald, R., & Norwood, W. D. (2000). Patterns of adjustment among children of battered women. *Journal of Consulting and Clinical Psychology, 68,* 84–94.

Guarnaccia, P. J. (1993). *Ataques de nervios* in Puerto Rico: Culture-bound syndrome or popular illness? *Medical Anthropology, 15*(2), 157–170.

Hinshaw, S. P., & Nigg, J. T. (1999). Behavior rating scales in the assessment of disruptive behavior disorders in childhood. In D. Shaffer, C. P. Lucas, & J. E. Richters (Eds.), *Assessment in child and adolescent psychopathology* (pp. 91–126). New York: Guilford Press.

Horowitz, M., Wilner, N., & Alvarez, W. (1979). Impact of Event Scale: A measure of subjective stress. *Psychosomatic Medicine, 41,* 209–218.

Jensen, P. S., Salzberg, A. D., Richters, J. E., & Watanabe, H. K. (1993). Scales, diagnoses, and child psychopathology: I. CBCL and DISC relationships. *Journal of the American Academy of Child and Adolescent Psychiatry, 32,* 397–406.

Jones, L., & Kafetsios, K. (2002). Assessing adolescent mental health in war-affected societies: The significance of symptoms. *Child Abuse and Neglect, 26,* 1059–1080.

Kaufman, J., Birmaher, B., Brent, D., Rao, U., Flynn, C., Moreci, P., et al. (1997). Schedule for Affective Disorder and Schizophrenia for School-Age Children— Present and Lifetime Version (K-SADS-PL): Initial reliability and validity data. *Journal of the American Academy of Child and Adolescent Psychiatry, 36,* 980–988.

Kilpatrick, D. G., Ruggiero, K. J., Acierno, R., Saunders, B. E., Resnick, H. S., & Best, C. L. (2003). Violence and risk of PTSD, major depression, substance abuse/ dependence, and comorbidity: Results from the National Survey of Adolescents. *Journal of Consulting and Clinical Psychology, 71,* 692–700.

Kleinman, A., & Good, B. (1986). *Culture and depression: Studies in anthropology and cross-cultural psychiatry of affect and disorder.* Los Angeles: University of California Press.

Laor, N., Wolmer, L., & Cohen, D. J. (2001). Mothers' functioning and children's symptoms 5 years after a SCUD missile attack. *American Journal of Psychiatry, 158*(7), 1020–1026.

Levendosky, A. A., Huth-Bocks, A. C., Semel, M. A., & Shapiro, D. L. (2002). Trauma symptoms in preschool-age children exposed to domestic violence. *Journal of Interpersonal Violence, 17,* 150–164.

Linley, P. A., & Joseph, S. (2004). Positive change following trauma and adversity: A review. *Journal of Traumatic Stress, 17,* 11–21.

Loeber, R., Green, S. M., Lahey, B. B., & Stouthamer-Loeber, M. (1991). Differences and similarities between children, mothers, and teachers as informants on disruptive child behavior. *Journal of Abnormal Child Psychology, 19*(1), 75–95.

McFarlane, A. C., Policansky, S. K., & Irwin, C. (1987). A longitudinal study of the psychological morbidity in children due to a natural disaster. *Psychological Medicine, 17*(3), 727—738.

McLeer, S. V., Dixon, J. F., Henry, D., Ruggiero, K., Escovitz, K., Niedda, T., et al. (1998). Psychopathology in non-clinically referred sexually abused children. *Journal of the American Academy of Child and Adolescent Psychiatry, 37,* 1326–1333.

Mollica, R. F., Caspi-Yavin, Y., Bollini, P., Truong, T., Tor, S., & Lavelle, J. (1992). The Harvard Trauma Questionnaire: Validating a cross-cultural instrument for measuring torture, trauma and posttraumatic stress disorder in Indochinese refugees. *Journal of Nervous and Mental Disease, 180,* 111–116.

Mollica, R. F., Cui, X., McInnes, K., & Massagli, M. P. (2002). Science-based policy for psychosocial interventions in refugee camps: A Cambodian example. *Journal of Nervous and Mental Disease, 190,* 158–166.

Murphy, L. L., Plake, B. S., Impara, J. C., & Spies, R. A. (2002). *Tests in print: VI. An index to tests, test reviews, and the literature on specific tests.* Lincoln: University of Nebraska Press.

Murray, L. K. (2006). HIV and child sexual abuse in Zambia: An intervention feasibility study (NIMH Grant No. K23 MH077532). Boston: Boston University School of Public Health Center for International Health.

Myers, K., & Winters, N. C. (2002). Ten-year review of rating scales: I. Overview of scale functioning, psychometric properties, and selection. *Journal of the American Academy of Child and Adolescent Psychiatry, 41*(2), 114–122.

Newman, E., Weathers, F. W., Nader, K., Kaloupek, D. G., Pynoos, R. S., Blake, D. D., et al. (2004). *Clinician-Administered PTSD Scale for Children and Adolescents (CAPS-CA).* Los Angeles: Western Psychological Services.

Norris, F. H., Friedman, M. J., Watson, P. J., Byrne, C. M., Diaz, E., & Kaniasty, K. (2002). 60,000 disaster victims speak: Part I. An empirical review of the empirical literature, 1981–2001. *Psychiatry, 65*(3), 207–239.

Ohan, J., Myers, K., & Collett, B. (2002). Ten-year review of rating scales: IV. Scales assessing trauma and its effects. *Journal of the American Academy of Child and Adolescent Psychiatry, 41,* 1401–1422.

Pfefferbaum, P. (1997). Posttraumatic stress disorder in children: A review of the past 10 years. *Journal of the American Academy of Child and Adolescent Psychiatry, 36*(11), 1503–1511.

Plake, B. S., Impara, J. C., & Spies, R. A. (2003). *The fifteenth mental measurements yearbook.* Lincoln, NE: Buros Institute of Mental Measurements.

Pynoos, R., & Eth, S. (1986). Witness to violence: The child interview. *Journal of the American Academy of Child Psychiatry, 25,* 306–319.

Pynoos, R., & Nader, K. (1991). Prevention of psychiatric morbidity in children after disaster. In S. Goldstein, J. Yaeger, C. Heinecke, & R. Pynoos (Eds.), *Prevention of mental health disturbances in children.* Washington, DC: American Psychiatric Association Press.

Pynoos, R., Rodriguez, N., Sternberg, A., Stauber, M., & Frederick, C. (1998). *UCLA PTSD Index for DSM-IV—Child Version.* Los Angeles: UCLA Trauma Psychiatry Service.

Pynoos, R. S., Frederick, C., Nader, K., Arroyo, W., Steinberg, A., Eth, S., et al. (1987). Life threat and posttraumatic stress in school-age children. *Archives of General Psychiatry, 44*(12), 1057–1063.

Pynoos, R. S., Goenjian, A., & Steinberg, A. M. (1998). A public mental health approach to the post-disaster treatment of children and adolescents. *Child and Adolescent Psychiatric Clinics of North America, 7,* 195–210.

Pynoos, R. S., Goenjian, A., Tashjian, M., Karakashian, M., Manjikian, R., Manoukian, G., et al. (1993). Post-traumatic stress reactions in children after the 1988 Armenian earthquake. *British Journal of Psychiatry, 163,* 239–247.

Reich, W., Leacock, N., & Shanfield, C. (1994). *Diagnostic Interview for Children and Adolescents—Revised (DICA-R).* St. Louis, MO: Washington University.

Rhee, H. (2003). Physical symptoms in children and adolescents. *Annual Review of Nursing Research, 21*, 95–122.

Rigamer, E. F. (1986). Psychological management of children in a national crisis. *Journal of the American Academy of Child Psychiatry, 25*, 364–369.

Sack, W. H., Clarke, G. N., Kinney, R., Belestos, G., Him, C., & Seeley, J. (1995). The Khmer Adolescent Project: II. Functional capacities in two generations of Cambodian refugees. *Journal of Nervous and Mental Disease, 183*(3), 177–181.

Sack, W. H., Seeley, J. R., Him, C., & Clarke, G. N. (1998). Psychometric properties of the Impact of Events Scale in traumatized Cambodian refugee youth. *Personality and Individual Differences, 25*(1), 57–67.

Saylor, C., & DeRoma, V. (2002). Assessment of children and adolescents exposed to disaster. In A. M. La Greca, W. K. Silverman, E. M. Vernberg, & M. C. Roberts (Eds.), *Helping children cope with disasters and terrorism* (pp. 35–53). Washington, DC: American Psychological Association.

Scheeringa, M. S., & Zeanah, C. H. (1994). *PTSD Semi-Structured Interview and Observational Record for Infants and Young Children.* New Orleans, LA: Department of Psychiatry and Neurology, Tulane University Health Sciences Center.

Scheeringa, M. S., Zeanah, C. H., Drell, M. J., & Larrieu, J. A. (1995). Two approaches to the diagnosis of posttraumatic stress disorder in infancy and early childhood. *Journal of the American Academy of Child and Adolescent Psychiatry, 34*(2), 191–200.

Shalev, A. Y., Tuval-Mashiach, R. , & Hadar, H. (2004). Posttraumatic stress disorder as a result of mass trauma. *Journal of Clinical Psychiatry, 65*(Suppl. 1), 4–10.

Smith, P., Perrin, S., Dyregrov, A., & Yule, W. (2002). Principal components analysis of the Impact of Event Scale with children in war. *Personality and Individual Differences, 34*, 315–322.

Smith, P., Perrin, S., Yule, W., & Rabe-Hesketh, S. (2001). War exposure and maternal reactions in the psychological adjustment of children from Bosnia–Hercegovina. *Journal of Child Psychology and Psychiatry, and Allied Disciplines, 42*(3), 395–404.

Tedeschi, R. G., Park, C. L., & Calhoun, L. G. (Eds.). (1998). *Posttraumatic growth: Positive changes in the aftermath of crisis.* Mahwah, NJ: Erlbaum.

Terr, L. (1988). What happens to early memories of trauma?: A study of twenty children under age five at the time of documented traumatic events. *Journal of the Academy of Child and Adolescent Psychiatry, 27*, 96–104.

Thienkrua, W., Cardozo, B. L., Chakkraband, M. L. S., Guadamuz, T. E., Pengjuntr, W., Tantipiwatanaskul, P., et al. (2006). Symptoms of posttraumatic stress disorder and depression among children in tsunami-affected areas in southern Thailand. *Journal of the American Medical Association, 296*, 549–559.

Weiss, D., & Marmar, C. (1997). The Impact of Event Scale—Revised. In J. P. Wilson & T. M. Keane (Eds.), *Assessing psychological trauma and PTSD.* New York: Guilford Press.

Yates, T. M., Dodds, M. F., Sroufe, A., & Egeland, B. (2003). Exposure to partner violence and child behavior problems: A prospective study controlling for child physical abuse and neglect, child cognitive ability, socioeconomic status, and life stress. *Development and Psychopathology, 15*, 199–218.

Yule, W. (1999). Post-traumatic stress disorder. *Archives of Disease in Childhood, 80*(2), 107–109.

Yule, W. (2001). Posttraumatic stress disorder in the general population and in children. *Journal of Clinical Psychiatry, 62*(Suppl. 17), 23–28.

PART II

EARLY INTERVENTIONS: TREATMENT OF ASD AND PREVENTION OF CHRONIC PTSD

CHAPTER 4

Psychological Debriefing for Adults

Jonathan I. Bisson, Alexander C. McFarlane,
Suzanna Rose, Josef I. Ruzek, and Patricia J. Watson

Critical incident stress debriefing (CISD), first described by Mitchell in 1983, stimulated the development of several similar interventions known collectively as psychological debriefing (PD). PD became widely used following traumatic events in the 1980s and 1990s, fueled by anecdotal reports of its effectiveness. In the mid-1990s researchers began to question the evidence base that proclaimed its effectiveness and called for randomized controlled trials (Bisson & Deahl, 1994; Raphael, Meldrum, & McFarlane 1995). This has resulted in the completion of several randomized controlled trials of PD, allowing a more confident evaluation of its true effectiveness (see Bisson, McFarlane, & Rose, 2000; National Collaborating Centre for Mental Health, 2005; Rose, Bisson, Churchill, & Wessely, 2005; Van Emmerick, Kamphuis, Hulsbosch, & Emmelkamp, 2002).

In the first edition of this volume, Bisson and colleagues (2000) concluded that the absence of rigorous research into early interventions was disappointing, and that it was essential that efforts be made to determine what, if anything, should be offered to individuals following traumatic events. A bias toward the more systematic study of individual PD as a stand-alone intervention was noted, as opposed to group PD as part of a more comprehensive traumatic stress management program. No evidence to support the preventive value of debriefing delivered in a single session was found. The authors recommended further randomized controlled trials, especially with group interventions (e.g., the efficacy of group PD as part of an overall traumatic stress management program, particularly in relation to emergency workers), children, multiple-session interventions, and methods of crisis intervention that do not involve intense reexposure to the traumatic event. In the last 6 years, several of these areas have been addressed. A number of randomized controlled trials of multiple-session interventions now exist (see Litz & Bryant, Chapter 6, this volume) and more randomized controlled trials of PD have been completed. This chapter reviews the current evidence base for PD.

Theoretical Context

Acute preventive interventions can only be implemented if there is broad acceptance of a notion of collective responsibility, and the value of group survival and care for individuals. Hence, the effectiveness and theoretical underpinnings of debriefing are critically dependent upon more general systems of leadership and the management of morale, and entail an essential series of beliefs about the dignity of the individual and his or her importance to the broader social group. The clinical practice of debriefing has often been driven by the immediacy of the imperative to help rather than the development of a sophisticated theory that is carefully applied and tested to establish its usefulness for widespread implementation. In many ways, acute preventive interventions may be seen to be as much products of social movements as they are interventions emerging from refinements in clinical practice. However, theoretical origins of debriefing appear to come from a variety of sources.

The Proximity, Immediacy, and Expectancy Model

The management of acute combat stress disorders is a school of treatment that emerged in World War I and was then rediscovered in World War II. The proximity, immediacy, and expectancy (PIE) model is based on these three principles described by Kardiner and Spiegel (1947) and also used in more recent conflicts (e.g., Israeli soldiers during the Lebanon War; see Solomon & Benbenishty, 1988) in which individuals were treated close to the battle zone (proximity), as soon as possible (immediacy), and with the expectation of returning to duty (expectancy).

The Narrative Tradition

During World War II, General Marshall (1944), the chief historian of the U.S. Army at that time, used and subsequently wrote about debriefing. He advocated holding debriefing sessions on the battlefield as soon as possible after the action, and estimated that 7 hours were needed to debrief one fighting day. Although one of the main functions of these meetings was information gathering, Marshall noted that the emotional effects of the debriefing were "spiritually purging," "morale-building" experiences that the men usually relished. Marshall's debriefing method provided a structured intervention that recognized and respected individuals' experiences, grief, and expression of emotional responses. He believed that the debriefing technique was relatively simple and could be performed by commanders without the need for specialist training. In a sense, his exploration of the events of battle gave the troops an opportunity to develop a narrative, or "internal verbal representation," of the experience.

Group Psychotherapy

Another paradigm employed in the CISD model is that of group psychotherapy. Lindy, Green, Grace, and Titchener (1983) have spoken of the "trauma membrane" that forms around a community involved in disaster. This notion refers to the mutual and tacit understanding that envelops people who have undergone similar suffering. These principles are central to the efficacy of group intervention. Groups use the therapeutic forces within the group, and the constructive support and interaction to heal people and modify their reactions. The adaptive outcome of the group is the primary aim, rather than the focus on individuals.

Crisis Intervention

Social psychiatry has a particular focus on the role of life events as a cause of psychiatric illness. Its accompanying arm of intervention is crisis intervention, as originally championed by Caplan (1961) and Lindemann (1944). Crisis intervention assumes that a clear precipitant exists and that the individual's distress is clear. It attempts to remove such distress from the domain of illness and presumes that the patient has experienced an offense that has caused this disequilibrium because of its suddenness, which has not allowed the individual time to master his or her emotional response. The essence of the intervention is that the temporary support of the mental health professional will bring about mastery. It is a model of intervention based on the premise that the event is over, and the symptoms exhibited by the patient are no longer appropriate. The therapist provides a reorganizing influence that assists the individual who is feeling overwhelmed. The critical dimension is to assist the person in reestablishing rational problem solving.

Grief Counseling

The concepts of crisis intervention rapidly extended into management of the bereaved. Lindemann's (1944) work after the Coconut Grove nightclub fire led to both an investigation of the stages of grief and interventions that might be helpful. Progressively, grief counseling grew away from crisis intervention as a separate discipline. First, Raphael's (1977) work with widows at high risk of negative outcomes following bereavement highlighted the value of interventions in this context. These therapies included an educational component aimed at normalizing the feelings and behaviors associated with grief. Second, the importance of expression of the range of complex emotions associated with loss was often assisted by visiting memorials and handling possessions of the dead person. Focusing on the relationship with the deceased allowed the development of the individual's new sense of identity and integrated self-concept. Raphael's use of this approach to assist the bereaved following the Granville train disaster led her to advocate for the importance of acute interventions and support following disasters.

Cognitive-Behavioral Therapies

Although behavior therapy only became a clinical practice in the last half of the 20th century, the learning principles underlying its development were well understood in the first half of the century. Two aspects have contributed particularly to debriefing. First, its procedures of desensitization and exposure provided an explicit rationale to include in debriefing a discussion of the trauma to reduce distress and to minimize avoidance in the immediate aftermath of traumatic experiences. A further contribution to emerge from cognitive-behavioral therapy has been the exploration of the cognitive schemas associated with traumatic memories. Cognitive-behavioral therapy for posttraumatic stress disorder (PTSD) emerged within the same time frame as early posttrauma preventive interventions. Therefore, this area of clinical practice has not seen full application to early intervention impact. However, the idea of manualized treatments was brought to psychotherapy research by behavioral therapy, and manualized debriefings have become an important component of this field.

Psychoeducation

In many regards, debriefing is a form of psychoeducation. This is an important component of many cognitive-behavioral treatments. It raises questions regarding the extent to which treatments of psychological trauma owe their treatment effects to simple provision of educational information as opposed to more specific factors. There appears to be little doubt that giving traumatized individuals a psychological map to help them understand their reactions does much to contain their distress and allow them to engage in a series of self-regulatory processes.

Catharsis

The expression of affect associated with the memory of an event is also a central component of debriefing. The notion of catharsis goes back to Breuer and Freud's (1893) first lecture, "On the Psychical Mechanism of Hysterical Phenomena: Preliminary Communication."

Key Issues

One of the intellectual questions that is important to debriefing and early intervention generally is whether symptoms arising in relation to an event simply reflect a distress response or are indicative of a more substantial psychiatric disorder. Some psychological models emphasize that social and intrapsychic factors are critical determinants of psychological symptoms. Implicit in this idea is the suggestion that efforts to shape an individual's processing of the event might help to minimize or prevent any prolonged distress or pathology. Biological model theorists argue that people with PTSD show an abnormal acute stress response of a biological nature (Yehuda, McFarlane, & Shalev, 1998). If individuals with a normal biological stress response do not develop PTSD, the question may be raised as to whether, for such individuals, interventions may modify the adaptive acute stress response in such a way as to increase the risk of PTSD. Given the dictum "First, do no harm," the challenge is to demonstrate that in individuals who have a predicted normal outcome, specific acute interventions do not interfere with processes of normal adaptation. In their separate domains, the theories that contribute to debriefing appear sound. However, the issue arises as to whether they have been applied in optimal ways, and whether the objectives of debriefing have been addressed in the most effective ways possible.

Another key issue is what outcomes are important. Most studies of early interventions have used "treatment" outcomes, primarily measuring efficacy or harm by whether they increase or decrease PTSD symptoms compared to natural recovery. It may be unrealistic to expect an early intervention to reduce PTSD symptoms and lead us to ignore other important, potential outcomes (Deahl, 2000), including return of function irrespective of symptom outcome (Ursano, Fullerton, & Norwood, 2003) and its screening function. Satisfaction of those who receive the early intervention is widely noted. Indeed, high levels of satisfaction have been reported, although it is difficult to determine whether this is specific to the early intervention, or whether it reflects the perception that contact with someone shortly after a traumatic event is helpful. It is also difficult to imagine that individuals in control groups would rate no intervention as satisfying.

Description of Techniques

CISD was first described by Mitchell (1983) as a group intervention for ambulance personnel following exposure to traumatic situations in their work. It was described as a form of crisis intervention as opposed to a form of psychological treatment; therefore, it does not have the same philosophy (i.e., debriefing does not explicitly treat a pathological response). CISD and other PD models have become recognized as semistructured interventions designed to reduce initial distress and to prevent the development of later psychological sequelae, such as PTSD following traumatic events, by promoting emotional processing through the ventilation and normalization of reactions, and preparation for possible future experiences. Further aims are to identify individuals who may benefit from more formalized treatment and to offer such treatment to them.

It has generally been considered that any individual exposed to the traumatic event is eligible for PD irrespective of the presence of psychological symptoms. It is, however, apparent that many participants of debriefings would have fulfilled the criteria for acute stress disorder or had symptoms of PTSD, anxiety, and depression. Debriefings have been used with survivors/victims, emergency workers, and providers of psychological care. The focus of PD is on current reactions of those involved in a trauma rather than earlier life experiences that may shape their individual reactions. Psychiatric "labeling" is avoided, and the emphasis is placed on normalization of the experience. The participants are assured that they are normal people who have experienced an abnormal event. Mitchell and Everly (1995) have argued that debriefing should be considered as one part of a comprehensive, systematic, multicomponent approach to the management of traumatic stress (critical incident stress management [CISM]), and that it should not be used as a one-time, stand-alone intervention. Despite this assertion, many practitioners have used debriefing as a stand-alone intervention.

Mitchell's (1983) CISD is a seven-phase technique. The *introduction* phase concerns explanation of the purpose of the debriefing, guidelines, and some introductions. During the *fact* phase, a factual description of exactly what happened is produced, with acknowledgment of accompanying emotions if they are expressed, but these are not considered in detail at this time. The *thought* phase considers participants' thoughts at the time of the incident. The *reaction* phase focuses on participants' emotions associated with the event. The *symptoms* phase aims to help move participants from the emotional reaction to a more cognitively oriented stage in which various trauma-related symptoms are discussed. The *teaching* phase flows from the symptoms phase and is led by the facilitators, who discuss typical symptoms and coping strategies for stress. The *reentry* phase clarifies issues, gives participants the opportunity to ask questions, provides a summary of the debriefing, and ends with closure.

Since Mitchell's initial description of CISD, several authors have described other, different forms of psychological debriefing (Rose, 1997). Dyregrov (1989) described PD, which represents his interpretation of Mitchell's technique and is indeed very similar, although it specifically includes discussion of sensory information experienced at the time. Dyregrov also appeared to devote more attention to individual reactions and to the normalization of reactions. The seven stages of PD, as described by Dyregrov, are detailed as follows:

1. *The introduction.* The debriefer(s) states that the purpose of the meeting is to review the participant(s) reactions to the trauma, to discuss them, and to identify methods of dealing with them to prevent future problems. The debriefer assumes control and specifies his or her own competence to inspire confidence in participants. Three rules are made explicit: (a) participants are under no obligation to say anything except why they have come and what their role was vis-à-vis the traumatic event; (b) confidentiality is emphasized in groups, and the members understand not to divulge outside the group what others have said; and (c) the focus of the discussions is on the impressions and reactions of participants.

2. *Expectations and facts.* The details of what actually happened are discussed in considerable detail, without focusing on thoughts, impressions, and emotional reactions. Participants are encouraged to describe their expectations (i.e., did they expect what happened?). Expectations are felt to be extremely important in certain situations; for example, unexpectedly encountering injured children can magnify the intensity of a traumatic situation. Discussion of expectation is believed to focus individuals on their experiences at the time and to help them understand why they reacted the way they did.

3. *Thoughts and impressions.* When the facts are being described, the debriefer elicits thoughts and impressions by asking questions, such as "What were your thoughts when you first realized you were injured?" and "What did you do?" This information aims to (a) construct a picture of what happened, (b) put individual reactions into perspective, and (c) help with the integration of traumatic experiences. Sensory impressions in all five modalities are elicited when the debriefer, for example, asks, "What did you see, hear, touch, smell, taste?" The aim is to produce a more realistic reconstruction of the trauma.

4. *Emotional reactions.* This is usually the longest stage in the PD. The earlier questions concerning thoughts and impressions lead to answers concerning emotions. The debriefer attempts to aid the release of emotions with questions about some of the common reactions during the trauma, such as fear, helplessness, frustration, self-reproach, anger, guilt, anxiety, and depression. Emotional reactions that participants have experienced since the event are also discussed.

5. *Normalization.* After participants' emotional reactions have been expressed, the debriefer aims to facilitate their acceptance by stressing that the reactions are entirely normal. When more than one person is present in the PD, it is likely that emotions will be shared. Acknowledgment of this universality of experience helps with normalization. The debriefer stresses that individuals do not have to experience all of the emotions that normally occur after a trauma, but it is normal to experience some reaction after a critical incident. The debriefer also describes common symptoms that individuals may experience in the future: intrusive thoughts and images; distress when reminded of what happened; attempts to avoid thoughts, feelings, and reminders; detachment from others; loss of interest in things that once gave

pleasure; anxiety and depressed mood; sleep disturbance, including night-mares; irritability and anger; shame and guilt; hypervigilance; and increased startle reactions.

6. *Future planning/coping.* This stage allows the debriefer to focus on ways of managing symptoms should they arise and to attempt to mobilize internal support mechanisms (e.g., discussion of coping mechanisms) and external supports (e.g., family and friends). Emphasis is on the importance of open discussion of feelings with family and friends, highlighting the possibility that additional support may be needed from them for a while.

7. *Disengagement.* In this stage, other topics are discussed. Leaflets describing normal reactions and how to cope with them may be distributed. Guidance is also given regarding the need for further help and where it may be obtained, if necessary. Participants are advised to seek further help, for example, if (a) psychological symptoms do not decrease after 4–6 weeks; (b) psychological symptoms increase over time; (c) there is ongoing loss of func-tion and occupation/family difficulties; or (d) others comment on marked personality changes.

Raphael (1986) described a psychological debriefing that although less structured than the Mitchell and Dyregrov models, still had much in com-mon with them, including the fact that it was designed as a group interven-tion for secondary rather than primary victims. She suggested particular topics for discussion that might be useful during the debriefing, including personally experienced disaster stressors, such as death encounter; survivor conflict, loss, and dislocation; positive and negative feelings; victims and their problems; and the special nature of disaster work and personal experiences.

Another model, the multiple stressor debriefing model (Armstrong, O'Callahan, & Marmar, 1991), designed for use with American Red Cross personnel, contains elements from the other debriefings but is the first model to focus on pretrauma strategies adopted by individuals to deal with stressful situations. Four stages are completed. The first stage, disclosure of events, is followed by the second, consideration of feelings and reactions. In the third stage, coping strategies are discussed, including the previous ways that indi-viduals have dealt with stressful events. Finally, the termination stage consid-ers what it will be like leaving the disaster, the positive work done, and the need to talk to significant others about experiences and feelings.

These group PD models have been modified for use with groups of pri-mary victims and also for development of interventions for individuals who have recently been exposed to a trauma (see, e.g., Hobbs, Mayou, Harrison, & Warlock, 1996; Lee, Slade, & Lygo, 1996). The individual debriefings described in the literature to date have adopted a seven-stage model very similar to that of Mitchell. With the group processes obviously missing, the debriefings focus directly on one individual's experiences and reactions. Some authors have commented that because group factors are of essential importance to the process of PD, the technique should not be transferred for use with individu-als (see, e.g., Dyregrov, 1998). In individual PD, the facilitator normalizes the individual's reactions by sharing information gained from previous trauma victims and the literature, rather than by highlighting common reactions within a group. Most reported individual debriefings have been for primary victims with physical injuries. When dealing with individuals who have sustained significant physical injury, attention has also centered on discussion of physical concerns, and possible emotions and reactions associated with disability/disfigurement (Bisson, Jenkins, Alexander, & Bannister, 1997).

In addition to describing an early, brief crisis intervention, the term "psychological debriefing" has also been used to describe a variety of other interventions. For example, Hayman and Scaturo (1992) described an eight-session "psychological debriefing" for military personnel following the Gulf War. Busuttil and colleagues (1995) described "debriefing" as an integral part of a group treatment package for chronic PTSD. Such diverse usage of the term has resulted in a somewhat confused literature, and these applications are beyond the scope of this chapter. Here, we use the term to denote a brief preventive technique that occurs within 1 month of a traumatic event.

Method of Collecting Data

This review primarily considers randomized controlled trials of PD. To identify all potential studies, the authors drew on the results of two systematic reviews of randomized controlled trials of brief, early psychological interventions following trauma that involved at least one author of this chapter (National Collaborating Centre for Mental Health, 2005; Rose et al., 2005), supplemented by trials subsequently identified. The independently performed systematic reviews included electronic searches in which we used standardized search strings of 16 databases (Biosis, Center Register of Controlled Trials [CCTR], Cumulative Index to Nursing and Allied Health Literature [CINAHL], Cochrane Library, EMBASE, LILACS, MEDLINE, National Research Register [NRR], Occupational Safety and Health, Pascal, Published International Literature on Traumatic Stress [PILOTS], PsycINFO, PsychLit, PSYNDEX, System for Information on Grey Literature in Europe [SIGLE], SOCIOFILE) and a hand search of the *Journal of Traumatic Stress*. We also contacted experts in the traumatic stress field and asked to identify other randomized controlled trials of which they were aware.

All potentially appropriate studies identified by the searches were obtained and critically read. The references of all identified articles were scrutinized and any relevant ones obtained to identify further randomized controlled trials. The Cochrane Review (Rose et al., 2005) included 15 studies, compared with seven studies included in the United Kingdom's National Institute of Health and Clinical Excellence (NICE) guidelines review (National Collaborating Centre for Mental Health, 2005). This reflects the stricter inclusion criteria used by the NICE guideline development group, resulting in the exclusion of studies of PD following childbirth and those that did not meet the required methodological standards. For the purpose of this review we have excluded childbirth studies but have included all other randomized controlled trials of PD or interventions similar to PD delivered within 1 month of a traumatic event with the potential to fulfill the DSM-IV (American Psychiatric Association, 1994) a criteria for PTSD.

To give the reader a wider knowledge of the literature in this area, controlled trials that have not been randomized are summarized in the second part of Table 4.1.

Literature Review

Thirteen randomized controlled trials that fulfilled the inclusion criteria were identified (Bisson et al., 1997; Bordow & Porritt, 1979; Bunn & Clarke, 1979; Campfield & Hills, 2001; Conlon, Fahy, & Conroy, 1999; Dolan, Bowyer, Freeman, & Little, 1999; Hobbs et al., 1996; Mayou, Ehlers, & Hobbs, 2000; Lee et al., 1996; Litz & Adler, 2005; Marchand et al., 2006; Rose, Brewin, Andrews, & Kirk, 1999; Sijbrandij, Olff, Reitsma, Carlier, & Gersons, 2006; Stevens & Adshead, 1996 [published in Hobbs & Adshead, 1996]). The studies covered a variety of traumatic events and are summarized in the first part of Table 4.1. Eleven of the studies compared PD with a nonintervention control group. Campfield and Hills (2001) compared psychological debriefing within 10 hours of the traumatic event, with psychological debriefing more than 48 hours after the traumatic event. Conlon and colleagues (1999) compared PD with the provision of advice and a leaflet. Sijbrandij and colleagues (2006) conducted a dismantling study in which emotional debriefing and psychoeducational debriefing were compared with a nonintervention control group.

In 12 studies the PD was delivered during a single session. Marchand and colleagues (2006) delivered the PD over two sessions. Whereas Litz and Adler (2005) conducted the only study of group PD, in the Campfield and Hills (2001) study, PDs were delivered individually or to small groups. In the Bisson and colleagues (1997) study, PDs were delivered individually or to couples. Three studies had additional control groups of social worker input over 3 months (Bordow & Porritt, 1979), education alone (Rose et al., 1999), and a stress education class (Litz & Adler, 2005).

Methodological Quality

Methodological quality varied considerably among the studies considered. The highest quality studies had several methodological strengths, including good sample sizes, concealed randomization, and use of well-validated outcome measures administered by assessors blind to the randomization. The lowest quality studies suffered from various methodological weaknesses, including small sample sizes, outcomes measured by the debriefer, and very short follow-up periods.

Results

Table 4.1 describes the results of the trials, including their effect sizes, when it was possible to calculate them. Of the 10 studies that compared individual PD with no intervention, 2 were positive, 5 were neutral, and 3 were negative. The one group PD study, conducted with active duty military personnel (Litz & Adler, 2005) was neutral. Campfield and Hills (2001) found a marked difference in favor of PD within 10 hours of the traumatic event in their study over PD delivered more than 48 hours after the traumatic event. Bordow and Porritt (1979) found that PD fared worse than did 3 months of social worker input. There was no difference between PD and education (Litz & Adler, 2005; Rose et al., 1999). Sijbrandij and colleagues (2006) found that emotional debriefing fared worse than psychoeducational debriefing and no intervention. Only two studies provided follow-up beyond 1 year, and both were negative (Bisson et al., 1997; Hobbs et al., 1996; Mayou et al., 2000). However, confounds may have accounted for the more severe symptoms in the debriefing groups, rather than an iatrogenic effect of the one-session intervention.

Despite randomization, the debriefing groups in the studies had more severe injuries, longer hospital stays, and, in one study, a more extensive prior history of exposure to traumatic events (Bisson et al., 1997).

Although many of the PD studies have methodological flaws, there are many possible theoretical explanations for both neutral and negative findings. For example, there is preliminary evidence that increased arousal in the immediate phases posttrauma is linked to long-term pathology, and it is possible that PD interventions with primary civilian survivors are too brief to allow for adequate emotional processing, that they increase arousal and anxiety levels, or that they inadvertently decrease the likelihood that individuals will pursue more intensive interventions. For this reason, an expert panel noted that the use of any intervention focused on emotional processing during the early period posttrauma may be contraindicated (Watson, 2004). There are particularly strong recommendations against its use in postdisaster settings involving mass trauma due to the chaotic postincident environment, the need for attention to pragmatic material needs, possible cultural and bereavement issues, and multiple recovery trajectories based on complex variables (Watson, Friedman, Ruzek, & Norris, 2002).

Nonrandomized Controlled Trial Evidence

More of the nonrandomized controlled trials shown in the second part of Table 4.1 reported positive results, although, in common with the randomized controlled trials, positive, neutral and negative results were reported. None of these studies adhered to the rigors of the randomized controlled trial, and they were also characterized by other methodological flaws, including those described in the previous section.

Text continues on page 98

TABLE 4.1. Summary of Randomized and Nonrandomized Controlled Trials of One-Off Early Psychological Interventions

Study	Target population[a]	Time posttrauma; length of sessions	Treatment(s); control[b]	Main outcome measure	Major findings	Between-group effect size	Within-group effect size
Randomized studies							
Bisson et al. (1997)	Acute burn trauma victims (N = 110)	2–19 days; 30–120 min	57 debriefing; 46 standard care	IES	Intervention group fared worse	0.22	Debriefing: 0.26; no intervention: 0.05
Bordow & Porritt (1979)	Motor vehicle accident (MVA) victims (N = 70)	< 1 wk; 60 min	10 immediate debriefing; 30 immediate debriefing and 3-month social worker input; 30 standard care	Traumatic neurosis symptoms	Social worker input fared best followed by immediate review	Insufficient data	Insufficient data
Bunn & Clarke (1979)	Relatives of seriously ill/injured (N = 30)	< 12 hr; 20 min	15 debriefing; 15 standard care	Composite of anxiety scores	Intervention group fared better	Insufficient data	Insufficient data
Campfield & Hills (2001)	Victims of robbery (N = 77)	< 10 hr or > 48 hr; 60–120 min	36 individual or small-group debriefing; 41 delayed debriefing	PDS	< 10-hr group fared better	Insufficient data	Insufficient data
Conlon et al. (1999)	MVA victims (N = 40)	< 14 days, 30 min	18 debriefing; 22 advice and leaflet	IES	No significant difference	−0.02	Debriefing: −0.87; advice and leaflet: −0.72
Dolan et al. (1999)	Accident and emergency attenders (N = 100)	< 14 days, 45–120 min	34 debriefing; 46 standard care	IES	No significant difference	0.04	Insufficient data

Hobbs et al. (1996)/Mayou et al. (2000)	MVA victims (N = 114)	24–48 hr, 60 min	59 debriefing; 55 standard care	IES	Intervention group fared worse	0.21	Debriefing: 0.07; no intervention: –0.18
Lee et al. (1996)	Miscarriage (N = 39)	14 days, 60 min	21 debriefing; 18 standard care	IES	No significant difference	–0.12	Debriefing: –0.26; no intervention: –0.27
Litz & Adler (2005)	Soldiers deployed on a peacekeeping mission (N = 1,050)	In Kosovo pre redeployment, 48–148 min	338 group CISD; 316 stress education class; 325 no intervention	PCL	No significant difference	Insufficient data	Insufficient data
Rose et al. (1999)	Victims of violence (N = 157)	< 1 mo, 60 min	45 debriefing; 46 education; 47 standard care	PSS	No significant difference	0.06	Psychological debriefing: –0.46; education: 0.40; no intervention: –0.28
Sijbrandij et al. (2006)	Civilian survivors of various traumatic events (N = 236)	11–19 days (median = 15); 45–60 min	63 emotional debriefing; 63 psychoeducational debriefing; 63 no intervention	SI-PTSD	No significant differences. Some evidence of worse outcome in emotional debriefing	Emotional debriefing: 0.18; emotional debriefing: –0.03	Emotional debriefing: –0.14; educational debriefing: –0.28; no intervention: –0.16
Stevens & Adshead (1996)	MVA, assault, or dog bite	< 24 hr, 60 min	Individual counseling	IES	No significant difference	Insufficient data	Insufficient data

(continued)

TABLE 4.1. *(continued)*

Study	Target population[a]	Time posttrauma; length of sessions	Treatment(s); control[b]	Main outcome measure	Major findings	Between-group effect size	Within-group effect size
Nonrandomized studies							
Carlier et al. (1998)	Airplane crash (N = 105)	"As soon as possible"; duration unknown	46 group debriefing; 59 standard care	DSM-III-R PTSD	No effect at 8 mo, worse at 18 mo	Insufficient data	Insufficient data
Carlier et al. (2000)	Police officers (N = 243)	24 hr, 1 mo, and 3 mo posttrauma	86 debriefing; 82 refused group debriefing; 75 group before group debriefing introduced	DTS IES	More reexperiencing in PD group at 1 wk; no differences at 6 mo	Insufficient data	Insufficient data
Deahl et al. (1994)	Gulf War dead body handling (N = 29)	Variable time posttrauma, unknown duration	14 standard care; 15 Dyregrov GPD	IES	No overall effect	Insufficient data	Insufficient data
Deahl et al. (2000)	Male military peacekeepers (N = 106)	End of 6-mo tour of duty, 2 hr	54 group CISD; 52 assessment-only control	IES, HADS	No difference in HADS or IES scores; SCL-90 scores and CAGE (alcohol) scores higher in the intervention group at 1 year	Insufficient data	Insufficient data
Eid et al. (2001)	Military personnel and firefighters exposed to car accident (N = 27)	1 day postaccident; 2.5 hr	Group interventions with or without PD	PTSS-10, IES, GHQ-30	Lower PTSS-10 score in group with PD, but no differences on IES or GHQ-30	Insufficient data	Insufficient data

Study	Population	Timing	Groups	Measure	Outcome		
Hytten & Hasle (1989)	Firefighters ($N = 58$)	"Soon after"; duration unknown	39 PD; 19 standard care	IES	No effect on outcome	Insufficient data	Insufficient data
Jenkins (1996)	Emergency service personnel ($N = 29$)	< 24 hr; unknown duration	14 standard care; 15 group CISD	SCL-90	Less depression and anxiety in CISD	Insufficient data	Insufficient data
Kenardy et al. (1996)	Emergency workers ($N = 195$)	Unknown	62 PD; 133 standard care	GHQ-12, IES	No effect overall	Insufficient data	Insufficient data
McFarlane (1988)	N.S. firefighters ($N =$ unknown)	"Soon after"; duration unknown	Standard care; PD	IES, GHQ	More acute PTSR, less delayed PTSR	Insufficient data	Insufficient data
Matthews (1998)	Assaulted direct care mental health workers ($N = 63$)	Unknown	14 PD; 18 offered but rejected PD; 31 not offered PD	9-item IES Satisfaction	Reduced IES scores in those offered PD; 57% said PD helped reduce stress; 43% said it did not	Insufficient data	Insufficient data
Wee et al. (1999)	Emergency medical service workers during Los Angeles civil disturbances ($N = 65$)	1–3 days, duration unknown	PD no details; selected not to have PD	FRI-A	Reduced symptoms with PD	Insufficient data	Insufficient data

Notes. CAGE, Cut Down, Annoyed by Criticism, Guilty, Eye-Opener Drinks; DTS, Davidson Trauma Scale; FRI-A, Frederick Reaction Index—Adult; GHQ-12, 12-item General Health Questionnaire; GHQ-30, 30-item General Health Questionnaire; GPD, group psychological debriefing; HADS, Hospital Anxiety and Depression Scale; IES, Impact of Events Scale; PCL, PTSD Checklist; PDS, Posttraumatic Stress Diagnostic Scale; PSS, PTSD Symptom Scale; PTSR, Post Traumatic Stress Reaction; PTSS-10, Post Traumatic Stress Syndrome 10-Questions Inventory; SI-PTSD, Structured Interview for PTSD; SCL-90, Symptom Checklist 90.

[a]$N =$ subjects starting study.

[b]$N =$ subjects in data analysis.

Results of Previous Systematic Reviews

The results of previous systematic reviews that have only included randomized controlled trials are consistent with the results of this review despite their differing inclusion criteria. The United Kingdom's NICE guidelines (National Collaborating Centre for Mental Health, 2005) found no difference between PD and no intervention groups on reducing the likelihood of having a PTSD diagnosis at 3- to 6-month follow-up, but a significant difference favoring the control over the PD group at 13-month follow-up, although this was based on the result of one study only (Bisson et al., 1997). *The Cochrane Review* (Rose et al., 2005) found no evidence of PD group reduction in PTSD severity greater than that in the no-intervention group at 1–4 months, 6–13 months, or at 3 years.

Another systematic review (Van Emmerick et al., 2002) included two nonrandomized controlled trials (Carlier, Voerman, & Gersons, 2000; Shalev, Peri, Rogel-Fuchs, Ursana, & Marlowe, 1998) among the seven that satisfied their strict inclusion criteria. They performed a meta-analysis of the effect sizes of the studies and concluded that PD did not improve natural recovery from psychological trauma. This contrasts with positive results reported in reviews that included other forms of evidence and focused on a broader definition of crisis intervention (e.g., Everly, Boyle, & Lating, 1999; Roberts & Everly, 2006).

Summary and Recommendations

Since the first edition of this volume was published, four new randomized controlled trials have been identified. With the exception of Campfield and Hills (2001), their findings support and strengthen the original conclusion that no evidence suggested that PD is effective in the prevention of PTSD symptoms shortly after a traumatic event or in the prevention of longer term psychological sequelae. Follow-up of the Hobbs and colleagues (1996), Mayou and colleagues (2000), and Sijbrandij and colleagues (2006) studies suggest that individual PD may exacerbate symptoms in some individuals. Their finding that more symptomatic individuals—increased intrusion and avoidance in Mayou and colleagues and increased hyperarousal in Sijbrandij and colleagues—fare worse following debriefing than those with less symptoms is particularly concerning because these individuals are at increased risk of developing longer term psychological sequelae (Brewin, Andrews, & Valentine, 2000).

The two positive studies (Bordow & Porritt, 1979; Bunn & Clarke, 1979) were conducted before PD was formally described, and thvwwe interventions appeared to involve less intensive reliving of the traumatic incident than occurs in CISD and PD. The Campfield and Hills (2001) results suggest that PD may be helpful for some people. Given the absence of a no-intervention control group, it is not possible to comment on whether their PD group would

have fared better than a no-intervention group, but the markedly better outcomes in those who received PD within 10 hours are striking, and it should
be noted that the only other study to implement a PD-like intervention within
12 hours posttrauma also obtained a positive result (Bunn & Clarke, 1979).
Campfield and Hills argued that their study supported the use of immediate
PD for civilian employees who were victims of robbery. However, the primary
investigator who conducted all debriefings reported that she may have been
biased in favor of immediate debriefing. Other studies have found no difference in outcome for different timings of PD (Marchand et al., 2006), or a
better outcome with those who received PD later (Bisson et al., 1997). However, in these two studies, no one was debriefed until several days after the
traumatic event. The results may also have been different in the Campfield
and Hills study because they included individuals with essentially less traumatizing events. Participants were selected on the basis of having been involved
in a robbery, but individuals in robberies in which a weapon was used were
excluded. The possibility that less traumatized individuals benefit more from
PD is supported by the childbirth literature on PD, in which the study with
the biggest effect size in favor of PD (Lavender & Walkinshaw, 1998) excluded
all instrumental childbirths.

    One of the major criticisms of systematic reviews of PD studies has been
that most of the randomized controlled trials have been of individual PD and
have not considered a group format or population as originally described by
Mitchell (1983). This is a valid criticism and one explicitly acknowledged in
the original chapter (Bisson et al., 2000), the Cochrane Review (Rose et al.,
2005), and the NICE guidelines (National Collaborating Centre for Mental
Health, 2005). The group delivery of PD to helpers has now been addressed
by the Litz and Adler (2005) study, which resulted in a neutral outcome.
Although active duty personnel rated their satisfaction with CISD as high
and exhibited a trend toward greater perceived command support at 9-month
follow-up, mental health outcomes at follow-up did not worsen as a result of
CISD, and there were no differences among the CISD, stress education, and
survey-only conditions on any behavioral health outcome, including PTSD,
depression, general well-being, aggressive behavior, marital satisfaction, perceived organizational support, or morale. Heart rate and blood pressure readings before and after the sessions did not indicate a change in physiological
stress, and subjective ratings of distress did not change pre- to postsession.

    It remains vital that we not overgeneralize research findings beyond the
particular situations or populations investigated. The results of studies regarding one form of intervention (e.g., PD), similarly, should not be overgeneralized to form conclusions about other forms of intervention, even though
related (Bisson, Brayne, Ochberg, & Everley, 2007). This has been a problem
in the past and is potentially very damaging for the prospects of dissemination of effective early interventions in the future. One of the most popular
daytime radio programs in the United Kingdom highlighted the "fact" that
no psychological interventions worked at all following traumatic events. The

authors of the Cochrane Review attempted to limit any damage caused by this false information by publicizing the early interventions that had been shown to be effective. They wrote to one of the main national newspapers in the United Kingdom, but their response was rejected. Several months later, their views were published in the *British Journal of Psychiatry*, with minimal impact on the general population (Rose, Bisson, & Wessely, 2003).

A further issue is that although the trials demonstrate no specific effect of particular methods of debriefing, they do not address nonspecific effects of the intervention. The assessment process and the control intervention, which may be no intervention, have the capacity to convey a significant amount of information to the participants and to imply a sense of care and concern. The current studies do not address the question of what the impact of no intervention at all would be. Answering this question is an important issue because the existence of a system of care may be a powerful form of communication.

Clinical Implications

Current evidence suggests that individual PD should not be used following traumatic events. There remains an absence of evidence with regard to group PD as one component of a package of care, although the Litz and Adler (2005) study of group PD alone suggests that there is unlikely to be a significant beneficial effect of group PD. Therefore, we do not advocate its use. Indeed even some of the staunchest advocates of debriefing do not now advocate it as a one-off intervention, and they argue instead that it should only be used as part of an overall CISM package, and then only after careful assessment (Everly & Mitchell, 1999). This is a far cry from its ongoing use in certain areas as a routine single-session, stand-alone intervention for anybody involved in a traumatic event.

The actual effectiveness of CISM and other models of early intervention, such as psychological first aid (National Child Traumatic Stress Network and National Center for PTSD, 2006; Ruzek et al., 2007) and trauma risk management (Jones, Roberts, & Greenberg, 2003), in preventing PTSD and reducing distress following traumatic events has yet to be determined but is worthy of further exploration. One impact of PD is to address issues of mental health literacy. Given the stigma and poor understanding of these issues in the general population, the question that remains is whether early interventions create an environment where there is a greater take-up of services if individuals become symptomatic. Early interventions have the potential to monitor a population, identify individuals at risk, and implement follow-up and early treatment for these individuals.

At present, however, early cognitive-behavioral interventions for symptomatic individuals appear to show the most promise for amelioration of distress and prevention of long-term psychopathology (see Litz & Bryant, Chapter 6, this volume; Ruzek, 2006).

Given the current evidence base, it is important to remember that the usual reaction following a traumatic event is a normal one that leads to recovery. We should not disrupt this process, but it may be helpful to consider five recent recommendations, the first two by Bisson and colleagues (2007) and the final three by Watson (2007):

1. Shortly after a traumatic event, it is important that those affected should be provided, in an empathic manner, with practical, pragmatic psychological support. Individuals should be provided with information about possible reactions; what they can do to help themselves (coping strategies); accessing support from those around them (particularly families and community); and how, where, and when to access further help, if necessary.

2. It is important to make provision for the appropriate early support of individuals following a traumatic event. However, any early intervention approach should be based on an accurate and current assessment of need prior to intervention. People cope with stress in differing ways. No formal intervention should be mandated for all exposed to trauma. Use of trauma support should be voluntary except in cases where event-related impairment is a threat to an individual's own safety or the safety of others.

3. Strive to make interventions culturally sensitive, developmentally appropriate, and related to the local formulation of problems and ways of coping.

4. Lack of distress and/or rapid recovery may not be a desired outcome. Ethnic, political, cultural, and economic factors may contribute to differing goals for functioning and identity, and providers should be sensitive to the particular motivations of each survivor.

5. Because of the dearth of evidence in early interventions, as much as possible, strive to evaluate whether early interventions are effective in ameliorating specific outcomes, or whether new interventions should be designed to accomplish such objectives.

Future Research

We can see little advantage in investing limited research resources into further evaluation of individual or group PD as a single-session intervention. It is probable that certain components of PD are helpful. Indeed, several components of PD, such as education, are included in interventions shown to be effective for treating established PTSD. The research focus should now be on the development of new approaches, with PD as a stand-alone intervention regarded as an intervention with good face validity and an appropriate subject for randomized controlled trials, but one that was not shown to be effective in either significantly reducing distress or preventing long-term psychopathology. The metaphorical baby should not be thrown out with the bathwater, however. The PD era should not only inform the development of new interventions but also serve as a stark reminder that psychological interventions can be extremely powerful and cause negative, as well as positive, effects. Therefore, future research efforts should focus on evaluating tailored, multilevel systems of care for high-risk populations, such as emergency services workers, as well as innovative applications of methods proven to be effective in other posttrauma settings, such as cognitive-behavioral interventions. If, in the future, early treatment is shown to be superior to late treatment, the argument for contact in the immediate posttrauma period to identify those at highest risk will be further strengthened.

References

American Psychiatric Association. (1994). *Diagnostic and statistical manual of mental disorders* (4th ed.). Washington, DC: Author.

Armstrong, K., O'Callahan, W., & Marmar, C. R. (1991). Debriefing Red Cross disaster personnel: The multiple stressor debriefing model. *Journal of Traumatic Stress, 4*, 581–593.

Bisson, J., & Deahl, M. (1994). Psychological debriefing and prevention of posttraumatic stress: More research is needed. *British Journal of Psychiatry, 165*, 717–720.

Bisson, J., Jenkins, P., Alexander, J., & Bannister, C. (1997). A randomised controlled trial of psychological debriefing for victims of acute burn trauma. *British Journal of Psychiatry, 171*, 78–81.

Bisson, J., McFarlane, A., & Rose, S. (2000). Psychological debriefing [Special issue: Guidelines for treatment of PTSD]. *Journal of Traumatic Stress, 4*, 555–558.

Bisson, J. I., Brayne, M., Ochberg, F., & Everley, G. (2007). Early psychosocial intervention following traumatic events. *American Journal of Psychiatry, 164*, 1016–1019.

Bordow, S., & Porritt, D. (1979). An experimental evaluation of crisis intervention. *Social Science and Medicine, 13a*, 251–256.

Breuer, J., & Freud, S. (1893). On the psychical mechanism of hysterical phenomena: Preliminary communication. In S. Freud & J. Breuer (Eds.), *Studies on hysteria* (pp. 53–69). London: Penguin.

Brewin, C. R., Andrews, B., & Valentine, J. D. (2000). Meta-analysis of risk factors for post-traumatic stress disorder in trauma-exposed adults. *Journal of Consulting and Clinical Psychology, 68*, 748–766.

Bunn, T., & Clarke, A. (1979). Crisis intervention: An experimental study of the effects of a brief period of counselling on the anxiety of relatives of seriously injured or ill hospital patients. *British Journal of Medical Psychology, 52*, 191–195.

Busuttil, W., Turnbull, G., Neal, L., Rollins, J., West, A., Bland, N., et al. (1995). Incorporating psychological debriefing techniques within a brief group psychotherapy programme for the treatment of posttraumatic stress disorder. *British Journal of Psychiatry, 167*, 495–502.

Campfield, K., & Hills, A. (2001). Effect of timing of critical incident stress debriefing (CISD) on posttraumatic symptoms. *Journal of Traumatic Stress, 14*(2), 327–340.

Caplan, G. (1961). *An approach to community mental health.* New York: Grune & Stratton.

Carlier, I., Lamberts, R. D., Uchelen, A. J., & Gersons, B. P. R. (1998). Disaster related stress in police officers: A field study of the impact of debriefing. *Stress Medicine, 14*, 143–148.

Carlier, I., Voerman, A., & Gersons, B. (2000). The influence of occupational debriefing on post-traumatic stress symptomatology in traumatized police officers. *British Journal of Medical Psychology, 73*, 87–98.

Conlon, L., Fahy, T., & Conroy, R. (1999). *PTSD in ambulant RTA victims: Prevalence, predictors and a randomized controlled trial of psychological debriefing in prophylaxis.* Unpublished manuscript.

Deahl, M. (2000). Psychological debriefing: Controversy and challenge. *Australian and New Zealand Journal of Psychiatry, 34,* 929–939.

Deahl, M. P., Gillham, A. B., Thomas, J., Searle, M. M., & Srinivasan, M. (1994). Psychological sequelae following the Gulf War: Factors associated with subsequent morbidity and the effectiveness of psychological debriefing. *British Journal of Psychiatry, 165,* 60–65.

Deahl, M. P., Srinivasan, M., Jones, N., Thomas, J., Neblett, C., & Jolly, A. (2000). Preventing psychological trauma in soldiers: The role of operational stress training and psychological debriefing. *British Journal of Medical Psychology, 73,* 77–85.

Dolan, L., Bowyer, D., Freeman, C., & Little, K. (1999). [Critical incident stress debriefing after trauma: Is it effective?] Unpublished raw data.

Dyregrov, A. (1989). Caring for helpers in disaster situations: Psychological debriefing. *Disaster Management, 2,* 25–30.

Dyregrov, A. (1998). Psychological debriefing—an effective method? *Traumatology, 4*(2), 6–15.

Eid, J., Johnsen, B. H., & Weisaeth, L. (2001). The effects of group psychological debriefing on acute stress reactions following a traffic accident: A quasi-experimental approach. *International Journal of Emergency Mental Health, 3,* 145–154.

Everly, G., Boyle, S., & Lating, J. (1999). The effectiveness of psychological debriefing with vicarious trauma: A meta-analysis. *Stress Medicine, 15,* 229–233.

Everly, G. S., Jr., & Mitchell, J. T. (1999). *Critical incident stress management (CISM): A new era and standard of care in crisis intervention.* Ellicott City, MD: Chevron.

Hayman, P. M., & Scaturo, D. J. (1992). *Psychological debriefing of returning military personnel: A protocol for post combat intervention.* Paper presented at the 25th International Congress of Psychology, Brussels, Belgium.

Hobbs, M., & Adshead, G. (1996). Preventive psychological intervention for road crash survivors. In M. Mitchell (Ed.), *The aftermath of road accidents: Psychological, social and legal perspectives* (pp. 159–171). London: Routledge.

Hobbs, M., Mayou, R., Harrison, B., & Warlock, P. (1996). A randomised trial of psychological debriefing for victims of road traffic accidents. *British Medical Journal, 313,* 1438–1439.

Hytten, K., & Hasle, A. (1989). Fire fighters: A study of stress and coping. *Acta Psychiatrica Scandinavica, 80*(Suppl. 355), 50–55.

Jenkins, S. R. (1996). Social support and debriefing efficacy among emergency medical workers after a mass shooting incident. *Journal of Social Behavior and Personality, 11,* 477–492.

Jones, N., Roberts, P., & Greenberg, N. (2003). Peer-group risk assessment: A posttraumatic management strategy for hierarchical organisations. *Occupational Medicine, 53,* 469–475.

Kardiner, A., & Spiegel, H. (1947). *War stress and neurotic illness.* New York: Paul B. Hoeber.

Kenardy, J. A., Webster, R. A., Lewin, T. J., Carr, V. J., Hazell, P. L., & Carter, G. L. (1996). Stress debriefing and patterns of recovery following a natural disaster. *Journal of Traumatic Stress, 9,* 37–49.

Lavender, T., & Walkinshaw, S. A. (1998). Can midwives reduce postpartum psychological morbidity?: A randomised trial. *Birth, 25,* 215–219.

Lee, C., Slade, P., & Lygo, V. (1996). The influence of psychological debriefing on emotional adaptation in women following early miscarriage: A preliminary study. *British Journal of Medical Psychology, 69,* 47–58.

Lindemann, E. (1944). Symptomatology and management of acute grief. *American Journal of Psychiatry, 101,* 141–148.

Lindy, J. D., Green, B. L., Grace, M., & Titchener, J. (1983). Psychotherapy with survivors of the Beverly Hills fire. *American Journal of Psychotherapy, 37,* 593–610.

Litz, B., & Adler, A. (2005). [A controlled trial of group debriefing.] Unpublished raw data.

Marchand, A., Guay, S., Boyer, R., Iucci, S., Martin, A., & St. Hilaire, M. (2006). A randomized controlled trial of an adapted form of individual critical incident stress debriefing for victims of an armed robbery. *Brief Treatment and Crisis Intervention, 6*(2), 122–129.

Marshall, S. L. (1944). *Island victory.* New York: Penguin Books.

Matthews, L. R. (1998). Effect of debriefing on posttraumatic stress symptoms after assaults by community housing residents. *Psychiatric Services, 49,* 207–212.

Mayou, R., Ehlers, A., & Hobbs, M. (2000). Psychological debriefing for road traffic accident victims: Three year follow-up of a randomised controlled trial. *British Journal of Psychiatry, 176,* 589–593.

McFarlane, A. C. (1988). The longitudinal course of posttraumatic morbidity: The range of outcomes and their predictors. *Journal of Nervous and Mental Disease, 176,* 30–39.

Mitchell, J. T. (1983). When disaster strikes. *Journal of Emergency Medical Services, 8,* 36–39.

Mitchell, J. T., & Everly, G. S. (1995). *Critical incident stress debriefing: An operations manual for the prevention of traumatic stress among emergency services and disaster workers.* Ellicott City, MD: Chevron.

National Child Traumatic Stress Network and National Center for PTSD. (2006). *Psychological first aid: Field operations guide* (2nd ed.). Los Angeles: Author.

National Collaborating Centre for Mental Health. (2005). *Post-traumatic stress disorder: The management of PTSD in adults and children in primary and secondary care.* London: Gaskell.

Nurmi, L. A. (1999). The sinking of *Estonia*: The effects of critical incident stress debriefing (CISD) on rescuers. *International Journal of Emergency Mental Health, 1,* 23–31.

Raphael, B. (1977). Preventive intervention with the recently bereaved. *Archives of General Psychiatry, 34,* 1450–1454.

Raphael, B., Meldrum, L., & McFarlane, A. C. (1995). Does debriefing after psychological trauma work? *British Medical Journal, 310,* 1479–1480.

Roberts, A., & Everly, G. (2006). A meta-analysis of 36 crisis intervention studies. *Brief Treatment and Crisis Intervention, 6*(1), 10–21.

Rose, S. (1997). Psychological debriefing: History and methods counselling. *Journal of the British Association of Counselling, 8*(1), 48–51.

Rose, S., Bisson, J., Churchill, R., & Wessely, S. (2005). *A systematic review of brief psychological interventions ("debriefing") for the treatment of immediate trauma related symptoms and the prevention of posttraumatic stress disorder* [CD-ROM]. Oxford, UK: Update Software.

Rose, S., Bisson, J., & Wessely, S. (2003). Counselling and psychotherapy: Media distortion. *British Journal of Psychiatry, 183,* 263–264.

Rose, S., Brewin, C. R., Andrews, A., & Kirk, M. (1999). A randomized controlled trial of psychological debriefing for victims of violent crime. *Psychological Medicine, 29,* 793–799.

Ruzek, J. I. (2006). Bringing cognitive-behavioral psychology to bear on early intervention with trauma survivors: Accident, assault, war, disaster, mass violence, and terrorism. In V. M. Follette & J. I. Ruzek (Eds.), *Cognitive-behavioral therapies for trauma* (2nd ed., pp. 433–462). New York: Guilford Press.

Ruzek, J. I., Brymer, M. J., Jacobs, A. K., Layne, C. M., Vernberg, E. M., & Watson, P. J. (2007). Psychological first aid. *Journal of Mental Health Counseling, 29,* 17–49.

Shalev, A., Peri, T., Rogel-Fuchs, Y., Ursana, R., & Marlowe, D. (1998). Historical group debriefing after combat exposure. *Military Medicine, 163,* 494–498.

Sijbrandij, M., Olff, M., Reitsma, J., Carlier, I., & Gersons, B. (2006). Emotional or educational debriefing after psychological trauma: Randomised controlled trial. *British Journal of Psychiatry, 189,* 150–155.

Solomon, Z., & Benbenishty, R. (1988). The role of proximity, immediacy and expectancy in frontline treatment of combat stress reaction among Israelis in the Lebanon War. *American Journal of Psychiatry, 143,* 613–617.

Ursano, R. J., Fullerton, C. S., & Norwood, A. E. (Eds.). (2003). *Terrorism and disasters: Individual and community mental health interventions.* Cambridge, UK: Cambridge University Press.

Van Emmerick, A., Kamphuis, J., Hulsbosch, A., & Emmelkamp, P. (2002). Single session debriefing after psychological trauma: A meta-analysis. *Lancet, 360,* 766–771.

Watson, P. (2004). Mental health interventions following mass violence. *Stresspoints, 12,* 4–5.

Watson, P. J. (2007). Early intervention for trauma-related problems following mass trauma. In R. J. Ursano, C. S. Fullerton, L. Weisaeth, & B. Raphael (Eds.), *Textbook of disaster psychiatry* (pp. 121–139). Cambridge, UK: Cambridge University Press.

Watson, P. J., Friedman, M. J., Ruzek, J. I., & Norris, F. H. (2002). Managing acute stress response to major trauma. *Current Psychiatry Reports, 4,* 247–253.

Wee, D. F., Mills, D. M., & Koehler, G. (1999). The effects of critical incident stress debriefing (CISD) on emergency medical services personnel following the Los Angeles civil disturbance. *International Journal of Emergency Mental Health, 1,* 33–37.

Yehuda, R., McFarlane, A. C., & Shalev, A. Y. (1998). Predicting the development of posttraumatic stress disorder from the acute response to a traumatic event. *Biological Psychiatry, 44,* 1305–1313.

CHAPTER 5

Acute Interventions for Children and Adolescents

Melissa J. Brymer, Alan M. Steinberg,
Eric M. Vernberg, Christopher M. Layne,
Patricia J. Watson, Anne K. Jacobs, Josef I. Ruzek,
and Robert S. Pynoos

Over the past several decades, a variety of acute interventions have been conducted among children after traumatic experiences. "Acute interventions" are defined in this chapter as interventions provided in the first 6 weeks after exposure. Such strategies have included psychoeducation; bereavement support; various forms of psychological debriefing; clarification of cognitive distortions; discussion of thoughts and feelings; reinforcing adaptive coping and safety behaviors, and use of support systems; structured and unstructured art and play activities; and massage. Interventions have been delivered using a variety of modalities, including individual, group, and classroom sessions; crisis intervention groups; provision of psychoeducational materials; and establishment of crisis hotlines.

Much of the material describing these efforts has been published not in mainstream psychological and psychiatric journals, but rather in journals devoted to other disciplines that have less stringent standards for methodological rigor. In addition, the majority of these reports provide only anecdotal findings, with relatively few using randomized designs with adequate control groups. This chapter presents two theoretical models for conceptualizing and addressing child traumatic stress, a review of current acute interventions for traumatized children, a critical review of selected published studies on acute interventions for children and adolescents, and future directions for the development and evaluation of acute interventions.

Theoretical Context

Developmental Framework

Over the past decade, a conceptual model of childhood traumatic stress has been progressively refined (Pynoos, Steinberg, & Wraith, 1995). The model assigns a tripartite etiology to acute posttraumatic reactions that arise from (1) aspects of the traumatic experience; (2) trauma and loss reminders; and (3) posttrauma stresses and adversities. Both objective and subjective features of traumatic experiences have been shown to predict severity of posttraumatic reaction (Goenjian et al., 2001). Trauma and loss reminders can include sights, sounds, places, smells, specific people, time of day, situations, or feelings (e.g., being afraid or anxious). They are associated with intense psychological and physiological reactivity, and serve to provoke and maintain distress. They also underlie avoidant behavior because children and adolescents restrict their activities to avoid confronting powerful reminders that evoke traumatic images and reactions. Traumatic events are commonly associated with a cascade of secondary adversities. These constitute additional sources of distress and increase the risk of comorbidity of posttraumatic stress reactions with other adverse reactions. Secondary adversities complicate efforts at adjustment, interfere with normal opportunities for development, and initiate maladaptive coping responses.

Theory on Stress, Coping, and Adaptation

The following five basic principles have received broad empirical support for facilitating positive adaptation following stress: (1) promoting a sense of safety; (2) promoting calming; (3) promoting a sense of self- and community efficacy; (4) promoting connectedness; and (5) instilling hope (Hobfoll et al., 2007).

Promoting a Sense of Safety

Physiological and psychological responses to trauma constitute alarm reactions, and trigger feelings of helplessness and concerns over safety. Traumatic events also interrupt young children's expectations of protection from parents/caregivers. Many early intervention strategies are intended to help children restore a sense of safety by managing and reducing these physiological and psychological responses, enhancing parent/caregiver capacity for protecting and responding to their children, reestablishing a family routine to increase predictability, and reducing exposure to further trauma.

Promoting Calming

Traumatic events create anxiety, fear, and emotional arousal that can interfere with sleep, attention, and concentration. For children who have serious difficulty orienting to the environment or managing overwhelming emotions, anxiety management techniques (e.g., grounding, breathing, muscle relaxation, cognitive restructuring) and problem-solving strategies are used to reduce the severity of these reactions and enhance children's ability to calm down. Establishing routines and encouraging normal child activities have also been used to promote a sense of calm for children.

Promoting a Sense of Self- and Community Efficacy

Disaster research has indicated that loss of personal, social, and economic resources is associated with diminished perception of self-efficacy and confidence in the community's ability to promote recovery (Galea et al., 2002; Norris & Kaniasty, 1996). To address issues of self-efficacy, intervention strategies include providing practical assistance, encouraging positive coping, assisting with problem solving, promoting proactive engagement in constructive activities, and linking with ancillary services.

Promoting Connectedness

The objective of connecting individuals and families with social supports is based on research indicating that social support is related to improved emotional well-being and recovery following trauma (Bleich, Gelkopf, & Solomon, 2003; Stein et al., 2004). Promoting social connectedness includes increasing different types of social support (e.g., emotional closeness, physical assistance, material support), and enhancing the range of sources of support and family cohesion (Layne et al., 2001). Many interventions promote connectedness by using group and family modalities, facilitating connections with loved ones, and identifying and assisting those who lack strong support.

Instilling Hope

Survivors who are likely to have more favorable outcomes are those who maintain optimism, positive expectancy, and a feeling of confidence that life and self are predictable (Carver, 1998). Many intervention strategies are designed to promote a sense of hopefulness about the future and expectations of recovery. These include connecting children and families with services to rebuild their lives, and encouraging proactive problem solving and prosocial community activities.

Acute Interventions

For a variety of reasons there is a paucity of rigorous intervention studies among children and adolescents in the early aftermath of disasters and terrorism (Steinberg, Brymer, Steinberg, & Pfefferbaum, 2006). Many of the lessons learned from the general stress literature have been applied to the design of acute interventions. These interventions fall into four major categories. First, there have been systemic approaches that include psychoeducation; consultation with school personnel, media, and parents; and establishment of crisis hotlines (e.g., Blaufarb & Levine, 1972; Echterling, 1989; Macy et al., 2004; Ponton & Bryant, 1991). Psychoeducation typically includes information about the nature and course of posttraumatic stress reactions, affirms that they are understandable and expectable; identifies and helps with ways to cope with trauma reminders; and discusses ways to manage distress. Psychoeducation has been geared to children, adolescents, parents, school personnel, and other child caregiving professionals. Macy and colleagues (2004) described a community-based continuum of response that includes the affected community in the design and implementation after a crisis or disaster. Such an approach includes community-based assessment and communitywide services for children, adolescents, families, and other child caregivers.

Second, art and massage therapies have been employed (e.g., Chapman, Morabito, Ladakakos, Schreier, & Knudson, 2001; Field, Seligman, Scafidi, & Schansberg, 1996). In the Chapman and colleagues (2001) study, children made successive drawings of aspects of their traumatic experiences and engaged in retelling the event to develop a trauma narrative. During this process, the researchers discussed misperceptions, rescue and revenge fantasies, blame, shame, and guilt, and coping strategies.

Third, trauma- and grief-focused cognitive-behavioral approaches have been used (e.g., Stubenbort, Donnelly, & Cohen, 2001). Cognitive-behavioral approaches have utilized components summarized by the acronym PRACTICE, including psychoeducation and parenting skills, relaxation, affective modulation, cognitive coping and processing, trauma narrative, *in vivo* mastery of trauma reminders, conjoint child–parent sessions, and enhancement of future safety and development (Cohen, Mannarino, & Deblinger, 2006). For further details on CBT for children and adolescents, see Cohen, Mannarino, Deblinger, and Berliner (Chapter 8, this volume).

Fourth, debriefing strategies have included reconstruction of the event, identification of thoughts and feelings about the event, psychoeducation and normalization, and information on coping (e.g., Morgan & White, 2003; Stallard et al., 2006; Vila, Porche, & Mouren-Simeoni, 1999; Yule, 1992). Over the past decade, research on the effectiveness of debriefing techniques, one of the most widely used acute interventions after a range of traumatic events, has been mixed (McNally, Bryant, & Ehlers, 2003). Additionally, there has been limited empirical support for other approaches, and a pressing need for a comprehensive operational guide for conducting acute interventions.

In response, the psychological first aid (PFA) approach has been endorsed as an acute intervention that is supportive and nonintrusive. The goal is not to force disclosure of traumatic details, but to respond to immediate needs and concerns, and provide information to survivors. As one example of a PFA approach, the National Child Traumatic Stress Network and the National Center for Posttraumatic Stress Disorder have developed *Psychological First Aid: Field Operations Guide, Second Edition* (Brymer et al., 2006), an evidence-informed modular approach for assisting children, adolescents, adults, and families in reducing the initial distress caused by catastrophic events, and fostering short- and long-term adaptive functioning. An overview of the eight core actions of PFA are presented in Table 5.1.

TABLE 5.1. Psychological First Aid Core Actions

1. Contact and engagement
    Goal: To respond to contacts initiated by survivors, or to initiate contacts in a non-intrusive, compassionate, and helpful manner.

2. Safety and comfort
    Goal: To enhance immediate and ongoing safety, and provide physical and emotional comfort.

3. Stabilization (if needed)
    Goal: To calm and orient emotionally overwhelmed or disoriented survivors.

4. Information gathering: Current needs and concerns
    Goal: To identify immediate needs and concerns, gather additional information, and tailor psychological first aid interventions.

5. Practical assistance
    Goal: To offer practical help to survivors in addressing immediate needs and concerns.

6. Connection with social supports
    Goal: To help establish brief or ongoing contacts with primary support persons and other sources of support, including family members, friends, and community helping resources.

7. Information on coping
    Goal: To provide information about stress reactions and coping to reduce distress and promote adaptive functioning.

8. Linkage with collaborative services
    Goal: To link survivors with available services needed at the time or in the future.

Note. These core actions of psychological first aid constitute the basic objectives of providing early assistance within days or weeks following an event. Providers should be flexible, basing the amount of time they spend on each core action on the survivors' specific needs and concerns.

Method of Collecting Data

We used five different search engines in the literature search: PsycINFO, Google Scholar, JSTOR (Journal Storage), Info Trac One File, and Criminal Justice Abstracts, using a combination of the following key words: "early intervention," "child trauma," "psychological first aid," "EMDR" (eye movement desensitization and reprocessing), and "debriefing." We consulted colleagues in the field and reviewed several book chapters.

Literature Review

The first part of Table 5.2 identifies three randomized controlled studies of acute posttrauma interventions among children and adolescents that include posttraumatic stress disorder (PTSD) as an outcome measure. In an early study of debriefing, Yule (1992) reported statistically lower scores on the Impact of Event Scale (IES) among 24 students receiving debriefing 10 days after the sinking of the *Jupiter* compared to 15 students who received no help until a year later. The significant difference in total IES score was attributable to lower scores on intrusion items. There was no effect on anxiety or depression. This study would have benefited from the collection of baseline data.

Chapman and colleagues (2001) conducted a randomized controlled study of the effectiveness of manualized art therapy compared with hospital care as usual. These subjects had experienced traumatic injuries that required hospitalization for a minimum of 24 hours. The experimental subjects were engaged in art therapy within days of the accident. There were no between-group differences in PTSD scores measured at 1 week and 1 month posttreatment. This study also failed to utilize a dose of exposure methodology and, surprisingly, did not provide statistical analyses to support the findings.

In a randomized control trial of debriefing, Stallard and colleagues (2006) compared outcomes for 82 experimental subjects and 76 controls. The experimental group was provided with a manualized debriefing intervention 4 weeks following road traffic accidents, whereas the control group was engaged in a non-accident-focused discussion. Children in both groups showed significant pre–post improvements in PTSD, depression, and anxiety, with the only difference being that children in the experimental group reported fewer behavioral and emotional problems. There were no between-group differences in PTSD diagnosis, depression, and anxiety at postintervention. The authors conclude that this form of early intervention is not effective. An important issue for this study, as well as many others, is the lack of control for level of exposure to the traumatic incident. For example, in this study, there were no specific analyses of subgroups within each condition that initially met diagnostic criteria for PTSD.

In regard to randomized controlled studies using other interventions, Field and colleagues (1996) compared eight sessions of massage therapy to a video–attention control condition provided to 60 grade-school-age children within the first month after being exposed to a hurricane. The findings indicated that children in the massage condition experienced greater reduction in anxiety, depression, and cortisol levels, and an increase in positive feelings. The lack of follow-up, and the absence of a postintervention PTSD assessment, are important limitations of this study.

The second part of Table 5.2 identifies one nonrandomized controlled study. In a quasi-experimental design, Vila and colleagues (1999) conducted two group debriefing sessions with 21 directly exposed children 24 hours and 6 weeks after a hostage-taking situation in their classroom. This group was compared with 21 students in another classroom in the school who were not directly exposed. Follow-up data were collected up to 18 months postevent. The findings indicated that debriefing did not prevent PTSD or anxiety disorders. Additionally, the directly exposed students who did not receive any treatment had worse outcomes. The lack of random assignment, subjects not receiving the same treatments (some subjects only received one debriefing session and others received individual treatment), and incomparability of the comparison group make this study difficult to interpret.

Summary and Recommendations

In reviewing the literature on acute interventions for children following traumatic events, most studies to date have been limited by small sample size, lack of adequate control/comparison groups, and absence of long-term follow-up. Some studies have geared evaluation metrics to specific intervention objectives, whereas others have used available child or adolescent measures. Such standardized instruments may not be adequately sensitive in detecting the benefits of the intervention, especially if these domains are not intervention targets. Another problem is the variability in the time posttrauma in which the intervention is delivered, making cross-study comparisons difficult.

Especially in disaster situations, their unpredictable nature and the chaos that typically permeates the postdisaster environment are undoubtedly severe obstacles to well-planned and -designed mental health research. In addition, because community systems, including school, health, and mental health systems, are responding to the event, it is difficult to utilize optimal research strategies while integrating research into these response activities (Steinberg et al., 2006). Nevertheless, especially in disaster-prone areas, preparatory training in acute interventions, preliminary design of study methods, metrics, and preapproved Institutional Review Board (IRB) protocols can set the stage for studies that may be implemented in the acute aftermath. Such preplanned studies can then provide more systematic and rigorous data to establish the evidence base for these interventions.

TABLE 5.2. A-Level and B-Level Studies: Randomized and Nonrandomized Controlled Trials

Treatment tested	Population	Comparison group	N	Duration of sessions	Main outcome measure	Within-group effect size	Between-group effect size[b]	Follow-up period	Results
Randomized controlled trials									
Modified Debriefing (Yule, 1992)	Cruise ship disaster survivors ages 14–16; 10 days postevent	Debriefing	24	1 day	Revised Impact of Events Scale (IES)	[a]	1.02	5–9 mo	• Significant between-group differences in IES Total scores and IES Intrusion subscale scores.
		Control	15						
Chapman art therapy treatment intervention (CATTI; Chapman et al., 2001)	Pediatric trauma patients ages 7–17; days after the trauma	CATTI	31	1 day	PTSD Reaction Index	[a]	[a]	6 mo	• No significant difference between CATTI and standard hospital treatment groups at 1-wk and 1-mo follow-up.
		Standard hospital care control	27						• No outcome data reported for no-PTSD group or 6-mo follow-up.
		No-PTSD control	27						

(continued)

113

TABLE 5.2. (continued)

Treatment tested	Population	Comparison group	N	Duration of sessions	Main outcome measure	Within-group effect size	Between-group effect size[b]	Follow-up period	Results
Modified debriefing (Stallard et al., 2006)	British road traffic accident survivors ages 7–18; approximately 4 wk postevent	Debriefing	82	1 day	Children's IES	0.42	0.05	8 mo	• No significant between-group differences in IES scores.
		Control	76			0.61			
Nonrandomized controlled trials									
Debriefing (Vila et al., 1999)	Students in a classroom that was taken hostage in France ages 6–9; within 24 hr and at 6 wk postevent	Students in the school but not in the classroom on the day of the hostage situation	21 students in each condition	2 days	IES			18 mo	• Debriefing did not prevent development of psychotraumatic disorders in debriefed children, but nondebriefed, nontreated directly exposed children had worse outcomes. • Some students in the debriefing group did not get both sessions and others received individual treatment, making the findings difficult to interpret.

[a]Insufficient information provided to calculate effect sizes.

[b]Positive effect size means greater drop in measurement outcome for the experimental group (vs. the control group).

114

In particular, the evidence base for PFA needs to be established in progressive stages that correspond to a number of basic research questions. These questions address issues ranging from the evaluation of training to assessment of short- and long-term PFA effectiveness. Among the overarching research questions are the following:

1. What types of training methods and resources are needed to disseminate PFA effectively?
2. Do trained PFA practitioners adhere to the PFA protocol?
3. Can PFA be delivered effectively by providers and effectively received by disaster survivors in actual disaster settings?
4. Does implementing the PFA protocol with fidelity assist in realization of each of the specific PFA objectives (internal evaluation)?
5. Does implementing the PFA protocol lead to improved outcomes compared to other intervention practices (external evaluation)?

References

Blaufarb, H., & Levine, J. (1972). Crisis intervention in an earthquake. *Social Work,* *17,* 16–19.

Bleich, A., Gelkopf, M., & Solomon, Z. (2003). Exposure to terrorism, stress-related mental health symptoms, and coping behaviors among a nationally representative sample in Israel. *Journal of the American Medical Association, 290*(5), 612–620.

Brymer, M., Jacobs, A., Layne, C., Pynoos, R., Ruzek J., Steinberg, A., et al. (2006). *Psychological first aid: Field operations guide, Second edition.* Los Angeles, CA & White River Junction, VT: National Child Traumatic Stress Network and National Center for PTSD. Available online at *www.nctsn.org* and *www.ncptsd.va.gov.*

Carver, C. S. (1998). Resilience and thriving: Issues, models and linkages. *Journal of Social Issues, 54,* 245–266.

Chapman, L., Morabito, D., Ladakakos, C., Schreier, H., & Knudson, M. (2001). The effectiveness of art therapy interventions in reducing post traumatic stress disorder (PTSD) symptoms in pediatric trauma patients. *Art Therapy, 18,* 100–104.

Cohen, J. A., Mannarino, A. P., & Deblinger, E. (2006). *Treating trauma and traumatic grief in children and adolescents.* New York: Guilford Press.

Echterling, L. G. (1989). An ark or prevention: Prevention school absenteeism after a flood. *Journal of Primary Prevention, 9,* 177–184.

Field, T., Seligman, S., Scafidi, F., & Schanberg, S. (1996). Alleviating posttraumatic stress in children following Hurricane Andrew. *Journal of Applied Developmental Psychology, 17,* 37–50.

Galea, S., Ahern, J., Resnick, H., Kilpatrick, D., Bucuvalas, M., Gold, J., et al. (2002). Psychological sequelae of the September 11 terrorist attacks in New York City. *New England Journal of Medicine, 346,* 982–987.

Goenjian, A. K., Molina, L., Steinberg, A. M., Fairbanks, L. A., Alvarez, M. L., Goenjian, H. A., et al. (2001). Posttraumatic stress and depressive reactions among Nicaraguan adolescents after Hurricane Mitch. *American Journal of Psychiatry, 158,* 788–794.

Hobfoll, S. E., Watson, P. E., Bell, C. C., Bryant, R. A., Brymer, M. J., Friedman, M. J., et al. (2007). Five essential elements of immediate and mid-term mass trauma intervention: Empirical evidence. *Psychiatry: Interpersonal and Biological Processes, 70*, 283–315.

Layne, C. M., Pynoos, R. S., Saltzman, W. R., Arslanagic, B., Black, M., Savjak, N., et al. (2001). Trauma/grief-focused group psychotherapy: School-based postwar intervention with traumatized Bosnian adolescents. *Group Dynamics: Theory, Research, and Practice, 5*, 277–290.

Macy, R. D., Behar, L., Paulson, R., Delman, J., Schmid, L., & Smith S. F. (2004). Community-based acute posttraumatic stress management: A description and evaluation of a psychosocial intervention continuum. *Harvard Review of Psychiatry, 12*, 217–228.

McNally, R. J., Bryant, R. A., & Ehlers, A. (2003). Does early psychological intervention promote recovery from posttraumatic stress? *Psychological Science in the Public Interest, 4*, 45–79.

Morgan, K. E., & White, P. R. (2003). The functions of art-making in CISD with children and youth. *International Journal of Emergency Mental Health, 5*, 61–76.

Norris, F. H., & Kaniasty, K. (1996). Received and perceived social support in times of stress: A test of the social support deterioration deterrence model. *Journal of Personality and Social Psychology, 71*, 498–511.

Ponton, L. E., & Bryant, E. C. (1991). After the earthquake: Organizing to respond to children and adolescents. *Psychiatric Annals, 21*, 539–546.

Pynoos, R. S., Steinberg, A. M., & Wraith, R. (1995). A developmental model of childhood traumatic stress. In D. Cicchetti & D. J. Cohen (Eds.), *Manual of developmental psychopathology* (pp. 72–93). New York: Wiley.

Stallard, P., Velleman, R., Salter, E., Howse, I., Yule, W., & Taylor, G. (2006). A randomised controlled trial to determine the effectiveness of an early psychological intervention with children involved in road traffic accidents. *Journal of Child Psychology and Psychiatry, and Applied Disciplines, 47*, 127–134.

Stein, B. D., Elliott, M. N., Jaycox, L. H., Collins, R. L., Berry, S. H., Klein, D. J., et al. (2004). A national longitudinal study of the psychological consequences of the September 11, 2001 terrorist attacks: Reactions, impairment, and help-seeking. *Psychiatry, 67*, 105–117.

Steinberg, A. M., Brymer, M. J., Steinberg, J. R., & Pfefferbaum, B. (2006). Conducting research on children and adolescents after mass trauma. In F. H. Norris, S. Galea, M. J. Friedman, & P. J. Watson (Eds.), *Methods for disaster mental health research* (pp. 243–253). New York: Guilford Press.

Stubenbort, K., Donnelly, G. R., & Cohen, J. A. (2001). Cognitive-behavioral group therapy for bereaved adults and children following an air disaster. *Group Dynamics: Theory, Research, and Practice, 5*, 261–276.

Vila, G., Porche, L., & Mouren-Simeoni, M. (1999). An 18-month longitudinal study of posttraumatic disorders in children who were taken hostage in their school. *Psychosomatic Medicine, 61*, 746–754.

Yule, W. (1992). Post traumatic stress disorders in child survivors of shipping disasters: The sinking of the *Jupiter. Psychotherapy and Psychosomatics, 57*, 200–205.

CHAPTER 6

Early Cognitive-Behavioral Interventions for Adults

Brett T. Litz and Richard A. Bryant

Theoretical Context

It is often presumed that there is a critical threshold or window of opportunity to help those who are vulnerable to development of chronic posttraumatic stress disorder (PTSD) in the early aftermath of trauma (e.g., Rothbaum, Foa, & Riggs, 1992). There is also convincing evidence that preventing chronic PTSD is imperative because PTSD can be pernicious and disabling for many people across the lifespan (e.g., Kessler, Sonnega, & Bromet, 1995; Kulka, Schlenger, & Fairbanks, 1990). Even more alarming, when individuals with chronic PTSD overcome various personal, familial, cultural, economic, and logistical barriers to care, they may still not get the care they need (e.g., Becker, Zayfert, & Anderson, 2004), their problems may be so entrenched that they fail to benefit from formal treatment (e.g., Kessler et al., 1995; Schnurr, Friedman, & Foy, 2003), or they may drop out of treatment prematurely (Tarrier, Pilgrim, & Sommerfield, 1999; Van Minnen, Arntz, & Keijsers, 2002). As a result, early intervention to prevent chronic PTSD and other problems brought about by exposure to trauma is a critical public health mandate (e.g., Litz & Gray, 2004).

In theory, if those trauma survivors most at risk for chronic PTSD can get early symptom relief and learn to manage various painful posttraumatic sequelae effectively, they may recover in lasting ways. Because trauma survivors in many instances are exposed to health care contexts or emergency services personnel in the hours, days, and weeks after trauma, this period is ripe for capturing those most at risk for serious posttraumatic difficulties and promoting recovery. However, longitudinal research has shown that early signs of distress or ineffective functioning are not necessarily indicative of a certain course of posttraumatic difficulties or resilience. Although many who are initially impaired recover effectively over time (e.g., Bonanno, 2005), the emergence of PTSD may be delayed (e.g., Buckley, Blanchard, & Hickling, 1996; Gray, Bolton, & Litz, 2004). Thus, another challenge for the field is to generate risk algorithms with the greatest predictive validity, so that those most in need are offered the scarce, early intervention resources.

The central question for this chapter is as follows: What is the state of evidence for early mental health intervention to prevent chronic PTSD and related disability for adult trauma survivors? There are two prevailing methods of early intervention for adults: "psychological debriefing" and "cognitive-behavioral therapy" (CBT; Litz, Gray, Bryant, & Adler, 2002). In Chapter 4 (this volume), Bisson, McFarlane, Rose, Ruzek, and Watson address the efficacy and appropriateness of debriefing. This chapter address the efficacy of CBT approaches. Although there are a variety of appropriate and worthy early intervention targets and goals (e.g., encouraging healthy coping and self-care, increasing social connectedness, preventing revictimization, addressing traumatic bereavement; Litz & Maguen, 2007), this chapter only reviews trials that attempt to prevent chronic PTSD using CBT. Open and uncontrolled trials are considerably less revealing because they capitalize on natural recovery trajectories; therefore, this chapter emphasizes evidence from A-rated randomized controlled trials (RCTs).

It should be underscored that best practice recommendations for early intervention depend not only on the quality and quantity (replicability) of efficacy trials but also on evidence of *effectiveness*. Factors that inform decisions about what intervention strategies to use, whom to target, who provides the intervention, and when the intervention is provided include the scope and impact of the traumatic events, the social and cultural context, the exigencies of different traumas (e.g., serious physical injury), the role(s) of survivors and survivor groups (e.g., first responders), resources (personal, social, governmental, professional), preclinical activities and preparatory activities (e.g., training, information in the posttrauma context), barriers to care (including beliefs that interfere with help seeking), and the current state of the individual or group (e.g., refugees in transit). Unfortunately, there are no early intervention, CBT-based effectiveness trials. Because trauma type and trauma context may vary a great deal, practitioners need to know whether CBT is an effective early intervention for the types of challenges their patients face. Accordingly, the CBT trials reviewed below are categorized according to the types of trauma survivors studied.

Description of Techniques

The CBT strategies used to target PTSD in the early intervention context generally mirror CBT techniques that have been found to ameliorate chronic PTSD symptoms in tertiary care (e.g., Foa et al., 1999). The CBT trials described below typically employed a family of CBT strategies (Keane & Barlow, 2002), including psychoeducation, stress management skills training, cognitive therapy (CT), and exposure therapy (ET). All of the CBT is collaborative, action-oriented and experiential, and utilizes homework and *in vivo* application of strategies learned in face-to-face therapy. Occasionally, a specific CBT strategy is tested in isolation, (usually CT; e.g., Ehlers, Mayou, & Bryant, 1998), and dismantling studies are rare. Unfortunately, all of the best RCTs (described in detail below) are, with the exception of effect size, incomparable due to procedural variations (e.g., length of intervention) and differences in the specific CBT techniques employed across studies.

There is no standardized content or process of delivering psychoeducation. Therapists commonly share information that (1) promotes understanding of the impact of trauma on functional capacities and psychological health and well-being, (2) helps patients explain the cause of their difficulties, commonly by employing a conditioning and learning frame, which also provides a cogent rationale for the intervention, and (3) provides accurate expectations about the demands and course of the treatment and positive expectancies about its efficacy. In the best trials, educational information is manualized to standardize presentation within RCTs. In trials, psychoeducation is always provided in the beginning of the first formal therapy session. In practice, psychoeducation can be an evolving process that occurs over the course of therapy as new challenges and experiences emerge.

There is also no standardized content or process for stress management. Typically, arousal and negative affect management skills are taught in some fashion. Deep, slow, diaphragmatic breathing is the most frequent technique employed, followed by progressive muscle relaxation. In most CBT trials, patients are not taught these skills to a criterion and the therapy time they receive is dwarfed by other components of CBT for PTSD: ET and CT.

Although CT techniques vary in the trials described below, the core strategies are shared by all CT (e.g., Hollon, Stewart, & Strunk, 2006): Provide experiential opportunities for patients to monitor, to examine critically, and to change the way they think about various trauma-related challenges and modify beliefs about the meaning and implication of the trauma as manifested in generalized expectations about the self and various outcomes. CT is highly effective in the treatment of chronic PTSD; however, there is no evidence that it is any more or less effective than other CBT-based interventions (e.g., Marks, Lovell, Noshirvani, Livanou, & Thrasher, 1998; Resick & Schnicke, 1992). In addition, virtually all CTs for PTSD incorporate an exposure component (e.g., *in vivo* confrontation of difficult situations, writing about the trauma).

ET comprises repeated presentations of trauma-related stimuli, typically in the patient's imagination, coupled with prevention of various avoidance behaviors and maneuvers (e.g., making sure that the patient focuses on dreaded feelings and events). The memories are processed in as rich and salient a way as possible; sensations, thoughts, beliefs, and especially feelings that arise during recall of the trauma are uncovered, disclosed, and managed many times. Patients are asked to close their eyes and describe an event in the first-person present tense to maximize vividness and experiential focus. They are taught how to rate subjective units of distress (SUDS), which are monitored repeatedly and act as a guide of patients' distress and a strategy to monitor reduction in negative affect. Sometimes, patients are provided an audiotape of the within-session experience (e.g., Foa et al., 1999); at other times, they are required simply to repeat as homework the exercise they learned in session (e.g., Bryant, Sackville, & Dang, 1999). Ideally, the result of these activities is in-session and across-session extinction of conditioned reactions. The ensuing cumulative and lasting reductions in aversive reactions to trauma reminders, in theory, can lead to various success experiences, enhanced self-efficacy, and symptom reduction. However, it should be emphasized that the necessary and sufficient change agents for ET's efficacy are uncertain. There is general agreement that nonreinforced exposure is an optimal and efficient method of providing a corrective experience that counteracts maladaptive ways of thinking about the meaning and implication of the trauma (the pain is not unbearable, arousal and negative affect peak, the person does not go crazy, others can understand and bear witness to their experience, etc.).

Method of Collecting Data

Table 6.1 provides a snapshot summary of the results of early intervention trials that used CBT strategies. The PILOTS database (Published International Literature on Traumatic Stress) PubMed, and PsycINFO were searched for the following terms: "early intervention," "acute stress disorder," "cognitive-behavioral therapy," and "posttraumatic stress." Trials were included if the goal was the prevention of chronic PTSD using some combination of CBT described earlier. The trials are grouped according to the following scheme: *mixed-gender motor vehicle accidents (MVAs) and industrial accidents*; *mixed-gender accidents and nonsexual assaults*; and *female-only sexual and nonsexual assaults*. Three trials targeted a single trauma type: MVAs (Ehlers, Clark, & Hackmann, 2003; Gidron et al., 2001) and sexual assault (Echeburúa, de Corral, & Sarasua, 1996); these were included under the mixed-gender accidents and female assault categories, respectively. The review that follows focuses on the trials that met most or all of the International Society for Traumatic Stress

TABLE 6.1. Summary of Early Intervention Trials Using CBT

Study	Treatment tested	Population	Comparison groups	N	Rating	Duration of trial	Main outcome measure	Within-group ES	Comparison	Between-N group ES ITT	Between-N group ES Completer	Results
Mixed-gender MVAs and industrial accidents												
Bryant et al. (1998)	CBT	MVA and industrial accident survivors	CBT	12	A	5 weeks	IES Intrusion	2.15	CBT vs. SC (IES Int)		1.21	CBT > SC, p < .01
							IES Avoidance	1.94	CBT vs. SC (IES Av)		1.82	CBT > SC, p < .001
			SC	12			IES Intrusion	1.58				
							IES Avoidance	0.56				
Ehlers et al. (2003)	CT	MVA	CT	28	A	12 weeks	CAPS Frequency	2.04	CT vs. SH (CAPS Freq)		0.99	CT > SH, p < .001
							CAPS Intensity	1.92	CT vs. SH (CAPS Int)		1.01	CT > SH, p < .001
			RA	29			CAPS Frequency	0.58	CT vs. RA (CAPS Freq)		1.22	CT > RA, p < .001
							CAPS Intensity	0.31	CT vs. RA (CAPS Int)		1.12	CT > RA, p < .001
			SH	28			CAPS Frequency	0.87	SH vs. RA (CAPS Freq)		0.21	NS
							CAPS Intensity	0.85	SH vs. RA (CAPS Int)		0.26	NS
Gidron et al. (2001)	MSI	MVA	MSI	8	A	2 telephone sessions	PDS		MSI vs. control		1.09	MSI > control, p < .05
			Supportive listening	9								
Turpin, Downs, & Mason (2005)	SH booklet	Physical injury	SH	75	A	Sent a booklet	PDS	0.12	SH vs. control		0.04	NS
			Wait-list control	67				0.06				

(continued)

121

TABLE 6.1. (continued)

Study	Treatment tested	Population	Comparison groups	N	Rating	Duration of trial	Main outcome measure	Within-group ES	Comparison	Between-N group ES ITT	Between-N group ES Completer	Results
Mixed-gender MVAs and nonsexual assault												
Andre et al. (1997)	CBT	Assault	CBT	65	A	1 to 6 weeks	IES	NA		NA	NA	CBT > standard care, $p < .05$
			Standard care	67				NA		NA	NA	
Bisson et al. (2004)	CBT	Physical injury	CBT	76	A	4 weeks	IES	2.12	CBT vs. standard care		0.27	NS
			Standard care	76				2.48				
Bryant et al. (1999)	CBT	MVA, nonsexual assault	PE	14	A	5 weeks	IES Intrusion	2.48	PE+AM vs. PE (IES Int)		0.35	NS
							IES Avoidance	2.09	PE+AM vs. PE (IES Av)		0.24	NS
			PE + AM	15			IES Intrusion	1.26	PE+AM vs. SC (IES Int)		0.71	PE + AM > SC
							IES Avoidance	1.79	PE+AM vs. SC (IES Av)		1.25	PE + AM > SC
			SC	16			IES Intrusion	0.49	SC vs. PE (IES Int)		1.55	PE > SC
							IES Avoidance	0.23	SC vs. PE (IES Av)		1.81	PE > SC
Bryant et al. (2003)	CBT	MVA and nonsexual assault with mild TBI	CBT	12	A	5 weeks	IES Intrusion	1.98	CBT vs. SC (IES Int)		0.88	CBT > SC, $p < .01$
							IES Avoidance	3.31	CBT vs. SC (IES Av)		1.58	CBT > SC, $p < .01$
			SC	12			IES Intrusion	0.65				
							IES Avoidance	-0.05				

122

Study	Treatment	Population	Condition	N (n)	Assessment	Time	Measure	Mean (SD)	Comparison	ES	ES	Significance
Bryant et al. (2005)	CBT	MVA, nonsexual assault	CBT	33 (24)	A	6 weeks	IES Intrusion	1.01 (1.59)	CBT vs. CBT+ (IES Int)	−0.46	−0.59	ITT: CBT+ > CBT, $p < .05$
							IES Avoidance	0.94 (1.72)	CBT vs. CBT+ (IES Av)	−0.31	0.38	NS
			CBT + hypnosis	30 (23)			IES Intrusion	1.49 (2.35)	CBT vs. SC (IES Int)	0.28	0.61	ITT: CBT > SC, $p < .05$. Completers: CBT > SC, $p < .05$
							IES Avoidance	0.8 (1.54)	CBT vs. SC (IES Av)	0.63	1.16	Completers: CBT > SC, $p < .001$
			SC	24 (22)			IES Intrusion	0.52 (0.55)	CBT+ vs. SC (IES Int)	0.85	1.38	ITT: CBT+ > SC, $p < .005$. Completers: CBT+ > SC, $p < .001$
							IES Avoidance	0.13 (0.14)	CBT+ vs. SC (IES Av)	0.28	0.81	Completers: CBT+ > SC, $p < .05$

Female sexual and nonsexual assault

Study	Treatment	Population	Condition	N (n)	Assessment	Time	Measure	Mean (SD)	Comparison	ES	ES	Significance
Echeburúa et al. (1996)	CT + coping skills training	Sexual assault	CT + coping skills training	10	A	5 weeks	SSPSDS	3.03	CT+ vs. PMR		0.79	NS
			PMR	10				1.78				
Foa, Zoellner, & Feeny (2006)	CBT	Sexual and nonsexual assault	CBT	31 (22)	A	4 weeks	PSS-I	[1.81]	B-CBT vs. AC	0.05		NS
			SC	29 (23)				[1.93]	B-CBT vs. SC	−0.33		NS
			RA	30 (20)				[1.37]	AC vs. SC	−0.37		NS

Note. Blank cells indicate values not calculated or calculable. AC, assessment condition; AM, anxiety management; B-CBT, Brief Cognitive Behavioral Intervention; CAPS, Clinician-Administered PTSD Scale; CBT, cognitive-behavioral therapy; CT, cognitive therapy; ES, effect size; IES, Impact of Events Scale; ITT, intention to treat; MSI, Memory Structuring Intervention; MVA, motor vehicle accident; NS, not significant; PDS, Post-Traumatic Diagnostic Scale; PE, prolonged exposure; PMR, progressive muscle relaxation; PSS-I, PTSD Symptom Scale—Interview; RA, repeated assessment; SC, supportive counseling; SH, self-help booklet; SSPSDS, Scale of Severity of Post-traumatic Stress Disorder Symptoms; TBI, traumatic brain injury.

123

Studies (ISTSS) guidelines intended to maximize internal validity in clinical trials (e.g., Foa & Meadows, 1997).

Literature Review

Mixed-Gender MVAs and Industrial Accidents

In one of the early, well-designed trials, Bryant, Harvey, and Dang (1998) compared five 90-minute weekly individual sessions of a heterogeneous set of CBT strategies (psychoeducation, relaxation training, CT, and imaginal and *in vivo* exposure) to the same amount of supportive counseling (SC), which included psychoeducation, general problem-solving skills training, and unconditional support. Far fewer participants receiving CBT met criteria for PTSD at posttreatment and at the 6-month follow-up. Moreover, the CBT arm led to impressive clinical and statistical reductions in avoidance, intrusive, and depressive symptomatology.

In each of their studies, Bryant and colleagues provided CBT within the first month of a trauma to individuals with acute stress disorder (ASD; American Psychiatric Association, 1994) to ensure that the intervention was provided to the individuals most at risk for chronic PTSD (e.g., Bryant & Harvey, 1997). Ehlers and colleagues (2003) reasoned that because MVA survivors have a steady recovery trajectory over several months (Ehlers et al., 1998), early intervention should be considered only for those survivors who have PTSD *several months* after the accident. Because the goal of early intervention is the prevention of chronic PTSD, which can become a lifelong struggle, this reasoning is sound. Ehlers and colleagues also posited correctly that because there was no untreated control group in previous early intervention CBT trials of accident survivors, they could not conclude that the CBT was effective per se; it might be that supportive counseling impedes recovery because it fails to offer specific change agents.

In their well-designed trial, Ehlers and colleagues (2003) targeted MVA survivors approximately 4 months after their accident, comparing a specific form of CBT, CT (up to 12 weekly and three monthly booster sessions), with a repeated assessment (no treatment) and a self-help booklet based on cognitive and behavioral principles. The results were unequivocally supportive of CT. Not only was the self-help booklet ineffective but no intervention produced higher end-state functioning at follow-up. This is consistent with another self-help booklet trial that was unequivocally negative (Turpin, Downs, & Mason, 2005). It appears that there is sufficient evidence not to recommend informational booklets as an early intervention for trauma, if the target of treatment is reduction of PTSD symptoms and enhancement of quality of life. On the other hand, informational materials about PTSD that also provide accurate, stigma-reducing expectations about what early intervention (and tertiary care) entails and information on obtaining help are arguably an important resource in settings where traumatized individuals are routinely processed (e.g., emergency rooms).

The rates of patients meeting PTSD criteria at follow-up were 11 and 17%, respectively, for the groups receiving CBT in the Ehlers and colleagues (2003) and Bryant and colleagues (1998) trials. These rates are extremely impressive in light of the rates for the control groups (e.g., 61% of the patients in the self-help arm in Ehlers and colleagues were PTSD cases at follow-up), and they represent small, absolute numbers in light of the size of the various arms of the studies. Because the criterion of functional impairment was not used to establish a PTSD diagnosis in either study, it is unclear what the PTSD diagnosis signifies posttreatment: It could very well be that the PTSD prevalence rates would be attenuated considerably.

The rates of PTSD at follow-up in these excellent and very positive trials nonetheless raise the question: What should the goal of early intervention be? It is unrealistic and conceptually baseless to expect an early intervention to prevent vulnerability for posttraumatic difficulties across the lifespan (especially in the event of certain horrific traumatic events; Litz & Gray, 2004). Because of the relatively arbitrary nature of diagnostic cut points, significant symptom reduction and enhanced functional capacities (and quality of life) are more valid indicators of efficacy (Litz, 2004). With the exception of the early trials with sexual assault victims, which employed behavioral indicators of change (e.g., Frank, Anderson, & Stewart, 1988; see also the trial by Echeburúa), efficacy trials have focused exclusively on medical model outcomes (e.g., prevalence and degree of self-disclosed disease burden, and comorbid conditions), without evaluating functional capacities. If posttraumatic functional impairment were routinely required for a diagnosis, using DSM-IV Criterion F, then the PTSD diagnosis in early intervention trials would have substantially more meaning.

Mixed-Gender Accidents and Nonsexual Assaults

No study in this category substantiated its reason for culling these two disparate trauma types, so the assumption is that this was done to meet study recruitment goals. These experiences are fundamentally different. Assaults introduce human maliciousness and betrayal of trust (most assaults are perpetrated by intimates), which adversely influence adaptation and create greater risk for chronic posttraumatic difficulties, especially interpersonal problems (e.g., Kessler et al., 1995; Norris, Friedman, & Watson, 2002). The evidence supporting the efficacy of CBT is, accordingly, less clear cut for trials that targeted both accident and assault survivors.

Bryant and colleagues (1999) examined the differential efficacy of five 90-minute sessions of ET plus anxiety management, ET alone, and SC provided to patients with ASD within 2 weeks of trauma exposure (the difference in intervention method makes this study somewhat incomparable to Bryant et al., 1998). The results were somewhat mixed. There were fewer PTSD cases for both active interventions at 6 months, but the three arms did not differ in their impact on intrusive reexperiencing symptoms (indexed by the Impact of Event Scale [IES]; Horowitz, Wilner, & Alvarez, 1979) at the 6-month follow-up (at posttreatment, SC differed from ET), and there were no differential effects for total PTSD severity, as indexed by the Clinician-Administered PTSD Scale (CAPS; Blake, Weathers, & Nagy, 1995). A 4-year follow-up of approximately 50% of those treated originally showed no impact on reports of intrusive symptoms, but the two CBT arms were highly different from SC on IES Avoidance scores, as they had been at 6 months (Bryant, Moulds, & Nixon, 2003). Notably, the CBT interventions did not affect depression across the follow-up intervals (indexed by the Beck Depression Inventory [BDI]; Beck, Steer, & Garbin, 1988).

In an optimally designed trial, Bryant, Moulds, and Guthrie (2005) examined whether the addition of elements of hypnosis would improve the CBT package used in Bryant and colleagues (1998), again, relative to SC. The group's exclusion of individuals who reported sexual abuse in childhood may have reduced external validity of the results. A completer analysis revealed fewer PTSD cases at the 6-month follow-up for both active treatments relative to SC; impressively, these effects were maintained at a 3-year follow-up (Bryant, Moulds, & Nixon, 2006). However, the attrition rate for CBT was greater than that for SC. Although CBT plus hypnosis led to quicker gains (at posttreatment), it had no long-term differential impact, and the intent-to-treat (ITT) analyses yielded an equal number of PTSD cases at the 6-month follow-up. There was also no differential effect of either the CBT arm or end-stage functioning, and differential effect sizes were more moderate relative to Ehlers and colleagues (2003) and Bryant and colleagues (1999)—although, relative to Bryant and colleagues, there was a stronger effect on Intrusions. It is worth noting that Bryant and colleagues (1999, 2003) required the presence of impairment for a diagnosis of PTSD and, accordingly, these studies do suggest that early provision of CBT does lead to less PTSD and related-impairment than does counseling.

In a well-powered study, Bisson, Shepherd, and Joy (2004) compared four 1-hour CBT sessions to no intervention, provided to individuals endorsing at least moderate PTSD symptoms 1–3 weeks after mild to moderate physical injury. There were no statistical differences in CAPS scores between the two treatment groups, and there was a relatively small effect size based on CAPS scores. The CBT did not affect symptoms of anxiety and depression.

Female-Only Sexual and Nonsexual Assaults

In their small study, Echeburúa and colleagues (1996) targeted treatment-seeking, female, sexual assault survivors with PTSD within 3 months of the assault. They examined the impact of five 1-hour sessions of cognitive therapy plus coping skills training (CT+) compared to progressive muscle relaxation only. Both arms led to highly significant change in PTSD diagnosis at 12-month follow-up, but relative to PTSD symptom severity at 12 months, the CT+ arm performed better. There were no differences between the two treatments in fears of assault-related situations, anxiety, depression, and functional abilities at 12 months. The fact that both groups improved considerably suggests that a no-intervention control group is needed.

As a follow-up to Foa, Hearst-Ikeda, and Perry's (1995) initial uncontrolled trial, Foa, Zoellner, and Feeny (2006) conducted a well-designed, state-of-the-art early intervention trial of women survivors of sexual and physical aggression. Their CBT was a mixture of exposure (imaginal and *in vivo*) and CT, with the addition of psychoeducation and breathing retraining, provided in four weekly, 2-hour meetings within 4 weeks of the assault. Unlike Foa and colleagues' (1995) treatment model for chronic PTSD, there was no emphasis on exposure above the other elements, and the therapy was briefer. Foa and colleagues (2006) compared CBT with SC (four weekly, 2-hour meetings) and four weekly, 2-hour repeated assessments of PTSD and current functioning (assessment only [AO]).

Foa and colleagues (2006) demonstrated that weekly, very thorough monitoring of symptoms and functioning by a caring, knowledgeable, and credible professional facilitates recovery and prevents chronic PTSD to the same degree as does CBT. At each posttreatment interval, the CBT and the AO arms did not differ on any outcome measure (70% of the AO group no longer had PTSD at the last follow-up). Consistent with Ehlers and colleagues' (2003) argument that elements of SC may delay or impede recovery, Foa and colleagues also showed that the SC arm led to worse outcomes at posttreatment, although, contrary to Ehlers and colleagues, these effect sizes were very low, and the differences disappeared at the last follow-up. In the CBT group, self-reported PTSD scores improved, but clinician ratings of PTSD scores did not when compared with SC at the postintervention interval and at the 3-month follow-up; there were no differences in depression, end-stage functioning, or clinically significant change. There were also no differences in end-stage functioning between the three arms at the last follow-up; 85% of the AO group, 87.5% of the SC group, and 91% of the CBT group demonstrated clinically significant change.

The results of Foa and colleagues' (2006) trial are surprising in light of the extensive evidence of CBT efficacy for chronic PTSD in female assault survivors (e.g., Foa, Rothbaum, & Riggs, 1991). The reasons for this are unclear. Foa and colleagues made homework optional in their early intervention trial (to make it sound less onerous), which is in contrast with their CBT package for patients with chronic PTSD. They argue that downplaying the necessity of *in vivo* exposure and homework-based imaginal exposure trials may have attenuated the effects of the CBT—a viable hypothesis.

If modification of the "fear structure" by varied means (experiential reductions in negative affect, unrealized catastrophic expectations, etc.) is the change agent in ET for physical and sexual assault in women, then the results of Foa and colleagues' (2006) trial are particularly inexplicable, because the *in vivo* and imaginal exposure components of their brief CBT should be effective and long-lasting in an early intervention framework; this is because the fear structure is less generalized and the maladaptive associations are less rigidly overlearned. In learning terms, extinction-based procedures, such as imaginal and *in vivo* ET, produce an inhibition of the conditioned response: The association between assault-related cues and danger is not eradicated; rather, it is lessened in retrieval strength (i.e., inhibited; Bouton & Swartzentruber, 1991). The retrieval strength of nondanger associations should be much stronger if therapeutic exposure occurs weeks after conditioning (assault) relative to years later. It could be that the AO and SC groups in Foa and colleagues' trial had similar positive outcomes because, over time, both treatments had natural, nonreinforced exposure to trauma-related cues, or because the CBT was not potent enough or optimally implemented. For example, it may be that the spacing and timing of prolonged exposure trials might need to be different in an early intervention frame (see Lang, Craske, & Bjork, 1999).

Summary and Recommendations

CBT should be employed routinely as an early intervention for survivors of relatively discrete accidents who endorse significant, enduring posttraumatic difficulties. The studies by Bryant and colleagues (1998) and Ehlers and colleagues (2003) stand out as definitive efforts, with very strong standardized effects. At present, it is unknown how much time should elapse after a traumatic experience before CBT is recommended to an individual as a course of treatment. If the intervention is provided too early (hours to days), the net will be cast too widely, and many individuals will be provided CBT who do not need this expensive and scarce form of expert care. In addition, if the CBT is provided too early, most traumatized individuals will be too distraught, bereft, or consumed with other pressing needs, and may be unable to abide by the various demands of the approach (e.g., homework; Litz et al., 2002). It is for this reason that numerous trials have not commenced early intervention before 2 weeks have passed since the traumatic event (Bryant et al., 1998, 1999, 2003). There now appears to be evidence that repeated monitoring of symptoms can hasten recovery in some and assist in the identification of those most in need; thus, it seems most prudent to follow the timing parameters and procedures very successfully employed by Ehlers and colleagues; that is, when feasible, clinicians should begin a process of self- or professional monitoring of impact soon after exposure to trauma and wait several months before offering formal CBT only to those whose symptoms either do not abate or arise anew. Whereas most accident survivors visit emergency rooms, such a policy could readily be part of a discharge plan (see Zatsick, Roy-Byrne, & Russo, 2001). The monitoring could be conducted efficiently with various Telehealth methods (e.g., automated telephoning, Internet-based monitoring). Clinically, the added benefit of routine monitoring within the first weeks is that it can also trigger self-referral to formal CBT, if symptoms or impairment are sufficiently severe.

It is difficult to draw definitive conclusions from studies that included both physical and sexual assault survivors, and it is problematic to compare these with accident-only trials. What is clear is that the efficacy data are considerably less strong and more focalized, and, in the case of female physical and sexual assault, disappointing. For mixed-gender accident and assault survivors, CBT appears to reduce avoidance behaviors successfully (e.g., Bryant et al., 1999), but it has little impact on other symptoms of PTSD and co-occurring depression. Trials that included assault survivors may have less positive results because adaptation to interpersonal violence, especially sexual violence, is more complicated and multifaceted. MVAs and industrial accidents are typically circumscribed, and CBT is well prepared to address anxiety and functioning in these contexts. The negative psychological and social impact of interpersonal violence is much more likely to generalize beyond the incident context, so experiences with human brutality and sadism, in contrast to MVAs and industrial accidents, are more likely to negatively affect core beliefs that otherwise sustain well-being. These factors may complicate early interventions using CBT, necessitate a unique set of targets and strategies, or require novel, yet-to-be-tested approaches.

CBT appears to hasten recovery in female assault survivors relative to supportive care, but supportive care also leads to marked improvement over time. In one of the best-designed studies to date, CBT did not confer any lasting advantage relative to a monitoring-only condition. At the very least, this underscores that assault survivors who endorse severe symptoms and difficulties in the first few weeks should be provided sustained, repeated, and credible symptom monitoring. Consistent with recommendations by Foa and colleagues (2006), the repeated monitoring should be conducted in a warm, empathic, careful, yet inquisitive context.

Until alternative CBT early intervention therapies can be developed and tested to outperform the results of repeated monitoring, it is prudent to recommend CBT for those women who fail to benefit from continued monitoring over several months given the strong efficacy of CBT for assault victims with enduring PTSD. It is also wise to prepare women assault survivors for the possibility of CBT during the monitoring phase. This would entail providing women with accurate expectations about what CBT would demand of them and where to get services. Once an individual considers seeking early intervention, it is appropriate to provide questions and answers that might enhance readiness and motivation for care, as well as to consider obstacles to intervention (e.g., no health insurance, stigma, a lack of family support). The dropout rates for CBT in existing trials are substantial, and because considerably less restrictive entry criteria are used in clinical contexts, active treatment should be avoided until obstacles to compliance and motivation are addressed.

Future early intervention trials should not only comply with all the recommendations made by the ISTSS for maximizing internal validity but also
include a repeated AO comparison group. Researchers might also consider
alternatives to SC, such as placebo control groups, because some evidence
suggests that SC impedes recovery, and at the very least, active interventions
outdoing inert therapies do not advance the field. Other good candidates for
comparison groups to CBT include behavioral interventions that target stress
and negative affect reduction/regulation only (with no traumatic memory
processing of any kind), and interventions designed only to target maintenance of self-care (sleep hygiene, eating properly and regularly, exercise) and
functioning in relationships and at work.

Future early intervention trials might also systematically evaluate indices
of functional capacities (work, leisure, self-care, relationship satisfaction) and
track these over time. Most CBT-based early interventions address what is generally labeled as "relapse prevention" at the end of treatment. Because this is
the least articulated aspect of care in published studies, it is unclear whether
sufficient attention is focused on plans for coping and managing inevitable
periods in the future, when a survivor is faced with particularly salient or sustained traumatic reminders. Because traumatic events may impose a lifetime
burden of symptom exacerbations, CBT is especially well suited to provide
survivors a *toolkit* of coping skills and the proper guidance to use them during times of stress. Given the considerable lifetime burden, an outcome is
successful if a person is able to maintain functioning over time in the face of
symptoms.

Researchers working with assault victims might consider the unique early
phenomenology and the initial challenges imposed by physical assaults, especially sexual assault. CBT models need to be designed and tested to address
these issues. Generally, CBT entails a variety of treatment strategies and
components, so it becomes important to examine the key mediators to positive outcomes. Likely candidates are self-efficacy, treatment outcome expectations, acceptance/meaning making, and the acquisition of a thoughtful
approach to self management over time. Dismantling studies are needed to
determine the elements necessary to promote recovery from different types
of traumatic events.

Formal, resource-intensive secondary prevention interventions should be
applied only to trauma survivors who are least likely to recover on their own;
but unfortunately, it is unclear at present how best to identify survivors most
at risk for chronic PTSD. Based on current knowledge, ASD is a reasonable
predictor of long-term outcome and impairment (and approximately 75%" of
individuals with ASD develop chronic PTSD). However, the utility of ASD has
been questioned (e.g., Harvey & Bryant, 2002). For example, the incremental validity of the dissociation symptoms, relative to an assessment of "early"
PTSD, appears to be questionable (Brewin, Andrews, & Rose, 2003). In future
research, it would be prudent to evaluate PTSD at each assessment interval

in early intervention trials. Ultimately, there are multiple, interrelated pathways to the development of chronic PTSD (e.g., Brewin, Andrews, & Valentin, 2000; King, Vogt, & King, 2004), and these factors vary across different trauma contexts. Unfortunately, to date, risk research has not informed decisions about early intervention (e.g., Litz et al., 2002).

Future research should examine different methods of determining who most needs care. For example, early posttraumatic depression and severe hyperarousal appear to increase risk for development of chronic PTSD (Freedman, Brandes, & Peri, 1999; Harvey & Bryant, 1999; Shalev, Freedman, & Peri, 1997). Prior exposure to trauma and personality traits (e.g., negative affectivity) are also good candidates to consider (Dougall, Herberman, Delahanty, Inslicht, & Baum, 2000; King, King, Foy, Keane, & Fairbank, 1999; Miller, 2004; Stretch, Knudson, & Durand, 1998). Clues to answer the question of who most needs care may be found by generating and testing moderators of intervention efficacy: Whom is the intervention most likely to benefit? What types of traumatic experiences, current social contexts, and personal characteristics attenuate outcomes? Unfortunately, most trials to date possess limited numbers of participants, a factor that makes it impossible to conduct valid mediator and moderator analyses.

Another critical and highly related research priority is to vary the timing of CBT initiation systematically in clinical trials. At present, there is no scientific basis to guide decision making about timing early intervention for trauma. Two highly divergent methods have been deployed successfully; intervening within approximately 2 weeks after trauma exposure (e.g., Bryant et al., 1998) and waiting several months (Ehlers et al., 2003). However, these strategies have not been compared empirically.

CBT is administered across multiple sessions, requires considerable therapist expertise, and is demanding of therapist and survivor time and resources. From a public health standpoint, individualized CBT will not reach the majority of individuals who most need intervention. As a result, it will prove fruitful to adapt various CBT technologies to a self-help or self-management framework (e.g., Lange, van de Ven, & Schrieken, 2001; Litz, Williams, Wang, & Engel, 2004). CBT is also not readily available to first-responder and other groups for whom trauma exposure represents an occupational hazard (e.g., the military). At present, debriefing models are attractive because they are cogent, face-valid, and especially well suited for the emergency services and employee assistance programs. It is relatively easy to learn debriefing and to be trained; the debriefing culture is egalitarian in the sense that one does not need professional preparation to be trained. Commanders, managers, and planners appreciate debriefing models because they deemphasize psychopathology and highlight the expectation of return to work/duty. CBT methods and technologies, especially stress management and stress inoculation, are highly amenable to work cultures, but more complete application will require attention to dissemination and to program development.

References

American Psychiatric Association. (1994). *Diagnostic and statistical manual of mental disorders* (4th ed.). Washington, DC: Author.

André, C., Lelord, F., Legeron, P., Reignier, A., & Delattre, A. (1997). Effectiveness of early intervention on 132 bus driver victims of aggressions: A controlled study. *L'Encéphale, 23,* 65–71.

Beck, A. T., Steer, R. A., & Garbin, M. G. (1988). Psychometric properties of the Beck Depression Inventory: Twenty-five years of evaluation. *Clinical Psychology Review, 8,* 77–100.

Becker, C. B., Zayfert, C., & Anderson, E. (2004). A survey of psychologists' attitudes towards and utilization of exposure therapy for PTSD. *Behaviour Research and Therapy, 42,* 277–292.

Bisson, J. I., Shepherd, J. P., & Joy, D. (2004). Early cognitive-behavioural therapy for post-traumatic stress symptoms after physical injury: Randomised controlled trial. *British Journal of Psychiatry, 184,* 63–69.

Blake, D. D., Weathers, F. W., & Nagy, L. M. (1995). The development of a Clinician-Administered PTSD Scale. *Journal of Traumatic Stress, 8,* 75–90.

Bonanno, G. A. (2005). Resilience in the face of potential trauma. *Current Directions in Psychological Science, 14,* 135–138.

Bouton, M. E., & Swartzentruber, D. (1991). Sources of relapse after extinction in Pavlovian and instrumental learning. *Clinical Psychology Review, 11,* 123–140.

Brewin, C. R., Andrews, B., & Rose, S. (2003). Diagnostic overlap between acute stress disorder and PTSD in victims of violent crime. *American Journal of Psychiatry, 160,* 783–785.

Brewin, C. R., Andrews, B., & Valentine, J. D. (2000). Meta-analysis of risk factors for posttraumatic stress disorder in trauma-exposed adults. *Journal of Consulting and Clinical Psychology, 68,* 748–766.

Bryant, R. A., & Harvey, A. G. (1997). Acute stress disorder: A critical review of diagnostic issues. *Clinical Psychology Review, 17,* 757–773.

Bryant, R. A., Harvey, A. G., & Dang, S. T. (1998). Treatment of acute stress disorder: A comparison of cognitive-behavioral therapy and supportive counseling. *Journal of Consulting and Clinical Psychology, 66,* 862–866.

Bryant, R. A., Moulds, M. L., & Guthrie, R. M. (2005). The additive benefit of hypnosis and cognitive-behavioral therapy in treating acute stress disorder. *Journal of Consulting and Clinical Psychology, 73,* 334–340.

Bryant, R. A., Moulds, M. L., & Nixon, R. D. (2003). Cognitive behaviour therapy of acute stress disorder: A four-year follow-up. *Behaviour Research and Therapy, 41,* 489–494.

Bryant, R. A., Moulds, M. L., & Nixon, R. D. V. (2006). Hypnotherapy and cognitive behaviour therapy of acute stress disorder: A 3-year follow-up. *Behaviour Research and Therapy, 44,* 1331–1335.

Bryant, R. A., Sackville, T., & Dang, S. T. (1999). Treating acute stress disorder: An evaluation of cognitive behavior therapy and supporting counseling techniques. *American Journal of Psychiatry, 156,* 1780–1786.

Buckley, T. C., Blanchard, E. B., & Hickling, E. J. (1996). A prospective examination of delayed onset PTSD secondary to motor vehicle accidents. *Journal of Abnormal Psychology, 105,* 617–625.

Dougall, A. L., Herberman, H. B., Delahanty, D. L., Inslicht, S. S., & Baum, A. (2000). Similarity of prior trauma exposure as a determinant of chronic stress responding to an airline disaster. *Journal of Consulting and Clinical Psychology, 68*, 290–295.

Echeburúa, E., de Corral, P., & Sarasua, B. (1996). Treatment of acute posttraumatic stress disorder in rape victims: An experimental study. *Journal of Anxiety Disorders, 10*, 185–199.

Ehlers, A., Clark, D. M., & Hackmann, A. (2003). A randomized controlled trial of cognitive therapy, a self-help booklet, and repeated assessments as early interventions for posttraumatic stress disorder. *Archives of General Psychiatry, 60*, 1024–1032.

Ehlers, A., Mayou, R. A., & Bryant, B. (1998). Psychological predictors of chronic posttraumatic stress disorder after motor vehicle accidents. *Journal of Abnormal Psychology, 107*, 508–519.

Foa, E. B., Dancu, C. V., Hembree, E. A., Jaycox, L. H., Meadows, E. A., & Street, G. P. (1999). A comparison of exposure therapy, stress inoculation training, and their combination for reducing posttraumatic stress disorder in female assault victims. *Journal of Consulting and Clinical Psychology, 67*, 194–200.

Foa, E. B., Hearst-Ikeda, D., & Perry, K. J. (1995). Evaluation of a brief cognitive behavioral program for the prevention of chronic PTSD in recent assault victims. *Journal of Consulting and Clinical Psychology, 63*, 948–955.

Foa, E. B., & Meadows, E. A. (1997). Psychosocial treatments for posttraumatic stress disorder: A critical review. *Annual Review of Psychology, 48*, 449–480.

Foa, E. B., Rothbaum, B. O., & Riggs, D. S. (1991). Treatment of posttraumatic stress disorder in rape victims: A comparison between cognitive-behavioral procedures and counseling. *Journal of Consulting and Clinical Psychology, 59*, 715–723.

Foa, E. B., Zoellner, L. A., & Feeny, N. C. (2006). An evaluation of three brief programs for facilitating recovery after assault. *Journal of Traumatic Stress, 19*, 29–43.

Frank, E., Anderson, B., & Stewart, B. D. (1988). Efficacy of cognitive behavior therapy and systematic desensitization in the treatment of rape trauma. *Behavior Therapy, 19*, 403–420.

Freedman, S. A., Brandes, D., & Peri, T. (1999). Predictors of chronic post-traumatic stress disorder: A prospective study. *British Journal of Psychiatry, 174*, 353–359.

Gidron, Y., Reuven, G., Freedman, S., Twiser, I., Lauden, A., Snir, Y., et al. (2001). Translating research findings to PTSD prevention: Results of a randomized-controlled pilot study. *Journal of Traumatic Stress, 14*, 773–780.

Gray, M. J., Bolton, E. E., & Litz, B. T. (2004). A longitudinal analysis of PTSD symptom course: Delayed-onset PTSD in Somalia peacekeepers. *Journal of Consulting and Clinical Psychology, 72*, 909–913.

Harvey, A. G., & Bryant, R. A. (1999). The relationship between acute stress disorder and posttraumatic stress disorder: A 2-year prospective evaluation. *Journal of Consulting and Clinical Psychology, 67*, 985–988.

Harvey, A. G., & Bryant, R. A. (2002). Acute stress disorder: A synthesis and critique. *Psychological Bulletin, 128*, 886–902.

Hollon, S. D., Stewart, M. O., & Strunk, D. (2006). Enduring effects for cognitive behavior therapy in the treatment of depression and anxiety. *Annual Review of Psychology, 57*, 285–315.

Horowitz, M. J., Wilner, N., & Alvarez, W. (1979). Impact of Event Scale: A measure of subjective stress. *Psychosomatic Medicine, 41*, 209–218.

Keane, T. M., & Barlow, D. H. (2002). Posttraumatic stress disorder. In D. Barlow (Ed.), *Anxiety and its disorders: The nature and treatment of anxiety and panic* (2nd ed., pp. 418–453). New York: Guilford Press.

Kessler, R. C., Sonnega, A., & Bromet, E. (1995). Posttraumatic stress disorder in the National Comorbidity Survey. *Archives of General Psychiatry, 52,* 1048–1060.

King, D. W., King, L. A., Foy, D. W., Keane, T. M., & Fairbank, J. A. (1999). Posttraumatic stress disorder in a national sample of female and male Vietnam veterans: Risk factors, war-zone stressors, and resilience-recovery variables. *Journal of Abnormal Psychology, 108,* 164–170.

King, D. W., Vogt, D. S., & King, L. A. (2004). Risk and resilience factors in the etiology of chronic posttraumatic stress disorder. In B. T. Litz (Ed.), *Early intervention for trauma and traumatic loss* (pp. 34–64). New York: Guilford Press.

Kulka, R. A., Schlenger, W. E., & Fairbank, J. A. (1990). *Trauma and the Vietnam War generation: Report of findings from the National Vietnam Veterans Readjustment Study.* Philadelphia: Brunner/Mazel.

Lang, A. J., Craske, M. G., & Bjork, R. (1999). Application of the new theory of disuse to long-term fear reduction. *Clinical Psychology: Science and Practice, 6,* 80–94.

Lange, A., van de Ven, J.-P., & Schrieken, B. (2001). Interapy: Treatment of posttraumatic stress through the Internet: A controlled trial. *Journal of Behavior Therapy and Experimental Psychiatry, 32,* 73–90.

Litz, B. T. (2004). Closing remarks. In B. Litz (Ed.), *Early intervention for trauma and traumatic loss* (pp. 319–326). New York: Guilford Press.

Litz, B. T., & Gray, M. J. (2004). Early intervention for trauma in adults: A framework for first aid and secondary prevention. In B. T. Litz (Ed.), *Early intervention for trauma and traumatic loss* (pp. 87–111). New York: Guilford Press.

Litz, B. T., Gray, M. J., Bryant, R., & Adler, A. B. (2002). Early intervention for trauma: Current status and future directions. *Clinical Psychology: Science and Practice, 9,* 112–134.

Litz, B. T., & Maguen, S. (2007). Early intervention for trauma. In M. J. Friedman, T. M. Keane, & P. A. Resick (Eds.), *Handbook of PTSD: Science and practice* (pp. 306–329). New York: Guilford Press.

Litz, B. T., Williams, L., Wang, J., & Engel, C. (2004). A therapist-assisted Internet self-help program for traumatic stress. *Professional Psychology: Research and Practice, 35,* 628–634.

Marks, I., Lovell, K., Noshirvani, H., Livanou, M., & Thrasher, S. (1998). Treatment of posttraumatic stress disorder by exposure and/or cognitive restructuring: A controlled study. *Archives of General Psychiatry, 55,* 317–325.

Miller, M. W. (2004). Personality and the development and expression of PTSD. *PTSD Research Quarterly, 15*(3), 1–7.

Norris, F. H., Friedman, M. J., & Watson, P. J. (2002). 60,000 disaster victims speak: Part I. An empirical review of the empirical literature, 1981–2001. *Psychiatry: Interpersonal and Biological Processes, 65,* 207–239.

Resick, P. A., & Schnicke, M. K. (1992). Cognitive processing therapy for sexual assault victims. *Journal of Consulting Clinical Psychology, 60,* 748–756.

Rothbaum, B. O., Foa, E. B., & Riggs, D. S. (1992). A prospective examination of posttraumatic stress disorder in rape victims. *Journal of Traumatic Stress, 5,* 455–475.

Schnurr, P. P., Friedman, M. J., & Foy, D. W. (2003). Randomized trial of trauma-focused group therapy for posttraumatic stress disorder: Results from a Department of Veterans Affairs Cooperative Study. *Archives of General Psychiatry, 60,* 481–489.

Shalev, A. Y., Freedman, S., & Peri, T. (1997). Predicting PTSD in trauma survivors: Prospective evaluation of self-report and clinician-administered instruments. *British Journal of Psychiatry, 170,* 558–564.

Stretch, R. H., Knudson, K. H., & Durand, D. (1998). Effects of premilitary and military trauma on the development of post-traumatic stress disorder symptoms in female and male active duty soldiers. *Military Medicine, 163,* 466–470.

Tarrier, N., Pilgrim, H., & Sommerfield, C. (1999). A randomized trial of cognitive therapy and imaginal exposure in the treatment of chronic posttraumatic stress disorder. *Journal of Consulting and Clinical Psychology, 67,* 13–18.

Turpin, G., Downs, M., & Mason, S. (2005). Effectiveness of providing self-help information following acute traumatic injury: Randomised controlled trial. *British Journal of Psychiatry, 187,* 76–82.

Van Minnen, A., Arntz, A., & Keijsers, G. P. J. (2002). Prolonged exposure in patients with chronic PTSD: Predictors of treatment outcome and dropout. *Behaviour Research and Therapy, 40,* 439–457.

Zatzick, D. F., Roy-Byrne, P., & Russo, J. E. (2001). Collaborative interventions for physically injured trauma survivors: A pilot randomized effectiveness trial. *General Hospital Psychiatry, 23,* 114–123.

PART III

TREATMENT FOR CHRONIC PTSD

CHAPTER 7

Cognitive-Behavioral Therapy for Adults

Shawn P. Cahill, Barbara Olasov Rothbaum,
Patricia A. Resick, and Victoria M. Follette

This chapter reviews the extant literature on cognitive-behavioral therapy (CBT) for chronic (duration of symptoms greater than 3 months) posttraumatic stress disorder (PTSD) among adults. Due to the strength of the literature base in this area, only published or "in press" empirical studies are included and only some studies are highlighted in the text. Based on this review, we offer suggestions regarding decision making for the use of CBT in the treatment of PTSD and future research. As in all of the chapters, the reader should consult the source documents or treatment manuals for more details.

Theoretical Context

CBT for PTSD encompasses numerous diverse techniques. Earlier therapies (systematic desensitization, relaxation training, biofeedback) focused primarily on Mowrer's (1960) two-factor theory of conditioned fear and operant avoidance. With the later development of other therapy procedures specifically focused on PTSD symptoms (prolonged exposure, stress inoculation training, cognitive therapy, cognitive processing therapy) emotional/ information-processing theories of PTSD predominated over learning theory. Social-cognitive theories focus on the content of cognitions within a social

139

context. Recently there have been efforts to integrate the two theories in Brewin's dual representation theory. There is supporting research evidence for all three theoretical approaches.

Contemporary learning theory attempts to account for much of the development and maintenance of the PTSD symptoms (Hayes, Follette, & Follette, 1995; Hayes, Wilson, Gifford, Follette, & Strosahl, 1996; Naugle & Follette, 1998). Reexperiencing and arousal symptoms are viewed as conditioned emotional responses that result from classical conditioning during the traumatic event, which are subsequently elicited by environmental stimuli. According to behavioral theory, although initial symptoms may be caused by the trauma, many current symptoms may represent attempts to manage trauma-induced distress. These attempts then respond to current situational contingencies and become functionally autonomous. Avoidance behaviors, behavioral excesses, and behavioral deficits are under operant control. Appropriate reinforcers in the environment may be lacking, or reinforcers may be ineffective or aversive. Clinical problems can also result from inappropriate stimulus control, whereby the response is appropriate but occurs under the wrong conditions. Problematic behavior is under the control of antecedent stimuli and reinforcing stimuli that affect the probability of the occurrence of the behavior. Thoughts, feelings, and physiological responses are classified as private events that can serve as antecedent stimuli or consequences. Therefore, as a result of applied behavior analysis, the focus for treatment may not necessarily be on the trauma itself, but on the maladaptive behavior that developed in the aftermath of the trauma. However, exposure to conditioned stimuli in the absence of the negative consequences is hypothesized to extinguish conditioned emotional reactions. Therefore, in behavioral theory, as well as information-processing theories, exposure is presumed to be the appropriate treatment for reexperiencing and arousal symptoms, whereas contingency management would be implemented for avoidance and other behavioral problems.

Emotional processing theory (Foa & Kozak, 1986) holds that PTSD emerges due to the development of a fear network in memory that elicits escape and avoidance behavior (Foa, Steketee, & Rothbaum, 1989). Mental fear structures include stimulus, responses, and meaning elements. Any information associated with the trauma is likely to activate the fear structure. The fear structure in people with PTSD is thought to include a particularly large number of stimulus elements; therefore, it is easily accessed. Attempts to avoid this activation result in the avoidance symptoms of PTSD. Emotional processing theory proposes that successful therapy involves correcting the pathological elements of the fear structure, and that this corrective process is the essence of emotional processing. Two conditions have been proposed to be required for fear reduction. First, the fear structure must be activated. Second, new information must be provided that includes elements incompatible with the existing pathological elements, so that they can be corrected. Exposure procedures consist of confronting the patient with trauma related information, thus activating the trauma memory. This activation constitutes an opportunity for the patient to integrate corrective information, thus modifying the pathological elements of the trauma memory. Of particular relevance to PTSD are studies demonstrating that fear activation during treatment promotes successful outcome (e.g., Foa, Riggs, Massie, & Yarczower, 1995; Pitman, Orr, Altman, & Longpre, 1996).

Several mechanisms are thought to be involved in the specific changes relevant to improvement of PTSD. First, repeated imaginal reliving of the trauma is thought to promote extinction of conditioned fear reactions (also called "habituation" in the theory), thus reducing anxiety previously associated with the trauma memory and correcting the patient's erroneous belief that anxiety stays forever unless avoidance or escape is realized. In fact, PTSD can be viewed as a failure of extinction to occur. Second, the process of deliberately confronting the feared memory blocks negative reinforcement of cognitive and behavioral avoidance of trauma-related thoughts, feelings, and reminders. Third, reliving the trauma in a therapeutic, supportive setting incorporates safety information into the trauma memory, thereby helping the patient to realize that remembering the trauma is not dangerous. Fourth, focusing on the trauma memory for a prolonged period helps the patient to differentiate the trauma event from other, nontraumatic events, thereby rendering the trauma as a specific occurrence rather than as a representation of a dangerous world and of an incompetent self. Fifth, the process of imaginal reliving helps to change the meaning of PTSD symptoms from being a sign of personal incompetence to one of mastery and courage. Sixth, prolonged, repeated reliving of the traumatic event affords the opportunity to focus on details central to negative self-evaluations, thereby allowing modification of those evaluations (Foa, Hembree, & Rothbaum, 2007). Many of these mechanisms also operate in exposure in vivo. However, the mechanisms most salient during in vivo exposure are the correction of erroneous probability estimates of danger and extinction of fearful responses to trauma-relevant stimuli.

The social-cognitive theories are also concerned with information processing, but they focus on the impact of trauma on a person's belief system and the adjustment that is necessary to reconcile the traumatic event with prior beliefs and expectations. These theories focus on a range of primary (fear, sadness, anger) and secondary (guilt, shame) emotions, and not just fear. They are the basis for cognitive therapies for PTSD. New information that is congruent with prior beliefs about self or world is assimilated quickly and without effort because the information matches schemas, and little attention is needed to incorporate it. However, when events occur that are schema-discrepant, individuals must reconcile the event with their beliefs about themselves and the world. Their schemas must be altered ("accommodation") to incorporate this new information. However, people often avoid this process because of the strong affect associated with the trauma and, frequently, because altering beliefs may leave people feeling more vulnerable to future traumatic events. Thus, rather than accommodating their beliefs to incorporate the trauma, victims may distort the trauma ("assimilation") to keep their beliefs intact.

An alternative to assimilation or accommodation is overaccommodation (Resick & Schnicke, 1992). In this case, trauma victims alter their belief structure to the extreme in an attempt to prevent future traumas. Overaccommodated beliefs may take the form of extreme distrust and poor regard for self and others. Prior traumatic events or negative preexisting beliefs contribute to "the evidence" that these extreme statements are true. Overaccommodated beliefs interfere with natural emotions that emanated from the event (e.g., fear, sadness), therefore preventing appropriate processing of the emotions and beliefs. Furthermore, overgeneralized negative statements can produce secondary emotions that originally might not have been associated with the event (e.g., shame, guilt). Given this social-cognitive model, affective expression is needed, not for habituation, but so that the trauma memory may be processed fully. It is assumed that natural affect, once accessed, will dissipate rather quickly, and that the work of accommodating the schemas with the new information can begin. Once faulty beliefs regarding the event and overaccommodated beliefs about oneself and the world are challenged, then secondary emotions also diminish, along with the intrusive reminders.

In an attempt to reconcile the theories of PTSD, Brewin, Dalgleish, and Joseph (1996) have proposed a dual representation theory that incorporates both the information-processing and social-cognitive theories. They proposed that sensory input is subject to both conscious and nonconscious processing. Dual representation theory describes two types of emotional reactions. One type, the primary reaction, is conditioned during the event (e.g., fear) and is activated along with reexperienced sensory and physiological information. Other, secondary, emotional reactions (e.g., anger, guilt) result from the consequences and implications of the trauma. Brewin and colleagues propose that emotional processing of the trauma has two elements: the activation of nonconscious memories (as suggested by the information-processing theories) and the conscious attempt to search for meaning, ascribe cause or blame, and to resolve conflicts between the event and prior expectations and beliefs. The goal of this process is to reduce the negative emotions and to restore a sense of relative safety and control in one's environment. This theory suggests that both exposure and cognitive therapy may be needed in some cases.

Description of Techniques

Seven different cognitive-behavioral treatments for PTSD are reviewed. A brief description of each treatment is provided below. The techniques are exposure therapy (EX), stress inoculation training (SIT), cognitive processing therapy (CPT), cognitive therapy (CT), relaxation training (RLX), dialectical behavior therapy (DBT), and acceptance and commitment therapy (ACT). In addition, many studies have evaluated treatments that combine elements of two or more of the preceding treatments, such as EX combined with SIT or CT. The previous edition of this volume (Rothbaum, Meadows, Resick, & Foy, 2000) included a review of the literature on systematic desensitization, assertiveness training, and biofeedback. Because there was very limited research support for these techniques at the time and no new, relevant research has been published since, we have not included them in this chapter.

Exposure Therapy

A variety of terms have been used to describe prolonged exposure to anxiety-provoking stimuli without relaxation or other anxiety-reducing methods. These include "flooding," "imaginal," *in vivo*, and "directed"; in this chapter, these are referred to collectively as "exposure therapy" (EX). EX typically begins with the development of an anxiety hierarchy. In some forms of EX (e.g., flooding), treatment sessions are begun with exposure to the highest rated item on the hierarchy; others begin with items rated as moderately anxiety-provoking. EX methods share the common feature of confrontation with frightening yet realistically safe stimuli that continues until the anxiety is reduced. By continuing to expose oneself to a frightening stimulus, anxiety diminishes, leading to a decrease in the escape and avoidance behaviors maintained via negative reinforcement (Mowrer, 1960). A more recent conceptualization of EX's mechanism of action was put forth by Foa and Kozak (1986), with the introduction of emotional processing theory for anxiety disorders in general, and by Foa and Rothbaum (1998) for PTSD in particular.

As noted earlier, there are several variants of EX. In imaginal exposure, patients confront their memories of the traumatic event. In some imaginal methods (e.g., Foa, Rothbaum, Riggs, & Murdock, 1991; Foa et al., 1999), patients provide their own narrative by discussing the trauma in detail in the present tense for prolonged periods of time (e.g., 45–60 minutes), with prompting by the therapist for omitted details. In other forms of imaginal exposure (e.g., Cooper & Clum, 1989; Keane, Fairbank, Caddell, & Zimering, 1989), the therapist presents a scene to the patient based on information gathered prior to the exposure exercise. Duration and number of exposure sessions have also varied, sometimes within the same study. Finally, most exposure treatments do not consist solely of exposure but include other components, such as psychoeducation or relaxation training. Some treatments that combine such components spend vastly more time on exposure than on these other components, which are often presented as preliminary ways of building up to the exposure. In such cases, we treat the program as a form of EX. Other treatments combine EX with more extensive use of the other elements, in which case we treat them as a combined (COMB) treatment. An exception is cognitive processing therapy, which in its original form is a combined treatment. But because it is a specific protocol that has been researched and can be implemented with or without the narrative accounts, we consider it separately from the combined treatments. Details on the implementation of exposure for PTSD are provided in Foa and colleagues (2007).

Stress Inoculation Training

Stress inoculation training (SIT) was developed by Meichenbaum (1974) as an anxiety management treatment. It was later modified by Kilpatrick, Veronen, and Resick (1982) to treat rape survivors, although this was prior to widespread use of the PTSD diagnosis to describe postrape symptomatology. The modified SIT program included education, muscle relaxation training, breathing retraining, role playing, covert modeling, guided self-dialogue, graduated *in vivo* exposure, and thought stopping. Some studies did not include some of the original SIT strategies, such as *in vivo* exposure, because these were included in the comparison treatments. The rationale underlying SIT focuses on anxiety that becomes conditioned at the time of the trauma and generalizes to many situations. Patients learn to manage this anxiety by using these new skills, thus decreasing avoidance and anxiety.

Cognitive Processing Therapy

Cognitive processing therapy (CPT), developed by Resick and Schnicke (1993), originally targeted rape-related PTSD in a group format. It incorporates elements of cognitive therapy (CT) and exposure, although it is predominantly a cognitive therapy. The trauma-focused CT component includes training to challenge problematic cognitions, particularly selfblame and attempts mentally to undo the traumatic event. Patients are asked first to challenge assimilated beliefs regarding the event itself, using the skills obtained in challenging thoughts and beliefs, and later to work on overgeneralized beliefs emanating from the rape. Among them are beliefs about safety, trust, power/control, esteem, and intimacy (McCann & Pearlman, 1990). The exposure component consists of writing a detailed account of the trauma and reading it back in the presence of the therapist and at home. Aside from the expression of affect, the account is used to generate the patient's "stuck points," moments during the assault that cause conflict with previously held beliefs or are particularly hard to accept. These points receive particular attention during CT. CPT has subsequently been applied to other trauma populations and has been studied as an individual or group treatment with or without the written accounts.

Cognitive Therapy

Cognitive therapy (CT) was initially developed by Beck and colleagues (Beck, 1976; Beck, Rush, Shaw, & Emery, 1979) to treat depression, then further developed as a treatment for anxiety and other disorders (Beck, Emery, & Greenberg, 1985; Clark, 1986). CT is based on Beck's (1976) theory that the interpretation of an event, rather than the event itself, is what determines emotional states. Thus, interpretations that are negatively biased lead to negative emotions. These erroneous or unhelpful interpretations are generally referred to as automatic ("dysfunctional") thoughts and are typically seen as either inaccurate or as too extreme for the situation that prompted them. Cognitive therapy aims to modify automatic thoughts. This occurs in steps wherein patients are taught to identify these dysfunctional thoughts, to challenge those thoughts evaluated as inaccurate or unhelpful, and finally to replace them with more logical or beneficial thoughts. Much attention is paid to trauma survivors' appraisals of safety/danger, trust, and views of themselves, which serve to maintain a continued sense of current threat (Ehlers & Clark, 2000).

Relaxation Training

Relaxation training (RLX) has been used to treat PTSD as part of a comprehensive program, such as SIT, and as a primary intervention used as a comparison condition for other treatments. As with other anxiety management methods, such as SIT, RLX is intended to provide a way for patients to reduce anxiety that may be elicited by trauma-related stimuli.

Dialectical Behavior Therapy

Dialectical behavior therapy (DBT; Linehan, 1993), a treatment approach first developed as an intervention for chronically suicidal people meeting criteria for borderline personality disorder (BPD), has subsequently been applied to other conditions. Within the DBT framework, the psychopathology associated with the diagnosis of BPD is conceptualized as the result of an interaction between biological factors that contribute to intense, long-lasting emotional reactions to environmental events and experiential factors, particularly an invalidating environment during childhood, that lead to deficits in emotion regulation skills. Because many individuals with PTSD also experience many of the difficulties associated with BPD, and many individuals with BPD also have PTSD, proponents have suggested that DBT may be useful in the treatment of PTSD and have advanced two approaches to applying DBT to PTSD (Wagner & Linehan, 2006). The first approach would be to utilize DBT as the primary intervention, in a manner similar to how it is implemented to treat BPD. The second approach would be to provide DBT skills training to facilitate the tolerability and efficacy of subsequent trauma-focused treatment, such as EX.

One of the distinguishing features of DBT is the explicit application of "dialectical theory," the recognition of the oppositional nature of reality (thesis–antithesis). The most important dialectical tension is between acceptance of the patient as he or she is and recognition of the need or desirability for change (Wagner & Linehan, 2006). Recognition of the tension between acceptance and change guides both conceptualization and technique selection; some interventions are designed to promote acceptance, whereas others foster change.

Acceptance and Commitment Therapy

Acceptance and commitment therapy (ACT) is theoretically based on an analysis of language from the perspective of functional contextualism (Follette, Palm, & Hall, 2004; Hayes, 1987; Hayes & Wilson, 1994). A central tenent of ACT (Hayes, Strosahl, & Wilson, 1999) is that much of human suffering is brought about by "experiential avoidance," the attempt to prevent or modify unwanted private experiences (e.g., the reexperiencing symptoms of PTSD). Such attempts are generally not very effective and, paradoxically, may result in more of the very thoughts and emotions the person was attempting to avoid. Faced with such failures, the person may then resort to increasingly dysfunctional means to achieve experiential avoidance (e.g., social isolation, substance abuse). Because the very attempt to control internal experiences is thought to be the problem from the ACT perspective, interventions are designed instead to promote the person's acceptance of internal experiences, whatever they might be, while acting in accord with his or her values.

Method of Collecting Data

We gathered information via PsychLIT, PsychINFO, and Published International Literature on Traumatic Stress (PILOTS) searches and analyzed relevant reference lists from articles, chapters, and books, and personal communication with PTSD researchers. We then examined individual studies to judge their methodology according to the nine features of well-controlled studies described in the introductory chapter (Foa, Keane, Friedman, & Cohen, Chapter 1, this volume) and added the results to the comprehensive summary. The methods and primary results are summarized in Table 7.1 for randomized controlled studies and in Table 7.2 for nonrandomized studies.

Seven of the features of well-controlled studies—(1) clearly defined target symptoms; (2) reliable and valid measures; (3) use of blind evaluators; (4) assessor training; (5) manualized, replicable, specific treatment programs; (6) unbiased assignment to treatment; and (7) treatment adherence—correspond to the "gold standards" for clinical research (Foa & Meadows, 1997) established in the previous edition of this volume and continue to serve as the core features addressed in our methodological critique of studies in the current review. The two added features, intent to treat (ITT) data analyses and "equipoise" or comparability of treatment conditions regarding therapist background and experience, allegiance, training, and supervision for all

Text continues on page 189

TABLE 7.1. Summary of Randomized Controlled Trials of CBT for PTSD

Study	Target population[a]	Time posttrauma and length of sessions	Treatment(s)/control[b]	Main outcome measure	Major findings	Within-group effect size (Hedges unbiased g)	Between-group effect size (Hedges unbiased g)
Basoglu et al. (2006)	31 male and female earthquake survivors with PTSD in Turkey	Study conducted between 12/2003 and 8/2005; earthquake occurred in 1999 (4–6 yr) Single-session treatment comprised 60 min of psychoeducation, rationale, and self-exposure instructions, followed by exposure in an earthquake simulator, lasting a mean of 33 min	*Intent to treat* (ITT) EX = 16 WL = 15	Clinician-Administered PTSD Scale (CAPS)	Intervention group statistically superior to control group on measures of PTSD, anxiety, depression, and functioning at assessments conducted 4 and 8 wk posttreatment; treatment gains maintained at follow-up 1–2 yr posttreatment	EX: 1.58 WL: 0.48	EX vs. WL: 0.86
Basoglu et al. (2005)	59 male and female earthquake survivors in Turkey	Study conducted between 2/2002 and 1/2004; index trauma occurred on 8/17/1999 (3–4 yr) Single-session treatment, a form of self-directed *in vivo* EX, was conducted in 1 session, 60 min in duration	*Intent to treat* EX = 31 WL = 28	CAPS	Intervention group statistically superior to control group on measures of PTSD, anxiety, depression, and functioning at assessments conducted 6 wk posttreatment; treatment gains maintained at follow-up 1–2 yr posttreatment	EX: 1.09 WL: 0.32	EX vs. WL: 0.44

(continued)

TABLE 7.1. (continued)

Study	Target population[a]	Time posttrauma and length of sessions	Treatment(s)/ control[b]	Main outcome measure	Major findings	Within-group effect size (Hedges unbiased g)	Between-group effect size (Hedges unbiased g)
Beck et al. (in press)	44 male and female survivors of motor vehicle accidents (MVAs) with chronic PTSD	Mean time since the index MVA was 52.9 months (median = 15.5 mo). Group COMB treatment was administered in 14 weekly sessions, 120 min each; WL participants received a telephone call every four weeks for the 14-week period	*Completers* COMB = 17 WL = 16	CAPS	Intervention group statistically superior to control group on measures of PTSD but not depression, anxiety, physical functioning, or pain severity; treatment gains were maintained at follow-up 3 mo posttreatment	COMB: 1.55 WL: 0.38	COMB vs. WL: 0.85
Bichescu et al. (2007)	18 male and female Romanian political detainees randomly selected from a larger sample from a previous study (Bichescu et al., 2005)	Average period of time elapsed since release from detention was 42.0 yr Narrative EX comprised 5 treatment sessions with a time period of 10 wk; sessions were weekly/ biweekly and 120 min per session; psychoeducation (EDU) comprised 1 session	*Intent to treat* EX = 9 EDU = 9	Composite International Diagnostic Interview— PTSD Module (CIDI-PTSD)	Intervention group statistically superior to control group on measures of PTSD and depression at assessment conducted 6 mo posttreatment	EX: 4.18 EDU: 0.40	EX vs. EDU: 1.41
Blanchard et al. (2003)	98 male and female survivors of MVAs with chronic PTSD (81) or subthreshold PTSD (17)	Target MVA occurred minimum of 6 mo prior to pretreatment evaluation Both CBT (COMB) and supportive counseling (SC) had a range of 8–12 weekly individual sessions (60 min each), averaging 9.8 sessions for COMB and 10.0 for SC	*Completers* COMB = 27 SC = 27 WL = 24	CAPS	On the CAPS, COMB treatment was superior to SC and WL in the ITT completers analyses; SC was superior to WL for completers analysis. COMB treatment was also superior to SC and WL on measures of depression and anxiety, and resulted in greater reduction in incidence of major depressive disorder	COMB: 1.79 SC: 0.95 WL: 0.43	COMB vs. WL: 1.14 SC vs. WL: 0.53 COMB vs. SC: 0.62

Study	Sample	Procedure	Completers	Measures	Results	Effect size
					(MDD) and generalized anxiety disorder (GAD) diagnoses. Treatment gains were maintained at 3-mo follow-up. Reanalysis of CAPS ITT data indicated that COMB was superior to SC and WL, and a trend for SC to be superior to WL.	—
Boudewyns & Hyer (1990)	51 male inpatient Vietnam War veterans	Study conducted between 12/1/1986 and 3/1/1988, veterans served in Southeast Asia theater between 8/5/1964 and 5/7/1975, as determined by the Medical Administration Service at the Augusta VA Medical Center (11–24 yr since service) EX was administered in 12–14 sessions, 50 min each; the control condition received treatment as usual (TAU)	*Completers* EX = 19 TAU = 19	*Physiological measures* Facial EMG, heart rate, skin conductance level *Psychological measures* MMPI, Veterans Adjustment Scale (VET), Mississippi Scale (MISS)	Means and standard deviations of PTSD measures not reported, therefore effect sizes (ESs) were not calculated. At follow-up, participants who displayed decreased physiological responding also showed improvement on community adjustment measures of anxiety/depression, alienation, vigor, and confidence in skills.	—
Bradley & Follingstad (2003)	49 incarcerated women with histories of childhood sexual abuse (CSA) and/ or physical abuse	Time since trauma not reported Group therapy comprising 9 sessions (2.5 hr each) of DBT exercises followed by 9 sessions focused on structured writing assignments, including description of trauma and impact on life	*Completers* DBT/EX = 13 WL = 18	Trauma Symptom Inventory (TSI)	Intervention group statistically superior to control group on 6 out of 7 TSI subscales (Depression, Anxious Arousal, Intrusive Experiences, Anger and Irritability, Dissociation, Impaired Self-Reference; no difference on Defensive Avoidance)	Intrusion DBT/EX: 0.96 WL: −0.16 Avoidance DBT/EX: 0.73 WL: 0.31 Intrusion DBT/EX vs. WL: 0.45 Avoidance DBT/EX vs. WL: −0.05

(continued)

149

TABLE 7.1. (continued)

Study	Target population[a]	Time posttrauma and length of sessions	Treatment(s)/ control[b]	Main outcome measure	Major findings	Within-group effect size (Hedges unbiased g)	Between-group effect size (Hedges unbiased g)
Bryant et al. (2003)	58 male and female survivors of physical assault (31) and MVAs (27)	Minimum of 3 mo since trauma Treatment with EX, EX plus CT (COMB), and SC comprised 8 weekly 90-min sessions	*Intent to treat* EX = 20 COMB = 20 SC = 18 *Completers* EX = 15 COMB = 15 SC = 15	CAPS	No differences among groups for ITT analyses. For completers analyses, EX superior to SC on PTSD (CAPS Intensity but not Frequency; IES Intrusions and Avoidance) and anxiety. COMB superior to SC on PTSD (CAPS Intensity and Frequency; IES Intrusions and Avoidance), depression, anxiety, and trauma-related cognitions. COMB superior to EX on IES Intrusions and Depression. Treatment gains were maintained at 6-mo follow-up.	*Intent to treat* Intensity EX: 1.31 COMB: 1.52 SC: 0.39 Frequency EX: 1.40 COMB: 1.46 SC: 0.60 *Completers* Intensity EX: 1.97 COMB: 2.46 SC: 0.75 Frequency EX: 2.03 COMB: 2.33 SC: 1.11	*Intent to treat* Intensity EX vs. SC: 0.65 COMB vs. SC: 0.83 EX vs. COMB: −0.26 Frequency EX vs. SC: 0.63 COMB vs. SC: 0.78 EX vs. COMB: −0.23 *Completers* Intensity EX vs. SC: 0.83 COMB vs. SC: 1.14 EX vs. COMB: −0.47 Frequency EX vs. SC: 0.76 COMB vs. SC: 1.10 EX vs. COMB: −0.44

Study	Sample	Treatment	Completers	Measures	Findings	Effect sizes	
Chard (2005)	71 women with PTSD from at least one episode of CSA	All index traumas occurred in childhood; the average age of participants was 32.8 yr

Cognitive processing therapy (CPT) for sexual abuse survivors was conducted in 17 wk individual and group therapy, with patients attending a 90-min group session each week and 60-min individual sessions for the first 9 wk and at week 17 | *Completers* CPT = 28 WL = 27 | CAPS | Intervention was superior to WL on measures of PTSD, depression, and dissociation. Treatment gains were maintained at 3- and 12-mo follow-up. | CPT: 2.75 WL: 0.19 | CPT vs. WL: 2.32 |
| Chemtob et al. (1997) | 28 male Vietnam War veterans with PTSD and clinically elevated anger scores | Time since trauma not reported

Stress inoculation training (SIT) for anger administered in 12 sessions, 60 min each | *Completers* SIT (anger) = 8 TAU = 7 | CAPS, Spielberger Anger Expression Scale (Ang-Ex) | Intervention was superior to TAU on measures of anger expression, depression, and frequency of PTSD reexperiencing symptoms. Treatment gains on anger were maintained at 1.5 yr posttreatment. | Ang-Ex SIT: 1.29 TAU: 0.08 | Ang-Ex SIT vs. TAU: 0.73 |
| Cloitre et al. (2002) | 58 women with PTSD related to CSA, physical abuse, or both | All index traumas occurred in childhood; the average age of participants was 34 yr | *Completers* DBT/EX = 22 WL = 24 | CAPS, Modified PTSD Symptom Scale Self-Report (MPSS-SR) | At the end of treatment, intervention was superior to WL on measures of PTSD, negative mood regulation, anger | Overall CAPS DBT/EX: 1.76 WL: 0.35 | Overall CAPS DBT/EX vs. WL: 1.27 |

(continued)

TABLE 7.1. (continued)

Study	Target population[a]	Time posttrauma and length of sessions	Treatment(s)/ control[b]	Main outcome measure	Major findings	Within-group effect size (Hedges unbiased g)	Between-group effect size (Hedges unbiased g)
Cloitre et al. (2002) (cont.)		Treatment comprised 16 individual sessions conducted over 12 wk. Skills training in affect and interpersonal *regulation*, based on DBT, comprised 8 weekly sessions, 60 min each; followed by imaginal EX, comprised 8 twice-weekly sessions, 90-min each.			expression, dissociation, alexithymia, depression, anxiety, social adjustment, and social support. Treatment gains were maintained or further gains obtained at follow-up 3- and 9-mo posttreatment. Reanalysis of ITT data revealed the same pattern of results. At the end of initial DBT, intervention was superior to WL on measures of negative mood regulation, anger expression, depression, and anxiety	MPSS-SR DBT/EX: 1.72 WL: 0.61 DBT only MPSS-SR DBT/EX: 0.40 WL: 0.27	MPSS-SR DBT/EX vs. WL: 1.01 DBT only MPSS-SR DBT/EX vs. WL: 0.23
Cooper & Clum (1989)	22 male Vietnam War combat veterans	Time since trauma not reported Treatment comprised once or twice weekly EX, up to 14 sessions, 90 min each, added to TAU; TAU was weekly individual therapy sessions, 60 min each, plus weekly group therapy sessions, 120 min each.	*Completers* EX = 7 TAU = 7	Hours of sleep/week, nightmares/ week, subjective anxiety during Behavioral Avoidance Task (BAT)	No standardized measures of PTSD administered; therefore ESs were not computed. Intervention was superior to TAU on measures of anxiety, sleep disturbances, nightmares, and subject anxiety during BAT. Treatment gains were maintained at follow-up 3-mo posttreatment.	—	—

152

Study	Sample	Treatment	N	Measures	Outcome	Effect size	Effect size
Davis & Wright (2007)	43 men and women who experienced a traumatic event and were having nightmares at least 1 time a week for the previous 3 mo; 27 (63%) met full criteria for PTSD	Time since trauma was not reported Three weekly sessions of exposure, relaxation, and rescripting therapy (ERRT; a COMB treatment), 120 min each. The treatment can be administered in either individual or group format, but treatment format for the present study is not reported.	*Intent to treat* COMB = 21 WL = 22 *Completers* COMB = 17 WL = 15	MPSS-SR, Pittsburgh Sleep Quality Index (PSQI)	Intervention was superior to WL on measures of PTSD, nightmares, sleep quality, and depression in both ITT and completers analyses. Treatment gains for completers were maintained at follow-up 3- and 6-mo posttreatment.	*Intent to treat* MPSS-SR COMB: 0.37 WL: −0.07 PSQI COMB: 0.64 WL: 0.23 *Completers* MPSS-SR COMB: 0.47 WL: −0.10 PSQI COMB: 0.90 WL: 0.35	*Intent to treat* MPSS-SR COMB vs. WL: 0.52 PSQI COMB vs. WL: 0.24 *Completers* MPSS-SR COMB vs. WL: 0.38 PSQI COMB vs. WL: 0.22
Difede, Cukor, et al. (2007)	21 men and women with PTSD related the September 11, 2001, terrorist attacks on the World Trade Center	Study was conducted between 2/2002 and 8/2005, minimum of 5 mo and maximum of 4 yr since trauma Number of weekly virtual reality–assisted EX sessions was flexible, up to 14 sessions, 75 min each; mean number of EX sessions was 7.5 (range = 6–13).	*Completers* EX = 10 WL = 8	CAPS	Intervention was superior to WL on PTSD but not depression. Additional analyses of PTSD scores indicates intervention was superior to WL for reexperiencing and avoidance/numbing but not hyperarousal. Treatment gains were maintained as follow-up 6-mo posttreatment.	EX: 0.95 WL: −0.28	EX. vs. WL: 1.60

(continued)

TABLE 7.1. (continued)

Study	Target population[a]	Time posttrauma and length of sessions	Treatment(s)/control[b]	Main outcome measure	Major findings	Within-group effect size (Hedges unbiased g)	Between-group effect size (Hedges unbiased g)
Difede, Malta, et al. (2007)	31 male and female disaster workers exposed to the September 11, 2001, terrorist attack on the World Trade Center or its aftermath meeting criteria for PTSD (21) or subthreshold (10) PTSD	Mean time since the attack was 21.2 mo. The COMB of EX plus SIT was administered in 12 weekly sessions, 75 min each. For TAU, participants were referred back to their original referral source.	*Intent to treat* COMB = 15 TAU = 16 *Completers* COMB = 7 TAU = 14	CAPS	No differences between intervention and TAU in the ITT analysis; intervention was superior to TAU on measures of PTSD, but not depression or alcohol consumption, among completers.	*Intent to treat* COMB: 0.52 TAU: 0.12 *Completers* COMB: 1.51 TAU: 0.14	*Intent to treat* COMB vs. TAU: 0.34 *Completers* COMB vs. TAU: 1.31
Duffy et al. (2007)	58 men and women with PTSD related to terrorism and civil conflict in Northern Ireland	Median time since index traumatic event was 8 yr for CT group and 5.4 yr for WL. The number of CT sessions was flexible, up to 12 weekly sessions, 90 min for the first session and 60 min for subsequent sessions, followed by a review and additional sessions if clinically warranted; mean of 7.8 sessions, 5.9 within the first 12 wk	*Intent to treat* CT = 29 WL = 29	Posttraumatic Stress Diagnostic Scale (PDS)	Intervention was superior to WL on measures of PTSD, depression, and social functioning in both ITT and completers analyses. Treatment gains were maintained at follow-up, up to 1 yr posttreatment.	CT: 1.10 WL: 0.35	CT vs. WL: 0.88

154

			Intent to treat / Completers	Scale of Severity of PTSD			
Echeburúa et al. (1997)	20 women with PTSD from either rape in adulthood (11) or CSA (9)	Mean time since trauma for rape survivors was 3.25 yr, for survivors of CSA mean time since trauma was 9.5 yr COMB of EX plus CT was conducted in weekly sessions over a 6-wk period for a total of 7 hr. RLX was also conducted in weekly sessions over 6 wk for a total of 4.15 hr.	*Intent to treat* COMB = 10 RLX = 10	Scale of Severity of PTSD—Interview	Intervention was superior to RLX on PTSD at posttreatment and 3-, 6-, and 12-mo follow-up; intervention was superior to RLX on depression at 12-mo follow-up.	COMB: 3.63 RLX: 1.66	COMB vs. RLX:1.44
Ehlers et al. (2003)	97 male and female MVA survivors entered a 3-wk self-monitoring phase; 85 participants still meeting PTSD randomized to study conditions	Self-monitoring began approximately 4 wk after MVA, study conditions began approximately 7 wk after MVA. CT was administered in up to 12 weekly sessions, 90 min for the first session and 60 min for subsequent sessions, plus up to 3 monthly booster sessions, 60 min each; patients received an average of 9 sessions and 2.4 booster sessions. In the self-help booklet (SELF) condition, participants received a self-help booklet and met with a therapist one time for 40 min.	*Completers* CT = 28 SELF = 25 WL = 27	CAPS	Intervention was superior to SELF and WL on measures of PTSD, depression, and anxiety both immediately posttreatment and at 9-mo follow-up. No differences between SELF and WL.	Frequency CT: 2.04 SELF: 0.87 WL: 0.58 Distress CT: 1.92 SELF: 0.85 WL: 0.31	Frequency CT vs. WL: 1.22 SELF vs. WL: 0.21 CT vs. SELF: 0.99 Distress CT vs. WL: 1.12 SELF vs. WL: 0.26 CT vs. SELF: 1.01

(continued)

TABLE 7.1. (continued)

Study	Target population[a]	Time posttrauma and length of sessions	Treatment(s)/control[b]	Main outcome measure	Major findings	Within-group effect size (Hedges unbiased g)	Between-group effect size (Hedges unbiased g)
Ehlers et al. (2005)	28 men and women with PTSD following civilian traumas, primarily MVAs (15)	Minimum time since trauma was 6 mo; median time since trauma was 11.5 mo for CT and 10.8 months for WL CT was administered in 4–12 weekly sessions, 90 min for the first session and 60 min for subsequent sessions, plus up to 3 monthly booster sessions, 60 min each; patients received an average of 10 weekly sessions and 2.9 booster sessions.	*Intent to treat* CT = 14 WL = 14 CAPS	CAPS	Intervention was superior to WL on measures of PTSD, depression, anxiety, and social functioning. Treatment gains were maintained at follow-up 3-mo posttreatment.	Frequency CT: 2.04 WL: −0.38 Distress CT: 1.91 WL: −0.20	Frequency CT vs. WL: 1.40 Distress CT vs. WL: 1.43
Falsetti et al. (2001)	22 women with comorbid PTSD and panic attacks	Minimum time since trauma was 3 mo Multiple-channel exposure therapy, a COMB of CPT and panic control treatment, was administered in a group format consisting of 12 weekly sessions, 90 min each.	*Completers* COMB = 12 WL = 15 (5 WL patients received delayed treatment and their results were included as part of the 12 COMB condition)	CAPS, Panic Module of the Anxiety Disorders Interview Schedule (ADIS-P), Physical Reactions Scale (PRS)	Means and/or standard deviations for outcome measures were not reported; ESs therefore could not be computed. Intervention was superior to WL on PTSD: Fewer subjects receiving COMB met criteria for PTSD following treatment (8.3%) than WL (66.7%). Intervention was also superior to WL on panic frequency (50% panic free vs. 6.7%), panic symptoms, and depression.	—	—

Study	Sample	N	Measure	Results	Within effect sizes	Between effect sizes
Fecteau & Nicki (1999)	23 men and women with PTSD following MVAs	*Completers* COMB = 10 WL = 10	CAPS	Intervention was superior to WL on measures of PTSD and anxiety, but not depression. Treatment gains were maintained at follow-up 3 and 6 mo posttreatment.	COMB: 1.31 WL: 0.11	COMB vs. WL: 1.28
	For the 20 completers, mean time since the accident was 18.8 mon (range 3–95 mo) COMB was administered in 4 weekly sessions, range 90–180 min each					
Foa et al. (1999)	96 female sexual and non-sexual-assault survivors with PTSD	*Completers* EX = 23 SIT=19 EX/SIT = 22 WL=15	PTSD Symptom Scale Interview (PSS-I)	In the ITT analysis, EX was superior to WL on measures of PTSD, depression and anxiety; SIT and EX/SIT were superior to WL on measures of PTSD and depression. In the completer analyses, all three treatments were superior to WL on PTSD, depression, and anxiety. Comparisons among treatments revealed that EX was superior to SIT on anxiety (ITT analysis), EX/SIT on depression (ITT analysis), EX/SIT on depression (ITT analysis) and anxiety (ITT analysis and completers analyses).	EX: 2.00 SIT: 1.83 COMB: 1.95 WL: 0.80	EX vs. WL: 1.91 SIT vs. WL: 1.57 COMB vs. WL: 1.45 EX vs. SIT: 0.14 EX vs. COMB: 0.22 SIT vs. COMB: 0.07
	Time since trauma not reported Treatments were administered in 9 twice-weekly sessions, 2 sessions of 120 min each and 7 sessions of 90 min each					
Foa et al. (2005)	179 female sexual and non-sexual-assault or CSA survivors	*Intent to treat* EX = 79 EX/CT = 74 WL = 26	PSS-I	In the ITT analyses, EX and EX/CT were each superior to WL on measures of PTSD and depression, but there were no differences between treatments. In the	*Intent to treat* EX: 1.45 COMB: 1.30 WL: 0.79	*Intent to treat* EX vs. WL: 0.66 COMB vs. WL: 0.80 EX vs. COMB: –0.08
	Minimum time since trauma was 3 mo, mean time was 9 yr Treatments were administered in 9–12 weekly sessions, 90–120 min each. Participants showing					

(continued)

TABLE 7.1. (continued)

Study	Target population[a]	Time posttrauma and length of sessions	Treatment(s)/control[b]	Main outcome measure	Major findings	Within-group effect size (Hedges unbiased g)	Between-group effect size (Hedges unbiased g)
Foa et al. (2005) (cont.)		a reduction of self-reported PTSD of ≥ 70% by Session 8 terminated treatment at Session 9; others were offered additional sessions, to a maximum of 12.	Completers EX = 52 EX/CT = 44 WL = 25		completer analyses, EX and EX/CT were superior to WL on measures of PTSD, depression, and social functioning, but there were no differences between treatments. Forty treatment completers (42%) terminated by session 9, 56 (58%) received additional sessions. Participants receiving additional sessions showed further improvement on self-reported PTSD from Session 8 to endpoint.	Completers EX: 3.31 COMB: 2.35 WL: 0.84	Completers EX vs. WL: 1.92 COMB vs. WL: 0.80 EX vs. COMB: 0.00
Foa et al. (1991)	55 female rape survivors	Minimum time since trauma was 3 mo; mean time was 6.2 yr Treatments were administered in 9 twice-weekly sessions, 90 min each.	Completers EX = 10 SIT = 14 SC = 11 WL = 10	PSS-I	All conditions showed significant improvement from pre- to posttreatment on measures of PTSD, depression, and anxiety. SIT was superior to SC and WL on PTSD. There were no differences between EX and SIT. Treatment gains were maintained at follow-up.	EX: 1.16 SIT: 2.39 SC: 0.88 WL: 0.78	EX vs. WL: 0.42 SIT vs. WL: 1.48 SC vs. WL: 0.19 EX vs. SIT: −0.54 EX vs. SC: 0.28 SIT vs. SC: 1.22

Study	Sample	Treatment details	N / Design	Measures	Results		
Frank et al. (1988)	167 women, 138 survivors of sexual assault and 29 nonvictimized controls; 99 sought immediate treatment, 39 sought delayed treatment; treatment participants were also compared with a repeated assessment condition from a separate sample (see Kilpatrick & Calhoun, 1988).	Average length of time for the "immediate" treatment seekers since assault was 20.1 days. Average time for the "delayed" treatment seekers was 128.7 days. Both CT and systematic desensitization (SD) were implemented in a 14-wk period.	*Completers* Immediate treatment (60): CT = 34 SD = 26 Delayed treatment (24): CT = 14 SD = 10	Beck Depression Inventory (BDI), State–Trait Anxiety Inventory— State Anxiety (STAI-S), Fear Survey Schedule (FSS)	No standardized measures of PTSD were administered; therefore ESs were not computed. SC and CT were superior to repeated assessment at posttreatment; no differences between treatments.	—	—
Frommberger et al. (2004)	21 men and women with chronic PTSD following civilian traumas	Mean time since trauma was 34 mo. COMB treatment was administered in 12 weekly sessions, 90–120 min each. Paroxetine (PAR) began at 10 mg/day and was increased to a maximum of 50 mg/day, with a mean maximum dose of 28 mg/day.	*Intent to treat* COMB = 10 PAR = 11	CAPS	Both interventions showed significant improvement on measures of PTSD, depression, and anxiety, with no differences between treatments. At follow-up, all COMB participants showed further numerical improvement, whereas some PAR participants showed numerical worsening, attributed by the researchers to the occurrence of adverse events.	COMB: 2.91 PAR: 2.18	COMB vs. PAR: 0.09

(continued)

TABLE 7.1. *(continued)*

Study	Target population[a]	Time posttrauma and length of sessions	Treatment(s)/control[b]	Main outcome measure	Major findings	Within-group effect size (Hedges unbiased g)	Between-group effect size (Hedges unbiased g)
Gersons et al. (2000)	42 male and female Dutch police officers with a primary diagnosis of PTSD	Mean time since trauma for the COMB group was 3 yr; mean time for the WL group was 5 yr. Brief eclectic psychotherapy, a form of COMB treatment, was implemented in 16 weekly sessions, 60 min each.	*Intent to treat* COMB = 22 WL = 20	Structured Interview for PTSD (SIP), translated into Dutch	Means and standard deviations for SIP were not reported; therefore ESs were not computed. Significantly fewer participants in COMB met criteria for PTSD at posttreatment (9%) and follow-up (4%) 3 mo following treatment than in WL (50% and 65% at posttreatment and follow-up, respectively).	—	—
Glynn et al. (1999)	42 male Vietnam War veterans with combat-related PTSD	Time since trauma not reported. COMB treatment (EX plus CT) was to be administered in 18 individual twice-weekly sessions, 90 min each (average of 17.6 session); after COMB treatment, some participants received 16 sessions of behavioral family therapy (BFT) that included the presence of one family member, 60 min each (average of 15.6 sessions). The WL condition was continued for 2 mo.	*Completers* COMB = 13 COMB/BFT = 12 WL = 17	Used factor analysis to construct separate indices of positive symptoms (SX+; e.g., reexperiencing and hypervigilence), and negative symptoms (SX–; e.g., avoidance and numbing).	The factor analysis was conducted on responses to the CAPS, Mississippi Scale for Military PTSD (M-PTSD), and IES. At the end of the EX phase, both CBT conditions were superior to WL on PTSD positive symptoms, but not negative symptoms. The addition of BFT resulted in superior results on a measure of problem solving compared to COMB alone.	SX+ COMB: 0.28 COMB/BFT: 0.68 WL: –0.08 SX– COMB: 0.66 COMB/BFT: 0.37 WL: 0.20	SX+ COMB vs. WL: 0.83 COMB/BFT vs. WL: 0.64 COMB vs. COMB/BFT: 0.07 SX– COMB vs. WL: 0.74 COMB/BFT vs. WL: 0.44 COMB vs. COMB/BFT: 0.19

160

| Hinton et al. (2005) | 40 male and female Cambodian refugees meeting criteria for PTSD and current neck-focused or orthostasis-triggered panic attacks; all participants had PTSD despite a minimum of 1 yr of treatment with an adequate dose of an SSRI medication plus supportive counseling. | Index traumas occurred in Cambodia between 1975 and 1979.

A COMB program, which incorporated interoceptive exposure, as well as imaginal and *in vivo* EX, CT, and SIT, was administered in 11 weekly sessions, duration of sessions not reported. Medication regimen was maintained constant during the study. | *Intent to treat* COMB = 20 WL = 20 | CAPS, Anxiety Sensitivity Index (ASI) | Intervention was superior to WL on measures of PTSD, anxiety sensitivity, neck- and orthostatic-focused panic, depression, and anxiety. Treatment gains were maintained at follow-up 20 wk posttreatment. | CAPS COMB: 1.99 WL: 0.27

ASI COMB: 2.61 WL: 0.17 | CAPS COMB vs. WL: 2.13

ASI COMB vs. WL: 3.70 |
| Hinton et al. (2004) | 12 male and female Cambodian and Vietnamese refugees with PTSD, most having panic episodes related to headaches and/or orthostatic cues; all participants had PTSD despite a minimum of 1 yr of treatment with an adequate dose of an SSRI medication plus supportive counseling. | Time since trauma was not reported.

A COMB program, which incorporated interoceptive exposure as well as imaginal and *in vivo* EX, CT, and SIT, was administered in 11 weekly sessions, duration of sessions not reported. Medication regimen was maintained constant during the study. | *Intent to treat* COMB = 6 WL = 6 | Harvard Trauma Questionnaire (HTQ), ASI | Intervention was superior to WL on measures of PTSD, anxiety sensitivity, depression, anxiety, and panic symptoms related to headaches and orthostatic cues. | HTQ COMB: 3.26 WL: −0.25

ASI COMB: 2.93 WL: −1.21 | HTQ COMB vs. WL: 2.21

ASI COMB vs. WL: 3.94 |

(continued)

TABLE 7.1. (continued)

Study	Target population[a]	Time postrauma and length of sessions	Treatment(s)/control[b]	Main outcome measure	Major findings	Within-group effect size (Hedges unbiased g)	Between-group effect size (Hedges unbiased g)
Hirai & Clum (2005)	36 men and women, mixture of college students seeking class credit and individuals from the larger community, who experienced civilian trauma with at least subclinical trauma symptoms (meeting reexperiencing and avoidance criteria)	For completers, average time since the trauma was 4.0 yr Self-help for traumatic event-related consequences, a COMB treatment, was an 8-wk intervention administered through the Internet.	*Completers* COMB = 13 WL = 14	Revised Impact of Events Scale (IES-R), Stressful Responses Questionnaire (SRQ)	Intervention was superior to WL on some measures of PTSD (SRQ Intrusions and Avoidance, but not SRQ arousal or IES-R) depression, anxiety, coping, and self-efficacy.	IES-R COMB: 1.80 WL: 0.74 SRQ-Intrusions COMB: 1.64 WL: 0.45 SRQ-Avoidance COMB: 0.93 WL: 0.32 SRQ-Arousal COMB: 0.91 WL: 0.34	IES-R COMB vs. WL: 0.77 SRQ-Intrusions COMB vs. WL: 1.28 SRQ-Avoidance COMB vs. WL: 0.70 SRQ-Arousal COMB vs. WL: 0.57
Hollifield et al. (2007)	84 men and women with PTSD	Mean age of participants was 42 yr, 62% of participants experienced trauma before age 12, 21% between ages 12 and 17, and 17% experienced trauma only as adult (18+). COMB treatment was administered in 12 weekly group therapy sessions, 120 min each; individual acupuncture (ACU) sessions were administered twice weekly, 60 min each.	*Intent to treat* COMB = 28 ACU = 29 WL = 27	PTSD Symptom Scale—Self-Report (PSS-SR)	Intervention with COMB or ACU was superior to WL on measures of PTSD, depression, anxiety, and functional impairment, and there were no differences between treatments. Treatment gains were maintained at follow-up.	COMB: 1.27 ACU: 1.40 WL: 0.26	COMB vs. WL: 0.92 ACU vs. WL: 0.68 COMB vs. ACU: 0.35

162

		Both interventions had a minimum of 15 min per day of assigned homework.				
Ironson, Freund, Strauss, & Williams (2002)	22 men and women with primary PTSD following civilian trauma, primarily interpersonal assault	Time since trauma was not reported Both EX and EMDR comprised 6 sessions, 90 min each. For both treatments, the first session was for evaluation, second and third sessions were preparatory, and fourth through sixth sessions were for active treatment. *In vivo* exposure implemented via homework assignments was incorporated into both treatments.	*Completers* EX = 9 EMDR = 10	PSS-SR	Both interventions showed significant improvement on measures of PTSD, depression, and anxiety, with no differences between treatments. Treatment gains were maintained at follow-up 3 mo posttreatment.	EX: 2.07 EMDR: 1.47 EX vs. EMDR: −0.62
Keane et al. (1989)	24 male Vietnam War veterans with PTSD	Time since trauma was not reported Imaginal EX was administered in 14 sessions, 90 min each; WL participants were reassessed an average of 4.5 mo after the initial evaluation. The original design included a SIT condition, but only 5 participants completed the treatment, and results were not reported.	*Intent to treat* EX = 11 WL = 13	PTSD Checklist (PCL), MMPI-PTSD Scale	Means and standard deviations were reported for the MMPI-PTSD scale but not the PCL. Intervention with EX was superior to WL on measures of depression and state-anxiety, as well as MMPI scales 1–3. Treatment gains were maintained at follow-up.	MMPI-PTSD EX: 0.56 WL: 0.46 MMPI-PTSD EX vs. WL: 0.22

(*continued*)

163

TABLE 7.1. (continued)

Study	Target population[a]	Time posttrauma and length of sessions	Treatment(s)/ control[b]	Main outcome measure	Major findings	Within-group effect size (Hedges unbiased g)	Between-group effect size (Hedges unbiased g)
Krakow, Hollifield, et al. (2001)	168 female sexual assault survivors with self-reported trauma symptoms; 83% had pretreatment CAPS scores > 65	Time since trauma was not reported but 90% reported physical, sexual, or emotional abuse in childhood; nightmare chronicity was 21.8 yr for treatment and 19.3 yr for WL. Imagery rehearsal therapy, a COMB therapy, was administered in a format of 3 individual therapy sessions; sessions 1 and 2 were 3 hr each, spaced 1 week apart. Session 3 was a 1-hr follow-up 3 wk later.	*Completers* COMB = 54 (CAPS available for 45 subjects; PSQI available for 53 subjects) WL = 60 (CAPS available for 52 subjects; PSQI available for 58 subjects)	CAPS, Pittsburgh Sleep Quality Index (PSQI)	Intervention was superior to WL on measures of PTSD, sleep quality, and nightmares 3- to 6-mo posttreatment.	CAPS COMB: 1.54 WL: 0.43 PSQI COMB: 0.71 WL: 0.12	CAPS COMB vs. WL: 0.72 PSQI COMB vs. WL: 1.04
Kubany et al. (2003)	37 female survivors of domestic violence	Minimum time since last incident of domestic violence was 30 days. Cognitive trauma therapy for battered women, a COMB treatment, was administered twice weekly in 8–11 sessions, 90 min each.	*Intent to treat* COMB = 19 WL = 18 *Completers* COMB = 18 WL = 14	CAPS	Intervention was superior to WL measures of PTSD, depression, trauma-related guilt, shame, and self-esteem. Treatment gains were maintained at follow-up 3-mo posttreatment.	*Intent to treat* COMB: 2.66 WL: 0.28 *Completers* COMB: 3.46 WL: 0.12	*Intent to treat* COMB vs. WL: 2.13 *Completers* COMB vs. WL: 2. 92
Kubany et al. (2004)	125 women survivors of domestic violence	Minimum time since last incident of domestic violence was 30 days, mean time was 5.0 yr	*Intent to treat* COMB = 63 WL = 62	CAPS	Intervention was superior to WL measures of PTSD, depression, trauma-related guilt, shame, and	*Intent to treat* COMB: 1.51 WL: 0.18	*Intent to treat* COMB: 1.45

Study	Description	Completers (N)	Measure	Findings	Completers	Completers
	Cognitive trauma therapy for battered women, a COMB treatment, was administered twice weekly in 8–11 sessions, 90 min each.	*Completers* COMB = 46 WL = 40		self-esteem. Treatment gains were maintained at follow-up 3- and 6-mo posttreatment.	*Completers* COMB: 3.43 WL: 0.24	*Completers* COMB vs. WL: 2.87
Lange et al. (2003)	184 men and women meeting criteria for mild to relatively severe PTSD following a range of civilian traumas; nearly twice as many participants were randomized to treatment (122) as to control (62).	*Completers* COMB = 69 WL = 32	IES	Intervention was superior to WL on measures of PTSD symptoms, depression, anxiety, somatization, and sleeping problems. Treatment gains were maintained at follow-up 6-wk posttreatment.	IES-I COMB: 1.07 WL: −0.24 IES-A COMB: 1.03 WL: −0.06	IES-I COMB vs. WL: 1.19 IES-A COMB vs. WL: 1.47
	Mean time since trauma was 9.0 yr Interapy, a COMB treatment, was administered through the Internet in 10 twice-weekly sessions, 45 min each. Participants received written feedback on their written assignments seven times from a study therapist.					
Lange et al. (2001)	30 male and female students with trauma-related symptoms following a range of civilian traumas, participating for course credit Mean time since trauma was 6.0 yr Interapy, a COMB treatment, was administered through the Internet in 10 twice-weekly sessions, 45 min each. Participants received written feedback on their written assignments seven times from a study therapist.	*Completers* COMB = 13 WL = 12	IES	Intervention was superior to WL on measures of PTSD symptoms, depression and fatigue. Treatment gains were maintained at follow-up 6-wk posttreatment.	IES-I COMB: 1.91 WL: 0.44 IES-A COMB: 1.44 WL: 0.35	IES-I COMB vs. WL: 0.49 IES-A COMB vs. WL: 1.05
Lee et al. (2002)	27 men and women with PTSD after 6-wk run-in phase; Time since the trauma ranged between 2 to 71 mo, mean time was 14.92 mo	*Completers* COMB = 12 EMDR = 12	SIP	Both interventions showed substantial improvement on measures of PTSD and depression. There	COMB: 1.50 EMDR: 1.64	COMB vs. EMDR: −0.60

(continued)

TABLE 7.1. (continued)

Study	Target population[a]	Time postrauma and length of sessions	Treatment(s)/ control[b]	Main outcome measure	Major findings	Within-group effect size (Hedges unbiased g)	Between-group effect size (Hedges unbiased g)
Lee et al. (2002) (cont.)	13 randomly assigned to each treatment condition; the final person was incarcerated	Treatment was administered in 7 weekly sessions, 90 min each.			were no differences between interventions at posttreatment, and treatment gains were maintained at follow-up. EMDR was superior to COMB at follow-up on both PTSD and depression.		
Lindauer, Gersons, et al. (2005)	24 men and women with primary PTSD from interpersonal violence, accidents, or disaster	Time since trauma was 2.7 yr for treatment condition and 6.1 yr for WL. Brief eclectic psychotherapy, a form of COMB treatment, was implemented in 16 weekly sessions, 45–60 min each.	*Intent to treat* COMB = 12 WL = 12	SIP, translated into Dutch	Intervention was superior to WL on PTSD reexperiencing and hyperarousal, but not avoidance symptoms, and superior to WL on anxiety but not depression.	Reexperiencing COMB: 1.72 WL: 0.55 Avoidance COMB: 1.28 WL: 0.22 Arousal COMB: 1.70 WL: 0.83	Reexperiencing COMB vs. WL: 1.11 Avoidance COMB vs. WL: 0.79 Arousal COMB vs. WL: 0.82
Lindauer, Vlieger, et al. (2005)	24 men and women with PTSD following civilian traumas	Time since trauma for 18 treatment completers was 3.2 yr Brief eclectic psychotherapy, a form of COMB treatment, was implemented in 16 weekly sessions, 45–60 min each.	*Completers* COMB = 9 WL = 9	SIP, translated into Dutch	Intervention was superior to WL on PTSD severity.	COMB: 1.93 WL: 0.61	COMB vs. WL: 0.88

166

Study	Sample	Treatment details	N	Measure	Outcome	Effect size (within)	Effect size (between)
Litz et al. (2007)	45 Department of Defense service members with PTSD as a result either of the Pentagon attack on September 11, 2001, or combat in Iraq/Afghanistan	Time since trauma not reported. COMB and SC interventions began with a 2-hour face-to-face meeting with a study therapist. Thereafter, the interventions were delivered via the internet over a period of 8 wk.	*Completers* COMB = 14 SC = 16	PSS-I	Both interventions showed significant improvement on measures of PTSD, depression, and anxiety. In the ITT analyses, there were no differences between groups at posttreatment; at 6-mo follow-up, COMB was superior to SC on PTSD, depression, and anxiety. In both the ITT and completer analyses, there were fewer participants with PTSD in the COMB condition than SC at posttreatment and follow-up.	COMB: 1.01 SC: 0.83	COMB vs. SC: 0.40
Maercker et al. (2006)	48 male and female survivors of MVAs with PTSD (22) or subsyndromal PTSD (20)	Mean time since the MVA was 63.1 mo for the COMB condition and 49.1 mo for WL. COMB comprised 8–12 individual weekly sessions, with therapists terminating treatment after Session 8 at their discretion; mean number of sessions was 11.4.	*Completers* CBT = 21 WL = 21	CAPS, German version	Intervention was superior to WL on measures of PTSD, depression, anxiety, and trauma-related cognitions. Treatment gains were maintained at follow-up 3-mo posttreatment. Reanalysis of the CAPS ITT data revealed the same pattern.	COMB: 1.52 WL: 0.32	COMB vs. WL: 0.79

(continued)

167

TABLE 7.1. (continued)

Study	Target population[a]	Time posttrauma and length of sessions	Treatment(s)/control[b]	Main outcome measure	Major findings	Within-group effect size (Hedges unbiased g)	Between-group effect size (Hedges unbiased g)
Marks et al. (1998)	87 men and women with chronic PTSD from a range of civilian traumas	All patients met PTSD criteria for a minimum of 6 mo All treatments administered in 10 "usually" weekly sessions, 90 min each, except EX plus CT sessions were 105 min each.	*Completers* EX = 20 CT = 19 EX/CT = 20 RLX = 18	CAPS	CBT interventions combined were superior to RLX on measures of PTSD, depression, and social adjustment, and treatment gains continued or were maintained during follow-up 1, 3, and 6 mo posttreatment. There were no differences among treatments. Reanalysis of ITT data generally revealed the same pattern of results.	EX: 1.00 CT: 1.53 COMB: 1.09 RLX: 0.92	EX vs RLX: 0.14 CT vs. RLX: 0.08 COMB vs. RLX: −0.23 EX vs. CT: 0.07 EX vs. COMB: 0.38 CT vs. COMB: 0.33
McDonagh et al. (2005)	74 women with PTSD and histories of CSA	Mean age at onset of childhood sexual abuse was 6.1 yr for COMB group, 7.6 yr for SC group, and 6.1 yr for WL; corresponding mean ages at time of treatment were 39.8, 39.6, and 42.0 yr Both COMB (EX plus CT) and present-centered therapy, a form of SC, were administered in 14 weekly sessions, the first 7 sessions, 120 min each; the final 7 sessions, 90 min each.	*Intent to treat* COMB = 29 SC = 22 WL = 23 *Completers* COMB = 17 SC = 20 WL = 20	CAPS	In the ITT analyses, the significant difference was that SC was superior to WL on reducing trauma-related cognitions. In the completer analyses, intervention with COMB and SC was superior to WL on measures of PTSD, anxiety, and trauma-related cognitions; COMB was superior to SC on anxiety. Treatment gains were maintained at follow-up 3- and 6-mo posttreatment.	*Intent to treat* COMB: 0.70 SC: 1.06 WL: 0.35 *Completers* COMB: 1.19 SC: 1.17 WL: 0.43	*Intent to treat* COMB vs. WL: 0.49 SC vs. WL: 0.88 COMB vs. SC: −0.22 *Completers* COMB vs. WL: 1.04 SC vs. WL: 0.87 COMB vs. SC: 0.25

Study	Sample	Design / N	Measure	Results	Within effect sizes	Between effect sizes
Monson et al. (2006)	60 male and female veterans with chronic military-related PTSD	Majority of participants (80%) served during the Vietnam War. CPT administered in 12 weekly sessions	*Intent to treat* CPT = 30, WL = 30	CAPS	Intervention was superior to WL on measures of PTSD and anxiety, but not depression. Treatment gains were maintained at follow-up 1-mo posttreatment.	CPT: 1.36, WL: 0.16	CPT vs. WL: 1.15
Mueser et al. (2008)	108 patients with comorbid severe mental illness (major depressive disorder, bipolar disorder, schizoaffective disorder, and schizophrenia) and PTSD following a range of civilian traumas, most commonly sexual (34%) or physical abuse in childhood (17%), sudden death of a loved one (15%), and adult sexual (13%) or physical assault (11%).	Time since trauma not reported. All patients received TAU: pharmacological management, case management, access to psychiatric rehabilitation services (e.g., vocational rehabilitation), and SC. The COMB treatment with a strong, but not exclusive focus on CT, was administered in 12–16 weekly sessions. Treatment completion was defined as completing a minimum of 12 sessions.	*Completers* COMB = 32, TAU = 27	CAPS	Intervention was superior to TAU on measures of PTSD, depression, anxiety, and trauma-related cognitions. Treatment gains were maintained at follow-up 3- and 6-mo posttreatment. Despite significant improvement, mean posttreatment scores were indicative of substantial residual symptoms.	COMB: 0.80, TAU: 0.37	COMB vs. TAU: 0.44
Neuner et al. (2004)	43 male and female Sudanese refugees diagnosed with	Mean time since the worst period of traumatic events was 7.5 yr	*Intent to treat* EX = 17, SC = 14, EDU = 12	PDS	EX was superior to SC and EDU on PTSD severity 1-yr posttreatment.	EX: 0.61, SC: 0.22, EDU: −0.08	EX vs. EDU: 0.10, SC vs EDU: 0.07, EX vs. SC: 0.06

(continued)

TABLE 7.1. (continued)

Study	Target population[a]	Time posttrauma and length of sessions	Treatment(s)/ control[b]	Main outcome measure	Major findings	Within-group effect size (Hedges unbiased g)	Between-group effect size (Hedges unbiased g)
Neuner et al. (2004) (cont.)	PTSD living in a Ugandan refugee settlement	Narrative exposure therapy, a form of EX, and SC comprised 4 sessions scheduled within 2 wk of each other. Duration was between 90–120 min. Psychoeducation (EDU) comprised a single session.					
Otto et al. (2003)	10 female Cambodian refugees with PTSD despite treatment with clonazepam in combination with an SSRI other than sertraline (SERT)	Index traumas occurred in Cambodia between 1975 and 1979. All participants began treatment with SERT, up to 200 mg/day. Final dose of SERT was 100 mg/day in the COMB treatment, 125 mg in the control condition. A COMB program, which incorporated interoceptive exposure, as well as imaginal and *in vivo* EX, CT, and SIT, was administered in 10 group therapy sessions.	*Intent to treat* SERT+COMB = 5 SERT = 5	CAPS, ASI	Inferential statistics were not reported. Based on consideration of the ESs for measures of PTSD, anxiety sensitivity, anxiety, and somatization, the authors concluded there was an advantage for the COMB condition.	CAPS— Reexperiencing COMB: 0.46 WL: −0.45 CAPS— Avoidance COMB: 0.73 WL: 0.04 CAPS—Arousal COMB: 0.19 WL: −0.07 ASI COMB: 0.67 WL: 0.20	CAPS— Reexperiencing COMB vs. WL: 0.23 CAPS— Avoidance COMB vs. WL: 0.46 CAPS—Arousal COMB vs. WL: 0.75 ASI COMB vs. WL: 1.78
Paunovic & Öst (2001)	20 male and female refugees with PTSD	Mean time since trauma was 7.8 yr	*Completers* EX = 9 COMB = 7	CAPS	Both interventions showed significant improvement on measures of PTSD,	EX: 2.54 COMB: 1.73	EX vs. COMB: 0.12

Study	Sample	Treatment	N	Measure	Results	Within effect size	Between effect size
		Both the EX and EX plus CT (COMB) interventions were administered in 16–20 sessions, 60–120 min each.			depression, anxiety, trauma-related cognitions, and quality of life; there were no differences between EX and COMB. Treatment gains were maintained at follow-up 6 mo posttreatment.		
Power et al. (2002)	105 men and women with PTSD from a range of civilian traumas	Mean time since the trauma was 180 wk for EMDR group, 155.4 wk for COMB group, and 259.5 wk for WL. Treatments were administered in up to 10 sessions, 90 min each. Mean number of sessions did not differ between COMB (EX plus CT; 6.4 sessions) and EMDR (4.2 sessions).	*Completers* COMB = 21 EMDR = 27 WL = 24	SIP, administered as self-report	Intervention was superior to WL on measures of PTSD, depression, and anxiety. There were few differences between treatments, although EMDR was superior to COMB on self-reported depression and social functioning at posttreatment and on interviewer-rated depression at follow-up 15-mo posttreatment.	COMB: 1.40 EMDR: 2.46 WL: 0.18	COMB vs. WL: 1.14 EMDR vs. WL: 1.69 COMB vs. EMDR: −0.51
Resick et al. (2008)	150 female assault survivors, sexual or nonsexual, occurring in childhood or adulthood	Mean time since trauma was 14.6 yr CPT with and without the trauma narrative (CPT-C) was administered in 12 twice-weekly sessions, 60 min each; the written account (WA) condition was administered in seven 2-hour sessions administered in 6 wk (2 wk in Week 1, weekly thereafter).	*Intent to treat* CPT = 53 CPT-C = 50 WA = 47	CAPS	All three interventions showed significant improvement from pre- to posttreatment on measures of PTSD, depression, anxiety, anger, trauma-related cognitions, guilt, and shame; treatment gains were maintained at follow-up 6-mo posttreatment. CPT-C was superior to WA on PTSD.	CPT: 1.62 CPT-C: 1.45 WA: 1.01	CPT vs. WA: 0.34 CPT-C vs. WA: 0.39 CPT vs. CPT-C: −0.10

(continued)

TABLE 7.1. (continued)

Study	Target population[a]	Time posttrauma and length of sessions	Treatment(s)/control[b]	Main outcome measure	Major findings	Within-group effect size (Hedges unbiased g)	Between-group effect size (Hedges unbiased g)
Resick et al. (2002)	171 female sexual assault survivors with PTSD	Average length of time since the assault was 8.5 yr EX was administered in one 60-min session followed by eight 90-min sessions over 6 wk; CPT was administered in 12 twice-weekly sessions, two sessions 90 min each and 10 sessions 60 min each.	*Intent to treat* EX = 62 CPT = 62 WL = 47 *Completers* EX = 40 CPT = 41 WL = 40	CAPS	Interventions were superior to WL on measures of PTSD, depression, and guilt; treatment gains were maintained at follow-up 3- and 6-mo posttreatment. CPT was superior to EX on two of four guilt measures.	*Intent to treat* EX: 1.15 CPT: 1.38 WL: 0.03 *Completers* EX: 2.36 CPT: 3.07 WL: 0.01	*Intent to treat* EX vs. WL: 0.86 CPT vs. WL: 1.13 EX vs. CPT: −0.18 *Completers* EX vs. WL: 2.04 CPT vs. WL: 2.78 EX vs. CPT: −0.24
Richards et al. (1994)	14 men and women with chronic PTSD following a range of civilian traumas	Mean time since trauma was 2 yr (range 6 months–8 yr) for completers Both treatments were administered in 8 weekly sessions, 60 min each. Four sessions focused on imaginal EX and four sessions focused on *in vivo* EX, administered in counterbalanced order.	*Completers* EX = 13 (combined across order of EX treatment)	PCL	Means and standard deviations were not reported separately for different EX groups. Both interventions showed significant improvement on measures of PTSD, depression, and social adjustment. There was an order effect, such that the treatment administered first was superior to the treatment administered second; imaginal and *in vivo* EX were equally effective except *in vivo* EX was superior to imaginal EX on anxiety during BAT.	EX: 3.02	—

Study	Sample	Treatment	N	Measure	Results	Effect size	Effect size
Rothbaum et al. (2005)	74 female rape survivors with chronic PTSD	Minimum time since trauma of 3 mo. EX and EMDR were delivered in 9 twice-weekly sessions, 90 min each.	*Completers* EX = 20 EMDR = 20 WL = 20	CAPS	Interventions were superior to WL on measures of PTSD, depression, anxiety, and dissociation; treatment gains were maintained at follow-up 6-mo posttreatment. More EX participants achieved good end-state functioning at follow-up than in EMDR; EMDR was superior to EX on dissociation at follow-up.	EX: 1.98 EMDR: 2.07 WL: 0.58	EX vs. WL: 2.00 EMDR vs. WL: 1.42 EX vs. EMDR: 0.43
Rothbaum et al. (2006)	Two-phase study, 88 men and women with chronic PTSD began Phase I of treatment; 65 participants randomized in Phase II	Mean time since index trauma for Phase II participants was 8.1 yr. Participants received open-label SERT for 10 wk, up to 200 mg/day; mean final dose of 173 mg/day. EX was administered in 10 twice-weekly sessions between Weeks 10–15, 90–120 min each.	*Phase II Intent to treat: Overall* SERT/EX = 34 SERT = 31 *Phase II Intent to treat: SERT Partial Responders* SERT/EX = 18 SERT = 15 *Phase II Intent to treat: SERT Excellent Responders* SERT/EX = 16 SERT = 16	SIP	Intervention with SERT resulted in significant improvement on PTSD, depression, and anxiety. The addition of EX resulted in further significant improvement on PTSD, but not depression or anxiety. In a post hoc analysis, participants were divided into partial and excellent medication responders based on their PTSD score at Week 10. The augmentation effect of adding EX to SERT was restricted to medication partial responders.	Overall SERT/EX: 2.78 SERT: 1.68 SERT Partial Responders SERT/EX: 2.33 SERT: 0.87 SERT Excellent Responders SERT/EX: 4.36	Overall SERT/EX: 0.38 SERT Partial Responders SERT/EX vs. SERT: 0.89 SERT Excellent Responders SERT/EX vs. SERT: –0.18

(continued)

TABLE 7.1. *(continued)*

Study	Target population[a]	Time posttrauma and length of sessions	Treatment(s)/control[b]	Main outcome measure	Major findings	Within-group effect size (Hedges unbiased g)	Between-group effect size (Hedges unbiased g)
Schauer et al. (2006)	32 survivors of organized violence, physical and sexual torture	Time since trauma not available to reviewers Narrative exposure therapy comprised 5–13 treatment sessions and was compared with TAU.	—	PDS	Intervention resulted in significant improvement on PTSD at the 6-mo follow-up, but not for TAU.	—	—
Schnurr et al. (2007)	284 female veterans with chronic PTSD	Minimum time since trauma of 3 mo; mean of 23.0 yr for EX group and 22.8 yr in comparison group. Both EX and present-centered therapy, a form of SC, were administered in 10 weekly sessions, 90 min each.	*Intent to treat* EX = 141 SC = 143	CAPS	Intervention resulted in significant improvement on PTSD, depression, and anxiety. EX was superior to SC on measures of PTSD, depression, and anxiety. Treatment gains were maintained at follow-up 3- and 6-mo posttreatment.	EX: 0.80 SC: 0.62	EX vs. SC: 0.27
Schnurr et al. (2003)	360 male Vietnam War veterans with combat-related PTSD	Time since trauma not specified Group COMB and group present-centered therapy, a form of SC, received 30 weekly sessions followed by 5 monthly booster sessions; treatment sessions were 90–120 min each. Group COMB also included monthly 15-min telephone calls during the booster phase.	*Intent to treat* EX = 162 SC = 163	CAPS	Intervention resulted in small but statistically significant improvement from pre- to posttreatment, with no differences between treatments in the ITT analyses. Among participants completing at least 24 active treatment sessions, EX was superior to SC.	EX: 0.40 SC: 0.38	EX vs. SC: 0.11

174

Study	Sample	Treatment	N	Measure	Results	Effect size	Between-group effect size
Tarrier et al. (1999)	72 men and women with chronic PTSD allocated to treatment after completing a 4-wk monitoring phase	34% of patients had trauma symptoms for less than 12 mo, 40% between 12–24 mo, 26% over 24 mo. CT and imaginal EX was administered in 16 60-min sessions	*Completers* IE = 29 CT = 33	CAPS	Both interventions resulted in significant improvement on measures of PTSD, depression, and anxiety. There were no differences between treatments, and treatment gains were maintained at follow-up.	EX: 0.90 CT: 1.33	EX vs. CT: 0.09
Taylor et al. (2003)	60 men and women, most (97%) with chronic PTSD	Mean time since trauma of 8.7 years. EX, EMDR, and RLX administered in eight 90-min sessions	*Completers* EX = 15 EMDR = 15 RLX = 15	CAPS	All three interventions resulted in significant improvement on measures of PTSD, depression, dissociation, guilt, and anger; treatment gains were maintained at follow-up 3-mo posttreatment. EX was superior to RLX on several measures, whereas EMDR was not superior to RLX on any measure. Reanalysis of self-reported PTSD ITT data found no differences between groups.	EX: 2.52 EMDR: 2.07 RLX: 1.10	EX vs. RLX: 0.70 EMDR vs. RLX: 0.15 EX vs. EMDR: 0.73
Vaughan et al. (1994)	36 men and women with PTSD	Mean time since trauma of 6.6 yr. All treatment conditions, image habituation training (a form of imaginal EX), EMDR, and RLX, were administered in 3–5 sessions (mean of 4.3	*Intent to treat:* Immediate Condition All Treatment Conditions = 19 WL = 17	SIP	Interventions combined were superior to WL on measures of PTSD and depression, and treatment gains were maintained at follow-up 3-mo posttreatment. There were no differences between active treatments.	Treatment: 0.77 WL: 0.22 EX: 0.59 EMDR: 1.34 RLX: 0.58	Treatment vs. WL: 0.76 EX vs. RLX: 0.01 EMDR vs. RLX: 0.62 EX vs. EMDR: −0.70

(continued)

TABLE 7.1. (continued)

Study	Target population[a]	Time posttrauma and length of sessions	Treatment(s)/ control[b]	Main outcome measure	Major findings	Within-group effect size (Hedges unbiased g)	Between-group effect size (Hedges unbiased g)
Vaughan et al. (1994) (cont.)		sessions) over 2–3 wk; sessions averaged 50 min each.	*Intent to treat:* Immediate and Delayed Treatment Conditions EX = 13 EMDR = 12 RLX = 11				
Zlotnick et al. (1997)	48 female CSA survivors with PTSD	Mean time since trauma not reported. All participants received individual psychotherapy and pharmacotherapy for at least 1 mo prior to beginning of study; these treatments were maintained for duration of the study. Affect management therapy, based on DBT, was administered in group therapy sessions over a 15-week period.	*Completers* DBT = 17 WL = 16	Davidson Trauma Scale (DTS)	Intervention was superior to WL on measures of PTSD and dissociation.	DBT: 0.72 WL: 0.06	DBT vs. WL: 0.83

Note. ACU, individual acupuncture; ADIS-P, panic module of the Anxiety Disorders Interview Schedule; Ang-Ex, Spielberg Anger Expression Scale; ASI, Anxiety Sensitivity Index; BAT, behavioral avoidance task; BDI, Beck Depression Inventory; BFT, behavioral family therapy; CAPS, Clinician-Administered PTSD Scale; CBT, cognitive-behavioral therapy; CIDI-PTSD, Composite International Diagnostic Interview—PTSD Module; COMB, combination CBT; CPT, cognitive processing therapy; CPT-C, CPT Cognitive; CSA, childhood sexual abuse; CT, cognitive therapy; DBT, dialectical behavior therapy; DTS, Davidson Trauma Scale; EDU, psychoeducation; EMDR, eye movement desensitization and reprocessing; EMG, electromyogram; ERRT, exposure, relaxation, and rescripting therapy; EX, exposure therapy; FSS, Fear Survey Schedule; HTQ, Harvard Trauma Questionnaire; IES, Impact of Events Scale; IES-R, Revised Impact of Events Scale; ITT, intent to treat; MISS, Mississippi Scale for Combat-Related PTSD; MMPI, Minnesota Multiphasic Personality Inventory; MPSS-SR, Modified PTSD Symptom Scale Self-Report; MVA, motor vehicle accident; PAR, paroxetine; PCL, PTSD Checklist; PDS, Posttraumatic Stress Diagnostic Scale; PRS, Physical Reactions Scale; PSQI, Pittsburg Sleep Quality Index; PSS-I, PTSD Symptom Scale Interview; PSS-SR, PTSD Symptom Scale Self-Report; RLX, relaxation training; SC, supportive counseling; SD, systematic desensitization; SELF, Self-Help Booklet; SERT, Sertraline; SIP, Structured Interview for PTSD; SIT, stress inoculation training; SRQ, Stressful Response Questionnaire; STAI-S, State–Trait Anxiety Inventory—State Anxiety; TAU, treatment as usual; VET, Veteran's Adjustment Scale; WA, written account; WL, wait list. [a]N = Ss starting study; [b] N = Ss in data analysis.

TABLE 7.2. Summary of Nonrandomized Trials of CBT for PTSD

Study	Target population[a]	Time posttrauma and length of sessions	Treatment(s)/ control[b]	Main outcome measure	Major findings	Within-group effect size (Hedges unbiased g)	Between-group effect size (Hedges unbiased g)
Basoglu et al. (2003)	10 females with PTSD symptoms, survivors of a 1999 earthquake in Turkey	Mean time since the earthquake was 20 months Treatment using an earthquake simulator was administered in one 60-min session.	*Completers* EX = 10	Clinician-Administered PTSD Scale (CAPS)	Significant improvement from pre- to posttreatment on measures of PTSD and depression; improvement was maintained at follow-up 12-wk posttreatment.	EX: 2.45	—
Basoglu, Livanou, Salcioglu, & Kalender (2003)	231 male and female survivors of 1999 earthquake in Turkey; 167 had PTSD, 64 had subsyndromal symptoms	Mean time since trauma was 13 months *In vivo* EX was administered without a predetermined number of sessions; mean number of sessions was 4.3. Sessions were planned to be weekly, but the average time between sessions was 16 days.	*Completers* EX = 155	Traumatic Stress Symptom Checklist (TSSC)	Significant improvement from pre- to posttreatment on measures of PTSD, depression, and social adjustment; improvement was maintained at follow-up 1–16-mo posttreatment (mean of 66 days).	EX: 1.92	—
Bolton et al. (2004)	105 male veterans with PTSD	Study was conducted between 1996 and 2001. 80% of participants were Vietnam War veterans, 8% WWII, 5% Korean War, 3% Gulf War, 4% other.	*Completers of each consecutive component* EDU = 105 SIT-Stress = 62 SIT-Anger = 30	PTSD Checklist (PCL)	Small but statistically significant reduction of PTSD reexperiencing during EDU; small but statistically significant reduction of depression during SIT-Stress; and	EDU: 0.12 SIT-Stress: 0.14 SIT-Anger: 0.00	— — —

(continued)

177

TABLE 7.2. *(continued)*

Study	Target population[a]	Time posttrauma and length of sessions	Treatment(s)/control[b]	Main outcome measure	Major findings	Within-group effect size (Hedges unbiased *g*)	Between-group effect size (Hedges unbiased *g*)
Bolton et al. (2004) *(cont.)*		Treatment comprised three sequential group treatments, each lasting 12 weeks: Education (EDU); stress management, similar to stress inoculation training (SIT); and anger management, also similar to SIT.			small but statistically significant improvement on general health and violence during SIT-Anger.		
Devilly & Spence (1999)	32 men and women meeting criteria for PTSD; the majority had civilian traumas	Minimum of 1 mo since trauma Trauma treatment protocol, a COMB treatment, comprised elements of SIT, EX, and CT; 9 weekly sessions, 90 min each, except Sessions 5–6, which lasted 120 min. EMDR administered in 8 weekly sessions, 90 min each. A block randomization procedure was used. The first 10 participants were assigned to COMB (randomly determined), the next 10 to EMDR; the remaining participants were alternately assigned to COMB or EMDR.	*Completers* COMB = 12 EMDR = 11	PTSD Interview (I-PTSD)	Significant improvement from pre- to posttreatment in both conditions on measures of PTSD, anxiety, and depression; greater improvement was observed for PTSD in the COMB condition; COMB was superior to EMDR on PTSD at follow-up 3-mo posttreatment.	COMB: 3.50 EMDR: 2.28	COMB vs. EMDR: 0.72

Study	Sample	Time since trauma / Treatment	Intent to treat / Completers	Measure	Results	Effect size
Ehlers et al. (2005)	20 men and women with PTSD following civilian traumas, primarily moter vehical accidents (MVAs; 13)	Median time since trauma 13.2 mo. No fixed number of sessions; CT administered in 4–20 weekly sessions (mean of 8.3 sessions), 90 min for the first session and 60 min for subsequent sessions each, plus up to 3 monthly booster sessions (mean of 2.1), 60 min each.	*Intent to treat* CT = 20	Posttraumatic Stress Diagnostic Scale (PDS)	Significant improvement from pre- to posttreatment on measures of PTSD and depression; improvement was maintained at follow-up 3- and 6-mo posttreatment.	CT: 2.66	—
Feske (2001)	10 African American women with chronic PTSD following physical or sexual assault	Time since trauma ranged from 4 mo to 32 yr, mean time since trauma of 8.7 yr. EX was administered in nine weekly sessions, 90–120 min.	*Completers* EX = 5	PDS	Significant improvement from pre- to posttreatment on measures of PTSD, depression, and anxiety, but not anger.	EX: 4.10	—
Forbes et al. (2001)	12 male Vietnam War veterans with chronic PTSD who completed an inpatient treatment program at least 6 mo prior to beginning study	Mean time since trauma not reported. Imagery rehearsal for nightmares, a COMB treatment, was administered in 6 weekly group therapy sessions, 90 min each.	*Completers* COMB = 12	Revised Impact of Events Scale (IES-R)	Significant improvement from pre- to posttreatment on measures of PTSD, depression, and nightmares.	COMB: 0.64	—
Frueh, Turner, Beidel, Mirabella, & Jones (1996)	15 male Vietnam War Veterans with chronic PTSD diagnosis	Mean time since trauma not reported. Trauma management therapy, a COMB treatment, comprised 29 sessions, 90 min each, administered over 17 wk; Sessions 1–15 (exposure phase) were administered individually, three times a week;	*Completers* COMB = 11	CAPS	Significant improvement from pre- to posttreatment on anxiety and self-monitored sleep, nightmares, and social activities.	COMB: 1.09	—

(continued)

179

TABLE 7.2. *(continued)*

Study	Target population[a]	Time posttrauma and length of sessions	Treatment(s)/control[b]	Main outcome measure	Major findings	Within-group effect size (Hedges unbiased *g*)	Between-group effect size (Hedges unbiased *g*)
Frueh et al. (1996) *(cont.)*		social and emotional rehabilitation sessions were administered in weekly small-group therapy (Session 16–29).					
Gillespie et al. (2002)	91 men and women who survived 1998 terrorist bombing in Omagh, Northern Ireland	Median time since trauma was 10 mo CT administered in weekly sessions with no fixed limit; median number was 8 sessions; 87% received < 20 sessions.	*Completers* CT = 78	PDS	Significant improvement from pre- to posttreatment on measures of self-reported PTSD, depression, and general psychiatric symptoms.	CT: 2.46	—
Hickling & Blanchard (1997)	12 men and women with PTSD following a MVA seen in a private psychological clinic	Minimum time since trauma was 6 mo, mean time since trauma was 52 wk COMB treatment was administered in 9–12 weekly sessions, 60 min each.	*Completers* COMB = 10	CAPS	Significant improvement from pre- to posttreatment on PTSD, depression, and anxiety that was maintained at follow-up at 3-mo posttreatment.	COMB: 2.22	—
Johnson & Zlotnick (2006)	18 women living in a shelter with PTSD or subthreshold PTSD following domestic violence in the preceding month	Last incident of domestic abuse occurred within 1 mo prior to entering the shelter; mean duration of PTSD was 25.6 mo. The COMB treatment, HOPE (Helping to Overcome PTSD with	*Intent to treat* COMB = 18	CAPS	Significant improvement from pre- to posttreatment on measures of PTSD, depression, effective use of resources and resource loss, and social adjustment that was maintained at follow-up 3 and 6 mo after leaving the shelter.	COMB: 1.05	—

			Completers			
		Empowerment), was administered in 9–12 twice-weekly sessions.				—
Kilpatrick et al. (1982)	Female rape survivors	Patients were offered choice of SIT, peer counseling, or systematic desensitization and each survivor received up to 20 hr of treatment; 70% selected SIT and 30% selected peer counseling; no one selected systematic desensitization.	—	—	No standardized measures of PTSD were administered. SIT was effective in reducing rape-related fear/anxiety/avoidance at post and 3-mo follow-up assessments.	—
Krakow, Johnston, et al. (2001)	62 male and female survivors of violent crime with PTSD	Minimum of 6 mo since the trauma, mean time since the trauma was 13 yr. Image rescripting therapy, was administered in 3 weekly individual sessions.	*Completers* COMB = 62	PDS, Pittsburgh Sleep Quality Index (PSQI)	Significant improvement from pre- to posttreatment on measures of PTSD, depression, anxiety, nightmares, and sleep quality that was maintained at follow-up 3-mo posttreatment.	PDS COMB: 0.71 PSQI COMB: 1.01
Lange et al. (2000)	24 college students who had a traumatic event and displayed symptoms of PTSD. Students participated for course credit.	Minimum time since trauma was 3 mo, mean time since trauma was not reported. Interapy, a COMB treatment, was administered through the Internet in 10 twice-weekly sessions, 45 min each. Participants received written feedback on their written assignments from a study therapist.	*Completers* COMB = 20	Impact of Events Scale (IES)	Significant improvement from pre- to posttreatment on measures of PTSD, depression, anxiety, somatization, and sleeping problems that were maintained at follow-up 6-wk posttreatment.	COMB: 1.32

181

(continued)

TABLE 7.2. (continued)

Study	Target population[a]	Time posttrauma and length of sessions	Treatment(s)/ control[b]	Main outcome measure	Major findings	Within-group effect size (Hedges unbiased g)	Between-group effect size (Hedges unbiased g)
Levitt et al. (2007)	59 men and women with PTSD symptoms related to the September 11, 2001, terrorist attacks	Minimum time since the trauma was 1 yr Treatment comprised DBT interventions followed by imaginal EX (DBT/ EX). Number of treatment sessions ranged between 12 and 25. On average, therapists completed 9 sessions of DBT and 9 of EX. Average time to complete treatment was 23 wk, with a range of 12–36 wk.	*Completers* DBT/EX = 38	Modified PTSD Symptom Scale—Self-Report (MPSS-SR)	Significant improvement from pre- to posttreatment on measures of PTSD, depression, hostility, interpersonal sensitivity, alcohol and drug use, negative mood regulation, social support, and social adjustment. Similar results were obtained for the ITT analyses.	DBT/EX: 1.75	—
Monson et al. (2005)	45 male veterans with PTSD	Time since trauma not reported; 80% were Vietnam War veterans, 11% were Korean War veterans, 5% were Gulf War veterans, and 4% were other war-zone veterans. Both trauma-focused group, a COMB treatment, and skills-focused group, a form of SIT, were administered in daily sessions, 60–90 min each, over a 3-wk period.	*Intent to treat* COMB = 18 SIT = 27	Short form of the Mississippi Scale for Combat-Related PTSD (MISS)	No change from pre- to posttreatment on PTSD, and no difference between groups.	Overall: 0.24 Means and standard deviations for separate groups not reported	—
Mueser et al. (2007)	80 participants with PTSD and a comorbid severe mental illness	Time since trauma was not reported Trauma recovery groups were conducted over 21 sessions, with group sizes of 6–8 patients	*Completers* COMB = 31	PCL	Significant improvement on PTSD, depression, and trauma-related cognitions that was maintained at follow-up 3-mo posttreatment.	COMB: 1.10	—

Study	Sample		Completers	Measure	Findings	Effect sizes	
Pitman et al. (1996)	20 male Vietnam War veterans with PTSD	Time since trauma was not reported Imaginal exposure (EX) was conducted on each of two memories for six 90–120 min sessions.	*Completers* EX on 1st memory = 20 EX on 2nd memory = 14	IES	Means and SDs for PTSD measures were not reported; therefore ESs were not computed. The study provided evidence of emotional processing, but only 13% overall decrease on outcome measures; 26% reduction in intrusive combat memories on self-monitoring.	—	—
Ready et al. (2008)	102 veterans (1 female) with chronic PTSD	Study was conducted between 1/17/2003 and 4/27/2005; time since treatment was not reported; 91% were Vietnam War veterans Group COMB treatment was administered in twice-weekly sessions, 180 min each, for 16–18 wk, depending on the size of the group, which ranged from 9–11 patients each.	*Completers* COMB = 98	CAPS	Significant improvement from pre- to posttreatment on multiple measures of PTSD; treatment gains were maintained at follow-up 6-mo posttreatment.	COMB: 1.36	—
Resick, Jordan, Girelli, Hutter, & Marhoefer-Dvorak (1988)	43 female survivors of sexual assault	Mean time since the trauma was 5.2 yr, with a range of 3 mo to 34 yr All treatments (SIT, assertiveness training, SC) were conducted in a group format over 6 wk, with sessions lasting 120 min. Assignment to treatment groups was nonrandom and WL was naturally occurring.	*Completers* SIT = 12 Assertiveness training (AT) = 13 SC = 12 WL = 13	IES	Significant improvement from pre- to posttreatment for all treatments but no change for WL. Treatment gains were maintained at 6-mo follow-up and no differences among treatments.	Intrusion SIT: 0.48 AT: 0.62 SC: 0.34 WL: 0.13 Avoidance SIT: 0.57 AT: 0.7 SC: 0.29 WL: −0.34	Intrusion SIT vs. WL: 0.07 AT vs. WL: 0.33 SC vs. WL: 0.19 SIT vs. SC: −0.30 AT vs. SC: −0.15 SIT vs. AT: 0.09 Avoidance SIT vs. WL: 0.60 AT vs. WL: 0.57 SC vs. WL: 0.50 SIT vs. SC: 0.07 AT vs. SC: 0.06 SIT vs. AT: 0.00

(continued)t

TABLE 7.2. (continued)

Study	Target population[a]	Time posttrauma and length of sessions	Treatment(s)/ control[b]	Main outcome measure	Major findings	Within-group effect size (Hedges unbiased g)	Between-group effect size (Hedges unbiased g)
Resick & Schnicke (1992)	41 female survivors of sexual assault	Mean time since the most recent rape was 6.4 yr CPT was administered in 12 weekly group therapy sessions, 90 min each. CPT was compared to a naturally occurring WL.	*Completers* CPT = 19 WL = 20	PSS-SR CPT group only, Symptom Checklist 90 (SCL-90)	CPT resulted in significant improvement on measures of PTSD, depression, and social adjustment, and treatment gains were maintained at follow-up 3- and 6-mo posttreatment. CPT was superior to WL on measures of PTSD and depression.	PSS-SR Re-Experiencing CPT: 0.92 Avoidance CPT: 1.09 Arousal CPT: 1.08 SCL-90 CPT: 0.89 WL: 0.02	— — — SCL-90 CPT vs. WL: 0.62
Rothbaum et al. (2001)	16 male Vietnam War veterans with PTSD	Time since the trauma was not reported. Virtual reality–assisted EX treatment was typically delivered in 8–16 twice-weekly sessions, 90 min each	*Completers* EX = 9	CAPS	Significant reduction on PTSD from pretreatment to 3-mo follow-up; significant reduction from pretreatment to 6-mo follow-up on PTSD and depression; trends toward reduction in PTSD and depression from pretreatment to posttreatment.	EX: 0.54	—
Schulz, Resick, Huber, & Griffin (2006)	53 male and female refugees from Afghanistan and the former Yugoslavia, receiving CPT in a community setting (archival data)	Time since the trauma was not reported. The number and duration of CPT sessions was flexible, averaging 17 sessions, 90–120 min in duration.	*Completer* CPT = 53 With interpreter = 25 No interpreter = 28	PTSD Symptom Scale Interview (PSS-I)	Significant reduction in PTSD from pre- to posttreatment. Patients requiring a translator, on average, had three more sessions than cases not using a translator, but there was no difference in outcome.	Overall CPT: 2.53 Interpreter CPT: 2.00 No Interpreter CPT: 3.35	— — —

184

Study	Sample	Treatment	Completers	Measure	Results	Effect size	
Taylor et al. (2001)	58 men and women with PTSD following MVAs, 92% met full criteria for chronic PTSD	Time since the target accident 2.4 yr. COMB treatment was administered in 12 weekly sessions of group therapy, 120 min each. Treatment included education, cognitive restructuring, applied relaxation, imaginal exposure, and *in vivo* exposure.	*Completers* COMB = 50	CAPS	Significant reduction in PTSD from pre- to posttreatment, maintained at follow-up. Cluster analysis revealed two distinct patterns: responders ($N = 30$) and partial-responders ($N = 20$). Partial responders reported greater pain, depression, and anger about the accident; lower levels of functioning; and greater use of medication during treatment than responders.	Reexperiencing COMB: 1.10 Avoidance COMB: 1.27 Numbing COMB: 0.65 Hyperarousal COMB: 1.21	—
Thompson, Charlton, Kerry, Lee, & Turner (1995)	24 men and women with PTSD symptoms following a range of traumas; 67% met full criteria for PTSD	Time since trauma not reported. Treatment with COMB (EX plus CT) was administered in 8-session blocks, so that some participants received 8 sessions while others received 16, depending on clinical judgment of progress. Sessions were weekly and of 90-min duration.	*Completers* COMB = 23	CAPS	Significant reduction of PTSD from pre- to posttreatment.	COMB: 0.83	—
Van Minnen, Arntz, & Keijsers (2002)	Two consecutive groups of men and women with chronic PTSD:	For Group 1, mean time since index trauma was 6 yr, 3 mo. For Group 2, the mean time was 9 yr, 7 mo.	*Completers* EX-Group 1 = 45 EX-Group 2 = 43	PTSD Symptom Scale Self-Report (PSS-SR)	Significant improvement from pre- to posttreatment on measures of PTSD, depression, and anxiety for both groups and	EX-Group 1 = 1.43 EX-Group 2 = 0.68	—

(*continued*)

185

TABLE 7.2. (continued)

Study	Target population[a]	Time posttrauma and length of sessions	Treatment(s)/ control[b]	Main outcome measure	Major findings	Within-group effect size (Hedges unbiased g)	Between-group effect size (Hedges unbiased g)
Van Minnen et al. (2002) (cont.)	Group 1, $N = 59$, Group 2, $N = 63$	For both groups, EX was administered in 9 weekly sessions, 90 min each.			treatment gains were maintained at follow-up 1-mo posttreatment. Pretreatment PTSD severity predicted posttreatment PTSD severity in both samples.		
Van Minnen & Foa (2006)	Two consecutive groups of men and women with chronic PTSD: Group 1 received 60 min of imaginal exposure in sessions (N = 60); Group 2 received 30 min of exposure in sessions (N = 32)	For Group 1 (EX-60) mean time since the trauma was 5 yr, 11 mo; for Group 2 (EX-30), the mean time since the trauma was 8 yr, 2 mo EX was administered in 10 weekly sessions, nine of which included prolonged imaginal exposure sessions. Treatments were identical except for length or sessions (90 vs. 60 min) and imaginal exposures during sessions (60 vs. 30 min).	*Intent to treat* EX-60 = 60 EX-30 = 32	PSS-SR, translated into Dutch	Significant improvement from pre- to posttreatment for both groups on measures of PTSD, depression, and anxiety. Although longer sessions was associated with more within-session habituation, both groups showed similar between-session habituation and there were no differences in treatment outcome.	EX-60: 1.04 EX-30: 1.23	— —
Van Minnen & Hagenaars (2002)	45 men and women with chronic PTSD	Average time since the trauma was 4 yr, 9 mon EX was administered in 10 weekly sessions	*Completers* EX = 34	PSS-SR, translated into Dutch	At the end of treatment 21 participants were improved, 13 were not improved, and 11 dropped out. Nonimproved patients had higher anxiety levels at the beginning of the first exposure session and	EX: 1.01	—

186

(continued)

Study	Sample	Intervention	Completers	Measures	Outcome	Effect size
Vaughan & Tarrier (1992)	10 men and women with PTSD from various traumas	Image habituation training, a form of imaginal EX, was administered in 10 sessions.	Completers EX = 8	IES	Significant improvement from pre- to posttreatment on measures of PTSD and depression that were maintained at follow-up at least 6-mo posttreatment. ... showed less within-session habituation during homework and less between-session habituation than improved patients. Dropouts were not different from completers on fear activation and within-session habituation.	EX: 1.31 —
Wald & Taylor (2007)	9 men and women with chronic PTSD	Minimum time since trauma was 3 mo; meant time since the trauma was not reported COMB treatment comprised 12 individual weekly sessions. The first four sessions were of interoceptive exposure (1st session was 90 min, remaining three were 60 min) followed by four 90-min sessions of imaginal exposure to the trauma memory, followed by four sessions of trauma-related in vivo exposure.	Completers COMB = 7	CAPS, Anxiety Sensitivity Index (ASI)	Inferential statistics were not reported, but there was substantial reduction from pre- to posttreatment on measures of PTSD, anxiety sensitivity, depression, anxiety, and trauma related cognitions. Notably, the rate of improvement on PTSD and anxiety sensitivity were similar and did not appear to vary as a function of the type of exposure (interoceptive vs. trauma-related exposure).	CAPS COMB: 2.14 ASI COMB: 2.70 — —

TABLE 7.2. *(continued)*

Study	Target population[a]	Time posttrauma and length of sessions	Treatment(s)/control[b]	Main outcome measure	Major findings	Within-group effect size (Hedges unbiased g)	Between-group effect size (Hedges unbiased g)
Wells & Sembi (2004)	6 individuals (5 women) with PTSD	Time since the trauma ranged between 3 and 10 mo After an initial 4-wk baseline period, patients began to receive metacognitive therapy intervention, a form of COMB treatment, administered over 8 wk.	*Completers* COMB = 6	Penn Inventory for PTSD (PENN)	Significant improvement from pre- to posttreatment on measures of PTSD, depression, and anxiety were maintained at follow-up.	COMB: 4.0	—

Note. ASI, Anxiety Sensitivity Index; AT, assertiveness training; CAPS, Clinician-Administered PTSD Scale; COMB, combination CBT; CPT, cognitive processing therapy; CT, cognitive therapy; DBT, dialectical behavior therapy; EDU, psychoeducation; EMDR, eye movement desensitization and reprocessing; EX, exposure therapy; HOPE, helping to overcome PTSD with empowerment; I-PTSD, PTSD Interview; IES, Impact of Events Scale; IES-R, Revised Impact of Events Scale; ITT, intent to treat; MISS, Mississippi Scale for Combat-Related PTSD; MPSS-SR, Modified PTSD Symptom Scale Self-Report; MVA, motor vehicle accident; PCL, PTSD Checklist; PDS, Posttraumatic Stress Diagnostic Scale; PENN, Penn Inventory for PTSD; PSQI, Pittsburg Sleep Quality Index; PSS-I, PTSD Symptom Scale Interview; PSS-SR, PTSD Symptom Scale Self-Report; SC, supportive counseling; SCL-90, Symptoms Checklist 90; TSSC, Traumatic Stress Symptoms Checklist. [a]N = Ss starting study; [b] N = Ss in data analysis.

treatments in comparative outcome studies—deserve some consideration at the outset. Of the 64 randomized controlled trials (RCTs) listed in Table 7.1, more than half (57%) reported ITT analyses, with a trend toward greater incidence of ITT analyses in more recent studies. For example, only 38% of studies published through 2000 (when the previous edition of this volume was published) reported ITT analyses, in comparison to 64% of studies published after 2000; and 75% of the most recent studies, published in 2007–2008 or currently in press, reported ITT analyses.

With regard to equipoise of treatment conditions, most studies directly comparing different CBT programs have adopted the strategy of using multiple therapists, describing the therapists or providing information about their level of education, having all therapists administer all treatments, providing specific training in the study treatments, and providing ongoing supervision over the course of the study. Indeed, 11 of the 18 studies comparing different CBT programs (including five studies comparing CBT to EMDR) met all four of these criteria, and three additional studies met at least three of the four. Six of the studies offered at least some additional information about the therapists' background or experience with the treatments prior to participation in the study, although much of this information seemed highly impressionistic. Only one study (Foa, Rothbaum, Riggs, & Murdock, 1991) reported having compared patient outcomes across therapists and found no significant differences. Another study (Foa et al., 2005) compared outcomes achieved among patients treated by doctoral-level therapists at the researchers' institution with those obtained by masters'-level therapists from the local rape crisis center who received training and ongoing supervision from the researchers: No significant differences in treatment response were observed between the two sites.

An alternative approach adopted by two large-scale, multisite studies comparing CBT and present-centered therapy (PCT) classified in this review as a form of supportive counseling. In these studies, the researchers used a large number of therapists and randomly assigned different groups of therapists to administer each of the two study treatments. The use of random assignments to allocate therapists to treatment conditions would be expected to balance therapist effects across the two treatment conditions (Schnurr et al., 2005; Schnurr, Friedman, Lavori, & Hsieh, 2001).

Literature Review

Exposure Therapy

Exposure therapy (EX) as a primary treatment for PTSD has been studied in 24 randomized trials and 9 nonrandomized studies with individual treatment. The populations that have been studied include male (5 studies) and female (1 study) veterans; female assault survivors (6 studies); mixed-gender and mixed-trauma survivors (12 studies); refugees (4 studies) and earthquake survivors (4 studies); and individuals affected by the September 11, 2001, attacks on the World Trade Center (1 study). To summarize, the overwhelming majority of studies found significant pre- to posttreatment changes on standardized measures of PTSD severity. Randomized controlled trials have compared EX to control conditions such as wait list (WL; 10 studies), supportive counseling (SC; 4 studies), RLX (3 studies), psychoeducation (2 studies), and treatment as usual (TAU; 3 studies). Consistently, EX has been more effective than the WL and the nonspecific control conditions. Comparative treatment studies in which two active PTSD treatments were compared have found no significant differences between EX and other forms of CBT for PTSD outcomes (SIT, CPT, CT, eye movement desensitization and reprocessing [EMDR]; 10 studies) and four of five studies that compared EX plus SIT or CT to EX alone were nonsignificant. However, it must be pointed out that most of these studies were not powered to find anything but large effect size differences (Schnurr, 2007). Given that the comparison of active and effective treatments would be expected to find only small to medium effect size differences, more research is needed to determine if there are differences between these active treatments or whether the addition of other components may be beneficial. Exposure therapy has been administered in different ways, including the combination of imaginal plus *in vivo* exposure, imaginal exposure alone, *in vivo* exposure alone, and exposure assisted by virtual reality or other technology.

Imaginal plus In Vivo Exposure

The combination of imaginal plus *in vivo* exposure has been studied in 12 randomized and four nonrandomized studies. Eight of the randomized and all four nonrandomized studies used variations of the prolonged exposure (PE) protocol developed by Foa and colleagues (2007). Except where noted, the PE protocol studies included nine 90-minute sessions once or twice weekly; the first two sessions were devoted to patient education and treatment planning, and the remaining sessions focused on conducting imaginal exposure. Homework comprised additional imaginal exposure via listening to audiotapes of the in-session imaginal exposures and implementing *in vivo* exposure. Among the randomized studies of PE, five had very similar designs, in which female survivors of assault (predominately rape) with chronic PTSD were randomly assigned to PE, WL, or another form of CBT, including SIT (Foa et al., 1991, 1999); PE combined with SIT (PE/SIT; Foa et al., 1999); PE combined with CT (PE/CT; Foa et al., 2005); CPT (Resick, Nishith, Weaver, Astin, & Feurer, 2002); or EMDR (Rothbaum, Astin, & Marsteller, 2005). These five studies met all seven "gold standards"; thus, strong conclusions may be drawn about the efficacy of PE. Results indicated that PE was associated with significant reductions in PTSD severity and was superior to WL in all studies except that of Foa and colleagues (1991), in which the improvement in PE was not statistically superior to that in WL, a finding that may be attributed to lack of power due to the small number of subjects (10 completers in each group). Treatment gains were maintained at follow-up assessments occurring 3–12 months after completion of treatment, and there were no significant PTSD severity differences between any of the comparison CBT conditions in any study either immediately after treatment or at follow-up. A unique feature of the Foa and colleagues (2005) study that compared PE and PE/CT with WL was the use of flexible dosing rule, in which participants who achieved at least 70% reduction in self-reported PTSD severity by session 8 were scheduled to terminate at session 9. The remaining participants were offered additional sessions, up to 12 total sessions. Among participants who received additional sessions (58% of the sample), additional improvement occurred between session 8 and the final session.

In a sixth landmark study that also met all seven "gold standards," female veterans and active duty personnel ($N = 284$) with chronic PTSD were randomly assigned to 10 sessions of PE or present-centered therapy (Schnurr et al., 2007). Most patients in this study were exposed to multiple traumatic events, but the most common trauma was sexual assault (93%), most of which occurred while the patient served in the service. Moreover, the type of trauma most frequently identified as the index trauma was sexual trauma (68%), followed by physical assault (16%) and war-zone exposure (6%). Overall, women who received PE experienced greater reduction in PTSD symptoms at posttreatment and 3-month follow-up, and were less likely to meet diagnostic criteria for PTSD and more likely to achieve remission. However, there were no significant differences at 6-month follow-up. Although dropout was higher for PE than for present-centered therapy, a similar percentage of dropouts receiving PE no longer met criteria for PTSD or achieved remission as dropouts receiving present-centered therapy (28 vs. 22% for loss of diagnosis, respectively; 10 vs. 9% for remission, respectively).

The remaining two randomized studies of PE included mixed-gender and mixed-trauma samples and failed to meet one or more of the "gold standards." In an innovative augmentation design, Rothbaum and colleagues (2006) provided 10 weeks of open-label treatment with sertraline, one of only two medications with U.S. Food and Drug Administration (FDA) indication for PTSD, to men and women with chronic PTSD, then randomly assigned patients either to continue on sertraline alone for 5 additional weeks ($N = 31$) or to continue sertraline and receive 10 PE sessions administered twice weekly ($N = 34$). Treatment with sertraline was associated with significant improvement during the first 10 weeks of treatment, followed by further improvement with the addition of PE, compared to maintenance of gains but no further improvement in the sertraline-only condition. Despite the differential pattern of improvement during the last 5 weeks of treatment, the difference between groups at the end of treatment was small and not statistically significant. A post hoc analysis that divided participants into groups based on their initial response to sertraline at Week 10 (excellent responders vs. partial responders) found that the augmentation effect was limited to medication partial

responders, for whom the addition of PE resulted in significantly better outcome than sertraline alone. This study met all of the "gold standards" except
for formally evaluating treatment fidelity for PE (pill counts were reported,
attesting to compliance with medication).

Utilizing a crossover design, Richards, Lovell, and Marks (1994) evaluated an EX program that provided four 60-minute sessions of *imaginal* exposure plus corresponding homework either preceded by or followed by four
60-minute sessions of *in vivo* exposure plus corresponding homework. Half of
the participants (male and female survivors of nonmilitary traumas) received
imaginal exposure sessions followed by *in vivo* exposure sessions, and the
remaining participants received the procedures in the reverse order (seven
participants per condition). Results indicated that both procedures were associated with improvement, and that improvement was greater for the first procedure administered, regardless of exposure modality, than for the second
procedure. The only difference between the exposure procedures was that
in vivo exposure produced a greater reduction in phobic avoidance than did
imaginal exposure. Outcome was evaluated via self-report measures or measures administered by the therapist, and assessment of treatment fidelity was
not reported. In a subsequent study, Marks, Lovell, Noshirvani, Livanou, and
Thrasher (1998) utilized an EX protocol of five weekly, 90-minute sessions
of imaginal exposure followed by five sessions devoted to *in vivo* exposure,
plus corresponding homework between sessions. Male and female survivors
of civilian traumas with chronic PTSD were randomly assigned to EX, CT, EX
plus CT, or RLX. Results for 77 completers revealed that all three active treatments led to more improvement than did RLX, but there were no differences
among active treatments. In a study by Taylor and colleagues (2003), four
weekly 90-minute sessions of imaginal exposure followed by four sessions of
in vivo exposure (plus corresponding homework) were compared with eight
90-minute sessions of EMDR or RLX. All three treatments were associated
with improvement. EX, but not EMDR, was found to be superior to RLX. The
studies by Marks and colleagues and Taylor and colleagues met all seven "gold
standards."

In the final randomized study, Paunovic and Öst (2001) found that 16–20
sessions (60–120 minutes' duration) of EX (imaginal exposure followed by *in
vivo* exposure) plus homework was as effective as EX plus CT among 20 political refugees (three females). All treatment in this study was administered by
a single therapist, who also administered all outcome measures, and assessment of treatment fidelity was not reported.

Imaginal Exposure Alone

Imaginal exposure without *in vivo* exposure has been examined in nine randomized studies and two nonrandomized studies. Four of these are older
studies that were conducted with male veterans, primarily from the Vietnam
War; four were conducted with mixed-gender/mixed-trauma civilian popu-

lations; and three were conducted with mixed-gender refugee populations. Keane and colleagues (1989) compared EX to a WL control for 24 veterans and found beneficial effects for reexperiencing symptoms. Cooper and Clum (1989) compared EX to standard treatment for 14 completers and found that EX improved self-report of symptoms directly related to the trauma. Boudewyns and Hyer (1990) compared EX to traditional counseling in 51 veterans and found that 75% of those designated as treatment successes had received exposure. None of these studies included independent evaluators, nor did they assess treatment fidelity.

Tarrier and colleagues (1999) compared 16 (60-minute) sessions of imaginal exposure to CT in a mixed-gender/mixed-trauma civilian sample of 72 participants with chronic PTSD and found that both treatments were equally effective in reducing symptoms from pre- to posttreatment. Bryant, Moulds, Guthrie, Dang, and Nixon (2003) compared imaginal exposure to imaginal exposure plus cognitive restructuring or supportive counseling in eight weekly 90-minute sessions in a sample of 58 civilians (males and females) with chronic PTSD. Results from the completer analyses, but not the ITT analyses, indicated that both exposure conditions led to more improvement than the counseling, with further advantages to the group that received the cognitive restructuring.

Two studies by Vaughan and colleagues (one randomized) utilized a variation of imaginal exposure called "image habituation training," in which participants create brief scripts related to specific images that are reexperienced, then tape-recorded and listened to repeatedly. Thus, image habituation training protocol differs in significant ways from how imaginal exposure was conducted in the studies described previously, which involve imaginal exposure to the full trauma memory in at least several sessions before focusing on isolated aspects of the memory. Vaughan and colleagues (1994) compared 3–5 sessions of image habituation training with EMDR and applied muscle relaxation in 36 male and female civilian participants (78% met full criteria for PTSD). All treatments led to significant but modest improvement that was comparable across treatments and was superior to WL. The researchers did not report the treatment fidelity.

Three randomized studies of four sessions of narrative EX among refugees and survivors of torture have been conducted. Narrative EX differs from typical EX in that patients are helped to construct narrative accounts of their entire lives, from birth to the present, including, but not limited to, a detailed account of specific traumatic events they have experienced over their lifetimes. Two of these studies were reported in English (Bichescu, Neuner, Schauer, & Elbert, 2007; Neuner, Schauer, Klaschik, Karunakara, & Elbert, 2004) and the third in German (Schauer et al., 2006). Neuner and colleagues (2004) compared four sessions of either narrative EX or SC to a single session of psychoeducation among 43 male and female Sudanese refugees with chronic PTSD, living in a Ugandan refugee settlement. At 1-year follow-up, participants receiving narrative EX had significantly less severe self-reported

PTSD symptoms than either of the other treatments. Compared to a single session of psychoeducation, the effect size (ES) for narrative EX immediately after treatment was 0.10, which increased to 0.42 at 4-month follow-up, and 1.29 at 1-year follow-up. Bichescu and colleagues (2007) compared five sessions of narrative EX with one session of psychoeducation among 18 former political detainees with PTSD of the Romanian Communist regime. At the 6-month follow-up assessment, there was a greater reduction in the number of PTSD symptoms, especially avoidance and hyperarousal symptoms, for narrative EX than for psychoeducation (ES = 1.41). Both studies met several of the "gold standards," although neither study reported on treatment fidelity. In a third randomized study, Schauer and colleagues (2006) compared nine sessions of narrative EX to TAU for 32 victims of organized violence or physical and sexual torture. At the 6-month follow-up, narrative EX had resulted in a significant reduction in self-reported PTSD severity, whereas TAU resulted in no change.[1]

In Vivo *Exposure*

We have already noted the Richards and colleagues (1994) crossover study designed to assess the relative contributions of imaginal and *in vivo* exposure, and the finding that both types of exposure were associated with improvement and that *in vivo* exposure resulted in somewhat greater reduction of phobic avoidance than imaginal exposure. Basoglu and colleagues conducted two studies (one randomized) of self-directed *in vivo* exposure in the treatment of PTSD symptoms among survivors of a 1999 earthquake in Turkey. The treatment was described to patients as a way to gain a sense of control over distressing trauma reminders and associated symptoms, and involved the development of a list of treatment targets and instruction in how to implement the self-exposures. In the randomized study (Basoglu, Salcioglu, Livanou, Kalender, & Gonul, 2005), which met all seven "gold standards," 59 male and female earthquake survivors with chronic PTSD were randomly assigned to WL or to one session of self-directed *in vivo* EX, then evaluated 6 weeks later. Treatment produced significantly greater reduction in PTSD severity than WL, and treatment gains were maintained or increased during the course of follow-up.

Technology-Assisted *Exposure*

Four studies (two randomized) have examined the use of technology to assist EX. Although not randomized, the first study to apply virtual reality (VR) EX for PTSD found it helpful for Vietnam War veterans (Rothbaum, Hodges, Ready, Graap, & Alarcon, 2001), and it is currently being used to treat veterans with PTSD from the current Iraq War (Gerardi, Rothbaum, Ressler, Heekin, & Rizzo, 2008). Difede, Cukor, and colleagues (2007) randomly assigned 21 individuals with chronic PTSD related to the September 11, 2001, attack on the World Trade Center to 6–13 sessions of graduated virtual reality exposure to images of the jets hitting the Twin Towers and their subsequent collapse or to WL. In both of these studies, virtual reality EX was associated with significant reductions in PTSD symptoms, and the randomized trial found significantly greater reduction in PTSD for treatment compared to WL; treatment gains in the randomized trial were maintained at 6-month follow-up. The randomized trial met all of the "gold standards" except assessment of treatment fidelity.

Basoglu and colleagues studied the use of an earthquake simulator, a small house based on a movable platform that simulated earth tremors, the intensity of which could be controlled by participants, to treat individuals with symptoms of PTSD and depression following an earthquake in Turkey. In their first (nonrandomized) study, Basoglu, Livanour, and Salcioglu (2003) administered one 60-minute session in the earthquake simulator to 10 female survivors, eight of whom had chronic PTSD. In their second study (Basoglu, Salcioglu, & Livanou, 2007), 31 male and female earthquake survivors with chronic PTSD were randomly assigned to WL or to one session of treatment comprising 60 minutes of education about the treatment rational plus 9–70 minutes ($M = 33$ minutes) in the simulator. Posttreatment assessments occurred 4 and 8 weeks after treatment. Both studies found significant reduction in PTSD severity associated with exposure in the earthquake simulator, and the randomized study found that PTSD severity was significantly lower for the treatment compared to the WL condition. There was either further improvement or maintenance of gains during follow-up, up to 1–2 years in the randomized study. The randomized study met all of the "gold standards" except for assessment of treatment fidelity.

Summary

The strongest evidence, based on the largest number of studies, is for the combination of imaginal plus *in vivo* exposure, although there is evidence that each component can be effective in at least some populations, and there have been more studies supporting the efficacy of imaginal exposure than for *in vivo* exposure. However, there is not adequate research to determine whether one modality is superior to the other, or whether the combination of imaginal plus *in vivo* exposure is superior to the individual modalities. EX has been compared with several other CBT programs, and a number of studies have evaluated whether adding other CBT interventions to EX enhances outcome. In general, treatment outcome for EX is comparable to that of other CBT programs, and the addition of other treatment components (SIT, CT) does not significantly enhance the efficacy of the combination of imaginal plus *in vivo* exposure, although the addition of CT may enhance the efficacy of imaginal exposure alone. However, as mentioned earlier, more studies that are powered for medium and small effect sizes (larger sample sizes or more assessment time points) or equivalence trials will be needed to determine if the lack of differences is due to methodological reasons. Research on technology to assist in the administration of EX is relatively new, but it shows promise, although the availability of such technology is limited at present and its relative efficacy compared to conventional therapy has not been studied.

Stress Inoculation Training

Eight studies (four randomized) have examined the efficacy of stress inoculation training (SIT), four with female sexual assault survivors and four with male veterans. As discussed earlier for EX, Foa and colleagues conducted two well-controlled studies of SIT in the treatment of female sexual assault victims with PTSD, comparing SIT to EX, SC, and WL in the first study (Foa et al., 1991); and comparing SIT alone to EX alone, EX plus SIT, and WL in the second study (Foa et al., 1999). Compared to WL, both studies found that nine 90-minute sessions of SIT were effective in reducing PTSD and related symptoms, and that SIT and EX were of comparable efficacy.

In a randomized study with veterans, Keane and colleagues (1989) reported in an end note that the original design of the study involved random assignment to EX, SIT, or WL. However, due to the low completion rate in the SIT condition, results for that condition were not included in the analyses. In the fourth, randomized study (Chemtob, Novaco, Hamada, & Gross, 1997), veterans with PTSD and high levels of anger received either 12 sessions of SIT focused on anger management (Novaco, 1994) or TAU for a comparable period of time. Compared to the control condition, SIT resulted in decreased anger, increased anger control, and fewer reexperiencing symptoms.

In summary, all four studies with female assault survivors found SIT to be effective, but only two studies were well controlled. One controlled study of individually administered SIT targeting the anger among male veterans found reductions in anger and PTSD reexperiencing symptoms. Thus, SIT has received mixed results, having its strongest support for female rape victims. More controlled research is needed on SIT, especially studies that include the *in vivo* exposure components that were originally part of the protocol.

Cognitive Processing Therapy

Six studies, four of which were randomized, have examined the efficacy of cognitive processing therapy (CPT). A study meeting all of the "gold standards" for a randomized clinical trial compared CPT, PE, and a WL control group (Resick et al., 2002) among female rape survivors. Participants in the WL condition were subsequently randomized into one of the two active conditions, allowing for a replication of the findings. There were no statistical differences between PE and CPT on PTSD, but both showed large improvement compared to the WL control group. CPT was statistically better than PE for two of four measures of guilt (intention-to-treat [ITT] ES advantages for CPT of 0.36 and 0.46 on the hindsight bias and lack of justification subscales, respectively, of the Trauma-Related Guilt Inventory; Kubany et al., 1996). Resick, Nishith, and Griffin (2003) subsequently conducted a secondary analysis to examine the effects of PE and CPT on symptoms of complex PTSD. There were no overall differences between the two therapies on a measure that assesses various aspects of complex PTSD, the Trauma Symptom Inventory (TSI; Briere, 1995). The sample was divided into rape victims with (41%) and without (59%) a history of child sexual abuse (CSA). Combining the two forms of treatment, the authors found no differences between the two trauma groups in PTSD and depression at pretreatment, and both groups displayed comparable improvement at posttreatment and maintained treatment gains at 9-month follow-up. Participants with a CSA history did score higher on several of the TSI subscales, both before and after treatment. With treatment, improvement of patients with a CSA history was marked and equal to that of patients without such histories, but because they started with higher scores, they ended with higher scores. When the pretreatment scores were covaried out, there were no significant differences between the two groups at the follow-up periods, indicating that even though participants who had experienced CSA had more complicated presentations, they too benefited from CPT and PE.

Chard (2005) developed an adaptation of CPT (CPT-SA) for victims of CSA and conducted a study that meets all the "gold standards." Despite the earlier Resick and colleagues (2003) results indicating that CPT is effective in reducing PTSD related to CSA, Chard and others propose that victims of CSA have a range of complex posttraumatic sequelae, as well as PTSD symptoms, that need to be addressed to profit more fully from evidence-based PTSD treatment. This adaptation of CPT includes a combination of group and individual treatment, with the processing of written exposures occurring in the individual treatment, and the cognitive interventions occurring primarily in the group context. The treatment protocol also adds modules that focus on developmental issues, communication skills, and seeking social support. In a trial comparing this 17-week treatment to WL, the treatment was highly efficacious, with a posttreatment ES of 1.52. There was also evidence that the participants continued to improve from posttreatment to 3-month assessment.

Resick and colleagues (2008) conducted an RCT meeting all of the "gold standards" to dismantle the components of CPT. Sexually and/or physically abused women were randomized to the full protocol, to the CT-only version of CPT (CPT-C), or a written account–only condition (WA). All three versions resulted in substantial reductions in PTSD scores and there was an overall group effect on the main analyses. On the primary analyses with mixed-effects regression analyses across treatment sessions as well as pretreatment, posttreatment, and follow-up scores, which allowed for enough power to detect differences, there was an overall group effect indicating that CPT-C was superior to WA on PTSD and depressive symptoms. There were no significant differences between full CPT and the WA condition or the CPT-C condition. Thus, adding the written account to cognitive therapy did not improve outcomes.

Monson and colleagues (2006) conducted a WL controlled study of CPT in male and female veterans with chronic military-related PTSD. CPT was superior to WL in reducing PTSD and comorbid symptoms; 40% of the ITT sample receiving CPT no longer met criteria for a PTSD diagnosis. They also found that PTSD-related disability status was not associated with the outcomes. This study met all of the "gold standards" for clinical research and, together with the Schnurr and colleagues (2007) study of PE, provides the most encouraging results to date in the treatment of veterans with military-related PTSD. In a report on effectiveness, Schultz, Resick, Huber, and Griffin (2006) examined archival data from a service-based community organization to evaluate CPT administered to 53 refugees (seven men) from Afghanistan and Bosnia–Herzegovina. All treatment was conducted in the client's native languages and an interpreter was necessary to facilitate treatment in approximately half of the cases. Treatment comprised an average of 17 90- to 120-minute sessions and was associated with a significant reduction in self-reported PTSD severity. Although treatment requiring the presence of an interpreter was associated with longer duration than treatment without an interpreter (33 vs. 41 hours), there was no difference in treatment outcome.

In summary, CPT has received consistent support in four studies meeting all the "gold standards" for clinical research and two nonrandomized studies. Study samples have been female victims of physical and sexual assault and CSA; male and female veterans; and male and female refugees.

Cognitive Therapy

Nine studies, seven randomized, have examined CT for trauma survivors, three of which were reviewed earlier (Marks et al., 1998; Resick et al., 2008; Tarrier et al., 1999). Marks and colleagues (1998) conducted a well-controlled study that met all seven "gold standards" and did not find differences between CT, EX, or the combination, but all three were more effective than RLX. As described earlier, CPT includes a strong cognitive component and the Resick and colleagues (2008) dismantling study indicated that the effectiveness of the CPT-C version was equal to full CPT and better than written accounts only. Tarrier and colleagues (1999) compared CT to imaginal EX for survivors of a variety of traumas and found them equally effective in producing improvement relative to pretreatment. Treatment gains were maintained at 5-year follow-up, and those who received CT did better than those who received imaginal exposure treatment (Tarrier & Sommerfield, 2004).

The CT program based on the Ehlers and Clark (2000) theory of PTSD, which incorporates a variety of interventions, including use of imaginal and *in vivo* exposure exercises, has been evaluated in three randomized (Duffy, Gillespie, & Clark, 2007; Ehlers et al., 2003; Ehlers, Clark, Hackmann, McManus, & Fennell, 2005) and two nonrandomized studies (Ehlers et al., 2005; Gillespie, Duffy, Hackmann, & Clark, 2002). In the first study, Gillespie and colleagues (2002) found that CT was associated with significant reductions in self-reported PTSD and depression among survivors of a terrorist bomb attack in Omagh, Northern Ireland. Duffy and colleagues (2007) subsequently conducted an RCT in Northern Ireland with men and women with terrorism- and civil-conflict-related PTSD. Compared to WL, CT resulted in significantly greater improvement on self-reported PTSD and depression.

Ehlers and colleagues (2003) conducted an RCT comparing CT or a self-help booklet to WL with motor vehicle accident (MVA) victims after a period of self-monitoring. They found that a small percentage of patients (12%) improved by self-monitoring alone. The remaining patients with PTSD were randomized into one of the three conditions approximately 3 months after the accident. Although the 64-page self-help booklet included cognitive-behavioral principles and education about PTSD, this condition was no different than the WL condition and both were less effective than CT. Indeed, CT was highly effective and had no dropouts. In a subsequent article, Ehlers and colleagues (2005) reported results first from a nonrandomized and second a randomized study in mixed-gender/trauma civilian samples. CT in both studies was associated with low dropout, significant improvement in PTSD severity, and maintenance of gains at follow-up, whereas WL in the controlled study resulted in no change on PTSD severity. Both of the nonrandomized and one of the randomized studies reported by Ehlers and her collaborators relied exclusively on self-report measures to assess treatment outcome. Only the two randomized studies reported by Ehlers and colleagues (2003, 2005) utilized a structured interview of PTSD severity administered by a blind, independent evaluator, and none of the studies reported on treatment fidelity.

In summary, different CT programs have been effective in reducing PTSD severity compared to WL (two studies), a self-help booklet (one study), and RLX (one study). Two studies found comparable outcomes immediately after treatment for CT and EX, and two studies found that CT alone was comparable to CT plus some kind of exposure.

Relaxation Training

Four randomized studies have utilized RLX as a comparison condition to evaluate the efficacy of some other CBT program. As discussed earlier, Marks and colleagues (1998) compared EX, CT, and EX plus CT to RLX and found that although RLX was associated with significant improvement, as a group, the CBT conditions produced greater improvement. Taylor and colleagues (2003) also found that EX, but not EMDR, was superior to RLX, and Echeburúa, de Corral, Zubizarreta, and Sarasua (1997) found that the combination of EX plus CT was superior to RLX. In the only study to include a WL control condition, Vaughan and colleagues (1994; discussed previously) found that active treatment (ET, EMDR, and RLX) was superior to WL control but did not report any comparisons of the individual treatments with WL. Thus, it is unknown whether RLX was superior to WL. Comparisons among treatments found no significant differences on overall PTSD severity. Although RLX may be a component of effective treatment for PTSD, the evidence does not support the use of RLX as a stand-alone treatment because other CBT interventions, such as exposure and combined treatments, have been found to be superior.

Dialectical Behavior Therapy

The effect of interventions based on dialectical behavior therapy (DBT), either alone or in combination with EX, on PTSD severity has been evaluated in three randomized studies and one nonrandomized study. Zlotnick and colleagues (1997) randomly assigned 48 female CSA survivors either to 15 weekly, 2-hour group therapy sessions or to a WL. The content of the group sessions comprised education and practice of various affect management skills, including emotion identification, anger management, self-soothing, and distress tolerance. The group treatment resulted in significant reductions in self-reported PTSD severity and dissociation, compared to no change in the WL condition. This study met five of the "gold standards," failing to use a clinician rating of PTSD severity administered by a blind evaluator at posttreatment and to report treatment fidelity.

Cloitre, Koenen, Cohen, and Han (2002) evaluated a two-phase treatment that comprised eight weekly individual therapy sessions teaching DBT-based affect and interpersonal regulation skills, followed by eight twice-weekly sessions of imaginal EX. Participants in the study were 58 adult female survivors of childhood physical and sexual abuse. The comparison condition was WL, and most assessment measures were obtained at pretreatment, midtreatment (between completion of two phases of treatment), and posttreatment. Unfortunately, the primary outcome measure, the Clinician-Administered PTSD Scale (CAPS), was not administered between the two phases. Thus the evaluation of the DBT component alone on PTSD severity was evaluated through self-report only. Overall, the two-phase treatment resulted in significantly greater reductions than WL on measures of PTSD severity, anger expression, dissociation, alexithymia, depression, and anxiety, along with increased ability to regulate negative affect. Analyses focused only on changes during the first phase revealed that the skills training component of treatment resulted in significant reductions in anger expression, depression, and anxiety, along with improvements in negative mood regulation, but no change in PTSD, dissociation, or alexithymia. There were no changes from pre- to midtreatment on any measure in the WL condition. This study met all of the "gold standards," although use of WL as the comparison condition precludes drawing strong conclusions regarding the effect of skills training on the acceptability or efficacy of the subsequent EX. In a nonrandomized study, Levitt, Malta, Martin, Davis, and Cloitre (2007) administered the same two-phase intervention to 59 men and women with PTSD symptoms related to the September 11, 2001, attacks on the World Trade Center. All participants were recruited at least 1 year after the attacks. The number of sessions administered in each session varied according to clinical judgment, but averaged 10 Phase 1 sessions and 9.1 Phase 2 sessions. Pre- to posttreatment improvement was observed on a range of outcome measures, and ESs for self-report measures of PTSD, depression, negative mood regulation, and functional impairment were similar to those reported by Cloitre and colleagues.

Bradley and Follingstad (2003) also used a two-phase treatment that comprised nine 2½-hour group sessions focused on education and teaching affect regulation skills, followed by 9 sessions focused on structured writing assignments among 49 incarcerated women with histories of exposure to interpersonal violence. In the writing assignments, participants were not required to write about any specific traumatic event, but they were encourage to write about their lives, including their experiences with violence, and to draw connections between past experiences and current feelings. Participants were randomly assigned to treatment or to WL conditions. Although no diagnostic measure of PTSD was administered, results revealed that treatment was associated with greater improvement than was WL on six out of seven subscales of the self-report TSI. Specific inclusion–exclusion criteria were not reported, the interventions were not well-described, and treatment fidelity was not reported.

In summary, the research on DBT-based interventions is limited at present. One well-conducted study (Cloitre et al., 2002) clearly indicated that the combination of DBT skills training, followed by imaginal exposure to the trauma memory, both delivered individually, was an effective treatment for PTSD and a range of concomitant problems. The success of this two-phase treatment was replicated in an uncontrolled study with a very different sample (victims of childhood abuse and survivors of the September 11, 2001, terrorist attacks, respectively). A midtreatment assessment in the Cloitre and colleagues (2002) study permitted isolation of the DBT component, which resulted in improvements relative to WL on some measures but not on PTSD severity. By contrast, the Zlotnick and colleagues (1997) study of group DBT-based treatment did result in significant reductions of PTSD severity. This difference in outcome may be due to differences in samples studied or differences in DBT protocols, such as format (individual vs. group therapy) and length of treatment (8 vs. 15 sessions). Although the rationale for phased treatment includes the idea that preliminary treatment with DBT skills training enhances implementation of subsequent EX, no published studies have evaluated this issue thus far.

Acceptance and Commitment Therapy (ACT)

At present, no published studies, randomized or nonrandomized, have evaluated the efficacy of ACT for the treatment of PTSD. Currently, however, there are ongoing evaluations of this treatment and several papers have documented experiential avoidance as a process in maintaining trauma-related symptoms (Batten, Orsillo, & Walser, 2005).

Combination Treatment

Forty-eight studies, 34 randomized and 14 nonrandomized, evaluated various combinations of EX, CT, or anxiety management training, not including studies of CPT (reviewed earlier) or EMDR (reviewed in Spates, Koch, Cusack, Pagoto, & Waller, Chapter 11, this volume), except those studies in which EMDR was directly compared with a combined CBT program (Devilly & Spence, 1999; Lee, Gavriel, Drummond, Richards, & Greenwald, 2002; Power et al., 2002). The randomized studies have compared the combination CBT treatments to WL (23 studies); to nonspecific control treatments, such as SC (five studies) and RLX (three studies); to TAU (two studies); and to other active treatments (nine studies). Most of these studies administered the treatment in individual therapy sessions. Populations included in the randomized studies of individual therapy include male and female MVA survivors (Blanchard et al., 2003; Fecteau & Nicki, 1999; Maercker, Zollner, Menning, Rabe, & Karl, 2006); female victims of sexual or nonsexual assault (Echeburúa et al., 1997; Foa et al., 1999, 2005) and CSA (Echeburúa et al., 1997; Foa et al., 2005; McDonagh et al., 2005) or domestic violence (Kubany, Hill, & Owens, 2003; Kubany et al., 2004); male veterans (Glynn et al., 1999); refugees (Hinton et al., 2004; Hinton, Chhean, et al., 2005; Otto et al., 2003; Paunovic & Öst, 2001); police officers (Gersons, Carlier, Lamberts, & van der Kolk, 2000), and rescue workers following the September 11, 2001, attacks on the World Trade Center (Difede, Malta, et al., 2007); and mixed-gender/trauma samples (Bryant et al., 2003; Frommberger et al., 2004; Lee et al., 2002; Lindauer, Gersons, et al., 2005; Marks et al., 1998; Power et al., 2002). Populations in the randomized studies of group treatment were male veterans (Schnurr et al., 2007), mixed-gender/trauma civilians (Hollifield, Sinclair-Lian, Warner, & Hammerschlag, 2007), and MVA victims (Beck, Coffey, Foy, Keane, & Blanchard, in press). Innovations examined in randomized studies include the development of treatments that (1) target PTSD samples with comorbid conditions such as panic disorder (e.g., Falsetti, Resnick, Davis, & Gallagher, 2001) or severe mental illness (Mueser et al., 2008) (for a more detailed discussion of comorbidity, including with substance use disorders, see Najavits et al., Chapter 21, this volume), (2) target nightmares (Davis & Wright, 2007; Krakow, Hollifield, et al., 2001), and (3) can be implemented via the Internet (Hirai & Clum, 2005; Lange, van de Ven, Schrieken, & Emmelkamp, 2001; Lange et al., 2003; Litz, Engel, Bryant, & Papa, 2007). In general, these studies found significant improvement from pre- to posttreatment and active CBT was more effective than WL or nonspecific control treatments.

Several studies have compared combined CBT programs with other active treatments. Three studies have compared a combined CBT program to EMDR. Power and colleagues (2002) compared EX plus CT to EMDR and WL in a mixed-gender/trauma sample. Compared to WL, both treatments were effective, and treatment gains were maintained at follow-up, with no significant differences between the two active treatments. Lee and colleagues (2002) compared EX combined with SIT to EMDR in a mixed-gender/trauma sample and found no significant differences at posttreatment, although greater improvement was observed for EMDR at follow-up. The Structured Clinical Interview for PTSD (SIP) severity was administered by the therapists rather than by a blind independent evaluator. Both of these studies utilized random assignment. A third study (Devilly & Spence, 1999), comparing EX combined with SIT and additional CT interventions to EMDR in a mixed-gender/trauma sample, utilized a block randomization procedure in which the first 10 participants received CBT (randomly determined), the next 10 received EMDR, and the remaining participants were assigned to their condition in an alternating fashion. Although both treatments were associated with improvement, CBT was found to be superior to EMDR both immediately after treatment and at follow-up.

Frommberger and colleagues (2004) randomly assigned participants (mixed-gender/trauma) to either EX plus SIT or to paroxetine, one of two medications with FDA indication of effectiveness for PTSD. Both groups showed significant improvement, with no differences between treatments. Although therapists in the study had been trained in EX by Foa, and therapists received supervision by experienced CBT therapists, no information was reported on assessment of treatment fidelity. Hollifield and colleagues (2007) compared a group combined CBT treatment program that incorporated education, behavioral activation, cognitive restructuring, image rehearsal therapy (discussed in more detail below), and systematic desensitization to acupuncture and WL. Compared to WL, both the combined CBT program and acupuncture resulted in significant reduction of self-reported PTSD severity, but the two treatments did not differ in terms of effectiveness.

Group Combination Therapy

Three studies (one randomized) have evaluated CBT programs combining EX with cognitive restructuring and/or coping skills training administered in groups of male veterans with chronic, military-related PTSD. Monson, Rodriguez, and Warner (2005) reported program evaluation results on 45 veterans who received group combination CBT ($N = 18$) or group skills training (anger, anxiety, and stress management, interpersonal skills). Group assignment was not conducted randomly. Neither treatment was associated with significant improvement in self-reported PTSD severity. By contrast, Ready and colleagues (2008) found that a group-administered combination CBT program did result in significant improvement on PTSD severity (ES = 1.35) and the treatment gains were maintained at 6-month follow-up. However, the average CAPS score at posttreatment and follow-up (both greater than 60) indicated that most patients continued to suffer significant PTSD despite completing treatment.

Schnurr and colleagues (2003) randomly assigned 360 male Vietnam War veterans to either group EX or to group present-centered therapy. Treatment comprised 30 weekly sessions plus five monthly booster sessions. They found a statistically significant but small reduction in PTSD severity for both groups, with an average change in CAPS scores of 6.4 points after 7 months, of treatment and 7.6 points after 1 year, with differences between groups. The randomized study met all seven of the "gold standards." As previously noted, Hollifield and colleagues (2007) found group CBT was more effective than WL in a mixed-gender/trauma nonveteran sample. Most recently, Beck and colleagues (in press) randomly assigned male and female MVA survivors to group-administered combination CBT to WL. Although both groups showed significant reductions in PTSD severity from pre- to posttreatment, improvement was significantly greater for the CBT condition (ES = 0.84).

Innovations

PTSD is highly comorbid with other disorders. For example, approximately 11% of individuals with PTSD also have comorbid panic disorder, compared to only about 4% prevalence of panic disorder in the general population (Kessler, Sonnega, Bromet, Hughes, & Nelson, 1995). Falsetti and colleagues (2001) integrated components of panic control therapy (Barlow & Craske, 1988, 1994), such as interoceptive and *in vivo* EX exercises, with CPT components of exposure to the trauma memory via writing and reading a trauma narrative, and CT. Result of this small study of 22 women (various traumas) indicated that treatment compared to WL was associated with a greater reduction in the percentage of women meeting criteria for PTSD and in panic symptoms.

Three small randomized studies of Cambodian and Vietnamese refugees were conducted by researchers at Massachusetts General Hospital (Hinton et al., 2004; Hinton, Cchean, et al., 2005; Otto et al., 2003). Frequently in this population, psychiatric distress manifests itself in "neck-focused" panic (Hinton et al., 2006) and orthostatically triggered (Hinton, Pollack, et al., 2005) panic. The treatment integrated interoceptive exposure exercises with imaginal and *in vivo* exposure, anxiety management training, cognitive restructuring, and training in cognitive flexibility. In all three studies, participants had continued to meet criteria for PTSD despite a history of treatment with an adequate dose of a serotonin reuptake inhibitor (SRI) plus supportive counseling. Participants were then randomly assigned to continuation on SRI medication alone or augmentation of the SRI medication with the combined CBT program. In all three studies, treatment was associated with substantial declines in PTSD severity and scores on the Anxiety Sensitivity Index compared to minimal improvement in these areas for the medication-only group. The same pattern was observed for PTSD severity in the two studies that included an appropriate measure. The lack of a PTSD treatment-only condition in these studies precludes definitive conclusions about the role of adding panic control treatment to treatment for PTSD because it is possible that PTSD treatment alone would also reduce panic symptoms. Similarly, the lack of a panic treatment-only condition in these studies precludes definitive conclusions about the role of adding PTSD treatment to treatment for panic because it is possible that panic treatment alone would also reduce PTSD symptoms. Wald and Taylor (2007) conducted a nonrandomized study of treatment that involved, sequentially, four sessions each of interoceptive exposure, imaginal exposure, and *in vivo* exposure. Assessment of PTSD severity and anxiety sensitivity at each treatment visit indicated gradual reductions across all three phases of the exposure treatment, suggesting that interoceptive exposure was as effective in reducing PTSD severity as imaginal or *in vivo* exposure, and that imaginal and *in vivo* exposure were as effective as interoceptive exposure in reducing anxiety sensitivity.

Individuals with severe mental illnesses, such as schizophrenia, schizoaffective disorder, severe major depression, and bipolar disorder, are at high risk for exposure to the kinds of traumatic events most likely to produce PTSD, such as sexual and physical assault (Goodman, Rosenberg, Mueser, & Drake, 1997). Mueser and colleagues (2007) developed and evaluated a CBT program for the treatment of PTSD among individuals with severe mental illness, many of whom also meet criteria for personality disorders and substance use disorders. The primary focus of the treatment is on cognitive restructuring, but the program also includes coping skills training. The treatment has been evaluated in two nonrandomized studies, in which CBT was delivered individually (Rosenberg, Mueser, Jankowski, Salyers, & Acker, 2004) and in a group format (Mueser et al., 2007). In a recently completed randomized study, Mueser and colleagues (2008) found individually administered CBT to be more effective than TAU across a range of outcome variables. Interestingly, treatment ESs for PTSD were larger among the more severely ill participants, and the amount of homework completed was associated with better outcome.

Nightmares and sleep disturbance are two common symptoms of PTSD. Krakow, Kellner, Pathak, and Lambert (1995, 1996; see also Kellner, Neidhardt, Krakow, & Pathak, 1992) developed image rehearsal therapy, which combines instruction in sleep hygiene, cognitive restructuring, and imaginal exposure with the content of the nightmare, which is intentionally altered in some way. Krakow, Johnston, and colleagues (2001) first administered three sessions of image rehearsal therapy in small groups to individuals with trauma-related nightmares in a nonrandomized study of male and female victims of sexual and nonsexual assault and found significant reductions in nightmares, sleep disruption, and PTSD. Krakow, Hollifield, and colleagues (2001) conducted a randomized study of image rehearsal therapy (three sessions, administered in small groups) in a group of female sexual assault victims. Compared to WL, treatment resulted in significant reductions in nightmares, sleep disruptions, and PTSD. Forbes, Phelps, and McHugh (2001) replicated the pattern of improvement on nightmares, sleep disruption, and PTSD severity in a nonrandomized study of six sessions of image rehearsal treatment administered in small groups of Vietnam War veterans. Davis and Wright (2007) slightly modified the image rescripting therapy by adding relaxation training, increased exposure to the trauma-related content through writing and talking about the nightmares, and education about common trauma-related themes typically explored in CPT. Treatment with this exposure, relaxation, and rescripting therapy (ERRT) was administered individually or in small groups for three weekly sessions. As with previous studies of image rehearsal therapy, treatment was associated with greater reductions in nightmares, sleep disruption, and PTSD severity than was WL.

Ready access to evidence-based treatment for PTSD is generally limited in the United States to large cities or those cities with medical schools or academic graduate training programs in clinical psychology. This situation is changing in the Department of Veterans Affairs (VA) system, in which recent initiatives actively promote the dissemination of evidence-based treatments to make them more widely available to veterans. Yet even in locations where CBT is available, some individuals may be particularly hesitant to seek mental health services due to concerns about stigmatization, for example active duty military personnel. One innovation in the delivery of treatment that has the potential to address these limitations is use of the Internet to administer treatment. Lange and his colleagues have developed a treatment program called Interapy, which uses writing assignments administered via the Internet to implement a combination of education, exposure, and cognitive restructuring. Participants complete their written assignments, then receive feedback from a therapist who has read the assignments. All screening and pre- and posttreatment assessments were also conducted via the Internet. In the first two studies of Interapy, one randomized (Lange et al., 2001) and one nonrandomized (Lange et al., 2000) study, participants were psychology undergraduate students who completed the treatment for course credit. All participants reported having experienced a traumatic event at least 3 months earlier and reported symptoms of posttraumatic stress. In a third study (Lange et al., 2003), also a randomized trial, participants were recruited more broadly from the population of Amsterdam ($N = 184$, although only 54% of the sample completed the posttreatment evaluation; rates of noncompletion were similar across conditions). All three studies found that Interapy was associated with significant reductions in PTSD symptoms, and the two randomized trials found greater improvement for Interapy compared to WL.

Hirai and Clum (2005) also evaluated a CBT program delivered via the Internet, which included instruction in anxiety management techniques, cognitive restructuring, and exposure via writing. Patients ($N = 36$) were recruited from both college psychology undergraduate students and the community at large. Initial screening was conducted by telephone interview, and the remaining pre- and posttreatment assessments were self-report measures collected either online or via regular mail. Participants were selected for having reported the experience of a traumatic event and the presence of PTSD symptoms; histories of CSA and combat were exclusionary criteria out of concern for suicide risk. Treatment resulted in significantly greater improvement on the Stressful Responses Questionnaire—Frequency scale (SRQ; Clum, 1999) for reexperiencing and avoidance but not arousal. On the more familiar Impact of Events Scale—Revised (IES-R), ESs on all three scales favored the treatment condition, but none of the comparisons achieved statistical significance.

In the methodologically most sophisticated study of Internet-delivered CBT, Litz and colleagues (2007) recruited Department of Defense service members with PTSD related to the September 11, 2001, attack on the Pentagon, and military personnel with PTSD related to combat in Iraq or Afghanistan ($N = 45$). The pretreatment assessment included a clinician-administered assessment of PTSD severity by the study therapists, and posttreatment assessment was administered by an independent evaluator, blind to the participants' study condition. Treatments comprised one face-to-face meeting with a study therapist, with the remainder of the intervention administered via the Internet. The CBT comprised a combination of anxiety management, cognitive restructuring, *in vivo* exposure, and exposure to the trauma memory via writing; the comparison condition was supportive counseling. There were no significant differences between groups in the ITT analysis, but CBT resulted in greater improvement among completers at the 6-month follow-up.

Taken together, these studies provide strong support for the use of several CBT programs for the treatment of PTSD, but there is no consistent evidence for clear superiority of one treatment over the others. We have noted innovations in the populations studied, such as explicitly targeting nightmares and addressing comorbid conditions, and in treatment delivery mechanisms that may make access to CBT more readily available.

Summary and Recommendations

The evidence in support of the effectiveness of individual CBT for the treatment of PTSD in adults is now quite compelling. Numerous such programs have been shown to work in well-controlled studies meeting high methodological standards. Considering both the quantity and quality of evidence supporting each treatment, EX has the most studies, with 24 randomized controlled studies that, with few exceptions, support its use across a wide range of traumatized populations. Across studies, EX has been effectively implemented in numerous ways, including imaginal exposure, *in vivo* exposure, and writing about the trauma, although the most frequent and, therefore, most supported method of implementing exposure is the combination of imaginal exposure to the trauma memory plus *in vivo* exposure to feared and avoided, but low-risk people, places, situations and activities. In fact, no other treatment modality has received as much support as EX.

The next most supported CBT approaches are variations of cognitive therapy and SIT. Among the cognitive therapies, Resick's CPT has received support from four randomized controlled trials across different trauma samples, including female survivors of rape and CSA, and male and female veterans; Ehlers and Clark's cognitive therapy has received support from three randomized controlled studies utilizing mixed-gender/trauma samples and individuals affected by terrorism in Northern Ireland; Beck's cognitive therapy is supported by four randomized studies with female assault survivors and mixed-gender/trauma samples. SIT for PTSD among female assault victims has support from two randomized studies but has not been found effective in the treatment of male combat veterans except in one study, in which anger was the target of intervention and there was some concomitant effect on PTSD reexperiencing symptoms.

Direct comparisons between different efficacious CBT programs (e.g., EX vs. CT) have generally found comparable outcomes across different treatments. Similarly, studies that have compared combined treatment programs with the constituent components (e.g., EX plus SIT vs. EX alone) found comparable outcomes for the individual treatments and the combination treatments. Accordingly, EX (the combination of imaginal plus *in vivo* exposure), CT, SIT, and several of the various combination programs (e.g., CPT) are assigned an Agency for Health Care Policy and Research (AHCPR) Level A rating and are recommended as first-line psychological treatments for PTSD. More research with larger samples, repeated assessments using longitudinal analysis methods, or equivalence analyses will be needed to determine if there are small effect size differences between two active treatments and to determine more definitively if the various techniques and components are truly equivalent.

CBT is intended to be a short-term treatment, and 8–15 sessions lasting 60–120 minutes once or twice weekly may be used as a general guideline for planning the duration of treatment. However, some patients may be responsive to fewer sessions and other patients with more complex conditions may require a somewhat longer course of treatment. Accordingly, it is recommended that treatment not be terminated arbitrarily based on the number of sessions. Rather, treatment duration should be determined by a combination of the patient's progress and current symptoms status: If the patient has shown improvement but continues to experience significant PTSD, then continued treatment is likely to result in further benefit. If the patient has not shown improvement with a particular CBT approach in this period of time, then the therapist may wish to consider one of the other evidence-based treatments (e.g., shift from EX to CT or SIT).

Most studies of CBT for PTSD have administered the treatment as individual therapy, and the studies that evaluated group-administered treatment have produced mixed results. Two of the three studies of group CBT with veterans found little or no improvement on PTSD, whereas better results were obtained with civilian samples. However, the treatment protocols also differed considerably across these studies, making it difficult to specify what accounts for the difference in outcome. In addition, no studies have directly compared group-administered treatment with the same treatment administered individually to determine the effect of the different treatment delivery methods. One particular CBT program that was effectively administered in a group format is imagery rehearsal therapy targeting nightmares. However, given the limited evidence base for this treatment relative to other CBT programs to date, imagery rehearsal therapy is not recommended as a first-line treatment for PTSD. It may be useful as an ancillary treatment if residual sleep problems remain after a course of other CBT.

Two recent technological innovations are the use of virtual reality technology to implement EX and delivery of CBT via the Internet. At present, the amount of research on these technologies is limited and it is currently unknown how virtual reality EX or CBT administered through the Internet compares to the same treatment administered in the more conventional manner. Practical considerations also limit the utility of these treatments at this time. Although virtual reality technology may make it feasible to implement certain kinds of exposure exercises that would be difficult to implement *in vivo* (e.g., riding in a military helicopter for Vietnam War veterans), there are practical limitations to its widespread use: The technology is still relatively expensive, few therapists have access to it, and treatment programs are available for only a limited number of traumas. Use of the Internet to deliver treatment has the potential to provide CBT to people in locations where it would otherwise not be available. However, use of a technology that allows a therapist to deliver treatment to someone he or she has never seen in person could very well mean providing treatment to someone in a different state or even country, raising ethical and legal issues that would need to be worked out prior to our making strong recommendations supporting the routine use of this service delivery mechanism.

The limited research on RLX indicates that it is less efficacious than other CBT programs and, based on the previous edition of this volume (Rothbaum et al., 2000), biofeedback and assertiveness training have not been found to be effective in the treatment of PTSD. Accordingly, such methods cannot be recommended as primary treatments for PTSD, although relaxation may be part of a combination CBT program, and assertiveness training may be useful as ancillary interventions for specific problems in certain patients with PTSD. The proposal that skills training in affect and interpersonal regulation, based on DBT, may play a useful role in the treatment of PTSD is supported in three randomized studies. In one study that employed group therapy with

DBT-based intervention as the primary mode of treatment, the intervention was found to be more effective than the WL condition. Given the limited evidence for the efficacy of DBT-based skills training as a primary treatment for PTSD in comparison to other CBT programs (i.e., EX, CT, and SIT) we cannot recommend routine use of this treatment modality for PTSD at this time. Two studies that employed DBT interventions as preparation for undergoing more trauma-focused interventions found this combination to be efficacious, although two considerations lead to us to conclude that *routine* application of DBT skills training prior to trauma-focused treatment is not recommended *at this time*. The first consideration is the strength of the evidence for other CBT interventions (i.e., EX, CT, and SIT) that have been helpful without such preliminary skills training. The second consideration is that, to date, no published studies have evaluated whether preliminary skills training enhances outcome for trauma-focused CBT. There are insufficient data to evaluate the efficacy of ACT at this time. Thus, we cannot recommend ACT as a first-line treatment for PTSD.

Future Directions

Research Methods

Our review has revealed three methodological limitations of much of the current research on treatment for PTSD. First, a significant minority of studies reported analyses only for treatment completers. As attrition from treatment may be related to treatment outcome (e.g., patients not responding well to treatment may be more likely to drop out), and attrition may be differential across study groups (e.g., dropout from CBT is higher than for control conditions; Hembree et al., 2003), completer analyses may yield biased results. This concern is supported by the observation that studies reporting both completer and ITT analyses typically find stronger treatment effects in the completer sample (e.g., Bryant et al., 2003; Foa et al., 2005; Resick et al., 2002). Although the proportion of studies reporting ITT analyses is increasing, 25% of studies published in 2007–2008 or currently "in press" exclusively reported completer analyses.

Second, most studies comparing different CBT programs did not have adequate samples to detect anything but large effect sizes. Thus, the general finding of comparable outcomes across different CBT programs may reflect low statistical power to detect small, but real, differences in efficacy. Future comparative outcome studies should be adequately powered to detect medium or even small effect sizes. And third, greater attention should be paid to the possible role of therapist effects (e.g., therapist background and allegiance) on treatment outcome, particularly in studies comparing active treatments. This may take the form of reporting greater detail about study therapists, using a large number of therapists and randomly assigning therapists to treatment conditions, and conducting analyses to evaluate variability in treatment outcome that may be related to therapist characteristics.

Comorbidity

Although most studies of CBT for PTSD include measures of common comorbid psychopathology, such as severity of depression and general anxiety, much less is known about effect of comorbidity on the efficacy of treatment for PTSD, and the effect of treatment for PTSD on comorbid conditions. Available evidence on such questions is limited and mixed. Although many studies have found reductions in depression diagnosis along with improvements in PTSD (e.g., Resick et al., 2002, 2008), there is evidence from the Tarrier and colleagues (1999) study of imaginal EX and CT that comorbidity with generalized anxiety disorder (GAD) is associated with worse outcome; yet, in contrast, the study of a combined CBT condition by Blanchard and colleagues (2003) found that treatment for PTSD reduced the incidence of GAD. To the extent that comorbidity reduces the efficacy of current treatments for PTSD, or that treatment for PTSD does not affect comorbidity, what are the optimal strategies for addressing comorbidity? The study by Falsetti and colleagues (2001) integrating panic control treatment with CPT provides one model for addressing common comorbidities, although additional research is needed to determine whether development or implementation of such integrated treatments is a necessary or optimal way to address comorbidity.

Related to the issue of comorbidity is the idea that certain trauma populations, such as victims of childhood abuse or domestic violence, have unique or additional needs that are not adequately addressed by certain CBT interventions, such as EX. For the most part, such recommendations are based on clinical judgment and research into matching patients with treatments or comparisons of the adapted treatments with the original treatment (e.g., EX with and without DBT skills or CPT-SA compared to CPT among CSA survivors) is needed.

Necessary, Sufficient, and Facilitating Conditions for Treating PTSD

As this review has demonstrated, a large number of studies has found a broad range of interventions to be effective in the treatment of PTSD, yet the sheer variety of treatment conditions that leads to improvement on PTSD (e.g., contrast the vast procedural differences among EX, CT, and SIT) indicates that although we have identified some of the *sufficient* conditions for the treatment of PTSD, we have not yet isolated the *necessary* conditions for its treatment, nor have we been able to specify which conditions, though not necessary for PTSD treatment, serve to facilitate it. Clear differentiation of the necessary, sufficient, and facilitatory conditions would be expected to streamline treatments by eliminating unnecessary components that neither contribute to overall efficacy nor maximize treatment outcome.

Mechanisms of Recovery from PTSD

Related to the preceding point is the observation that different CBT treatments, historically, were predicated on somewhat different theoretical formulations but appear to have similar efficacy. This raises the question of whether different mechanisms of recovery operate in different treatments that coincidentally yield similar results, or whether these seemingly different treatments actually tap into the same mechanisms. If the latter is the case, what are these mechanisms, and what is their relationship to natural recovery? We expect that a greater understanding of the mechanisms responsible for recovery from PTSD will lead to enhanced interventions for the treatment and prevention of chronic PTSD.

Enhancing Treatment Outcome

Our focus in this review has been on evidence for the efficacy of CBT for PTSD. Yet even among the best outcomes achieved in the treatment studies considered here, some participants receive little benefit, and many others have at least some residual symptoms of PTSD. The principal strategy employed thus far to enhance outcome has been to combine different treatment strategies, such as adding CT or SIT to EX, yet results of the few studies that have specifically studied this strategy have yielded generally disappointing results. What may be needed is the use of more creative research designs that isolate individuals who do not respond adequately to one of the currently supported treatments to identify needed alternative or additional interventions to achieve good outcome. Along these lines, studies of predictors of treatment outcome may lead to treatment matching that could facilitate outcomes.

Making Evidence-Based Treatment Widely Available

Evidence-based treatments for PTSD are of little use to trauma survivors if therapists who see these patients are not trained in, or for other reasons do not use, them. Creating innovative treatment delivery systems, such as the use of the Internet to deliver therapy, is one way to make treatments more available. Another approach is to identify and address the barriers that may exist for therapists in learning and using these treatments. Specifically, research needs to identify the most effective and efficient ways to train therapists in the use of evidence-based treatments, and to motivate them to use these treatments. Research on dissemination and implementation of evidence-based treatments may be one of the most important next-generation topics.

Acknowledgments

We gratefully acknowledge (in alphabetical order) the assistance of Kathryn C. Adair, Kallio Hunnicutt-Ferguson, James Marinchak, and Sofia Talbott.

Note

1. Because this study was published in German, the preceding description is based on a brief summary by Schauer (personal communication, September 30, 2007), and the current reviewers are not able to provide an independent evaluation of the quality of the study.

References

Barlow, D. H., & Craske, M. G. (1988). *Mastery of your anxiety and panic: Treatment manual.* Albany, NY: Graywind.

Barlow, D. H., & Craske, M. G. (1994). *Mastery of your anxiety and panic II: Treatment manual.* Albany, NY: Graywind.

Basoglu, E., Livanou, M., & Salcioglu, M. (2003). A single session with an earthquake simulator for traumatic stress in earthquake survivors. *American Journal of Psychiatry, 4,* 788–790.

Basoglu, E., Livanou, M., Salcioglu, M., & Kalender, D. (2003). A brief behavioral treatment of chronic post-traumatic stress disorder in earthquake survivors: Results from an open clinical trial. *Psychological Medicine, 33,* 647–654.

Basoglu, M., Salcioglu, E., & Livanou, M. (2007). A randomized controlled study of single- session behavioral treatment of earthquake-related post-traumatic stress disorder using an earthquake simulator. *Psychological Medicine, 37,* 203–213.

Basoglu, M., Salcioglu, E., Livanou, M., Kalender, D., & Gonul, A. (2005). Single-session behavioral treatment of earthquake-related posttraumatic stress disorder: A randomized waiting list controlled trial. *Journal of Traumatic Stress, 18,* 1–11.

Batten, S. V., Orsillo, S. M., & Walser, D. (2005). Acceptance and mindfulness based approaches to the treatment of posttraumatic stress disorder. In S. M. Orsillo & L. Roemer (Eds.), *Acceptance and mindfulness based approaches to anxiety: Conceptualization and treatment* (pp. 241–269). New York: Plenum Press.

Beck, A. T. (1976). *Cognitive therapy and the emotional disorders.* New York: International Universities Press.

Beck, A. T., Emery, G., & Greenberg, R. L. (1985). *Anxiety disorders and phobias.* New York: Basic Books.

Beck, A. T., Rush, A. J., Shaw, B. F., & Emery, G. (1979). *Cognitive therapy of depression.* New York: Guilford Press.

Beck, J. G., Coffey, S. F., Foy, D. W., Keane, T. M., & Blanchard, E. B. (in press). Group cognitive behavior therapy for chronic posttraumatic stress disorder: An initial randomized pilot study. *Behavior Therapy.*

Bichescu, D., Neuner, F., Schauer, M., & Elbert, T. (2007). Narrative exposure therapy of political imprisonment-related chronic trauma-spectrum disorders. *Behaviour Research and Therapy, 45,* 2212–2220.

Bichescu, D., Schauer, M., Saleptsi, E., Neculau, A., Elbert, T., & Neuner, F. (2005). Long-term consequences of traumatic experiences: An assessment of former political detainees in Romania. *Clinical Practice and Epidemiology in Mental Health, 1,* 17.

Blanchard, E. B., Hickling, E. J., Trishul, D., Veazey, C. H., Galovski, T. E., Mundy, E., et al. (2003). A controlled evaluation of cognitive behavioral therapy for posttraumatic stress in motor vehicle accident survivors. *Behaviour Research and Therapy, 41,* 79–96.

Bolton, E. E., Lambert, J. F., Wolf, E., Raja, S., Varra, A. A., & Fisher, L. M. (2004). Evaluating a cognitive-behavioral group treatment program for veterans with posttraumatic stress disorder. *Psychological Services, 1,* 140–146.

Boudewyns, P. A., & Hyer, L. (1990). Physiological response to combat memories and preliminary treatment outcome in Vietnam veterans PTSD patients treated with direct therapeutic exposure. *Behavior Therapy, 21,* 63–87.

Bradley, R. G., & Follingstad, D. R. (2003). Group therapy for incarcerated women who experienced interpersonal violence: A pilot study. *Journal of Traumatic Stress, 16,* 337–340.

Brewin, C. R., Dalgleish, T., & Joseph, S. (1996). A dual representational theory of posttraumatic stress disorder. *Psychological Review, 103,* 670–686.

Briere, J. (1995). *The Trauma Symptom Inventory (TSI): Professional manual.* Odessa, FL: Psychological Assessment Resources.

Bryant, R. A., Moulds, M. L., Guthrie, R. M., Dang, S. T., & Nixon, R. D. V. (2003). Imaginal exposure alone and imaginal exposure with cognitive restructuring in treatment of posttraumatic stress disorder. *Journal of Consulting and Clinical Psychology, 71,* 706–712.

Chard, K. M. (2005). An evaluation of cognitive processing therapy for the treatment of posttraumatic stress disorder related to childhood sexual abuse. *Journal of Consulting and Clinical Psychology, 73,* 965–971.

Chemtob, C. M., Novaco, R. W., Hamada, R. S., & Gross, D. M. (1997). Cognitive-behavioral treatment of severe anger in posttraumatic stress disorder. *Journal of Consulting and Clinical Psychology, 65,* 184–189.

Clark, D. M. (1986). A cognitive approach to panic. *Behaviour Research and Therapy, 24,* 461–470.

Cloitre, M., Koenen, K. C., Cohen, L. R., & Han, H. (2002). Skills training in affective and interpersonal regulation followed by exposure: A phase-based treatment for PTSD related to childhood abuse. *Journal of Consulting and Clinical Psychology, 70,* 1067–1074.

Clum, G. A. (1999). [Development of PTSD measures]. Unpublished raw data.

Cooper, N. A., & Clum, G. A. (1989). Imaginal flooding as a supplementary treatment for PTSD in combat veterans: A controlled study. *Behavior Therapy, 3,* 381–391.

Davis, J. L., & Wright, D. C. (2007). Randomized clinical trial for treatment of chronic nightmares in trauma-exposed adults. *Journal of Traumatic Stress, 20,* 123–133.

Devilly, G. J., & Spence, S. H., (1999). The relative efficacy and treatment distress of EMDR and a cognitive-behavior trauma treat protocol in the amelioration of posttraumatic stress disorder. *Journal of Anxiety Disorders, 13,* 131–157.

Difede, J., Cukor, J., Jayasinghe, N., Patt, I., Jedel, S., Spielman, L., et al. (2007). Virtual reality exposure therapy for the treatment of posttraumatic stress disorder following September 11, 2001. *Journal of Clinical Psychiatry, 68,* 1639–1647.

Difede, J., Malta, L. S., Best, S., Henn-Haase, C., Metzler, T., Bryant, R., et al. (2007). A randomized controlled clinical treatment trial for World Trade Center attack–related PTSD in disaster workers. *Journal of Nervous and Mental Disorders, 195,* 861–865.

Duffy, M., Gillespie, K., & Clark, D. M. (2007). Post-traumatic stress disorder in the context of terrorism and other civil conflict in Northern Ireland: Randomised controlled trial. *British Medical Journal, 334,* 1147–1150.

Echeburúa, E., de Corral, P., Zubizarreta, I., & Sarasua, B. (1997). Psychological treatment of chronic posttraumatic stress disorder in victims of sexual aggression. *Behavior Modification, 21,* 433–456.

Ehlers, A., & Clark, D. M. (2000). A cognitive model of posttraumatic stress disorder. *Behaviour Research and Therapy, 38,* 319–345.

Ehlers, A., Clark, D. M., Hackmann, A., McManus, F., & Fennell, M. (2005). Cognitive therapy for post-traumatic stress disorder: Development and evaluation. *Behaviour Research and Therapy, 43,* 413–431.

Ehlers, A., Clark, D. M., Hackmann, A., McManus, F., Fennell, M., Herbert, C., et al. (2003). A randomized controlled trial of cognitive therapy, a self-help booklet, and repeated assessment as early interventions for posttraumatic stress disorder. *Archives of General Psychiatry, 60,* 1024–1032.

Falsetti, S. A., Resnick, H. S., Davis, J., & Gallagher, N. G. (2001). Treatment of post-traumatic stress disorder with comorbid panic attacks: Combining cognitive processing therapy with panic control treatment techniques. *Group Dynamics: Theory, Research, and Practice, 5,* 252–260.

Fecteau, G., & Nicki, R. (1999). Cognitive behavioural treatment of post traumatic stress disorder after motor vehicle accident. *Behavioural and Cognitive Psychotherapy, 27,* 201–214.

Feske, U. (2001). Treating low-income and African-American women with posttraumatic stress disorder: A case series. *Behavior Therapy, 32,* 585–601.

Foa, E. B., Dancu, C. V., Hembree, E. A., Jaycox, L. H., Meadows, E. A., & Street, G. P. (1999). The efficacy of exposure therapy, stress inoculation training and their combination in ameliorating PTSD for female victims of assault. *Journal of Consulting and Clinical Psychology, 67,* 194–200.

Foa, E. B., Hembree, E. A., Cahill, S. P., Rauch, S. A., Riggs, D. S., Feeny, N. C., et al. (2005). Randomized trial of prolonged exposure for PTSD with and without cognitive restructuring: Outcome at academic and community clinics. *Journal of Consulting and Clinical Psychology, 73,* 953–964.

Foa, E. B., Hembree, E. A., & Rothbaum, B. O. (2007). *Prolonged exposure therapy for PTSD: Emotional processing of traumatic experiences.* New York: Oxford University Press.

Foa, E. B., & Kozak, M. J. (1986). Emotional processing of fear: Exposure to corrective information. *Psychological Bulletin, 99,* 20–35.

Foa, E. B., & Meadows, E. A. (1997). Psychosocial treatments for post-traumatic stress disorder: A critical review. In J. Spence, J. M. Darley, & D. J. Foss (Eds.), *Annual review of psychology* (Vol. 48, pp. 449–480). Palo Alto, CA: Annual Reviews.

Foa, E. B., Riggs, D. S., Massie, E. D., & Yarczower, M. (1995). The impact of fear activation and anger on the efficacy of exposure treatment for PTSD. *Behavior Therapy, 26,* 487–499.

Foa, E. B., & Rothbaum, B. O. (1998). *Treating the trauma of rape: A cognitive-behavioral therapy for PTSD.* New York: Guilford Press.

Foa, E. B., Rothbaum, B. O., Riggs, D., & Murdock, T. (1991). Treatment of post-traumatic stress disorder in rape victims: A comparison between cognitivebehavioral procedures and counseling. *Journal of Consulting and Clinical Psychology, 59,* 715–723.

Foa, E. B., Steketee, G., & Rothbaum, B. O. (1989). Behavioral/cognitive conceptualizations of post-traumatic stress disorder. *Behavior Therapy, 20,* 155–176.

Follette, V. M., Palm, K. M., & Hall, R. L. (2004). Acceptance, mindfulness and trauma. In S. C. Hayes, V. M. Follette, & M. M. Linehan (Eds.), *Mindfulness and acceptance: Expanding the cognitive-behavioral tradition* (pp. 192–208). New York: Guilford Press.

Forbes, D., Phelps A., & McHugh, T. (2001). Treatment of combat-related nightmares using imagery rehearsal: A pilot study. *Journal of Traumatic Stress, 14,* 433–442.

Frank, E., Anderson, B., Stewart, B. D., Dancu, C., Hughes, C., & West, D. (1988). Efficacy of cognitive behavior therapy and systematic desensitization in the treatment of rape trauma. *Behavior Therapy, 19,* 403–420.

Frommberger, U., Stieglitz, R. D., Nyberg, E., Richter, H., Novelli-Fischer, U., Angenendt, J., et al. (2004). Comparison between paroxetine and behaviour therapy in patients with posttraumatic stress disorder (PTSD): A pilot study. *International Journal of Psychiatry in Clinical Practice, 8,* 19–23.

Frueh, B. C., Turner, S. M., Beidel, D. C., Mirabella, R. F., & Jones, W. J. (1996). Trauma management therapy: A preliminary evaluation of a multicomponent behavioral treatment for chronic combatrelated PTSD. *Behaviour Research and Therapy, 34,* 533–543.

Gerardi, M., Rothbaum, B. O., Ressler, K., Heekin, M., & Rizzo, A. (2008). Virtual reality exposure therapy using a virtual Iraq: Case report. *Journal of Traumatic Stress, 21,* 209–213.

Gersons, B. P. R., Carlier, I. V. E., Lamberts, R. D., & van der Kolk, B. A. (2000). Randomized clinical trial of brief eclectic psychotherapy for police officers with posttraumatic stress disorder. *Journal of Traumatic Stress, 13,* 333–347.

Gillespie, K., Duffy, M., Hackmann, A., & Clark, D. M. (2002). Community based cognitive therapy in the treatment of post-traumatic stress disorder following the Omagh bomb. *Behaviour Research and Therapy, 40,* 345–357.

Glynn, S. M., Eth, S., Randolph, E. T., Foy, D. W., Urbatis, M., Boxer, L., et al. (1999). A test of behavioral family therapy to augment exposure for combatrelated PTSD. *Journal of Consulting and Clinical Psychology, 67,* 243–251.

Goodman, L. A., Rosenberg, S. D., Mueser, K. T., & Drake, R. E. (1997). Physical and sexual assault history in women with serious mental illness: Prevalence, correlates, treatment, and future directions. *Schizophrenia Bulletin, 23,* 685–696.

Hayes, S. C. (1987). A contextual approach to therapeutic change. In N. S. Jacobson (Ed.), *Psychotherapists in clinical practice: Cognitive and behavioral perspectives* (pp. 327–387). New York: Guilford Press.

Hayes, S. C., Follette, W. C., & Follette, V. M. (1995). Behavior therapy: A contextual approach. In A. S. Gurman & S. B. Messer (Eds.), *Essential psychotherapies: Theory and practice* (pp. 128–181). New York: Guilford Press.

Hayes, S. C., Strosahl, K. D., & Wilson, K. G. (1999). *Acceptance and commitment therapy: An experiential approach to behavior change.* New York: Guilford Press.

Hayes, S. C., & Wilson, K. G. (1994). Acceptance and commitment therapy: Altering the verbal support for experiential avoidance. *Behavior Analyst, 17*, 289–303.

Hayes, S. C., Wilson, K. G., Gifford, E., Follette, V. M., & Strosahl, K. D. (1996). Emotional avoidance and behavioral disorders: A functional dimensional approach to diagnosis and treatment. *Journal of Consulting and Clinical Psychology, 64*, 1152–1168.

Hembree, E. A., Foa, E. B., Dorfan, N. M., Street, G. P., Kowalski, J., & Tu, X. (2003). Do patients drop out prematurely from exposure therapy for PTSD? *Journal of Traumatic Stress, 16*, 555–562.

Hickling, E. J., & Blanchard, E. B. (1997). The private practice psychologist and manual-based treatments: Post-traumatic stress disorder secondary to motor vehicle accidents. *Behaviour Research and Therapy, 35*, 191–203.

Hinton, D. E., Chhean, D., Pich, V., Safren, S. A., Hofmann, S. G., & Pollack, M. H. (2005). A randomized controlled trial of cognitive-behavior therapy for Cambodian refugees with treatment-resistant PTSD and panic attack: A cross-over design. *Journal of Traumatic Stress, 18*, 617–629.

Hinton, D. E., Chhean, D., Pich, V., Um, K., Fama, J. M., & Pollack, M. H. (2006). Neck-focused panic attacks among Cambodian refugees: A logistic and linear regression analysis. *Journal of Anxiety Disorders, 20*, 119–138.

Hinton, D. E., Pham, T., Tran, M., Safren, S. A., Otto, M. W., & Pollack, M. H. (2004). CBT for Vietnamese refugees with treatment-resistant PTSD and panic attacks: A pilot study. *Journal of Traumatic Stress, 17*, 429–433.

Hinton, D. E., Pollack, M. H., Pich, V., Fama, J. M., & Barlow, D. H. (2005). Orthostatically induced panic attacks among Cambodian refugees: Flashbacks, catastrophic cognitions, and associated psychopathology. *Cognitive and Behavioral Practice, 12*, 301–311.

Hirai, M., & Clum, G. A. (2005). An Internet-based self-change program for traumatic event related fear, distress, and maladaptive coping. *Journal of Traumatic Stress, 18*, 631–636.

Hollifield, M., Sinclair-Lian, N., Warner, T. D., & Hammerschlag, R. (2007). Acupuncture for posttraumatic stress disorder: A randomized controlled pilot trial. *Journal of Nervous and Mental Disease, 195*, 504–513.

Ironson, G., Freund, B., Strauss, J. L., & Williams, J. (2002). Comparison of two treatments for traumatic stress: A community-based study of EMDR and prolonged exposure. *Journal of Clinical Psychology, 58*, 113–128.

Johnson, D. M., & Zlotnick, C. (2006). A cognitive-behavioral treatment for battered women with PTSD in shelters: Findings from a pilot study. *Journal of Traumatic Stress, 19*, 559–564.

Keane, T. M., Fairbank, J. A., Caddell, J. M., & Zimering, R. T. (1989). Implosive (flooding) therapy reduces symptoms of PTSD in Vietnam combat veterans. *Behavior Therapy, 20*, 245–260.

Kellner, R., Neidhardt, J., Krakow, B., & Pathak, D. (1992). Changes in chronic nightmares after one session of desensitization or rehearsal instructions. *American Journal of Psychiatry, 149*, 659–663.

Kessler, R. C., Sonnega, A., Bromet, E., Hughes, M., & Nelson, C. B. (1995). Posttraumatic stress disorder in the National Comorbidity Survey. *Archives of General Psychiatry, 52*, 1048–1060.

Kilpatrick, D. G., Veronen, L. J., & Resick, P. A. (1982). Psychological sequelae to rape:

Assessment and treatment strategies. In D. M. Dolays & R. L. Meredith (Eds.), *Behavioral medicine: Assessment and treatment strategies* (pp. 473–497). New York: Plenum Press.

Krakow, B., Hollifield, M., Johnston, L., Koss, M., Schrader, R., Warner, T. D., et al. (2001). Imagery rehearsal therapy for chronic nightmares in sexual assault survivors with posttraumatic stress disorder: A randomized controlled trial. *Journal of the American Medical Association, 286,* 537–545.

Krakow, B., Johnston, L., Melendrez, D., Hollifield, M., Warner, T. D., Chavez-Kennedy, D., et al. (2001). An open-label trial of evidence-based cognitive behavior therapy for nightmares and insomnia in crime victims with PTSD. *American Journal of Psychiatry, 158,* 2043–2047.

Krakow, B., Kellner, R., Pathak, D., & Lambert, L. (1995). Imagery rehearsal treatment for chronic nightmares. *Behavioural Research and Therapy, 33,* 837–843.

Krakow, B., Kellner, R., Pathak, D., & Lambert, L. (1996). Long-term reductions in nightmares treated with imagery rehearsal. *Behavioural and Cognitive Psychotherapy, 24,* 135–148.

Kubany, E. S., Haynes, S. N., Abueg, F. R., Manke, F. P., Brennan, J. M., & Stahura, C. (1996). Development and validation of the Trauma-Related Guilt Inventory (TRGI). *Psychological Assessment, 8,* 428–444.

Kubany, E. S., Hill, E. E., & Owens, J. A. (2003). Cognitive trauma therapy for battered women with PTSD: Preliminary findings. *Journal of Traumatic Stress, 16,* 81–91.

Kubany, E. S., Hill, E. E., Owens, J. A., Iannce-Spencer, C., McCaig, M. A., Tremayne, K. J., et al. (2004). Cognitive trauma therapy for battered women with PTSA (CTT-BW). *Journal of Counseling and Clinical Psychology, 72,* 3–18.

Lange, A., Rietdijk, D., Hudcovicova, M., van de Ven, J. P., Schrieken, B., & Emmelkamp, P. M. G. (2003). Interapy: A controlled randomized trial of the standardized treatment of posttraumatic stress through the internet. *Journal of Consulting and Clinical Psychology, 71,* 901–909.

Lange, A., Schrieken, B., van de Ven, J. P., Bredeweg, B., Emmelkamp, P. M. G., van der Kolk, J., et al. (2000). "Interapy": The effects of a short protocolled treatment of posttraumatic stress and pathological grief through the Internet. *Behavioural and Cognitive Psychotherapy, 28,* 175–192.

Lange, A., van de Ven, J., Schrieken, B., & Emmelkamp, P. M. G. (2001). Interapy: Treatment of posttraumatic stress through the internet: A controlled trial. *Journal of Behavior Therapy and Experimental Psychiatry, 32,* 73–90.

Lee, C., Gavriel, H., Drummond, P., Richards, J., & Greenwald, R. (2002). Treatment of PTSD: Stress inoculation training with prolonged exposure compared to EMDR. *Journal of Clinical Psychology, 58,* 1071–1089.

Levitt, J. T., Malta, L. S., Martin, A., Davis, L., & Cloitre, M. (2007). The flexible application of a manualized treatment for PTSD symptoms and functional impairment related to the 9/11 World Trade Center attack. *Behaviour Research and Therapy, 45,* 1419–1433.

Lindauer, R. J. L., Gersons, B. P. R., van Meijel, E. P. M., Blom, K., Carlier, I. V. E., Vrijlandt, I., et al. (2005). Effects of brief eclectic psychotherapy in-patient with posttraumatic stress disorder: Randomized clinical trial. *Journal of Traumatic Stress, 18,* 205–212.

Lindauer, R. J. L., Vlieger, E. J., Jalink, M., Olff, M., Carlier, I. V. E., Majoie, C., et al. (2005). Effects of psychotherapy on hippocampal volume in out-patients with post-traumatic stress disorder: A MRI investigation. *Psychological Medicine, 35,* 1421–1431.

Linehan, M. M. (1993). *Cognitive-behavioral treatment of borderline personality disorder.* New York: Guilford Press.

Litz, B. T., Engel, C. C., Bryant, R. A., & Papa, A. (2007). A randomized, controlled proof-of-concept trial of an Internet-based, therapist-assisted self-management treatment for posttraumatic stress disorder. *American Journal of Psychiatry, 164,* 1676–1683.

Maercker, A., Zollner, T., Menning, H., Rabe, S., & Karl, A. (2006). Dresden PTSD Treatment Study: Randomized controlled trial of motor vehicle accident survivors. *BMC Psychiatry, 6,* 1–8.

Marks, I., Lovell, K., Noshirvani, H., Livanou, M., & Thrasher, S. (1998). Treatment of posttraumatic stress disorder by exposure and/or cognitive restructuring: A controlled study. *Archives of General Psychiatry, 55,* 317–325.

McCann, I. L., & Pearlman, L. A. (1990). *Psychological trauma and the adult survivor: Theory, therapy, and transformation.* New York: Brunner/Mazel.

McDonagh, A., Friedman, M., McHugo, G., Ford, J., Sengupta, A., Mueser, K., et al. (2005). Randomized trial of cognitive-behavioral therapy for chronic posttraumatic stress disorder in adult female survivors of childhood sexual abuse. *Journal of Counseling and Clinical Psychology, 73,* 515–524.

Meichenbaum, D. (1974). Selfinstructional methods. In F. H. Kanfer & A. P. Goldstein (Eds.), *Helping people change* (pp. 357–391). New York: Pergamon Press.

Monson, C. M., Rodriguez, B. F., & Warner, R. (2005). Cognitive-behavioral therapy for PTSD in the real world: Do interpersonal relationships make a difference? *Journal of Clinical Psychology, 61,* 751–761.

Monson, C. M., Schnurr, P. P., Resick, P. A., Friedman, M. J., Young-Xu, Y., & Stevens, S. P. (2006). Cognitive processing therapy for veterans with military-related posttraumatic stress disorder. *Journal of Consulting and Clinical Psychology, 74,* 898–907.

Mowrer, O. A. (1960). *Learning theory and behavior.* New York: Wiley.

Mueser, K. T., Bolton, E., Carty, P. C., Bradley, M. J., Ahlgren, K. F., DiStaso, D. R., et al. (2007). The trauma recovery group: A cognitive-behavioral program for posttraumatic stress disorder in persons with severe mental illness. *Community Mental Health Journal, 43,* 281–304.

Mueser, K. T., Rosenberg, S. D., Xie, H., Jankowski, M. K., Bolton, E. E., Lu, W., et al. (2008). A randomized controlled trial of cognitive-behavioral treatment for posttraumatic stress disorder in severe mental illness. *Journal of Consulting and Clinical Psychology, 76,* 259–271.

Naugle, A. E., & Follette, W. C. (1998). A functional analysis of trauma symptoms. In V. M. Follette, J. I. Ruzek, & F. R. Abueg (Eds.), *Cognitivebehavioral therapies for trauma* (pp. 48–73). New York: Guilford Press.

Neuner, F., Schauer, M., Klaschik, C., Karunakara, U., & Elbert, T. (2004) A comparison of narrative exposure therapy, supportive counseling, and psychoeducation for treating posttraumatic stress disorder in an African refugee settlement. *Journal of Consulting and Clinical Psychology, 72,* 579–587.

Novaco, R. W. (1994). Clinical problems of anger and its assessment and regulation through a stress coping skills approach. In W. O'Donohue & L. Krasner (Eds.), *Handbook of psychological skills training: Clinical techniques and applications* (pp. 320–338). Boston: Allyn & Bacon.

Otto, M. W., Hinton, D., Korbly, N. B., Chea, A., Ba, P., Gershuny, B. S., et al. (2003). Treatment of pharmacotherapy-refractory posttraumatic stress disorder among Cambodian refugees: A pilot study of combination treatment with cognitive-behavior therapy vs. sertraline alone. *Behaviour Research and Therapy, 41*, 1271–1276.

Paunovic, N., & Öst, L. G. (2001). Cognitive-behavior therapy vs. exposure therapy in the treatment of PTSD in refugees. *Behaviour Research and Therapy, 39*, 1183–1197.

Pitman, R. K., Orr, S. P., Altman, B., & Longpre, R. E. (1996). Emotional processing and outcome of imaginal flooding therapy in Vietnam veterans with chronic posttraumatic stress disorder. *Comprehensive Psychiatry, 37*, 409–418.

Power, K., McGoldrick, T., Brown, K., Buchanan, R., Sharp, D., Swanson, V., et al. (2002). A controlled comparison of eye movement desensitization and reprocessing versus exposure plus cognitive restructuring versus waiting list in the treatment of post-traumatic stress disorder. *Clinical Psychology and Psychotherapy, 9*, 299–318.

Ready, D. J., Thomas, K. R., Worley, V., Backscheider, A. G., Harvey, L. A. C., Baltzell, D., et al. (2008). A field test of group based exposure therapy with 102 veterans with war-related posttraumatic stress disorder. *Journal of Traumatic Stress, 21*, 150–157.

Resick, P. A., Galovski, T. E., Uhlmansiek, M. O., Scher, C. D., Clum, G. A., & Young-Xu, Y. (2008). A randomized clinical trial to dismantle components of cognitive processing therapy for posttraumatic stress disorder in female victims of interpersonal violence. *Journal of Consulting and Clinical Psychology, 76*, 243–258.

Resick, P. A., Jordan, C. G., Girelli, S. A., Hutter, C. K., & Marhoefer-Dvorak, S. (1988). A comparative victim study of behavioral group therapy for sexual assault victims. *Behavior Therapy, 19*, 385–401.

Resick, P. A., Nishith, P., & Griffin, M. G. (2003). How well does cognitive-behavioral therapy treat symptoms of complex PTSD?: An examination of child sexual abuse survivors within a clinical trial. *CNS Spectrums, 8*, 340–342, 351–355.

Resick, P. A., Nishith, P., Weaver, T. L., Astin, M. C., & Feurer, C. A. (2002). A comparison of cognitive-processing therapy with prolonged exposure and a waiting condition for the treatment of chronic posttraumatic stress disorder in female rape victims. *Journal of Consulting and Clinical Psychology, 70*, 867–879.

Resick, P. A., & Schnicke, M. K. (1992). Cognitive processing therapy for sexual assault victims. *Journal of Consulting and Clinical Psychology, 60*, 748–756.

Resick, P. A., & Schnicke, M. K. (1993). *Cognitive processing therapy for rape victims: A treatment manual.* Newbury Park, CA: Sage.

Richards, D. A., Lovell, K., & Marks, I. M. (1994). Posttraumatic stress disorder: Evaluation of a behavioral treatment program. *Journal of Traumatic Stress, 7*, 669–680.

Rosenberg, S. D., Mueser, K. T., Jankowski, M. K., Salyers, M. P., & Acker, K. (2004). Cognitive-behavioral treatment of PTSD in severe mental illness: Results of a pilot study. *American Journal of Psychiatric Rehabilitation, 7*, 171–186.

Rothbaum, B. O., Astin, M. C., & Marsteller, F. (2005). Prolonged exposure versus eye movement desensitization and reprocessing (EMDR) for PTSD rape victims. *Journal of Traumatic Stress, 18*, 607–616.

Rothbaum, B. O., Cahill, S. P., Foa, E. B., Davidson, J. R. T., Compton, J., Connor, K., et al. (2006). Augmentation of sertraline with prolonged exposure in the treatment of PTSD. *Journal of Traumatic Stress, 19*, 625–638.

Rothbaum, B. O., Hodges, L., Ready, D., Graap, K., & Alarcon, R. (2001). Virtual reality exposure therapy for Vietnam veterans with posttraumatic stress disorder. *Journal of Clinical Psychiatry, 62*, 617–622.

Rothbaum, B. O., Meadows, E. A., Resick, P., & Foy, D. W. (2000). Cognitive-behavioral therapy. In E. B. Foa, T. M. Keane, & M. J. Friedman (Eds.), *Effective treatments for PTSD: Practice guidelines from the International Society for Traumatic Stress Studies* (pp. 60–83). New York: Guilford Press.

Schauer, M., Elbert, T., Gotthardt, S., Rockstroh, B., Odenwald, M., & Neuner, F. (2006). Wiedererfahrung durch Psychotherapie modifiziert Geist und Gehirn [Imaginary reliving in psychotherapy modifies mind and brain]. *Verhaltenstherapie, 16*, 96–103.

Schnurr, P. P. (2007). The rocks and hard places in psychotherapy outcome research. *Journal of Traumatic Stress, 20*, 779–792.

Schnurr, P. P., Friedman, M. J., Engel, C. C., Foa, E. B., Shea, M. T., Resick, P. A., et al. (2005). Issues in the design of multisite clinical trials of psychotherapy: VA Cooperative Study No. 494 as an example. *Contemporary Clinical Trials, 26*, 626–636.

Schnurr, P. P., Friedman, M. J., Engel, C. C., Foa, E. B., Shea, M. T., Resick, P. A., et al. (2007). Cognitive behavioral therapy for posttraumatic stress disorder in women: A randomized controlled trial. *Journal of the America Medical Association, 297*, 820–830.

Schnurr, P. P., Friedman, M. J., Foy, D. W., Shea, M. T., Hsieh, F. Y., Lavori, P. W., et al. (2003). Randomized trial of trauma-focused group therapy for posttraumatic stress disorder: Results from a Department of Veterans Affairs Cooperative Study. *Archives of General Psychiatry, 60*, 481–489.

Schnurr, P. P., Friedman, M. J., Lavori, P. W., & Hsieh, F. Y. (2001). Design of Department of Veterans Affairs Cooperative Study No. 420: Group treatment of posttraumatic stress disorder. *Contemporary Clinical Trials, 22*, 74–88.

Schultz, P. M., Resick, P. A., Huber, L. C., & Griffin, M. G. (2006). The effectiveness of cognitive processing therapy for PTSD with refugees in a community setting. *Cognitive and Behavioral Practice, 13*, 322–331.

Tarrier, N., Pilgrim, H., Sommerfield, C., Faragher, B., Reynolds, M., Graham, E., et al. (1999). A randomised trial of cognitive therapy and imaginal exposure in the treatment of chronic post traumatic stress disorder. *Journal of Consulting and Clinical Psychology, 67*, 13–18.

Tarrier, N., & Sommerfield, C. (2004). Treatment of chronic PTSD by cognitive therapy and exposure: 5-year follow-up. *Behavior Therapy, 35*, 231–246.

Taylor, S., Koch, W. J., Fecteau, G., Fedoroff, I. C., Thordarson, D. S., & Nicki, R. M. (2001). Posttraumatic stress disorder arising after road traffic collisions: Patterns of response to cognitive-behavior therapy. *Journal of Consulting and Clinical Psychology, 69*, 541–551.

Taylor, S., Thordarson, D. S., Maxfield, L., Federoff, I. C., Lovell, K., & Ogrodniczuk, J. (2003). Efficacy, speed, and adverse effects of three PTSD treatments: Exposure therapy, relaxation training, and EMDR. *Journal of Consulting and Clinical Psychology, 71*, 330–338.

Thompson, J. A., Charlton, P. F. C., Kerry, R., Lee, D., & Turner, S. W. (1995). An open trial of exposure therapy based on deconditioning for posttraumatic stress disorder. *British Journal of Clinical Psychology, 34*, 407–416.

Van Minnen, A., Arntz, A., & Keijsers, G. P. J. (2002). Prolonged exposure in patients with chronic PTSD: Predictors of treatment outcome and dropout. *Behaviour Research and Therapy, 40*, 439–457.

Van Minnen, A., & Foa, E. B. (2006). The effect of imaginal exposure length on outcome of treatment for PTSD. *Journal of Traumatic Stress, 19*, 427–438.

Van Minnen, A., & Hagenaars, M. (2002). Fear activation and habituation patters as early process predictors of response to prolonged exposure treatment in PTSD. *Journal of Traumatic Stress, 15*, 359–367.

Vaughan, K., Armstrong, M. S., Gold, R., O'Connor, N., Jenneke, W., & Tarrier, N. (1994). A trial of eye movement desensitization compared to image habituation training and applied muscle relaxation in posttraumatic stress disorder. *Journal of Behavior Therapy and Experimental Psychiatry, 25*, 283–291.

Vaughan, K., & Tarrier, N. (1992). The use of image habituation training with post-traumatic stress disorder. *British Journal of Psychiatry, 161*, 658–664.

Wagner, A. W., & Linehan, M. M. (2006). Applications of dialectical behavior therapy to posttraumatic stress disorder and related problems. In V. M. Follette & J. I. Ruzek (Eds.), *Cognitive-behavioral therapies for trauma* (2nd ed., pp. 117–145). New York: Guilford Press.

Wald, J., & Taylor, S. (2007). Efficacy of interoceptive exposure therapy combined with trauma-related exposure therapy for posttraumatic stress disorder: A pilot study. *Journal of Anxiety Disorders, 21*, 1050–1060.

Wells, A., & Sembi, S. (2004). Metacognitive therapy for PTSD: A preliminary investigation of a new brief treatment. *Journal of Behavior Therapy and Experimental Psychiatry, 35*, 307–318.

Zlotnick, C., Shea, T. M., Rosen, K., Simpson, E., Mulrenin, K., Begin, A., et al. (1997). An affect management group for women with posttraumatic stress disorder and histories of childhood sexual abuse. *Journal of Traumatic Stress, 10*, 425–436.

CHAPTER 8

Cognitive-Behavioral Therapy for Children and Adolescents

Judith A. Cohen, Anthony P. Mannarino,
Esther Deblinger, and Lucy Berliner

Theoretical Context

Children who experience traumatic life events may develop a wide variety of problems, including symptoms of anxiety, depression, behavioral dysregulation, substance use, and/or posttraumatic stress disorder (PTSD). Many children are also resilient and do not develop any lasting mental health problems. This chapter describes trauma-specific cognitive-behavioral therapies (CBTs) that are typically provided in settings other than schools. In this chapter we focus on how trauma-specific CBT treats PTSD symptoms. However, it is important to remember that children develop many other difficulties in response to trauma, and that trauma-specific CBT can effectively target problems other than PTSD.

By definition, upon exposure to a traumatic experience, children experience upsetting "affective states" or emotions: fear, terror, abhorrence. Children may feel other negative emotions, such as sadness, anger, and rage. These feelings may be mixed with positive feelings, such as excitement or arousal, if aspects of the experience were stimulating or pleasurable; such mixed feelings can contribute to confusion and increased guilt or shame. In the course of growing up, children experience numerous new and anxiety-provoking situations that once mastered are either forgotten or remembered as troubling, but successful, experiences. Children's memories of traumatic events differ from these ordinary, anxiety-provoking memories; because of the manner in which traumatic memories are encoded, reminders may trigger a recurrence of the emotions associated with the original traumatic experience. A traumatic reminder may be any person, place, thing, or situation that reminds the child of the original trauma. One of the hallmarks of PTSD is children's generalization of trauma reminders, such that innocuous environmental cues automatically trigger both memories and the negative emotions associated with previous traumatic events. When children remember the traumatic event in this way, they may reexperience the same affective responses they experienced at the time of the original trauma. Generalization of trauma reminders leads to triggering of trauma memories and the associated feelings by increasing the number of inherently innocuous cues (e.g., for a child who was sexually abused in her bathroom, any bathroom may become a traumatic reminder; simply entering a bathroom may lead to overwhelming trauma memories and the fearful feelings she experienced during the original sexual abuse). Over time such a child may become overwhelmed with negative affect and develop major depression, generalized anxiety, or panic disorder. Other children may develop marked instability of affect, or difficulty with "affective regulation" (easily losing their temper, crying with minimal provocation, etc.) as more and more cues in the environment trigger traumatic memories and the associated negative emotions.

The classic form of "behavioral dysregulation" in childhood PTSD is avoidance of trauma reminders, in which children avoid people, places, situations, and things that remind them of the traumatic event. Because children may have idiosyncratic memories of the trauma and/or trauma perpetrator, these reminders may be difficult to connect with the original trauma, particularly in the case of very young or developmentally challenged children. Very young children have difficulties at times distinguishing fantasy from reality and may refer to a violent perpetrator as a monster, ultimately developing stress reactions to other people, characters, or objects that they associate with "monsters." As with affective reminders, children's generalization of avoidant behaviors may range from avoiding the specific environment in which the trauma took place to avoiding even innocuous cues. For example, the girl in the previous paragraph who was sexually abused in the bathroom may at first avoid the bathroom where the abuse occurred, but as her fear response becomes generalized, as described earlier, her behavioral avoidance may also become generalized, such that she also avoids other bathrooms, for example, bathrooms at school. Such a girl might be at risk for developing secondary problems, such as enuresis or school refusal. If her parents do not understand the basis for these behaviors, then they might punish her, which might result in this child developing additional oppositional behavioral difficulties. As affective dysregulation becomes more uncomfortable, and avoidant strategies become less effective in keeping away trauma reminders, some children may turn to stronger methods of avoidance, such as using drugs or alcohol temporarily to manage their upsetting affective states. As in adults, substance abuse can lead to behavioral difficulties while children are under the influence, and/or when they are attempting to obtain drugs or alcohol. Particularly because many youth do not have independent financial means through which to buy drugs, they often need to steal money or turn to prostitution to obtain them. This in turn exposes these youth both to increased risky behaviors and to peers who engage in antisocial acts.

Body (physiological) dysregulation occurs in children with PTSD, as described elsewhere in this book (see Donnelly, Chapter 10, this volume).

Cognitive distortions may develop when children do not understand why bad things have happened to them. Because younger children have natural cognitive tendencies toward egocentrism, overgeneralizing, and identifying the simplest explanation for events, they may be particularly vulnerable to development of cognitive distortions following trauma ("Daddy beat Mommy because she is bad"). In their natural attempts to make sense of their world, and partially as a result of their developmentally normative belief in prevalent moral ("Things should be fair") and social ideals (i.e., "Wrongdoing gets punished"), many traumatized children may come to believe that they did something to "deserve" or cause the traumatic event they experienced, or that they could or should have done something to prevent the traumatic event. This idea of self-blame or guilt is one common cognitive distortion. Another is shame (i.e., that there is something inherently wrong, bad, or damaged about the child) related to the traumatic event, which either caused the event or came about as a result of the traumatic event and now cannot be taken away. In some cases the child may develop these distorted cognitions in direct response to the perpetrator of the traumatic event (i.e., the person who is abusing the child, or battering the child's mother, may directly tell the child, "This is your fault" or blame the nonoffending parent for these actions). In such a scenario the child may take the perpetrator at his or her word and accept responsibility for the trauma. Due to their natural tendency to overgeneralize, traumatized children may conclude that they are inalterably damaged (poor self-esteem), that no one believes or trusts what they say, and that they in turn cannot trust others (impaired interpersonal trust) and are in a deep sense different from those around them (alienation).

Trauma-specific CBT for children and parents targets these difficulties through specific interventions described in the following section. Whereas some of these components may be closely identified with CBT treatment (e.g., use of the cognitive triangle to help children understand relationships among thoughts, feelings, and behaviors; or creation of a trauma narrative to desensitize children gradually to trauma reminders), other trauma-specific CBT components may overlap considerably with more general types of child trauma treatment (e.g., affective expression and modulation skills). As would be expected, there is also some degree of overlap between the theoretical bases of CBT interventions and other interventions for treating PTSD symptoms in children. The theoretical bases for using these CBT interventions include the following:

1. Dysregulation of affect, behavior, physiology, and/or cognitions is conditioned or learned; therefore, it can be extinguished or unlearned through exposure techniques.
2. Inaccurate and/or unhelpful thoughts about the traumatic experience may be learned through modeling from the perpetrator of the traumatic experience, as described earlier, from a well-meaning adult (e.g., a parent who becomes overprotective, thus giving the message that the child is unsafe or unable to protect herself), or from the larger social context (through "victim blaming," etc.). These cognitive distortions can be corrected through cognitive and contextualizing techniques.
3. Providing skills building in affect modulation, stress management, cognitive coping, and effective parenting strategies early in treatment builds competency and self-confidence to face the more challenging and trauma-specific components of this model (i.e., directly talking about the child's personal traumatic experiences and cognitive processing of these experiences).
4. Inclusion of parents in treatment is important to provide support to children with PTSD symptoms, to reinforce the skills and active coping (as opposed to avoidant coping) strategies provided in treatment, to enhance effective parenting for behaviorally dysregulated children, and to address parents' own vicarious or direct trauma responses.
5. The therapeutic relationship is critically important in providing trauma- specific CBT interventions; a trusting relationship is enhanced in part by communicating to the child and parent that the therapist believes in their ability to master trauma reminders, without needing to rely primarily on avoidant strategies.

Additional aspects of trauma-specific CBT from other types of child trauma treatment include the following qualities:

1. *Collaborative empiricism:* The therapist works collaboratively and respectfully with the child and parents to explore a variety of ways of implementing the following interventions in order to see which ones result in better outcomes. This includes asking for ongoing suggestions and feedback from the child and parent, and using information from psychometrically sound instruments to assess symptoms on an ongoing basis when appropriate.
2. *Use of a strength- and skills-building approach:* Later components build upon skills that were learned and at least partially mastered earlier in therapy.
3. *Use of cognitive-behavioral methods to implement treatment components:* Modeling, rehearsal and practice of new skills, and extinction of avoidance through graduated exposure techniques are used throughout therapy.
4. *The therapist's active and directive role in treatment:* Therapists address "specific components treatment," a specific preferential order in

which components progress and the child develops a preference for some interventions (i.e., PRACTICE components in the following section) over others (i.e., nondirective therapeutic techniques). These are balanced by recognition of the centrality of the therapeutic relationship and sensitivity to child–parent issues and needs in therapy.

Description of Techniques

Although several different trauma-specific CBT models are currently in use, they all share common components that can be summarized by the acronym PRACTICE (Cohen, Mannarino, & Deblinger, 2006). Some CBT models for childhood PTSD do not include every component in this acronym; others include additional components and/or ancillary services in addition to child and parent psychotherapy (e.g., case management). The PRACTICE acronym stands for the following components, each of which are described below: A Parental treatment component, including parenting skills; Psychoeducation; Relaxation and stress management skills; Affective expression and modulation skills; Cognitive coping skills; Trauma narrative and cognitive processing of the child's traumatic experiences; *In vivo* desensitization to trauma reminders; Conjoint child–parent sessions; and Enhancing safety and future development.

Parental Treatment Component, Including Parenting Skills

The parental treatment components generally parallel the child components, which are described below (i.e., parents learn about the interventions their children receive for all of these components and are encouraged to reinforce their practice and use between treatment sessions). When appropriate, parents learn in therapy to adapt these interventions for their personal use (e.g., relaxation, affective modulation, cognitive coping). Effective parenting skills are also taught and practiced in treatment, for example, the use of positive praise, selective attention, time-out, and behavioral contingency reinforcement programs. These are tailored for the individual child and family's needs. Children with more serious behavioral problems may need more intensive interventions, either in conjunction with CBT treatment or instead of this treatment, if the behavioral problems are more prominent than PTSD symptoms.

Psychoeducation

The child and parent receive information about the type(s) of trauma experienced (e.g., how many children experience this type of trauma; the fact that it impacts many children, not just themselves; education about typical reactions to traumatic experiences, including what PTSD is; normalizing the child's and parents' reactions to the traumatic experience; and providing ongoing information to correct cognitive distortions throughout the course of treatment). Thus, psychoeducation continues throughout trauma-specific CBT therapy.

Relaxation Skills

Relaxation skills are provided in a variety of different ways in different trauma-specific CBT models. Most include individualized interventions, whereby children and parents are encouraged to develop ways of self-monitoring and regulating physiological tension through the use of skills, such as progressive muscle relaxation, deep or focused breathing, mindfulness exercises, biofeedback, dance, physical exercise, and so forth. The goal of all of these skills is to enhance children's ability to recognize their own physical tension, stress or anxiety, and to take active, productive steps to reduce these. Parents are also encouraged to learn and practice these skills between treatment sessions, both personally and with their children.

Affective Modulation Skills

In addition to relaxation skills, other ways of modulating distressing affective states, such as anxiety, anger, sadness, and emptiness, are addressed in trauma-specific CBT. Therapists use games and therapeutic activities to encourage the child's affective expression skills (i.e., accurately describing a range of different feelings and situations in which the child is likely to experience them). The therapist then assists the child in developing an individualized plan to identify the most difficult feelings and how to cope with situations in which these arise. For some children, this may entail seeking adult support; for others, it may involve using relaxation skills or cognitive coping (described below); for still others it may require leaving the situation. Some children may need to learn to disengage from activities that lead to negative affective states, learn how to make friends and to find activities they enjoy, and so forth. Many children need to learn all of these coping strategies, as well as how to choose selectively which skill to use in a given situation. For children who are severely affectively dysregulated, the affective modulation component may take many sessions. Parents are also encouraged to learn affective modulation skills, both for themselves and to assist and encourage their children to use these skills between treatment sessions.

Cognitive Coping Skills

"Cognitive coping" refers to understanding the connections among thoughts, feelings, and behaviors. Therapists also help children and parents to recognize that upsetting feelings often originate from *inaccurate* or *unhelpful* thoughts (Seligman, Reivich, Jaycox, & Gillham, 1995).

When children experience a distressing feeling or engages in a dysfunctional behavior, the therapist encourages them to learn to identify the thought that preceded the feeling or behavior. By changing to more accurate and/or helpful thoughts, children develop more soothing feelings and more positive behaviors. In the early stages of treatment, cognitive coping is used as a general stress management tool (i.e., to assist children in managing generally upsetting affective states rather than to change trauma-specific cognitive distortions). Later in therapy, after children have developed a narrative of their trauma experiences, these same strategies are used to explore and to reframe inaccurate and unhelpful cognitions related to children's traumatic experiences.

For example, the therapist might ask a child about any upsetting feelings he or she had during the past week. The child might say, "I was mad because I was climbing on the monkey bars and a kid bumped into me and I fell off." The therapist would clarify that the child was feeling "mad" and ask, "What was your thought that made you feel mad?" The child might say, "I knew he bumped into me on purpose." The therapist could then explore whether this thought was accurate (i.e., what is the evidence that this was true? For example, did the other child say he was sorry? If so, maybe it was an accident), and whether the thought was helpful. Might there be another thought that would make the child feel better, even if this were true ("I was almost to the top. I'm getting pretty good at climbing this monkey bar!"). The therapist might then help the child explore how each of these thoughts would make him or her feel, and understand that he or she can choose among all of these thoughts in this situation. Parents are also encouraged to learn cognitive coping skills, both for their personal use and to encourage their child to use them between sessions.

Trauma Narrative and Cognitive Processing of the Child's Traumatic Experiences

Once the child has gained some degree of ability to use these stress management skills, the therapist introduces the more trauma-specific components of this treatment model. The therapist first encourages the child to describe his or her personal traumatic experiences and to gradually include increasing details, until the child has described the "worst moment" or most terrifying aspects of the trauma. For children who have experienced multiple traumas, this may entail weaving several traumatic events into a single narrative or, alternatively, creating separate narratives for different traumas. Therapists liberally use praise and encouragement, and carefully calibrate how much exposure the child can tolerate during this exposure component of therapy, so that he or she is neither overwhelmed with traumatic memories nor inadvertently encouraged to use avoidant strategies "not to talk about it."

Once children have described detailed aspects of their traumatic experiences (including not only what they remember happening but also their thoughts, feelings, and bodily sensations both at the time of the trauma and when they are retelling it), the therapist encourages the child to examine these thoughts to evaluate whether they are accurate and helpful. This cognitive processing of the child's traumatic experiences echoes the cognitive process-ing of everyday events that the child learned earlier in therapy, and empha-sizes why mastering the early, skills-based components prior to introducing the trauma-specific components is optimal in this treatment approach. It is not uncommon for the child's idiosyncratic cognitive distortions to be identi-fied for the first time through the creation of the trauma narrative. Thus, it may be that the child previously denied self-blame for the traumatic event, but a self-blaming statement appeared as part of the trauma narrative. When reading through the narrative, the therapist can ask the child about this sen-tence, and whether it is an accurate and/or helpful thought, and help the child to explore what is behind this, in the context of the larger narrative.

In addition to allowing the child to process what has occurred, the trauma narrative allows the child to contextualize the traumatic event(s) he or she has experienced into the larger framework of his or her whole life. "Telling the story" of how the event(s) came to occur allows the child to see that a long time elapsed in his or her life before this event(s) occurred, and that in the time since then, the child has played, had friends, gone to school, and done other "normal kid things." The therapist can use this to help the child reframe the experience as one event (or a series of events) rather than as the defining experience of the child's life (i.e., that he or she can be more than a trauma survivor, and can instead be a normal child to whom some-thing bad happened). This perspective can also be helpful to parents, who hear the child's trauma narrative in individual sessions as the child is writing it and cognitively process their own feelings and thoughts about what their child (and they, either directly or vicariously) experienced as a result of the child's traumatic exposure.

In Vivo *Desensitization to Trauma Reminders*

If children are avoidant of inherently innocuous cues, they can benefit from *in vivo* desensitization, or graduated exposure. This is described elsewhere (Cohen, Mannarino & Deblinger, 2006). Parents must fully support these procedures to help children stop avoiding the feared situation.

Conjoint Child–Parent Sessions

Toward the end of treatment, the child and parents meet in joint sessions so that the child may share the trauma narrative directly with the parents (who already have heard this in their individual sessions with the therapist and are able to be supportive of the child) and engage in communication-building tasks, safety-enhancement tasks, and other interventions meant to transfer the child's ability to openly communicate any remaining questions, concerns, and feelings about the traumatic experience from the therapist to the parent as the end of therapy draws near. Should these concerns arise in the future, the hope is that the child knows that the parent is comfortable discussing this information with him or her in an open manner. Conjoint sessions may also be held earlier in treatment if indicated, to address behavioral communication or other issues.

Enhancing Safety and Future Development

Safety planning is an important part of treatment following trauma exposure, both to reverse children's typical sense of lost security and safety in the aftermath of traumatic events and to proactively optimize children's ability to protect themselves from dangerous situations, as well as to tell trusted adults if future traumatic events occur. Enhancing future development includes strengthening children's abilities in needed areas, such as social skills, problem solving, anger management, and in situations that might place the child at future risk for traumatic exposure. Parents are integrally involved in safety planning and are encouraged to reinforce children's safety skills between sessions, as well as after treatment termination.

Method of Collecting Data

We conducted a literature review using the following Medical Subject Headings (MeSH) terms in PubMed: "stress disorders," "Posttraumatic" *and* "randomized controlled trials" *and* "individual therapy"; Limits: "All children 0–18 years"; "only items with abstracts," "English," "randomized controlled trial," *or* "randomized" *and* "controlled" *and* "trials, male, female, humans." This search resulted in 104 abstracts. In our search of PsycINFO we used the following thesaurus terms: "Posttraumatic stress disorder"; Limit 1: "treatment outcome/randomized clinical trial"; Limit 2: "childhood or adolescence." This resulted in 24 abstracts. In a third search, the Published International Literature on Traumatic Stress (PILOTS) database, we used the terms "child *and* adolescent *and* clinical trials," which resulted in 20 abstracts. These searches were conducted in 2006. The abstracts were augmented by a search of the National Child Traumatic Stress Network (*www.nctsn.org*) website and personal communications with researchers in the child trauma field. We examined individual studies in detail and evaluated them for methodology. Child trauma-specific CBT interventions which are provided primarily in group or school settings, are included in Jaycox, Stein, and Amaya-Jackson (Chapter 13, this volume). Additional selected group or family treatments, which are not typically provided in school settings (e.g., because the content is related to substance abuse, cancer, or sexual abuse issues), are also included in this chapter. Only published or in press CBT treatment studies for traumatized children including an instrument that assessed children's PTSD symptoms were considered for inclusion in either of the tables of this review. Table 8.1 includes A-level studies (randomized controlled trials); Table 8.2 includes B-level studies.

Text continues on page 235

TABLE 8.1. Studies with Control or Comparison Groups

Study	Target population[a]	Number/length of sessions	Treatment/control[b]	Major findings	Between-group effect sizes	Within-group effect sizes
Deblinger, Lippmann, & Steer (1998b)	Sexually abused U.S. children 8–14 years; N = 100	12; 1.5 hr	*TF-CBT* 22 TF-CBT parent only 24 TF-CBT child only 22 TF-CBT P + C 22 community control	TF-CBT provided to child (combined groups) significantly superior to control for improving PTSD symptoms; TF-CBT provided to parents (combined groups) significantly superior to control for improving child depression, behavior problems, and parenting skills.	*K-SADS* Parent vs. Control 0.62 Child vs. Control 0.85 P + C vs. Control 0.99 Child vs. Parent 0.42 Child vs. P + C 0.04 Parent vs. P + C 0.33	*K-SADS* 1.56 1.69 2.18 1.08
Cohen & Mannarino (1996)	Sexually abused U.S. preschool children, 3–6 years; N = 86	12; 1.5 hr	*TF-CBT* 39 TF-CBT 28 nondirective supportive therapy (NST)	TF-CBT superior to NST in improving PTSD, internalizing, and sexual behavior symptoms.	*Weekly Behavior Report* Completer: 0.57	*Weekly Behavior Report* 1.18 0.64
Cohen, Deblinger, Mannarino, & Steer (2004a)	Sexually abused, multiply traumatized U.S. children, 8–14 years; N = 203	12; 1.5 hr	*TF-CBT* 89 TF-CBT 91 child-centered therapy (CCT)	TF-CBT significantly superior to CCT in improving PTSD, depressive, behavior, and shame symptoms in children and a number of parenting problems in participating parents.	*K-SADS* Intention to treat: 0.61	*K-SADS* 2.13 1.25

Study	Sample	Sessions; duration	Treatment groups	Results	Effect size	Effect size
King et al. (2000)	Sexually abused Australian children, 5–17 years; $N = 36$	20; 100 min	*TF-CBT* 12 TF-CBT child 12 TF-CBT family 12 wait list (WL)	TF-CBT significantly superior to WL in improving PTSD symptoms; inclusion of family only minimally improved child outcomes.	*ADIS* Child vs. WL: 1.09 Family vs. WL: 1.24 Child vs. Family: 0.21	*ADIS* 1.58 1.86 0.63
Cohen & Mannarino (1998)	Sexually abused U.S. children, 8–14 years (PTSD symptoms not required for entry); $N = 82$	12; 1.5 hr	*TF-CBT* 30 TF-CBT 19 NST	TF-CBT superior[c] to NST in improving depression and social competence at posttreatment and in improving PTSD and dissociation at 12-mo follow-up among treatment completers.	*TSCC* Completer: 0.22	*TSCC* 0.37 0.16
Smith et al. (2007)	U.K. children exposed to single-episode trauma, 8–18 years; $N = 24$	10; 1 hr	*Cognitive-based CBT* 12 CBT 12 WL	CBT significantly superior to WL for PTSD diagnosis; improvement in cognitive distortions partially mediated improvements in CBT group.	*CAPS-CA* Completer: 1.59	*CAPS-CA* 3.47 0.87
Najavits, Gallop, & Weiss (2006)	Adolescents with PTSD and substance use disorder (SUD); $N = 28$	25; 1.5 hr	*Seeking Safety* 15 Seeking Safety 13 treatment as usual (TAU)	Seeking Safety superior to TAU at 5-mo follow-up for many domains.	*TSCC* Completer: 0.12	*TSCC* 1.11 0.28

Notes. ADIS, Anxiety Disorders Interview Schedule; CAPS-CA, Clinician-Administered PTSD Scale for Children and Adolescents; K-SADS, Schedule for Affective Disorders and Schizophrenia for School-Age Children; TF-CBT, trauma-focused cognitive-behavioral therapy; TSCC, Traumatic Stress Symptom Checklist.

[a]N = subjects starting study or treatment.

[b]N = subjects in data analyses.

[c]Based on $p < .05$.

TABLE 8.2. Studies without Control or Comparison Conditions

Study	Target population[a]	Number/length of treatment sessions	Treatment orientation[b]	Major findings	Effect size[c]
Deblinger, McLeer, & Henry (1990)	Sexually abused U.S. children, age 8–14 years; N = 19	12 wk, 1.5 hr	*TF-CBT* N = 19	TF-CBT effective in reducing PTSD, depression, and behavior problems.	*K-SADS:* 2.80
Cohen, Mannarino, & Knudsen (2004)	Children with traumatic grief, age 6–17 years; N = 22	16 wk, 1.5 hr	*TG-CBT* N = 22	TG-CBT effective in improving PTSD, traumatic grief, and depressive symptoms in traumatically bereaved children and PTSD symptoms in their participating parents.	*CPSS:* 0.81
Cohen, Mannarino, & Staron (2006)	Children with traumatic grief, age 6–17 years; N = 51	12 wk, 1.5 hr	*TG-CBT* N = 39	TG-CBT effective in improving PTSD and traumatic grief symptoms in traumatically bereaved children and PTSD symptoms in their participating parents.	*CPSS:* 0.87
Saxe, Ellis, Folger, Hansen, & Sorkin (2005)	Traumatized children with complex needs, age 5–20 years; N = 110	3 mo; unspecified (variable)	*Trauma systems therapy* (TST) N = 110	TST effective in improving PTSD symptoms.	*CANS-TEA-PTSD:* 0.31

Notes. CANS-PTSD, Child and Adolescent's Needs and Strengths—PTSD; CPSS, Child PTSD Symptom Scale; K-SADS, Schedule for Affective Disorders and Schizophrenia for School-Age Children; TF-CBT, trauma-focused cognitive-behavioral therapy; TG-CBT, traumatic grief cognitive-behavioral therapy.

[a]N = subjects starting treatment.

[b]N = subjects in data analyses.

[c]Within-group effect size only.

Literature Review

Three individual PTSD-targeted CBT models for children or adolescents have been tested in randomized controlled trials (RCTs). Other individual models have been evaluated in less rigorous study designs. Because so few models have been subjected to the most rigorous level of testing, this review includes less well-controlled studies as well. Because conclusions drawn from these studies are less strong, they have received a lower rating on the Agency for Health Care Policy and Research (AHCPR) scale described by Foa, Keane, and Friedman (Chapter 1, this volume).

Trauma-Focused CBT

Individual trauma-focused CBT (TF-CBT) includes all of the PRACTICE components described earlier (Cohen, Mannarino & Deblinger, 2006; Deblinger & Heflin, 1996). TF-CBT particularly emphasizes the use of gradual exposure throughout treatment. Each PRACTICE component is incorporated incrementally by increasing discussion about the type of trauma(s) the child has experienced, so the child and parent gradually become more able to tolerate trauma reminders without feeling physically or psychologically overwhelmed. Since this process occurs gradually, the child masters skills and is well prepared by the time the trauma-specific components are introduced. TF-CBT is the most thoroughly studied treatment for traumatized children to date, with six randomized controlled treatment trials completed by three initially independent research teams (two have since united to conduct collaborative treatment outcome research). Of the five trials that assessed PTSD symptoms, four included PTSD symptoms as an inclusionary criterion to enter the study. All of these studies showed TF-CBT to be superior to other active treatments or wait-list control conditions with regard to improvement of PTSD symptoms, as well as a variety of other symptoms. The fifth study did not include PTSD symptoms as an inclusionary criterion but found differential treatment effects for PTSD at follow-up.

Deblinger, McLeer, and Henry (1990), in an initial pilot study, demonstrated the promising effectiveness of the TF-CBT model. Based on this preliminary work, Deblinger, Lippmann, and Steer (1996) randomly assigned 100 sexually abused children, ages 8–14 years, with PTSD symptoms to one of four conditions: TF-CBT provided to sexually abused children alone, TF-CBT provided to parents of sexually abused children alone, TF-CBT provided to sexually abused children and their parents, or community treatment as usual (TAU). Children receiving TF-CBT experienced significantly greater improvement in PTSD symptoms. Additional findings indicated that parental inclusion in treatment led to significantly greater improvement in child behavior problems and depressive symptoms, as well as parenting practices.

Cohen and Mannarino (1996) randomly assigned sexually abused preschool children, ages 3–7 years, to TF-CBT or nondirective supportive therapy

(NST). Because a validated interview assessment for PTSD in preschoolers was not available when this study was conducted, the Weekly Behavior Report (WBR) was used to assess PTSD symptoms. A cutoff level of symptoms on this instrument was established for entry into the study. The WBR measured reexperiencing symptoms (primarily sexually inappropriate behaviors), avoidance of feared situations, and hyperarousal symptoms in young children via parent report. Children receiving TF-CBT experienced significantly greater improvement in WBR scores than those receiving NST during the 1-year follow-up. An additional advantage of TF-CBT was significantly greater improvement in internalized and externalized behavioral symptoms.

In a multisite study, Cohen, Deblinger, Mannarino, and Steer (2004) randomly assigned 229 sexually abused children to TF-CBT or child-centered therapy (CCT), and demonstrated that children receiving TF-CBT experienced significantly greater improvement in all three PTSD clusters and in total PTSD symptoms at posttreatment. Children assigned to the CCT condition who had experienced multiple traumas and/or had higher (as opposed to lower) initial levels of depression were significantly more likely to have PTSD symptoms at posttreatment and/or follow-up, but these associations were not found for those assigned to the TF-CBT condition (Deblinger, Cohen, Mannarino, & Steer, 2006). The children assigned to TF-CBT also experienced significantly greater improvement in depression, anxiety, shame, and behavior problems than children assigned to the CCT condition in this study (Cohen, Deblinger, et al., 2004).

King and colleagues (2000) randomly assigned sexually abused 5- to 17-year-old sexually abused Australian children to one of three groups: TF-CBT provided individually; TF-CBT provided to children and parents; or a wait-list control group. Both TF-CBT conditions improved significantly more than the control condition with regard to PTSD symptoms; inclusion of parents resulted in significantly less fear at 3-month follow-up.

Cohen and Mannarino (1998) randomized eighty-two 8- to 14-year-old sexually abused children to TF-CBT or NST. Unlike the studies described earlier, PTSD symptoms were not required for entry into this project. At posttreatment there were no significant differences between the two groups with regard to PTSD symptoms, as measured by the Trauma Symptom Checklist for Children (TSCC) PTSD scale, but at 12-month follow-up, PTSD symptoms had improved significantly more in the TF-CBT condition. Additional benefits in the TF-CBT condition included significantly greater improvement in depression and social competence at posttreatment, and significantly less depression, sexualized behaviors, anxiety, and dissociation at 1-year follow-up (Cohen, Mannarino, & Knudsen, 2005).

Two forms of CBT were used in the Child and Adolescent Trauma Treatment and Services (CATS) Project, which provided treatment to New York City children and adolescents with PTSD symptoms related to the terrorist attacks of September 11, 2001. The final sample included 589 predominantly low-income Latino children. Children with moderate to severe PTSD symptoms received CBT (N = 445). Children with mild to moderate PTSD received only the PRAC components ("Enhanced Services," ES; N = 112). Children with very mild PTSD symptoms received treatment as usual (TAU; N = 32). Due to the small number receiving TAU these children were included in the ES group for data analyses. Children in both groups (CBT vs. ES/TAU) experienced significant improvement with no significant differences between the two groups, demonstrating that matching treatments according to initial symptom severity is a feasible model for allocating care after community disasters. Reliable improvement in the CBT group was greater over 6 months, with a mean of 9.7 points on the UCLA PTSD Reaction Index compared to 3.8 points for the comparison group, despite the CBT group starting with more severe PTSD scores, more multiple traumatizations, and more family adversity (Hoagwood et al., in press).

TF-CBT has been adapted for use in children experiencing childhood traumatic grief (CTG). This revised model, traumatic grief CBT (TG-CBT) adds grief-focused interventions to the standard TF-CBT components described earlier. In two open (uncontrolled) trials of TG-CBT, children experienced significant improvement in PTSD symptoms, as measured by the Children's PTSD Symptom Scale (CPSS), as well as in CTG symptoms and a variety of other psychological outcomes. Participating parents also experienced significant improvement in their personal PTSD symptoms (Cohen, Mannarino, & Knudsen, 2005; Cohen, Mannarino, & Staron, 2006).

Cultural Considerations

Cultural issues are included as part of the TF-CBT model, with particular emphasis in the traumatic grief components. TF-CBT has been adapted for Latino children and this version, culturally modified TF-CBT (CM-TF-CBT) has been evaluated in children of predominantly Mexican migrant workers with positive results (DeArellano et al., 2005). TF-CBT is being culturally modified and evaluated for African children who have experienced sexual abuse, domestic violence, traumatic loss, and/or HIV infection; and in Norway, Germany, the Netherlands, Cambodia, and other countries.

Cognitive-Based TF-CBT

Another individual form of trauma-focused CBT has been tested in a pilot RCT for children exposed to single-incident traumatic events (motor vehicle accidents [MVAs], interpersonal trauma, or witnessing violence) (Smith et al., 2007). This model includes the following components: psychoeducation, imaginal reliving of the traumatic event, cognitive restructuring, integration of the cognitive restructuring into the reliving, revisiting the site of the trauma, stimulus discrimination regarding trauma reminders, direct work with nightmares, image transformation techniques, behavioral experiments, and work with parents that includes joint parent–child sessions, if needed. No relaxation interventions are included in this model. The Smith and colleagues (2007) pilot RCT compared this model to a wait-list control and found large effect sizes for PTSD, anxiety, and depression. The positive effects of CBT were partially mediated by improvements in maladaptive cognitions, as predicted by cognitive models of PTSD.

Cultural Considerations

Cultural issues are included as part of the cognitive processing component of this model. Cognitive CBT has been tested only among English-speaking children to date.

Seeking Safety

Seeking Safety (Najavits, 2002), an integrated treatment model for comorbid PTSD and substance use disorder (SUD), was originally developed and tested for adults and has recently been studied in an RCT for adolescents (Najavits, Gallop, & Weiss, 2006). Seeking Safety can be provided individually or in a group format. It incorporates most of the PRACTICE components. Direct exposure techniques are not typically included (but can be done adjunctively). Key features include safety as the overarching goal; a focus on ideals to counteract the loss of ideals in both PTSD and substance abuse; simple, engaging language; and a high degree of flexibility (e.g., the number and order of treatment topics can vary, and Seeking Safety can be conducted by counselors without a formal degree in mental health). Examples of the model's 25 treatment topics include PTSD: Taking Back Your Power; Honesty; Asking for Help; Setting Boundaries in Relationships; and Grounding. The RCT of Seeking Safety for adolescents compared it to TAU for 33 outpatient girls. Participants in Seeking Safety evidenced significantly better outcomes than those in TAU in various domains at posttreatment, including substance use and associated problems, trauma-related symptoms, cognitions related to PTSD and SUD, psychiatric functioning, and several additional areas of pathology not targeted in the treatment (e.g., anorexia, somatization, generalized anxiety). Some gains were sustained at 3-month follow-up.

Cultural Considerations

Cultural issues and spirituality are addressed as part of the Seeking Safety model. Seeking Safety has been used on a limited basis in adolescents, but its adult parent model has been culturally adapted for Spanish-speaking adults, female veterans, and prison populations. This suggests that the model has broad acceptability among diverse groups with comorbid PTSD and SUD.

Surviving Cancer Competently Intervention Program and SCIPP— Newly Diagnosed

The Surviving Cancer Competently Intervention Program (SCIPP) is a cognitive- and family-based treatment for adolescents who have survived cancer. It has been provided in a four-session, 1-day intervention. Sessions 1 and 2 are group sessions provided separately to adolescents and parents. Components include psychoeducation; discussion of trauma-related events; identifying trauma memories; and providing coping skills, including affective expression, cognitive processing, and stress management. Sessions 3 and 4 include multiple-family groups to apply the materials from Sessions 1 and 2 within family contexts. Content included psychoeducation, cognitive processing, and functional family therapy. An RCT comparing SCIPP to a wait-list control for 150 adolescents and their mothers, fathers, and adolescent siblings showed significantly greater improvement in arousal symptoms of adolescent survivors who received SCIPP than in those in the wait-list condition (Kazak et al., 2004). Differences in overall PTSD symptoms were not found between the groups. Multiple imputation analyses suggested that if more families had been retained for follow-up, greater differences would likely have been detected between the groups. A preliminary trial of this intervention was tested in an RCT for 19 families of children with newly diagnosed cancer. Families were randomized to SCIPP—Newly Diagnosed (SCIPP-ND) or TAU subsequent to learning about their child's illness. Preliminary outcome data showed no significant differences, but trends were in the expected direction with regard to reduction of anxiety and parental PTSD symptoms (Kazak et al., 2005).

Cultural Considerations

Cultural and spirituality issues are included as part of the SCIPP model. SCIPP has been tested in U.S. adolescents.

Trauma Systems Therapy

Trauma systems therapy (TST) integrates CBT interventions with systems-based interventions for severely affectively dysregulated children (Saxe, Ellis, Fogler, Hansen, & Sorkin, 2005). TST has five phases of treatment: surviving, stabilizing, enduring, understanding, and transcending. In addition to PRACTICE components, TST also provides home-based services to stabilize the child and family environment, as well as pharmacological and advocacy services as needed. In addition, children receive case management coordination services and level of care consistent with their needs (up to and including inpatient admission). An open trial of TST demonstrated significant improvement in PTSD symptoms in 110 children at 3-month follow-up (Saxe et al., 2005).

Cultural Considerations

TST includes a strong cultural focus, with incorporation of faith-based support as a key component. TST has been tested with U.S. children.

KIDNET

A child-friendly version of narrative exposure therapy (NET)—KIDNET (Ruf et al., 2007)—has been developed and recently evaluated. NET was specifically developed to treat survivors of multiple and severe trauma (e.g., organized trauma, such as war and torture, or chronic severe trauma, such as domestic violence or repeated sexual violence). KIDNET begins with psychoeducation about the importance of reconstructing a life narrative. The therapist takes an empathic approach to assist the child in re-creating a complete unfragmented life narrative, which includes both pleasant life events and traumatic ones. There is a strong focus on child and human rights to help the child regain dignity and acknowledge what has been experienced. Cognitive processing is also included. KIDNET has been tested in one RCT, in which 25 refugee children were randomly assigned to KIDNET or to a wait-list control condition. This study was published in German in a book chapter and presented at a peer-reviewed conference, both in 2007. The study author communicated that KIDNET was superior to wait list ($p < .01$) (Dr. Maggie Schauer, commentary to International Society for Traumatic Stress Studies [ISTSS] Guidelines, posted September 30, 2007) but we were unable to review the study for calculation of effect size. For this reason KIDNET is not included in Table 8.1.

Cultural Considerations

KIDNET was developed in Germany and includes cultural issues as a core feature. KIDNET has been implemented with refugee child populations, including Somali, Ugandan, Rwandan, and others.

Life Skills/Life Story

Life Skills/Life Story is a two-module group or individual intervention to relieve PTSD, depression, and dissociation for girls who have experienced complex, multiple, and/or sustained trauma. This model includes all of the CBT components described earlier, but it devotes a longer period of time to the earlier stress management components to stabilize the often severe affective dysregulation in these adolescents. It has been used for girls, ages 12–21 years, who have experienced sexual or physical abuse, community or domestic violence, or sexual assault. An RCT in a residential school setting is ongoing.

Cultural Considerations

Life Skills/Life Story includes cultural issues as an important component. It has been used with diverse U.S. cultural groups.

Structured Psychotherapy for Adolescents Recovering from Chronic Stress

The Structured Psychotherapy for Adolescents Recovering from Chronic Stress (SPARCS) model is a 22-session group intervention designed specifically to address the needs of chronically traumatized adolescents who may still be living with ongoing trauma or stress. It focuses on 12- to 19-year-olds exposed to chronic abuse and violence, including interpersonal abuse, domestic or community violence, or medical trauma. This model includes the early stress management components (psychoeducation, relaxation, affective modulation, mindfulness, and cognitive processing) and also emphasizes enhancing personal safety but does not include direct exposure techniques. It has been extensively piloted in schools and outpatient settings in several states. An open study of SPARCS indicated that adolescents experienced significant improvement in interpersonal relationships, functional impairment, and behavioral symptoms (Habib & Ross, 2006). PTSD was not assessed in this study.

Cultural Considerations

SPARCS includes cultural issues, and spirituality is a core component of the SPARCS model. SPARCS has been implemented with diverse U.S. populations.

CBT Interventions Utilizing Single PRACTICE Components

Some models of trauma treatment have focused on providing a single PRACTICE component, such as relaxation in the form of massage therapy (Field, Seligman, Scafedi & Schanberg, 1996) or imaginal desensitization (Saigh, 1989, 1992). There are no data regarding the effect size of these single-component treatments for childhood PTSD symptoms; thus, at the present time there is stronger support for use of the entire TF-CBT package than for a single component. A TF-CBT deconstruction study is currently underway to assess the relative benefits and risks of including the trauma narrative and cognitive processing components for addressing PTSD symptoms in young children (4–11 years) (Deblinger, Mannarino, Cohen, & Steer, 2003).

Summary and Recommendations

Several TF-CBT models for children and adolescents have "A" or "B" level evidence of efficacy for improving PTSD, as well as other psychological symptoms. These models share many overlapping components but also have some distinct features. The field has made significant progress in a relatively short time in developing and testing effective ways of addressing a variety of difficulties for children traumatized by different types of events, presenting with a variety of complex clinical pictures across the developmental spectrum. Perhaps even more impressive are the inroads made in the acceptability CBT interventions have gained among therapists in community settings and for children of diverse cultural backgrounds. The unprecedented usage of TF-CBTWeb (*www.musc.edu/tfcbt*), a free, online TF-CBT training course, for which more than 30,000 primarily master's-level community-based learners from more than 60 countries registered during its first 3 years of availability, suggests that evidence-based CBT approaches for traumatized children may be broadly acceptable to therapists in settings where traumatized children are most likely to be served. This very promising development merits further research. At the present time, TF-CBT interventions are among the most effective in relieving PTSD and a variety of other symptoms in traumatized children and adolescents.

References

Cohen, J. A., Deblinger, E., Mannarino, A. P., & Steer, R. A. (2004). A multisite randomized controlled trial for children with sexual abuse-related PTSD symptoms. *Journal of the American Academy of Child and Adolescent Psychiatry, 43*, 393–402.

Cohen, J. A., & Mannarino, A. P. (1996). A treatment outcome study for sexually abused preschool children: Initial findings. *Journal of the American Academy of Child and Adolescent Psychiatry, 35*, 42–50.

Cohen, J. A., & Mannarino, A. P. (1998). Interventions for sexually abused children: Initial treatment findings. *Child Maltreatment, 3*, 17–26.

Cohen, J. A., Mannarino, A. P., & Deblinger, E. (2006). *Treating trauma and traumatic grief in children and adolescents.* New York: Guilford Press.

Cohen, J. A., Mannarino, A. P., & Knudsen, K. (2004). Treating childhood traumatic grief: A pilot study. *Journal of the American Academy of Child and Adolescent Psychiatry, 43*, 1225–1233.

Cohen, J. A., Mannarino, A. P., & Knudsen, K. (2005). Treating sexually abused children: 1 year follow up of a randomized controlled trial. *Child Abuse and Neglect, 29*, 135–145.

Cohen, J. A., Mannarino, A. P., & Staron, V. R. (2006). A pilot study of modified cognitive-behavioral therapy for childhood traumatic grief (CBT-CTG). *American Academy of Child and Adolescent Psychiatry, 45*, 1465–1473.

DeArellano, M. A., Waldrop, A. E., Deblinger, E., Cohen, J. A., Danielson, C. K., & Mannarino, A. P. (2005). Community outreach program for child victims of traumatic events: A community-based project for underserved populations. *Behavior Modification, 29,* 130–155.

Deblinger, E., & Heflin, A. (1996). *Treating sexually abused children and their non-offending caretakers.* Thousand Oaks, CA: Sage.

Deblinger, E., Lippman, J., & Steer, R. A. (1996). Sexually abused children suffering posttraumatic stress symptoms: Initial treatment outcome findings. *Child Maltreatment, 3,* 310–321.

Deblinger, E., Mannarino, A. P., Cohen, J. A., & Steer, R. (2003). *Young sexually abused children: Optimal CBT strategies.* Washington, DC: National Institute of Mental Health.

Deblinger, E., Mannarino, A. P., Cohen, J. A., & Steer, R. A. (2006). A follow up study of a multi-site, randomized, controlled trial for children with sexual abuse related PTSD symptoms. *Journal of the American Academy of Child and Adolescent Psychiatry, 45,* 1474–1484.

Deblinger, E., McLeer, S. V., & Henry, D. (1990). Cognitive behavioral treatment for sexually abused children suffering posttraumatic stress: Preliminary findings. *Journal of the American Academy of Child and Adolescent Psychiatry, 29,* 747–752.

Field, T., Seligman, S., Scafadi, S., & Schanberg, S. (1996). Alleviating posttraumatic stress in children following Hurricane Andrew. *Journal of Applied Developmental Psychology, 17,* 37–50.

Habib, M., & Ross, L. A. (2006). *Igniting SPARCS of change in treatment: An experiential introduction to a promising practice.* Presented at the 22nd Annual Meeting of the ISTSS, Hollywood, CA.

Hoagwood, K. E., and the CATS Consortium. (in press). Impact of CBT for traumatized children and adolescents affected by the World Trade Center disaster. *Journal of Clinical Child and Adolescent Psychology.*

Kazak, A. E., Alderfer, M. A., Streisand, R., Simms, S., Rourke, M. T., Barakat, L. P., et al. (2004). Treatment of posttraumatic stress symptoms in adolescent survivors of childhood cancer and their families: A randomized clinical trial. *Journal of Family Psychology, 18,* 493–504.

Kazak, A. E., Simms, S., Alderfer, M. A., Rourke, M. T., Crump, T., McClure, K., et al. (2005). Feasiblity and preliminary outcomes from a pilot study of a brief psychological intervention for families of children newly diagnosed with cancer. *Journal of Pediatric Psychology, 30,* 644–655.

King, N. J., Tonge, B. J., Mullen, P., Myerson, N., Heyne, D., Rollings, S., et al. (2000). Treating sexually abused children with posttraumatic stress symptoms: A randomized clinical trial. *Journal of the American Academy of Child and Adolescent Psychiatry, 39,* 1347–1355.

Layne, C. M., Pynoos, R. S, Saltzman, W. S., Arslanagic, B., & Black, M. (2001). Trauma/grief focused group psychotherapy: School based post-war intervention with traumatized Bosnian adolescents. *Group Dynamics, 5,* 277–290.

Najavits, L. M. (2002). *Seeking safety: A treatment manual for PTSD and substance abuse.* New York: Guilford Press.

Najavits, L. M., Gallop, R. J., & Weiss, R. D. (2006). Seeking safety therapy for adolescent girls with PTSD and substance use disorder: A randomized controlled trial. *Journal of Behavioral Health Services Research, 33,* 453–463. Available online at *www. seekingsafety.org*

Ruf, M., Schauer, M., Neuner, F., Schauer, E., Catani, C., Schauer, E., et al. (2007).

KIDNET—a highly effective treatment approach for traumatized refugee children. Paper presented at the European Conference on Traumatic Stress, Opatja, Croatia.

Saigh, P. (1989). The use of *in vitro* flooding package in the treatment of traumatized adolescents. *Developmental and Behavioral Pediatrics, 10,* 17–21.

Saigh, P. (1992). The behavioral treatment of child and adolescent posttraumatic stress disorder. *Advances in Behaviour Research and Therapy, 14,* 247–275.

Saxe, G. N., Ellis, H., Fogler, J., Hansen, S., & Sorkin, B. (2005). Comprehensive care for traumatized children: An open trial examines treatment using trauma systems therapy. *Psychiatric Annals, 53,* 443–448.

Seligman, M. E. P., Reivich, K., Jaycox, L., & Gillham, J. (1995). *The optimistic child.* Boston: Houghton Mifflin.

Smith, P., Yule, W., Perrin, S., Tranah, T., Dalgleish, T., & Clark, D. (2007). Cognitive behavior therapy for PTSD in children and adolescents: A preliminary randomized controlled trial. *Journal of the American Academy of Child and Adolescent Psychiatry, 46,* 1051–1061.

CHAPTER 9

Psychopharmacotherapy for Adults

Matthew J. Friedman, Jonathan R. T. Davidson, and Dan J. Stein

Theoretical Context

Posttraumatic stress disorder (PTSD) appears to be a very complex disorder associated with stable and profound alterations in many psychobiological systems that have evolved for coping, adaptation, and survival of the human species (Charney, 2004; Friedman & Davidson, 2007; Southwick et al., 2007). Table 9.1 summarizes current knowledge regarding psychobiological abnormalities in PTSD that involve specific neurotransmitter, neurohormonal, or neuroendocrine systems. Such information is relevant to understanding why certain medications might be effective therapeutic agents. It might also guide the development of future drugs designed specifically for use in PTSD. Ideally such an approach would lead to rational pharmacotherapy in which specific classes of drugs are selected because of their actions on specific psychobiological systems. As we consider PTSD from this conceptual perspective, the reader should keep in mind that most of our current information about pharmacotherapy for PTSD is based on empirical trials with established antidepressant, anxiolytic, and other medications, rather than agents specifically targeting putative neurobiological mechanisms underlying the pathophysiology of PTSD or targeting variations between individuals in these mechanisms.

TABLE 9.1. Psychobiological Abnormalities Possibly Associated with PTSD

Proposed psychobiological abnormality	Possible clinical effect
Adrenergic hyperreactivity	Hyperarousal, reexperiencing dissociation, rage/aggression Abnormal information/memory processes Panic/anxiety
Elevated CRF levels	Hyperarousal, reexperiencing Panic/anxiety
HPA dysregulation/enhanced negative feedback	Stress intolerance
Opioid dysregulation	Numbing
Limbic sensitization/kindling	Hyperarousal, reexperiencing
Inadequate serotonergic function	Numbing, reexperiencing Hyperarousal Poorly modulated stress responses Associated symptoms[a]
Glutamatergic dysregulation	Dissociation Impaired information and memory processing Resistance to extinction of conditioned fear
Inadequate GABA-ergic function	Excessive arousal Poorly modulated stress responses

Notes. [a]Rage, aggression, impulsivity, depression, panic/anxiety, obsessional thoughts, chemical abuse/dependency.
HPA, hypothalamic–pituitary–adrenocortical; CRF, corticotropin-releasing factor; GABA, gamma-aminobutyric acid.

Description of Techniques

The major techniques in pharmacotherapy involve the following:

1. Selecting a drug whose pharmacological actions might be expected to normalize the psychobiological abnormalities associated with a specific disorder.
2. Choosing the most appropriate therapeutic agent based on proven efficacy against the disorder itself, a specific symptom, cluster of symptoms, and/or comorbid disorder.

3. Monitoring and readjusting the dosage to optimize therapeutic efficacy and onset of action, while minimizing the likelihood of side effects.
4. Knowing when there has been an adequate therapeutic trial of a given drug to supplement treatment with an additional drug or to switch to a different agent.
5. Being aware of the therapeutic context within which a medication is being prescribed, including the patient's explanatory models of the disorder, to optimize the chances of a successful treatment.

There is a strong rationale for pharmacotherapy as an important treatment in PTSD. As noted previously, a number of neurobiological mechanisms seem pertinent to this disorder. In addition, patients with PTSD exhibit abnormalities in several key neurobiological systems (see Table 9.1). Furthermore, there is considerable overlap of symptoms among PTSD, depression, and other anxiety disorders. Finally, PTSD is frequently comorbid with psychiatric disorders that are responsive to drug treatment (e.g., major depression and panic disorder). Medication is one of the most feasible treatments for PTSD. It is generally accepted by most patients, although the occurrence of side effects, lack of patient compliance with prescribed drug regimens, patient and family concerns about pharmacotherapy, and the high commercial cost of new therapeutic agents lessen their full impact.

The cost of medication treatment is difficult to compare with the cost of psychotherapy because it depends on the duration of treatment, the cost of the drug itself, and many other factors. Because maintaining the benefits of pharmacotherapy in PTSD (as in depression and other anxiety disorders) generally requires continuous treatment, medication expenses are ongoing. Compliance with treatment is generally good during the initial weeks of treatment; it may remain high, if there is clinical improvement, but it may not do so, even if there is a favorable response to medication. Finally, although it is very easy to disseminate the necessary information about drug treatment to prescribing physicians, it is quite difficult to detect and correct improper prescribing practices.

PTSD is often associated with at least one comorbid psychiatric disorder (e.g., depression, other anxiety disorders and/or chemical abuse/dependency). It is often also associated with disruptive symptoms that are clinically significant (e.g., impulsivity, mood lability, irritability, aggressiveness and/or suicidal behavior). Some of the medications reviewed in this practice guideline have proven or probable efficacy in ameliorating some of these comorbid disorders or associated symptoms. Ideally, a practicing pharmacotherapist selects an agent that might be expected to ameliorate such comorbid disorders and associated symptoms at the same time that it reduces PTSD symptom severity (see Najavits, Ryngala, Back, Bolton, Mueser, & Brady, Chapter 21, this volume). This is pharmacotherapeutic technique at its best.

Method of Collecting Data

This practice guideline was developed after a comprehensive literature review of all randomized clinical trials (RCTs), open trials, and case reports on pharmacotherapy for PTSD published through 2006, included in the National Center for PTSD's PILOTS (Published International Literature on Traumatic Stress) bibliographical database. We conducted the search using the following key words: "PTSD," "pharmacotherapy," "antidepressants," "anxiolytics," "antiadrenergic agents," "anticonvulsants," and "antipsychotics," as well as the specific names of each drug mentioned in this report. Data from RCTs were given the greatest weight, and such findings and effect sizes for each RCT are summarized in Table 9.2. Table 9.3 is much more inclusive and summarizes results from all medication trials because of both the theoretical and clinical interest generated by such data. Table 9.3 also presents our recommendations on drug treatment, strength of the published evidence, and indications and contraindications. We produced the initial drafts; the final draft was submitted to the International Society for Traumatic Stress Studies (ISTSS) Practice Guidelines Task Force for approval, after which it was submitted to the full ISTSS Board of Directors.

Literature Review

Evidence from RCTs

As shown in Table 9.2, 34 RCTs have been published. Nine industry-sponsored, large-scale, multisite trials published since 2000 account for the vast majority of participants. These trials have focused primarily on selective serotonin reuptake inhibitors (SSRIs; sertraline, paroxetine, and fluoxetine) and a serotonin–norepinephrine reuptake inhibitor (SNRI; venlafaxine-ER [extended release]). Successful trials with sertraline (Brady et al., 2000; Davidson, Rothbaum, van der Kolk, Sikes, & Farfel, 2001) and paroxetine (Marshall, Beebe, Oldham, & Zaninelli, 2001; Tucker et al., 2001) have led to approval of both SSRIs as treatments for PTSD by the U.S. Food and Drug Administration (FDA). It is worth noting that samples in all four of these RCTs were recruited from the civilian sector and comprised mostly white, middle-aged women with PTSD caused by childhood or adult sexual abuse).

In contrast, a negative multisite sertraline RCT (conducted approximately 10 years ago but published recently) was carried out on male (mostly Vietnam War) combat veterans receiving treatment in Department of Veterans Affairs (VA) hospitals (Friedman, Marmar, Baker, Sikes, & Farfel, 2007). These negative findings set off speculation that women were more responsive than men to SSRI treatment; and that PTSD due to sexual trauma was more responsive

Text continues on page 259

TABLE 9.2. Randomized Clinical Trials of Medications for PTSD

Study	Target population[a]	Duration of trial	Treatments/ control[b]	Major findings	Between-group effect sizes	Within-group effect sizes
Sertraline						
Brady et al. (2000)	187 male and female civilians with PTSD	12 weeks	94 sertraline 93 placebo	Sertraline significantly better than placebo in reducing PTSD symptom severity	0.30; $p < .02$	1.90—sertraline; 1.31—placebo
Davidson, Rothbaum, et al. (2001)	202 male and female civilians with PTSD	12 weeks	98 sertraline 104 placebo	Sertraline > placebo	0.28; $p < .04$	2.04—sertraline; 1.63—placebo
Zohar et al. (2002)	42 male Israeli veterans with PTSD	10 weeks	23 sertraline 19 placebo	No difference	0.35 NS	1.41—sertraline; 1.15—placebo
Friedman et al. (2007)	169 male Vietnam veterans with PTSD	12 weeks	86 sertraline 83 placebo	No difference	−0.03 NS	0.69—sertraline; 0.78—placebo
Paroxetine						
Marshall et al. (2001)	547 males and females (mostly civilians) with PTSD	12 weeks	183—20 mg paroxetine 182—40 mg paroxetine 186 placebo	20 mg paroxetine > placebo 40 mg paroxetine > placebo	0.84 $p < .01$ 0.81 $p < .01$	2.46—paroxetine 20 mg; 1.59—placebo; 2.43—paroxetine 40 mg; 1.59—placebo
Tucker et al. (2001)	307 males and females with PTSD (mostly civilians)	12 weeks	151 paroxetine 150 placebo	Paroxetine > placebo	0.58 $p < .001$	2.06—paroxetine; 1.52—placebo

(continued)

TABLE 9.2. (continued)

Study	Target population[a]	Duration of trial	Treatments/control[b]	Major findings	Between-group effect sizes	Within-group effect sizes
Fluoxetine						
Connor et al. (1999)	50 male and female civilians with PTSD	12 weeks	26 fluoxetine 24 placebo	Fluoxetine > placebo	0.90 p < .005	2.40—fluoxetine; 1.20—placebo
van der Kolk et al. (1994)	33 male and female civilians with PTSD	5 weeks	33 fluoxetine Placebo not reported	Fluoxetine > placebo	0.77 p < .005	0.77—fluoxetine; placebo (unreported)
	31 male veterans with PTSD	5 weeks	31 fluoxetine Placebo not reported	No difference	0.26 NS	0.26—fluoxetine; placebo (unreported)
Fluoxetine						
Martenyi et al. (2002)	301 male veterans with PTSD	12 weeks	226 fluoxetine 75 placebo	Fluoxetine > placebo	0.49 p < .006	2.58—fluoxetine; 2.22—placebo
Venlafaxine						
Davidson, Rothabuam, et al. (2006)	531 male and female civilians with PTSD	12 weeks	179 venlafaxine 173 sertraline 179 placebo	Venlafaxine > placebo Sertraline vs. placebo NS (near significant) Venlafaxine vs. sertraline	0.27 p < .015 0.19 p < .081 0.08 NS	Unavailable— venlafaxine; unavailable— placebo; unavailable— sertraline
Davidson, Pearlstein, et al. (2006)	329 male and female civilians with PTSD	6 months	161 venlafaxine 168 placebo	Venlafaxine > placebo	0.32 p < .006	3.54—venlafaxine; 2.89—placebo

Nefazodone						
Saygin et al. (2002)	54 Turkish civilians with PTSD	6 months	24 nefazodone 30 sertraline	No difference	0.28 NS	3.28—nefazodone; 3.61—sertraline
McRae et al. (2004)	26 civilians with PTSD	12 weeks	13 nefazodone 13 sertraline	No difference	0.01 NS	5.21—nefazodone; 2.73—sertraline
Davis et al. (2000)	41 male veterans with PTSD	12 weeks	26 nefazodone 15 placebo	Nefazodone > placebo	0.41 $p < .04$	0.86—nefazodone; 0.79—placebo
Mirtazapine						
Davidson et al. (2003)	26 male and female civilians with PTSD	8 weeks	17 mirtazapine 9 placebo	No difference	0.81 NS	1.55—mirtazapine; 0.78—placebo
Chung et al. (2004)	100 male and female Korean civilians with PTSD	6 weeks	51 mirtazapine 49 sertraline	No difference	0.15 NS	1.84—mirtazapine; 1.39—sertraline
Imipramine						
Kosten et al. (1991)	41 male Vietnam War combat veterans with PTSD	8 weeks	23 imipramine 18 placebo	Imipramine > placebo	0.66 $p < .05$	0.54—imipramine; 0.09—placebo
Amitriptyline						
Davidson et al. (1990)	46 male Vietnam War combat veterans with PTSD	8 weeks	25 amitriptyline 21 placebo	Amitriptyline > placebo (near significant)	0.91 $p < .08$	0.80—amitriptyline; 0.54—placebo

(continued)

251

TABLE 9.2. (continued)

Study	Target population[a]	Duration of trial	Treatments/control[b]	Major findings	Between-group effect sizes	Within-group effect sizes
Desipramine						
Reist et al. (1989)	18 male Vietnam War combat veterans with PTSD	4 weeks (crossover)	18 desipramine 18 placebo	No difference (intrusion)	0.13 NS	0.14—desipramine; 0.05—placebo
				No difference (avoidance)	0.16 NS	0.04—desipramine; −0.10—placebo
Phenelzine						
Kosten et al. (1991)	37 male Vietnam War veterans with PTSD	8 weeks	19 phenelzine 18 placebo	Phenelzine > placebo	0.79 $p < .05$	0.84—phenelzine; 0.09—placebo
Shestatzky et al. (1988)	13 male combat veterans	4 weeks (crossover)	13 phenelzine 13 placebo	No difference	0.13 NS	0.09—phenelzine; 0.32—placebo
Brofaromine						
Baker et al. (1995)	114 male and female veterans and civilians	12 weeks	56 brofaromine 58 placebo	No difference	0.01 NS	1.67—brofaromine; 1.50—placebo
Katz et al. (1995)	45 male and female civilians and veterans	14 weeks	22 brofaromine 23 placebo	Brofaromine > placebo (near significant)	0.60 $p < .07$	1.95—brofaromine; 1.45—placebo
Prazosin						
Raskind et al. (2003)	10 male Vietnam War veterans	20 weeks (crossover)	10 prazosin 10 placebo	Prazosin > placebo	1.38 $p < .01$	1.28—prazosin; −0.16—placebo
Raskind et al. (2007)	34 male Vietnam War veterans	8 weeks	17 prazosin 17 placebo	No difference	0.30 NS	0.60—prazosin; 0.40—placebo

	Sample	Duration	N	Outcome	Statistic	Effect size/dose
Guanfacine						
Neylan et al. (2006)	63 male Vietnam War veterans	8 weeks	29 guanfacine 34 placebo	No difference	−0.01 NS	0.20—guanfacine; 0.30—placebo
Risperidone						
Monnelly et al. (2003)	15 male combat veterans	6 weeks	7 risperidone 8 placebo	Risperidone > placebo	Not available $p < .02$	Not available
Reich et al. (2004)	21 female civilians	8 weeks	12 risperidone 9 placebo	Risperidone > placebo	0.82 $p < .015$	1.70—risperidone; 1.35—placebo
Bartzokis et al. (2005)	48 male Vietnam War veterans	16 weeks	22 risperidone 26 placebo	Risperidone > placebo	0.43 $p < .05$	1.20—risperidone; 0.29—placebo
Hamner et al. (2003)	37 male Vietnam War veterans	5 weeks	19 risperidone 18 placebo	No difference	−0.05 NS	0.39—risperidone; 0.83—placebo
Olanzapine						
Stein et al. (2002)	19 male Vietnam War veterans	8 weeks	10 olanzapine 9 placebo	Olanzapine > placebo	1.02 $p < .05$	0.67—olanzapine; 0.17—placebo
Alprazolam						
Braun et al. (1990)	10 male and female civilians	12 weeks (crossover)	10 alprazolam 10 placebo	No difference	0.28 NS	0.51—alprazolam; 0.13—placebo
Lamotrigine						
Hertzberg et al. (1999)	14 male and female civilians	12 weeks	10 lamotrigine 4 placebo	Suggestive findings in favor of lamotrigine	Not available	50% response—lamotrigine; 25% response—placebo

(continued)

TABLE 9.2. *(continued)*

Study	Target population[a]	Duration of trial	Treatments/control[b]	Major findings	Between-group effect sizes	Within-group effect sizes
Tiagabine						
Davidson et al. (2007)	232 male and female civilians	12 weeks	116 tiagabine 116 placebo	No difference	−0.05 NS	1.94—tiagabine; 2.10—placebo
Cyproheptadine						
Jacobs-Rebhun et al. (2000)	69 male combat veterans	2 weeks	35 cyproheptadine 34 placebo	Difference (placebo group did better)	Not available NS	Not available
Inositol						
Kaplan e al. (1996)	13 male and female civilians	4 weeks (crossover)	13 inositol 13 placebo	No difference	0.25 NS	0.70—inositol; −0.03—placebo

[a]N = subjects starting study.
[b]N = subjects in data analysis.

254

TABLE 9.3. Medications for PTSD: Indications and Contraindications

Class	Medication	Strength of evidence[a]	Daily dose	Indications	Contraindications
Selective serotonin reuptake inhibitors (SSRIs)	Paroxetine[a] Sertraline[b] Fluoxetine Citalopram Fluvoxamine	A A A F B	10–60 mg 50–200 mg 20–80 mg 20–60 mg 50–300 mg	• Reduce B, C, and D symptoms • Produce clinical global improvement • Effective treatment for depression, panic disorder, social phobia, and obsessive–compulsive disorder • Reduce associated symptoms (rage, aggression, impulsivity, suicidal thoughts)	• May produce insomnia, restlessness, nausea, decreased appetite, daytime sedation, nervousness, and anxiety • May produce sexual dysfunction, decreased libido, delayed orgasm, or anorgasmia • Clinically significant interactions for people prescribed monoamine oxidase inhibitors (MAOIs) • Significant interactions with hepatic enzymes produce other drug interactions
Other serotonergic antidepressants	Nefazodone Trazodone	A C	200–600 mg 150–600 mg	• Superior to placebo in male combat veterans • Effective antidepressants • Trazodone has limited efficacy by itself but is synergistic with SSRIs and may reduce SSRI-induced insomnia	• May be too sedating, rare priapism • Reports of hepatotoxicity associated with nefazodone treatment
Other serotonergic agents	Cyproheptadine Buspirone	A F		• Not recommended • Make PTSD symptoms worse • May reduce PTSD symptoms • May potentiate SSRI treatment	• Drowsiness, weight gain • Few side effects • Rare dizziness, headache, and nausea
Other second-generation antidepressants	Venlafaxine[c] Mirtazepine[c]	A A	75–225 mg 15–45 mg	• Effective antidepressants • Efficacy in PTSD has been demonstrated	• Venlafaxine may exacerbate hypertension • Mirtazapine may produce somnolence, increased appetite, and weight gain
	Buproprion	C	200–450 mg	• Possibly effective	• Buproprion may exacerbate seizure disorder

(continued)

TABLE 9.3. (continued)

Class	Medication	Strength of evidence[a]	Daily dose	Indications	Contraindications
Monoamine oxidase inhibitors (MAOIs)	Phenelzine	A	15–90 mg	• Reduces B symptoms • Produces global improvement • Effective agents for depression, panic, and social phobia Efficacy in PTSD has not been demonstrated for other MAOIs	• Risk of hypertensive crisis makes it necessary for patients to follow a strict dietary regimen • Contraindicated in combination with most other antidepressants, central nervous system (CNS) stimulants and decongestants • Contraindicated in patients with alcohol/substance abuse/dependency • May produce insomnia, hypotension, anticholinergic and severe liver toxicity
Tricyclic antidepressants (TCAs)	Imipramine[d] Amitriptyline Desipramine	A A A	150–300 mg 150–300 mg 100–300 mg	• Reduce B symptoms • Produce global improvement • Effective antidepressant and antipanic agents • Imipramine prevented onset of PTSD in pediatric burn patient • Desipramine ineffective in one randomized clinical trial Other TCAs have not been tested in PTSD	• Anticholinergic side effects (dry mouth, rapid pulse, blurred vision, constipation) • May produce ventricular arrhythmias • May produce orthostatic hypotension, sedation, or arousal
Antiadrenergic agents	Propranolol[d] Prazosin Clonidine[c] Guanfacine[c]	B A C A	40–160 mg 6–10 mg 0.2–0.6 mg 1–3 mg	• Reduce B and D symptoms • Produce global improvement • Prazosin shown to have marked efficacy for PTSD nightmares and insomnia • Propranolol reduced physiological hyperreactivity in acutely traumatized individuals • A recent RCT showed that guanfacine was ineffective, although positive results have been seen in open trials	• May produce hypotension or bradycardia • Use cautiously with hypotensive patients • Titrate prazosin starting at 1 mg at bedtime and monitor blood pressure • Propranolol may produce depressive symptoms, psychomotor slowing, or bronchospasm

Category	Drug		Dose	Effects	Side effects
Glucocorticoids	Hydrocortisone[d]	A	5–30 mg	• Prevents later development of PTSD in septic shock patients and post cardiac surgery	• Immunosuppression, osteopenia, hyperglycemia, hypertension
Anticonvulsants	Carbamazepine[c]	B	400–1,600 mg	• Effective on B and D symptoms • Effective in bipolar affective disorder • Possibly effective in reducing impulsive, aggressive, and violent behavior	• Neurological symptoms, ataxia, drowsiness, low sodium, leukopenia
	Valproate[c]	B	750–1,750 mg	• Effective on C and D symptoms • Effective in bipolar affective disorder	• Gastrointestinal problems, sedation, tremor, and thrombocytopenia • Valproate is teratogenic and should not be used in pregnancy
	Gabapentin[c]	F	300–3,600 mg	• Small trials suggesting favorable effects of gabapentin and lamotrigine	• Gabapentin—sedation and ataxia
	Lamotrigine[c]	A/B	50–400 mg		• Lamotrigine—Stevens–Johnson syndrome, skin rash, and fatigue
	Topiramate[c]	B	200–400 mg	• Efficacy of topiramate has not been demonstrated in PTSD	• Topiramate—glaucoma, sedation, dizziness, and ataxia
	Tiagabine[c]	A	4–12 mg	• Tiagabine was ineffective in a large randomized trial	• Tiagabine—dizziness, somnolence, tremor, and seizures
	Vigabatrin[c]	F	250–500 mg		• Vigabatrin—constriction of visual fields
Glutamatergic agent	Cycloserine[e]	A	250–1,000 mg	• Reduction in PTSD severity • Improved cognition	• Somnolence, headache, tremor, dysarthria, vertigo, confusion, nervousness, irritability, psychotic reactions, hyperreflexia, and seizures
Gamma-aminobutyric acid–B agent	Baclofen[c]	F	30–80 mg	• Improvement in PTSD severity	• Sedation, CNS depression

(continued)

TABLE 9.3. (continued)

Class	Medication	Strength of evidence[a]	Daily dose	Indications	Contraindications
Benzodiazepines	Alprazolam	A	0.5–6 mg	• Not recommended	• Sedation, memory impairment, ataxia
	Clonazepam	B	1–8 mg	• Do not reduce core B and C symptoms	• Not recommended for patients with past or present alcohol/drug abuse/dependency because of risk for dependence
				• Effective only for general anxiety and insomnia	• May exacerbate depressive symptoms
				Other benzodiazepines have not been tested in PTSD	• Alprazolam may produce rebound anxiety
Conventional antipsychotics	Thioridazine	F	20–800 mg	Not recommended	• Sedation, orthostatic hypotension, anticholinergic, extrapyramidal effects, tardive dyskinesia, neuroleptic malignant syndrome, endocrinopathies, EKG abnormalities, blood dyscrasias, hepatotoxicity
	Chlorpromazine	F	30–800 mg		
	Haloperidol	F	1–20 mg		
Atypical antipsychotics	Risperidone[e]	A	4–16 mg	• Preliminary data suggests effectiveness against PTSD symptom clusters and aggression	• Weight gain with all agents
	Olanzapine[e]	A	5–20 mg		• Risk of type 2 diabetes with olanzapine
	Quetiapine	B	50–750 mg	• May have a role as augmentation treatment for partial responders to other agents	

Notes. RCT, randomized clinical trial; B, symptoms, intrusive recollections; C symptoms, avoidance/numbing; D symptoms, hyperarousal. From Friedman and Davidson (2007). Copyright 2007 by The Guilford Press. Adapted by permission.

[a]Level A, randomized clinical trials; Level B, well-designed clinical studies without randomization or placebo comparison; Level C, service and naturalistic clinical studies, combined with clinical observations that are sufficiently compelling to warrant use of this drug; Level F, a few observations that have not been subjected to clinical or empirical tests.

[b]FDA approval as indicated treatment for PTSD.

[c]The only data are from small trials and case reports.

[d]RCT to prevent PTSD.

[e]Utilized as adjunctive agent with prolonged exposure therapy.

than combat trauma to SSRIs. Neither of these speculations appears to be valid. First, men responded as well as women in the two large-scale paroxetine trials (Marshall et al., 2001; Tucker et al., 2001). Second, men with military trauma responded as well as women with sexual trauma and men with non-combat trauma in both of the aforementioned paroxetine RCTs, as well as a large fluoxetine trial (Martenyi, Brown, Zhang, Koke, & Prakash, 2002) with combat veterans of recent wars. In reviewing these findings, as well as negative results from earlier RCTs conducted with Vietnam veterans in VA hospital settings, Friedman (1997; Friedman et al., 2007) has argued that veterans who remain symptomatic after decades of VA treatment comprise a chronic, treatment-refractory cohort that is representative of neither men in general nor male veterans with PTSD. We await new SSRI trials with younger veterans of the recent wars in Afghanistan and Iraq to have a better understanding of this matter. (The issue of chronicity among VA patients may also account for the recent negative RCT with guanfacine; discussed below.)

Two other mostly negative sertraline trials are also shown in Table 9.2, one with Israeli veterans (Zohar et al., 2002) and the other with civilians as part of a venlafaxine trial (Davidson, Rothbaum, et al., 2006).

Three other important findings concerning SSRI treatment should guide practitioner decisions about evidence-based pharmacotherapy. First, although most people receiving SSRIs have shown improvement in PTSD symptom severity, only 30% have achieved complete remission after 12 weeks of treatment (Brady et al., 2000; Davidson, Rothbaum, et al., 2001; Marshall et al., 2001; Tucker et al., 2001). Second, when SSRI treatment is extended for another 24 weeks, more than half (55% of the partial responders) of the participants exhibit complete remission after a longer course of treatment (Londborg et al., 2001). Third, discontinuation of SSRIs following successful treatment is likely to result in relapse (Davidson, Pearlstein, et al., 2001; Davidson et al., 2005; Martenyi & Soldatenkova, 2006). In this regard, PTSD is no different than affective or other anxiety disorders because positive responders to pharmacotherapy generally need to remain on medication to maintain their clinical improvement.

Venlafaxine-ER (an SNRI), has proved superior to placebo and comparable to sertraline in two large-scale RCTs (Davidson, Baldwin, et al., 2006). Based on current evidence, it appears that this medication can be recommended, along with SSRIs, as a first-line treatment for PTSD.

Small trials with nefazodone have shown greater efficacy than placebo and equal efficacy to sertraline. Unfortunately, the original brand form of the medication has been withdrawn from the market by its manufacturer because of hepatotoxicity, although generic forms still exist.

Mirtazapine is the last of the newer antidepressants to have been tested. Results from small studies suggest that it is superior to placebo and comparable to sertraline (see Table 9.2).

There have not been any new RCTs with older antidepressants (e.g., tricyclic antidepressants [TCAs] and monoamine oxidase inhibitors [MAOIs]) since the first edition of this book was published in 2000. This is undoubtedly due to concern about the greater likelihood of side effects with these older agents, as well as lack of interest by pharmaceutical companies, for whom such medications are much less profitable. Because clinicians successfully utilized such agents for many years (side effects notwithstanding) before the development of SSRIs and newer medications, and these agents have proven generally to be as effective as the newer agents and much less expensive, and because only 30% of SSRI-treated patients achieve complete remission within 12 weeks, we strongly urge clinicians to keep TCAs and MAOIs in mind as legitimate treatment options for patients who fail SSRI/SNRI treatment.

As we shift attention to nonantidepressant medications that have been tested in RCTs (Table 9.2), comments are in order about antiadrenergics, atypical antipsychotics, anticonvulsants, and benzodiazepines.

Medications that reduce adrenergic activity would be expected to show efficacy in PTSD given the adrenergic hyperactivity associated with this disorder (see Table 9.1). A small, single-site trial has indicated that augmentation of an antidepressant with the alpha-1 adrenergic antagonist prazosin reduces overall PTSD symptom severity, with specific efficacy against traumatic nightmares (Raskind, Peskind, et al., 2003). In a second study by the same group (Raskind et al., 2007), prazosin was not superior to placebo with regard to overall PTSD symptom severity, although it significantly reduced insomnia and traumatic nightmares. A multisite VA study, currently in progress, should shed further light on the utility of this medication. Propranolol has also been tested as a prophylactic agent to prevent the later development of PTSD (see Friedman & Davidson, 2007; Pitman et al., 2002). On the other hand, in a study with Vietnam War veterans in a VA hospital setting, the alpha-2 adrenergic agonist guanfacine, which reduces presynaptic release of norepinephrine, failed to exhibit beneficial effects compared to placebo (Neylan et al., 2006).

Two RCTs have been conducted with anticonvulsants. One was a small trial with lamotrigine, in which 5 out of 10 patients exhibited symptomatic improvement (Hertzberg et al., 1999), although this positive interpretation has been challenged (Berlant, 2003). The second was a negative RCT in which tiagabine performed no better than placebo (Davidson, Brady, Mellman, Stein, & Pollack, 2007). Given the emerging recognition of the importance of glutamatergic and gamma-aminobutyric acid (GABA)-ergic mechanisms in PTSD, the wide variety of anticonvulsant agents that affect these systems, and the promising open-label findings with these agents, further investigations with this class of medications should be very important in the future.

Atypical antipsychotic medications (risperidone and olanzapine) have been tested in small RCTs as adjunctive agents to SSRIs for (mostly VA) patients who failed to respond to an adequate clinical trial with SSRIs. Results have been promising, especially because many patients in these studies exhibit chronic, severe, and treatment-refractory PTSD. A multisite VA study testing adjunctive risperidone treatment is currently in progress.

We remind the reader that the only RCT utilizing a benzodiazepine (Braun, Greenberg, Dasberg, & Lerer, 1990) was negative. In addition, one double-blind trial of clonazepam versus placebo (Cates, Bishop, Davis, Lowe, & Wolley, 2004) failed to show a benzodiazepine benefit relative to sleep disturbance in PTSD. Given that there are now a number of effective medications for PTSD, there is little justification for prescribing benzodiazepines.

Finally, other RCTs have shown the ineffectiveness of the serotonin receptor (5-HT$_2$) antagonist cyproheptadine and the second messenger inositol.

Other Evidence: Open Trials and Case Reports

A fair number of open trials and case reports has been published in addition to randomized clinical trials. Table 9.3 summarizes published evidence for the efficacy of all medications tested in PTSD. In some cases, the only information comes from open trials and case reports. The strength of this evidence [Levels A–F] is also shown. In the case of alprazolam and cyproheptadine, there is excellent evidence (Level A) that neither agent is effective in PTSD. Because of space limitations, we provide only a brief discussion of these findings. A more comprehensive review may be found elsewhere (Friedman & Davidson, 2007; Stein, Ipser, & Seedat, 2006).

Selective Serotonin Reuptake Inhibitors

In addition to large RCTs with SSRIs sertraline, paroxetine, and fluoxetine, a number of successful open trials and case reports have been published concerning fluoxetine, sertraline, paroxetine, and fluvoxamine (for references, see Friedman & Davidson, 2007). SSRIs are relatively well-tolerated, promote clinical global improvement and enhanced quality of life, are effective against comorbid disorders, and ameliorate associated symptoms, such as impulsive, suicidal, and aggressive behavior.

Other Serotonergic Agents

Although nefazodone, an SSRI plus 5-HT$_2$ antagonist, has been effective in 3 RCTs (see Table 9.2) and in open-label trials, the brand form has been withdrawn from the market by its manufacturer because of hepatotoxicity. Trazodone (which is also an SSRI plus 5-HT$_2$ antagonist) has shown only modest effectiveness against PTSD symptoms in a small open trial, but it has been prescribed mostly because of its capacity to reverse the insomnia caused by SSRI agents (see Friedman & Davidson, 2007).

As mentioned previously, an RCT showed that cyproheptadine, a 5-HT$_2$ antagonist for which there were anecdotal reports of efficacy against traumatic nightmares and flashbacks, was less effective than placebo. Buspirone is a partial 5-HT$_{1A}$ agonist generally prescribed as an anxiolytic agent. A few open trials and case reports have had inconsistent results with regard to its effectiveness in PTSD.

Newer Antidepressants

Venlafaxine appears to be a first-line treatment for PTSD based on large multisite RCTs reviewed previously. Small RCTs with mirtazapine, as well as an open-label trial in Korea, suggest that this is a promising medication. There is also an interesting case report describing the effectiveness of mirtazapine for reducing traumatic nightmares among refugees who had not achieved relief from other medications. Finally, open-label trials with bupropion have also been encouraging (see Friedman & Davidson, 2007).

Antiadrenergic Agents: Propranolol, Clonidine, and Guanfacine

Although it is well established that adrenergic dysregulation is associated with chronic PTSD (see Friedman & Davidson, 2007) there has been little research with this class of pharmacological agents. In addition to the aforementioned successful RCT with prazosin, the beta-adrenergic antagonist propranolol has been beneficial in an A-B-A (6 weeks off–6 weeks on–6 weeks off) design study with children (Famularo, Kinscherff, & Fenton, 1988).

A recent RCT with guanfacine (Neylan et al., 2006) had negative results that might have been due to problems of chronicity among veterans in VA settings, as discussed previously. On the other hand, four open trials in veterans, with the alpha-2 agonists clonidine and guanfacine have been promising (for references, see Friedman & Southwick, 1995).

Monoamine Oxidase Inhibitors

In addition to the randomized clinical trials reported previously, there have been two successful open trials, a number of positive case reports, and one negative open trial with phenelzine (see Friedman & Davidson, 2007). A comprehensive review of published findings on MAOI treatment (Southwick, Yehuda, Giller, & Charney, 1994) found that MAOIs produced moderate-to-good global improvement in 82% of patients, primarily due to reduction in reexperiencing symptoms.

The use of MAOIs has traditionally been limited when there are legitimate concerns that patients might ingest alcohol or pharmacologically contraindicated illicit drugs, or that they might not adhere to necessary dietary restrictions. One serious consequence of lack of compliance is a hypertensive crisis, which is a medical emergency. Such concerns do not generally apply to reversible monoamine oxidase A (MAOA) inhibitors such as moclobemide. Indeed, moclobemide produced significant reductions in PTSD reexperiencing and avoidant symptoms in a small open trial with 20 patients (Neal, Shapland, & Fox, 1997).

Tricyclic Antidepressants

In addition to the randomized clinical trials (showing positive results with imipramine and amitriptyline, and negative results with desipramine) reported previously, there are numerous case reports and open trials with TCAs (for references, see Ver Ellen & van Kammen, 1990). Results have been mixed and generally modest in magnitude. In their analysis of 15 randomized trials, open trials, and case reports involving TCA treatment for PTSD, Southwick and associates (1994) found that 45% of patients showed moderate-to-good global improvement following treatment and reduction in reexperiencing rather than avoidant/numbing or arousal symptoms.

Benzodiazepines

The evidence does not support benzodiazepines as an appropriate treatment for PTSD. In addition to the negative RCT with alprazolam reported previously (Braun et al., 1990), poor results have been observed in open trials with alprazolam and clonazepam. In two studies, with recently traumatized emergency room patients, benzodiazepines did not prevent the later development of PTSD (Gelpin, Bonne, Peri, Brandes, & Shalev, 1996; Mellman, Bustamante, David, & Fins, 2002).

Anticonvulsants

Interest in this class of pharmacological agents has begun to develop not only because of its antikindling properties but also its diverse actions on glutamatergic and GABA-ergic mechanisms. A detailed review of publications regarding carbamazepine, valproate, gabapentin, lamotrigine, topiramate, tiagabine, and vigabatrin may be found elsewhere (Friedman & Davidson, 2007). Despite promising open-label studies, an RCT with tiagabine was negative and another, with lamotrigine, was inconclusive (see previous discussion and Table 9.2).

Antipsychotic Agents

As mentioned earlier, a number of positive RCTs with atypical antipsychotics as adjunctive treatment for SSRI nonresponders has stimulated considerable interest in this class of medications. Case reports suggest that atypical antipsychotics may have a unique niche as adjunctive agents for not only chronic, treatment-refractory patients but also PTSD patients who exhibit extreme hypervigilance/paranoia, physical aggression, social isolation, and trauma-related hallucinations. On the other hand, there is no evidence to support the use of conventional antipsychotic agents for patients with PTSD, especially in view of potentially serious side effects, especially tardive dyskinesia (see Friedman & Davidson, 2007).

Summary and Recommendations

Currently, we know five things about pharmacotherapy for PTSD:

1. Many people are receiving medication.
2. Clinical trials usually show that some patients benefit greatly short term and then later from maintained pharmacotherapy.
3. SSRIs and SNRIs are currently the best-established drug treatment for PTSD and can be recommended as a first-line treatment.
4. Adjunctive treatment with atypical antipsychotics for SSRI/SNRI-refractory patients appears to be warranted.
5. Much more research is needed, including work on children and adolescents, individual predictors of response, PTSD prophylaxis, new approaches for treatment-refractory PTSD, outcomes with combined pharmacotherapy and cognitive-behavioral therapy (CBT), and adjunctive D-cycloserine to potentiate CBT treatment (see Friedman & Davidson, 2007).

Medications seem to have at least three potential benefits for patients with PTSD: amelioration of PTSD symptoms; treatment of comorbid disorders; and reduction of associated symptoms that interfere with psychotherapy and/ or daily function. There is good reason to anticipate exciting breakthroughs in the foreseeable future that equip clinicians with a greater variety of effective medications that benefit patients with PTSD.

References

Baker, D. G., Diamond, B. I., Gillette, G., Hamner, K., Katzelnick, D., Keller, T., et al. (1995). A double-blind, randomized placebo-controlled multi-center study of brofaromine in the treatment of post-traumatic stress disorder. *Psychopharmacology, 122,* 386–389.

Bartzokis, G., Lu, P. H., Turner, J., Mintz, J., & Saunders, C. S. (2005). Adjunctive risperidone in the treatment of chronic combat-related posttraumatic stress disorder. *Biological Psychiatry, 57,* 474–479.

Berlant, J. L. (2003). Antiepileptic treatment of posttraumatic stress disorder. *Primary Psychiatry, 10,* 41–49.

Brady, K., Pearlstein, T., Asnis, G. M., Baker, D., Rothbaum, B., Sikes, C. R., et al. (2000). Efficacy and safety of sertraline treatment of posttraumatic stress disorder. *Journal of the American Medical Association, 283,* 1837–1844.

Braun, P., Greenberg, D., Dasberg, H., & Lerer, B. (1990). Core symptoms of posttraumatic stress disorder unimproved by alprazolam treatment. *Journal of Clinical Psychiatry, 51,* 236–238.

Cates, M. E., Bishop, M. H., Davis, L. L., Lowe, J. S., & Wolley, T. W. (2004). Clonazepam for treatment of sleep disturbances associated with combat-related posttraumatic stress disorder. *Annals of Pharmacotherapy, 38,* 1395–1399.

Charney, D. S. (2004). Psychobiological mechanisms of resilience and vulnerability: Implication is for the successful adaptation to extreme stress. *American Journal of Psychiatry, 161*, 195–216.

Chung, M. Y., Min, K. J., Jun, Y. J., Kim, S. S., Kim, W. C., & Jun, E. M. (2004). Efficacy and tolerability of mirtazapine and sertraline in Korean veterans with posttraumatic stress disorder. *Human Psychopharmacology, 19*, 489–494.

Connor, K. M., Sutherland, S. M., Tupler, L. A., Malik, M. L., & Davidson, J. R. T (1999). Fluoxetine in post-traumatic stress disorder: Randomised, double-blind study. *British Journal of Psychiatry, 175*, 17–22.

Davidson, J. R. T., Baldwin, D. S., Stein, D. J., Kuper, E., Benattia, I., Ahmed, S., et al. (2006). Treatment of posttraumatic stress disorder with venlafaxine extended release: A 6-month randomized, controlled trial. *Archives of General Psychiatry, 63*, 1158–1165.

Davidson, J. R. T., Brady, K., Mellman, T. A., Stein, M. B., & Pollack, M. H. (2007). The efficacy and tolerability of tiagabine in adult patients with post-traumatic stress disorder. *Journal of Clinical Psychopharmacology, 27*, 1–4.

Davidson, J. R. T., Connor, K. M., Hertzberg, M. A., Weisler, R. H., Wilson, W. H., & Payne, V. M. (2005). Maintenance therapy with fluoxetine in posttraumatic stress disorder: A placebo-controlled discontinuation study. *Journal of Clinical Psychopharmacology, 25*, 166–169.

Davidson, J. R. T., Kudler, H., Smith, R., Mahorney, S. L., Lipper, S., Hammett, E. B., et al. (1990). Treatment of post-traumatic stress disorder with amitriptyline and placebo. *Archives of General Psychiatry, 47*, 259–266.

Davidson, J. R. T., Pearlstein, T., Londborg, P., Brady, K. T., Rothbaum, B. O., Bell, J., et al. (2001). Efficacy of sertraline in preventing relapse of posttraumatic stress disorder: Results of a 28-week double-blind, placebo-controlled study. *American Journal of Psychiatry, 158*, 1974–1981.

Davidson, J. R. T., Rothbaum, B. O., Tucker, P., Asnis, G., Benattia, I., & Musgnung, M. T. (2006). Venlafaxine extended release in posttraumatic stress disorder: A sertraline and placebo-controlled study. *Journal of Clinical Psychopharmacology, 26*, 259–267.

Davidson, J. R. T., Rothbaum, B. O., van der Kolk, B. A., Sikes, C. R., & Farfel, G. M. (2001). Multicenter, double-blind comparison of sertraline and placebo in the treatment of posttraumatic stress disorder. *Archives of General Psychiatry, 58*, 485–492.

Davidson, J. R. T., Weisler, R. H., Butterfield, M. I., Casat, C. D., Connor, K. M., Barnett, S., et al. (2003). Mirtazapine vs. placebo in posttraumatic stress disorder: A pilot trial. *Biological Psychiatry, 53*, 188–191.

Davis, L. L., Nugent, A. L., Murray, J., Kramer, G. L., & Petty, F. (2000). Nefazodone treatment for chronic posttraumatic stress disorder: An open trial. *Journal of Clinical Psychopharmacology, 20*, 159–164.

Famularo, R., Kinscherff, R., & Fenton, T. (1988). Propranolol treatment for childhood posttraumatic stress disorder, acute type. *American Journal of Diseases of Children, 142*, 1244–1247.

Friedman, M. J. (1997). Drug treatment for PTSD: Answers and questions. *Annals of the New York Academy of Sciences, 821*, 359–371.

Friedman, M. J., & Davidson, J. R. T. (2007). Pharmacotherapy for PTSD. In M. J. Friedman, T. M. Keane, & P. A. Resick (Eds.), *Handbook of PTSD: Science and practice* (pp. 376–405). New York: Guilford Press.

Friedman, M. J., Marmar, C. R., Baker, D. G., Sikes, C. R., & Farfel, G. (2007). Randomized double-blind comparison of sertraline and placebo for post-traumatic stress disorder in a Department of Veterans Affairs setting. *Journal of Clinical Psychiatry, 68,* 711–720.

Friedman, M. J., & Southwick, S. M. (1995). Towards pharmacotherapy for post-traumatic stress disorder. In M. J. Friedman, D. S. Charney, & A. Y. Deutch (Eds.), *Neurobiological and clinical consequences of stress: From normal adaptation to post-traumatic stress disorder* (pp. 465–482). Philadelphia: Lippincott-Raven.

Gelpin, E., Bonne, O., Peri, T., Brandes, D., & Shalev, A. Y. (1996). Treatment of recent trauma survivors with benzodiazepines: A prospective study. *Journal of Clinical Psychiatry, 57,* 390–394.

Hamner, M. B., Faldowski, R. A., Ulmer, H. G., Frueh, B. C., Huber, M. G., & Arana, G. W. (2003). Adjunctive rispiridone treatment in post-traumatic stress disorder: A preliminary controlled trial of effects of comorbid psychotic symptoms. *International Clinical Psychopharmacology, 18,* 1–8.

Hertzberg, M. A., Butterfield, M. I., Feldman, M. E., Beckham, J. C., Sutherland, S. M., Connor, K. M., et al. (1999). A preliminary study of lamotrigine for the treatment of posttraumatic stress disorder. *Biological Psychiatry, 45,* 1226–1229.

Jacobs-Rebhun, S., Schnurr, P. P., Friedman, M. J., Peck, R. E., Brophy, M. H., & Fuller, D. (2000). Posttraumatic stress disorder and sleep difficulty [Letter]. *American Journal of Psychiatry, 157,* 1525–1526.

Kaplan, Z., Amin, M., Swartz, M., & Levine, J. (1996). Inositol treatment of posttraumatic stress disorder. *Anxiety, 2,* 51–52.

Katz, R. J., Lott, M. H., Arbus, P., Croca, L., Herlobsen, P., Lingjaerde, O., et al. (1995). Pharmacotherapy of post-traumatic stress disorder with a novel psychotropic. *Anxiety, 1,* 169–174.

Kosten, T. R., Frank, J. B., Dan, E., McDougle, C. J., & Giller, E. L. (1991). Pharmacotherapy for post-traumatic stress disorder using phenelzine or imipramine. *Journal of Nervous and Mental Disease, 179,* 366–370.

Londborg, P. D., Hegel, M. T., Goldstein, S., Goldstein, D., Himmelhoch, J. M., Maddock, R., et al. (2001). Sertraline treatment of posttraumatic stress disorder: Results of weeks of open-label continuation treatment. *Journal of Clinical Psychiatry, 62,* 325–331.

Marshall, R. D., Beebe, K. L., Oldham, M., & Zaninelli, R. (2001). Efficacy and safety of paroxetine treatment for chronic PTSD: A fixed-dose placebo-controlled study. *American Journal of Psychiatry, 158,* 1982–1988.

Martenyi, F., Brown, E. B., Zhang, H., Koke, S. C., & Prakash, A. (2002). Fluoxetine versus placebo in posttraumatic stress disorder. *Journal of Clinical Psychiatry, 63,* 199–206.

Martenyi, F., & Soblatenkova, V. (2006). Fluoxetine in the acute treatment and relapse prevention of combat-related post-traumatic stress disorder: Analysis of a veteran group of a placebo-controlled randomized clinical trial. *European Neuropsychopharmacology, 16,* 340–349.

McCrae, A. L., Brady, K. T., Mellman, T. A., Sonne, S. C., Killeen, T. K., Timmerman, M. A., et al. (2004). Comparison of nefazadone and sertraline for the treatment of posttraumatic stress disorder. *Depression and Anxiety, 19,* 190–196.

Mellman, T. A., Bustamante, V., David, D., & Fins, A. I. (2002). Hypnotic medication in the aftermath of trauma [Letter]. *Journal of Clinical Psychiatry, 63,* 1183–1184.

Monnelly, E. P., Ciraulo, D. A., Knapp, C., & Keane, T. (2003). Low-dose risperidone as adjunctive therapy for irritable aggression in posttraumatic stress disorder. *Journal of Clinical Psychopharmacology, 19*, 377–378.

Neal, L. A., Shapland, W., & Fox, C. (1997). An open trial of moclobemide in the treatment of post-traumatic stress disorder. *International Journal of Clinical Psychopharmacology, 12*, 231–232.

Neylan, T. C., Lenoci, M., Franklin, K. W., Metzler, T. J., Henn-Haase, C., Hierholzer, R. W., et al. (2006). No improvement of posttraumatic stress disorder symptoms with guanfacine treatment. *American Journal of Psychiatry, 163*, 2186–2188.

Pitman, R. K., Sanders, K. M., Zusman, R. M., Healy, A., Cheema, F., Lasko, N., et al. (2002). Pilot study of secondary prevention of posttraumatic stress disorder with propranolol. *Biological Psychiatry, 51*, 189–192.

Raskind, M. A., Peskind, E. R., Hoff, D. J., Hart, K. L., Holmes, H. A., Warren, D., et al. (2007). A parallel group placebo-controlled study of prazosin for trauma nightmares and sleep disturbance in combat veterans with posttraumatic stress disorder. *Biological Psychiatry, 61*, 928–934.

Raskind, M. A., Peskind, E. R., Kanter, E. D., Petrie, E. C., Radant, A., Thompson, C. E., et al. (2003). Reduction of nightmares and other PTSD symptoms in combat veterans by prazosin: A placebo-controlled study. *American Journal of Psychiatry, 160*(2), 371–373.

Reich, D. B., Winternitz, S., Hennen, J., Watts, T., & Stanculescu, C. (2004). A preliminary study of risperidone in the treatment of posttraumatic stress disorder related to childhood abuse in women. *Journal of Clinical Psychiatry, 65*, 1601–1606.

Reist, C., Kauffman, C. D., Haier, R. J., Sangdahl, C., DeMet, E. M., Chicz-DeMet, A., et al. (1989). A controlled trial of desipramine in 18 men with post-traumatic stress disorder. *American Journal of Psychiatry, 146*, 513–516.

Saygin, M. Z., Sungur, M. Z., Sabol, E. U., & Cetinkaya, P. (2002). Nefazadone versus sertraline in treatment of posttraumatic stress disorder. *Bulletin of Clinical Psychopharmacology, 12*, 1–5.

Shestatzky, M., Greenberg, D., & Lerer, B. (1988). A controlled trial of phenelzine in posttraumatic stress disorder. *Psychiatry Research, 24*, 149–155.

Southwick, S. M., Davis, L. L., Aikins, D. E., Rasmusson, A., Barron, J., & Morgan, C. A., III. (2007). Neurobiological alterations associated with PTSD. In M. J. Friedman, T. M. Keane, & P. A. Resick (Eds.), *Handbook of PTSD: Science and practice* (pp. 166–189). New York: Guilford Press.

Southwick, S. M., Yehuda, R., Giller, E. L., & Charney, D. S. (1994). Use of tricyclics and monoamine oxidase inhibitors in the treatment of PTSD: A quantitative review. In M. M. Murburg (Ed.), *Catecholamine function in post-traumatic stress disorder: Emerging concepts* (pp. 293–305). Washington, DC: American Psychiatry Press.

Stein, D. J., Ipser, J., & Seedat, S. (2006). Pharmacotherapy for post-traumatic stress disorder (PTSD). *Cochrane Database of Systematic Reviews, 1*, CD002795.

Stein, M. B., Kline, N. A., & Matloff, J. L. (2002). Adjunctive olanzapine for SSRI-resistant combat-related PTSD: A double-blind, placebo-controlled study. *American Journal of Psychiatry, 159*, 1777–1779.

Tucker, P., Zaninelli, R., Yehuda, R., Ruggiero, L., Dillingham, K., & Pitts, C. D. (2001). Paroxetine in the treatment of chronic posttraumatic stress disorder: Results of a placebo-controlled, flexible-dosage trial. *Journal of Clinical Psychiatry, 62*, 860–868.

van der Kolk, B. A., Dreyfuss, D., Michaels, M., Shera, D., Berkowitz, R., Fisler, R., et al. (1994). Fluoxetine versus placebo in posttraumatic stress disorder. *Journal of Clinical Psychiatry, 55*, 517–522.

Ver Ellen, P., & van Kammen, D. P. (1990). The biological findings in post-traumatic stress disorder: A review. *Journal of Applied Social Psychology, 20*(21, Pt. 1), 1789–1821.

Zohar, J., Amital, D., Miodownik, C., Kotler, M., Bleich, A., Lane, R. M., et al. (2002). Double-blind placebo-controlled pilot study of sertraline in military veterans with posttraumatic stress disorder. *Journal of Clinical Psychopharmacology, 22*, 190–195.

CHAPTER 10

Psychopharmacotherapy for Children and Adolescents

Craig L. Donnelly

Posttraumatic stress disorder (PTSD), a common cause of distress and dysfunction in children and adolescents, occurs with high rates of psychiatric comorbidity. There are few controlled trials to guide practitioners. Medication may play an important role in targeting specific PTSD symptoms and associated disorders, helping to improve functioning in day-to-day life. A reasonable first approach in highly symptomatic children is to begin with a broad-spectrum agent such as a selective serotonin reuptake inhibitor (SSRI), which should target anxiety, mood, and reexperiencing symptoms. Adrenergic agents, medications for attention-deficit/hyperactivity disorder (ADHD), mood stabilizers, or atypical neuroleptics, used either alone or in combination with an SSRI, may be useful interventions to target severe symptoms and/or comorbid conditions. Reduction in even one disabling symptom through pharmacotherapy may have a positive ripple effect on a child's overall functioning.

Theoretical Context

Children's responses to stress and trauma, though similar to those of adults, have been less well characterized and studied than adult reactions. Children are especially vulnerable to stress in the environment and in their caretakers. Given exposure to identical traumatic experiences, children are more sensitive than adults to the effects of trauma (Amaya-Jackson & March, 1993).

There are few well-conducted, controlled trials of medication treatments of PTSD in childhood, yet medication treatment has a role to play in the disorder in this age group.

PTSD Symptom Complexity and Comorbidity

Childhood and adolescent PTSD is an extremely heterogeneous disorder. The DSM-IV-TR (American Psychiatric Association, 2000) criteria set allows for at least 1,750 possible symptom combinations in meeting minimum criteria for a diagnosis of PTSD (i.e., one in five B criteria, plus three in five C criteria, plus two in five D criteria yields 1,750 possible symptom combinations). Given this complexity, appropriate use of medication to treat children with PTSD entails segregating and specifying diagnoses and target symptoms. Traumatized children frequently have symptoms of disorders other than PTSD, and children with other disorders often have trauma histories or PTSD as a comorbid diagnosis (Famularo, Kinscherff, & Fenton, 1992; Ford et al., 2000; Seedat, Kaminer, Lockhat, & Stein, 2000).

Neurobiology and Rationale for Pharmacotherapy

Of the three symptom clusters in PTSD—reexperiencing, avoidance, and hyperarousal—the symptoms of hyperarousal (e.g., sleep disturbances, irritability, difficulty concentrating, hypervigilance, exaggerated startle responses, and outbursts of aggression) may be the most amenable to pharmacological intervention (Perry, 1994). Difficulty falling asleep, sleepwalking, and night terrors are not uncommon in children with PTSD, and may adversely affect mood states, learning, and behavior in school.

Hypervigilance and exaggerated startle responses may lead to chronic anxiety and may seriously alter self-concept and self-confidence. Finally, hyperarousal may lead to difficulty in modulating aggression and can make children act more irritable, oppositional, and explosive.

Method of Collecting Data

Literature reviewed for pharmacological treatments of PTSD in children and adolescents involved a search of PubMed (1966–June 2006) for articles with the Medical Subject Heading (MeSH) "stress disorders, traumatic/drug therapy" and limited to the age group "all child: 0–18 years."

Special Considerations in Child and Adolescent Populations

Certainly the initial step in the treatment of PTSD is psychoeducation of the child, parents, and adult caregivers. Treatment should never be a mystery.

Reviews of empirical evidence on the effectiveness of pharmacotherapeutic agents in children with PTSD (Famularo et al., 1992; Putnam & Hulsmann, 2002) and textbooks of pediatric psychopharmacology, as well as guidelines and reviews (Cohen, 1998; Kutcher, 2002; Pfefferbaum, 1997), clearly lag behind the adult literature. As a general principle, clinicians are advised to "start low and go slow" with medication dosages and titration schedules because children are not simply "small adults." Cognitive-behavioral therapy (CBT) in school-age and older children and adolescents is likely to be the treatment of first choice (Cohen, 1998; Cohen, Mannarino, Perel, & Staron, 2007). Many experts use a blend of cognitive, behavioral, dynamic, and family-based interventions for childhood PTSD.

Literature Review

Medication Use in Child and Adolescent PTSD

Despite the lack of data, medication use in children with PTSD has become a standard of care (Cohen, Mannarino, & Rogal, 2001). The acceptability of pharmacotherapy to the patient and parent is one criterion on which to base the decision to prescribe medication. Another is the presence of severe comorbid psychiatric conditions that are responsive to medications that also treat PTSD. Medication may be favored as a first-line choice when the intensity of PTSD is interfering with a child's ability to engage in psychotherapy. Finally, medication treatment may also be indicated when there is no access to psychotherapy.

Medication algorithms have been developed for such a stepwise approach in both adults and children (Donnelly & Amaya-Jackson, 2002). Medication should decrease intrusions, avoidance, and anxious arousal; minimize impulsivity; improve sleep; treat secondary disorders; facilitate cognitive-behavioral psychotherapies; and improve functioning in daily life. Effective treatment of even one symptom in children with PTSD (e.g., improvement of a sleep-onset disturbance) can have a positive effect, enhancing multiple domains of functioning. No medication currently has a U.S. Food and Drug Administration (FDA) label indication for the treatment of PTSD in childhood. The scant literature is not sufficiently rigorous to allow comparison of effect sizes.

Specific Medications for Use in PTSD

Adrenergic Agents

The alpha-2 agonists clonidine and guanfacine, and the beta-antagonist propranolol reduce sympathetic tone and may be effective in treating the symptoms of hyperarousal, impulsivity, activation, sleep problems, and nightmares seen in PTSD (Horrigan, 1996; Marmar, Foy, Kagan, & Pynoos, 1993).

Perry (1994), using clonidine in an open-label trial involving 17 children with PTSD, found significant improvement in anxiety arousal, concentration, mood, and behavioral impulsivity using relatively low doses. Harmon and Riggs (1996) reported on the effectiveness of the transdermal clonidine patch in reducing PTSD symptoms in all seven patients in their open-label trial. Horrigan (1996), in a single-case study, reported on the effectiveness of guanfacine in reducing PTSD-associated nightmares in a 7-year-old. In one of the first studies of medication treatment in childhood PTSD, propranolol was shown to reduce arousal symptoms in survivors of childhood sexual abuse. In this uncontrolled A-B-A design study of children with PTSD, Famularo, Kinscherff, and Fenton (1988) group found that propranolol significantly reduced PTSD symptoms over the 5 weeks of treatment (2.5 mg/kg/day) in 8 of 11 abused children. Intrusion and arousal symptoms appeared to be most responsive to treatment in this study. Lustig and colleagues (2002) reported an ongoing randomized clinical trial on an inpatient unit, using clonidine for youngsters with intrusive symptoms of PTSD.

Use of adrenergic agents to reduce central nervous system adrenergic tone to target reexperiencing and hyperarousal symptoms is a rational treatment strategy in PTSD. Additionally, the alpha-2 adrenergic agents may be more effective than the psychostimulants for ADHD symptoms in maltreated or sexually abused children with PTSD (DeBellis et al., 1994).

Dopaminergic Agents

Horrigan and Barnhill (1999), in an uncontrolled design, used risperidone to treat 18 children with PTSD who had high rates of comorbid psychiatric disorders (e.g., 83% with comorbid ADHD, and 35% with comorbid bipolar disorder). Thirteen of the 18 subjects in this study experienced remission of their PTSD symptoms. More recently, Stathis, Martin, and McKenna (2005) reported a case series of six juveniles, ages 15–17 years, in a youth detention center who met criteria for PTSD and were treated with quetiapine (50–200 mg/day). Using the Traumatic Symptom Checklist for Children, they found significant improvements in dissociation, anxiety, depression, and anger over the 6-week treatment period. Nighttime sedation was the chief side effect. All patients opted to continue treatment beyond the 6-week trial period. Clozapine was reported to be effective in a case series of six adolescents with chronic posttraumatic stress disorder and psychotic symptoms (Wheatley, Plant, Reader, Brown, & Cahill, 2004). Four of six patients exhibited improvement in psychiatric symptoms, behavioral observations, and self-reports. In a chart review of a mixed residential population of adolescents, Kant, Chalansani, Chengappa, and Dieringer (2004) reported that clozapine (mean daily dose = 102 mg) was effective in reducing polypharmacy in 19 of 39 youth who had diagnoses of PTSD, though they noted that clozapine is associated with serious side effects.

With scant evidence as to their utility in PTSD symptoms per se, the atypical neuroleptics are currently reserved for patients with refractory PTSD or for those who exhibit paranoid behavior, parahallucinatory phenomena or intense flashbacks, self-destructive behavior, explosive or overwhelming anger, or psychotic symptoms.

Serotonergic Agents

The neurotransmitter serotonin (5-hydroxytryptamine [5-HT]) may be associated with PTSD and symptoms such as aggression, obsessive/intrusive thoughts, alcohol and substance abuse, and suicidal behavior. Suicidal behavior is known to be associated with both childhood maltreatment and low 5-HT functioning.

Two medications, the SSRIs sertraline and paroxetine, have FDA indications for PTSD in adults, but none have approval for use in children. In children, SSRIs are approved for use in depression (fluoxetine) and in obsessive–compulsive disorder (fluoxetine, sertraline, and fluvoxamine). SSRIs may be useful for children with PTSD because of the variety of symptoms associated with serotonergic dysregulation, including anxiety, depressed mood, obsessional thinking, compulsive behaviors, affective impulsivity, rage, and alcohol or substance abuse.

The SSRIs have received the most clinical attention and are likely first-line choices for children because of their "broad-spectrum" activity. Seedat, Lockhat, Kaminer, Zungu-Dirwayi, and Stein (2001; see also Seedat, Kaminer, Lockhat, & Stein, 2000) reported the effectiveness of citalopram in a 12-week open-label trial in eight adolescents with moderate to severe PTSD. Subjects in their trial exhibited a 38% reduction in PTSD symptoms at the end of treatment, although, curiously, self-reported depressive symptoms failed to improve. In a second study comparing responses of children/adolescents versus adults, also using citalopram (20–40 mg/day), Seedat and colleagues (2002) found no differences in outcome between adults and children after 8 weeks of open-label treatment. Both groups exhibited significant reductions is mean Clinician-Administered PTSD Scale (CAPS) scores and Clinical Global Improvement (CGI) ratings at endpoint. Recently, in perhaps the best medication study completed to date, Cohen and colleagues (2007) found comparable results in twenty-four 10- to 17-year-olds treated with either trauma-focused CBT (TF-CBT) plus sertraline or TF-CBT plus placebo. Both groups experienced significant PTSD symptom relief.

The SSRIs are generally safe and well tolerated, notwithstanding the FDA's recent black box warning about increased suicidal ideation and behavior rates in depressed children treated with these medications.

Nefazodone, a serotonergic antagonist antidepressant, has been reported to be helpful in PTSD and associated irritability and disruptive behavior in adolescents in an uncontrolled case series reported by Domon and Anderson

(2000). It should be noted that nefazodone and Serzone have been withdrawn from the market, although the generic form is still available; as such, it is not used in childhood populations. Mirtazapine, a serotonin and norepinephrine active antidepressant, has shown promise in case reports either alone or in combination with an SSRI for the treatment of PTSD (Conner, Davidson, Weisler, & Ahearn, 1999; Good & Peterson, 2001).

Buspirone, a nonbenzodiazepine anxiolytic 5-HT$_{1A}$ partial agonist, may have a role in reducing anxiety, flashbacks, and insomnia (Wells, Chu, & Johnson, 1991), although no controlled studies of this agent have been published in child populations.

Cyproheptadine is an antihistaminic 5-HT antagonist that has limited utility in reducing traumatic nightmares. Because of its sedative action and generally safe side effect profile, many clinicians use this agent for sleep-onset problems and nightmares in children with PTSD, although there is no empirical support for this practice. Agents such as trazodone, a sedating serotonergic antagonist antidepressant, and cyproheptadine, used alone or in conjunction with the SSRIs, may be particularly useful in sleep dysregulation and trauma-related nightmares that frequently occur in patients with PTSD.

Adrenergic and Serotonergic Agents: Tricyclic Antidepressants, Venlafaxine

Tricyclic antidepressants such as imipramine and desipramine have been largely supplanted in child and adolescent psychiatry by the newer antidepressant agents owing to unwanted side effects and potential cardiotoxicity. Robert, Blakeney, Villarreal, Rosenberg, and Meyer (2000) reported the use of low-dose imipramine (1 mg/kg) to treat symptoms of acute stress disorder (ASD) in children with burn injuries. In this study, 25 children, ages 2–19 years, were randomized to receive either chloral hydrate or imipramine for 7 days. Ten of 12 subjects receiving imipramine experienced from half to full remission of ASD symptoms, whereas 5 of 13 subjects responded to chloral hydrate. Sleep-related flashbacks and insomnia appeared to be particularly responsive to treatment. In a retrospective chart review of 128 intensive care unit (ICU) pediatric burn patients, Tcheung and colleagues (2005) reported that 114 of 128 patients (89%) responded to either imipramine or fluoxetine in terms of ASD symptoms: 84 of 104 patients responded to initial treatment with imipramine, and 18 of 24 patients responded to fluoxetine. Of 26 nonresponders to initial treatment, 12 patients responded to the alternative medication.

Gamma-Aminobutyric Acid (GABA)-Ergic/Benzodiazepine Agents

There are few, if any, data to support benzodiazepine effectiveness in the core symptoms of PTSD. These agents (e.g., clonazepam, lorazepam) may have a minor role to play in reducing acute and intense symptoms of anxiety or agitation, or as short-term adjunctive treatment to facilitate exposure tasks in psychotherapy.

Opioid Antagonists

Opioid antagonists have been utilized with mixed results in adults with PTSD. No clinical trials with these agents have been published in children and adolescents with PTSD.

Miscellaneous Agents/Agents Affecting Multiple Neurotransmitters

A number of successful open label trials have been conducted with anti-kindling/anticonvulsive or mood stabilizing agents with adult patients with PTSD. Lithium, valproate, and carbamazepine may reduce extreme mood lability and anger dyscontrol. Loof, Grimley, Kuller, Martin, and Shonfield (1995) reported the use of carbamazepine (300–1,200 mg/day, serum levels 10.0–11.5 µg/ml) in 28 children and adolescents with sexual abuse histories. By treatment end 22 of 28 patients were asymptomatic regarding PTSD symptoms. The remaining six patients improved significantly in all PTSD symptoms except for continued abuse-related nightmares. Half of this cohort was comorbid for ADHD, depression, oppositional defiant disorder, or polysubstance abuse, and was treated with concomitant medications (e.g., methylphenidate, clonidine, sertraline, fluoxetine, or imipramine).

Anecdotal experience suggests that traumatized children in fact have favorable responses to reduction of hyperactivity, impulse dyscontrol, and attention impairment, with ADHD medications such as methylphenidate, dextroamphetamine, or atomoxetine. Similarly, bupropion is often considered a second-line agent for ADHD symptoms and may be a useful agent when affect dysregulation or depressed mood co-occurs with ADHD symptoms (Daviss, 1999).

Summary and Recommendations

The state of knowledge regarding medication treatments for children and adolescents continues to lag woefully behind that for adults. Medication may play a role in reducing debilitating symptoms of PTSD in their day-to-day lives and provide relief as children confront difficult material in therapy.

Broad-spectrum agents such as the SSRIs are a good first choice. Comorbid conditions such as ADHD or aggressive behavior should, of course, be targeted with pharmacotherapy that is known to be effective. Reduction in even one disabling symptom, such as insomnia or hyperarousal, may have a positive ripple effect on a child's overall functioning.

References

Amaya-Jackson, L., & March, J. (1993). Post-traumatic stress disorder in children and adolescents. In H. L. Leonard (Ed.), *Child psychiatric clinics of North America: Vol. 2. Anxiety disorders* (pp. 639–654). New York: Saunders.

American Psychiatric Association. (2004). *Diagnostic and statistical manual of mental disorders* (4th ed., text rev.). Washington, DC: Author.

Cohen, J. A. (1998). Practice parameters for the assessment and treatment of children and adolescents with posttraumatic stress disorder. *Journal of the American Academy of Child and Adolescent Psychiatry, 37*(Suppl.), 4s–26s.

Cohen, J. A., Mannarino, A. P., Perel, J. M., & Staron, V. (2007). A pilot randomized controlled trial of combined trauma-focused CBT and sertraline for childhood PTSD symptoms. *Journal of the American Academy of Child and Adolescent Psychiatry, 46*, 811–819.

Cohen, J. A., Mannarino, A. P., & Rogal, S. (2001). Treatment practices for childhood posttraumatic stress disorder. *Child Abuse and Neglect, 25*, 123–135.

Conner, K. M., Davidson, J. R., Weisler, R. H., & Ahearn, E. (1999). A pilot study of mirtazapine in post-traumatic stress disorder. *International Clinical Psychopharmacology, 14*, 29–31.

Daviss, W. B. (1999). Efficacy and tolerability of bupropion in boys with ADHD and major depression or dysthymic disorder. *Child and Adolescent Psychopharmacology Update, 1*(5), 1–6.

De Bellis, M. D., Chrousos, G. P., Dorn, L. D., Burke, L., Helmers, K., King, M. A., et al. (1994). Hypothalamic–pituitary–adrenal axis dysregulation in sexually abused girls. *Journal of Clinical Endocrinology and Metabolism, 78*, 249–255.

Domon, S. E., & Anderson, M. S. (2000). Nefazodone for PTSD. *Journal of the American Academy of Child and Adolescent Psychiatry, 39*, 942–943.

Donnelly, C. L., & Amaya-Jackson, L. (2002). Post-traumatic stress disorder in children and adolescents: Epidemiology, diagnosis and treatment options. *Pediatric Drugs, 4*(3), 159–170.

Famularo, R., Kinscherff, R., & Fenton, T. (1988). Propranolol treatment for childhood posttraumatic stress disorder, acute type. *American Journal of Diseases of Children, 142*, 1244–1247.

Famularo, R., Kinscherff, R., & Fenton, T. (1992). Psychiatric diagnoses of maltreated children: Preliminary findings. *Journal of the American Academy of Child and Adolescent Psychiatry, 31*, 863–867.

Ford, J. D., Racusin, R., Ellis, C. G., Daviss, W. B., Reiser, J., Fleischer, A., et al. (2000). Child maltreatment, other trauma exposure, and posttraumatic symptomatology among children with oppositional defiant and attention deficit hyperactivity disorders. *Child Maltreatment, 5*, 205–217.

Good, C., & Peterson, C. (2001). SSRI and mirtazapine in PTSD. *Journal of the American Academy of Child and Adolescent Psychiatry, 40*, 263–264.

Harmon, R. J., & Riggs, P. D. (1996). Clinical perspectives: Clonidine for posttraumatic stress disorder in preschool children. *Journal of the American Academy of Child and Adolescent Psychiatry, 35*, 1247–1249.

Horrigan, J. P. (1996). Guanfacine for posttraumatic stress disorder nightmares [Letter]. *Journal of the American Academy of Child and Adolescent Psychiatry, 35*, 975–976.

Horrigan, J. P., & Barnhill, L. J. (1999). Risperidone and PTSD in boys. *Journal of Neuropsychiatry and Clinical Neurosciences, 11*, 126–127.

Kant, R., Chalansani, R., Chengappa, K. N., & Dieringer, M. (2004). The off-label use of clozapine in adolescents with bipolar disorder, intermittent explosive disorder, or posttraumatic stress disorder. *Journal of Child and Adolescent Psychopharmacology, 14*(1), 57–63.

Kutcher, S. P. (2002). *Practical child and adolescent psychopharmacology*. Cambridge, UK: Cambridge University Press.

Loof, D., Grimley, P., Kuller, F., Martin, A., & Shonfield, L. (1995). Carbamazepine for PTSD. *Journal of the American Academy of Child and Adolescent Psychiatry, 34*, 703–704.

Lustig, S. L., Botelho, C., Lynch, L., Nelson, W. J., Eichelberger, W. J., & Vaughan, B. L. (2002). Implementing a randomized clinical trial on a pediatric psychiatric inpatient unit at a children's hospital: The case of clonidine for post traumatic stress. *General Hospital Psychiatry, 24*(6), 422–429.

Marmar, C. R., Foy, D., Kagan, B., & Pynoos, R. S. (1993). An integrated approach for treating post-traumatic stress. In R. S. Pynoos (Ed.), *Post-traumatic stress disorder: A clinical review* (pp. 239–272). Lutherville, MD: Sidran Press.

Perry, B. D. (1994). Neurobiological sequelae of childhood trauma: PTSD in children. In M. Murburgh (Ed.), *Catecholamine function in PTSD: Emerging concepts* (pp. 233–255). Washington, DC: American Psychiatric Press.

Pfefferbaum, B. (1997). Posttraumatic stress disorder in children: A review of the past 10 years. *Journal of the American Academy of Child and Adolescent Psychiatry, 36*, 1503–1511.

Putnam, F. W., & Hulsmann, J. E. (2002). Pharmacotherapy for survivors of childhood trauma. *Seminars in Clinical Neuropsychiatry, 7*(2), 129–136.

Robert, R., Blakeney, P. E., Villarreal, C., Rosenberg, L., & Meyer, W. J. (2000). Imipramine treatment in pediatric burn patients with symptoms of acute stress disorder: A pilot study. *Journal of the American Academy of Child and Adolescent Psychiatry, 39*(1), 11–12.

Seedat, S., Kaminer, D., Lockhat, R., & Stein, D. J. (2000). An overview of post-traumatic stress disorder in children and adolescents. *Primary Care Psychiatry, 6*, 43–48.

Seedat, S., Lockhat, R., Kaminer, D., Zungu-Dirwayi, N., & Stein, D. J. (2001). An open trial of citalopram in adolescents with post-traumatic stress disorder. *International Clinical Psychopharmacology, 16*, 21–25.

Seedat, S., Stein, D. J., Ziervogel, C., Middleton, T., Kaminer, D., Emsley, R., et al. (2002). Comparison of response to a selective serotonin reuptake inhibitor in children, adolescents and adults with posttraumatic stress disorder. *Journal of Child and Adolescent Psychopharmacology, 12*(1), 37–46.

Stathis, S., Martin, G., & McKenna, J. G. (2005). A preliminary case series on the use of quetiapine for posttraumatic stress disorder in juveniles within a youth detention center. *Journal of Clinical Psychopharmacology, 25*(6), 539–544.

Tcheung, W. J., Robert, R., Rosenberg, L., Rosenberg, M., Villarreal, C., Thomas, C., et al. (2005). Early treatment of acute stress disorder in children with major burn injury. *Pediatric Critical Care Medicine, 6*(6), 676–681.

Wells, G. B., Chu, C., & Johnson, R. (1991). Buspirone in the treatment of post-traumatic stress disorder. *Journal of Clinical Psychiatry, 55,* 517–522.

Wheatley, M., Plant, J., Reader, H., Brown, G., & Cahill, C. (2004). Clozapine treatment of adolescents with posttraumatic stress disorder and psychotic symptoms. *Journal of Clinical Psychopharmacology, 24*(2), 167–173.

CHAPTER 11

Eye Movement Desensitization and Reprocessing

C. Richard Spates, Ellen Koch, Karen Cusack,
Sherry Pagoto, and Stacey Waller

Theoretical Context

This chapter critically summarizes state-of-the-art knowledge relevant to the use of eye movement desensitization and reprocessing (EMDR) treatment for traumatic stress. We review empirical evidence and pertinent meta-analyses since the first edition of this volume was published. Data pertaining to EMDR treatment of both adults and children are incorporated. We also examined the evidence for its bearing on "questions in need of further research" from the previous update to determine whether the recommended research questions have been addressed. Finally, we raise a number of questions for continuing research relevant to EMDR and, more generally, the treatment of posttraumatic stress disorder (PTSD), in which the evidence points to opportunities for emerging, empirically supported practice.

EMDR, an intervention initially proposed for the treatment of traumatic stress (Shapiro, 1989a, 1989b), has existed, as of this writing, for over 15 years. EMDR treatment has been widely popularized, and research bearing on its use has moved from largely case analyses and uncontrolled open trials (Herbert & Mueser, 1992) to better controlled investigations of its efficacy (e.g., see Davidson & Parker, 2001; Van Etten & Taylor, 1998). A number of early investigators also sought, through dismantling research strategies, to account for the role of the most unusual feature of this treatment; namely, the saccadic eye movements, on treatment outcome (Devilly, Spence, & Rapee, 1998; Pitman et al., 1996; Renfrey & Spates, 1994). This was a salient target for investigation given that in early writings the creator of EMDR suggested that the eye movements (or alternating stimulation) play an essential role in achieving beneficial treatment outcomes. In light of the dismantling research, that insistence was modified by the mid-1990s (Shapiro, 1995).

In this chapter we address the empirical foundation of EMDR in terms of efficacy, comparative effectiveness, and durability. We also present evidence bearing on the conceptual framework, at least insofar as procedural components are concerned.

Description of the Technique

We first summarize the EMDR technique as described by its developer, then provide a brief overview of the putative underlying theory. Short mention is made of the history of the technique as reported by Shapiro (1989b). The technique is said to incorporate the following eight stages (the reader is referred to Shapiro & Maxfield, 2002, for a detailed description of protocols utilizing this technique):

1. *Patient history and treatment planning.* In this stage assessment of the patient's readiness and barriers to treatment is made, along with any dysfunctional behaviors, specific symptoms, and other illness characteristics.

2. *Preparation.* In this stage the therapeutic alliance is developed and fostered, patient education regarding trauma is provided, and the treatment technique is reviewed and explained, along with suggestions for coping with trauma reactions that might occur during treatment. Perspective taking in the face of trauma reactivation is also taught.

3. *Assessment.* This stage involves a careful and highly specific assessment of the trauma memory. The patient is asked to identify the distressing images in memory, the associated negative cognitions, an alternative positive cognition, and to rate the validity of the positive cognition, identify emotions associated with the trauma memory, rate the subjective level of disturbance associated with the traumatic memory, and identify trauma-relevant physical sensations and their respective bodily locations. This process, achieved via very careful interviewing, is quantified by use of subjective indicators and measures.

4. *Desensitization and reprocessing.* In this stage the patient is asked to hold the distressing image in mind, along with the negative cognition and associated bodily sensations, while tracking the therapist's fingers across the patient's complete field of vision in rhythmic sweeps of one full back-and-forth sweep per second. At the end of approximately 20 seconds (or 20 back-

and-forth sweeps) the patient is asked to "blank it out," which means to let go of the memory, to take a deep breath, and to note and provide feedback to the therapist of any changes in image, sensations, thoughts, or emotions that might have occurred. After noting the patient's verbal descriptions during feedback, the therapist instructs the patient as to what to attend to next, which initiates the next set of saccadic eye movements following a similar pattern. The procedure is modified slightly to adapt to exigencies such as blocked progress due to a number of factors. Additionally, researchers' substitution of alternative sources of parallel stimulation, aside from eye movements, have been found to be successful, as has the elimination of any parallel rhythmic activity (i.e., merely having the patient repeatedly hold the disturbing image in mind and doing nothing else simultaneously, but otherwise following the protocol as outlined).

5. *Installation of positive cognition.* Once the disturbing images have been desensitized (the subjective units of distress [SUDs] scale report by the patient indicates little or no distress [0–2 points on the 11-point scale]), the patient is instructed to hold the positive or desired cognition in mind while tracking the therapist's fingers as described earlier. The patient is not asked to report on changes in thoughts, feelings, and images during this phase, but to report on changes in the validity of cognition (VoC) utilizing a 7-point scale in which 7 is *completely valid* and 1 is *not valid at all*, in terms of the patient's personal experience of the positive cognition.

6. *Body scan.* In this stage the patient is requested to identify any continuing bodily tensions or discomfort, and if these are reported, is asked to attend to each of them in turn while tracking the therapist's fingers in saccadic fashion, as previously described.

7. *Closure.* In this stage the patient is provided with coping techniques, such as relaxation skills or positive visualization, to address emergent distressing emotions or memories. Journaling with regard to thoughts, dreams, and feelings is also emphasized as needed for use between sessions.

8. *Reevaluation.* In this stage the therapist evaluates whether treatment goals are being met and maintained. This is done at each session, and additional sessions are scheduled as needed to target further trauma memories and/or skills development.

Clearly, only Stages 4–6 are unique to EMDR treatment; the other stages are parts of many other forms of therapy.

When EMDR is applied to children, greater emphasis is placed upon establishing a safe place that evokes positive emotions prior to the procedure. Practitioners are encouraged to follow the previously described protocol as closely as possible, making adjustments only as needed, based on the child's developmental level. In younger children, typical modifications involve adjustments to the eye movements or replacing them with other forms of bilateral stimulation, modifying or omitting the cognitive elements, replacing the SUDs scale with a visual or physical means of indicating the magnitude of emotions, or omitting the body scan. EMDR sessions tend to be shorter for children than for adults and to vary based on individual children's attention spans. Older children and adolescents are typically able to follow the adult protocol. The reader is referred to Tinker and Wilson (1999) for additional recommendations on modifying the protocol for children.

Overall, EMDR is set against a theoretical backdrop referred to as "adaptive information processing" (Shapiro & Maxfield, 2002). According to this theory, which is intended to guide clinical practice of EMDR, trauma sets the stage in some individuals for incomplete information processing. Much of this information is physiological and is believed to be stored in memory networks that contain related thoughts, images, emotions, and sensations. The theory proposes that "if distressing memories remain unprocessed, they become the basis of current dysfunctional reactions" (Shapiro & Maxfield, 2002, p. 935). The suggestion is that EMDR, via the use of eye movements or other "dual attention" stimulation, facilitates information processing, relieving the patient of distress, distorted perceptions, and dysfunctional reactions. It is further suggested that during the treatment process "as the image becomes less salient, clients are better able to access and attend to more adaptive information, forging new connections within the memory networks" (p. 935). EMDR therapy is believed to supply some of this adaptive information through several of the phases of treatment identified earlier.

EMDR treatment was introduced by Shapiro in 1989, reportedly following a personal experience involving distressing memories. It was later applied to a series of clinical cases and ultimately to the first quasi-controlled experiment by Shapiro (1989a). Many early reports were in fact case studies. That early literature was critiqued methodologically by Herbert and Mueser (1992). Since that time there has been a substantial improvement in the quality of research on the efficacy of EMDR, and outcomes of the treatment have been generally positive. As reported in several meta-analytic investigations (Davidson & Parker, 2001; Van Etten & Taylor, 1998) as well as well-controlled randomized clinical trials (RCTs), the quality of research has provided empirical support for EMDR; in the last International Society for Traumatic Stress Studies (ISTSS)–sponsored guideline (Foa, Keane, & Friedman, 2000) as applied to adults with PTSD, it received an Agency for Health Care Policy and Research (AHCPR) rating of A/B.

As noted earlier, in this chapter we review empirical studies conducted since the last update in 2000, and examine the degree to which continuing investigations have been responsive to recommendations from that report.

Method of Collecting Data

We identified RCTs and meta-analyses of EMDR using an electronic search of PsycINFO and MEDLINE, and a manual review of articles for referenced studies. Articles comprising primary investigations were included if they met the following criteria: The study (1) treated individuals diagnosed with PTSD; (2) was published in a peer-reviewed journal; (3) employed a control or comparison treatment condition; (4) utilized random assignment; and (5) included at least one standard measure of PTSD. Studies involving use of EMDR treatment with children are included. Furthermore, we only included studies not covered in the previous review by Chemtob, Tolin, van der Kolk, and Pitman (2000). Finally, meta-analyses of EMDR studies or of PTSD studies including EMDR were also included.

Literature Review

Studies Comparing EMDR to Exposure Therapy

Earlier studies evaluated EMDR's efficacy relative to wait list, placebo, or other active treatments for PTSD (see Chemtob et al., 2000). However, these comparative treatments did not include the most empirically supported intervention for PTSD, prolonged exposure (PE; Foa et al., 2000), nor did they include pharmacological treatments. Studies comparing EMDR to PE and to medications are important steps in evaluation of the efficacy of EMDR. Since the previous edition of the ISTSS treatment guidelines, one study compared EMDR to a pharmacological agent, and six studies evaluated EMDR and PE or a primarily exposure-based procedure (see Table 11.1 for information regarding these studies).

In the previous edition of the ISTSS treatment guidelines, EMDR received an AHCPR rating of A/B. These conclusions derived largely from methodologically sound studies comparing the efficacy of EMDR to other forms of treatment in clinical RCTs. Studies cited to substantiate this very high rating include Vaughan and colleagues (1994), who compared EMDR to image habituation training and to relaxation training. All three treatments improved PTSD symptom ratings, but the effects on intrusive thoughts (i.e., nightmares and flashbacks) were stronger for patients receiving EMDR. In addition, Marcus, Marquis, and Sakai (1997) examined EMDR versus standard clinical care in a health maintenance organization (HMO). Again within the context of an RCT, these authors found faster and greater improvement on measures of PTSD, anxiety, and depression. At posttreatment, 75% of patients receiving EMDR no longer met diagnostic criteria for PTSD, compared to 50% of the comparison group. Carlson, Chemtob, Rusnak, Hedlund, and Muraoka (1998) also found that 75% of combat veterans with PTSD treated with EMDR and applied relaxation did not meet criteria for PTSD diagnosis at the 9-month follow-up.

Chemtob and colleagues (2000) noted that the earliest studies in general found large treatment effect sizes. The authors recognized the need for more extensive comparison conditions, and that EMDR needed to be compared to other extant PTSD treatments. It was on the basis of the well-conducted trials that the high rating of A/B was conferred.

TABLE 11.1. EMDR Adult Treatment Studies Reviewed

Study	Population	Comparison groups	N	Duration of trial	Main outcome measure	Within-group ES	Comparison	Between-N group ES ITT	Between-N group ES Completer	Results
van der Kolk et al. (2007)	Male and female, mixed trauma	EMDR FLU PLA	29 (24) 30 (26) 29 (26)	8 weekly sessions	CAPS	1.99 (2.38)[a] 1.68 (1.91)[a] 1.43 (1.87)[a]	EMDR vs. PLA	0.48 0.04 0.45	0.59 0.06 0.51	EMDR > PLA, $p < .05$[b] FLU > PLA, ns[c] EMDR > FLU, ns[c]
Taylor et al. (2003)[d]	Male and female, mixed traumas	EMDR PE REL	19 (15) 22 (15) 19 (15)	8 weekly sessions	CAPS	1.60 (2.35) 1.33 (2.47) 1.01 (1.62)	EMDR vs. REL E vs. REL EMDR vs. EXP	0.15 0.37 −0.27	0.04 0.61 −0.67	EMDR > REL, ns[c] EXP > REL, ns[c] EMDR < EXP, ns[c]
Rothbaum et al. (2005)[d]	Female sexual assault survivors	EMDR PE WL	25 (20) 23 (20) 24 (20)	9 biweekly sessions	CAPS	(2.07) (1.98) (0.58)	EMDR vs. WL PE vs. WL EMDR vs. PE		1.42 2.00 −0.43	EMDR > WL, $p < .001$ PE > WL, $p < .001$ EMDR < PE,[e] ns
Power et al. (2002)	Male and female, mixed traumas	EMDR EXP+CR WL	39 (27) 37 (21) 29 (24)	10 weekly sessions	IES	(2.54) (1.41) (0.38)	EMDR vs. WL EXP+CR vs. WL EMDR vs. EXP+CR		1.66 0.97 0.60	EMDR > WL, $p < .001$ EXP+CR > WL, $p < .05$ EMDR > EXP+CR, ns

Study	Sample	Comparison groups	n	Sessions	Outcome measure	(SD)	Comparison	ES	Results
Lee et al. (2002)	Male and female, mixed traumas	EMDR SIT+PE	13 (12) 13 (12)	7 weekly sessions	SI-PTSD	(2.00) (1.50)	EMDR vs. SIT+PE	0.60	EMDR > SIT+PE, *ns*
Ironson et al. (2002)	Male and female, mixed traumas	EMDR+IVE PE	10 (10) 12 (9)	5 weekly sessions[f]	PSS-SR	(1.47) (2.07)	EMDR vs. PE	0.62	EMDR > PE, *ns*
Rogers et al. (1999)	Male combat veterans	EMDR EXP	(6) (6)	1 session	IES-R	(0.79) (0.18)	EMDR vs. EXP	1.04	EMDR > EXP, *ns*

Notes. ES, effect size; ITT, intention to treat, *Comparison groups:* EMDR, eye movement desensitization and reprocessing; FLU, fluoxetine; PLA, pill placebo; PE, prolonged exposure; REL, relaxation; WL, wait list; EXP+CR, exposure plus cognitive restructing; SIT+PE, stress inoculation training with prolonged exposure; EMDR+IVE, EMDR plus *in vivo* exposure; EXP, exposure. Completer sample values in parentheses. *Main outcome measures:* CAPS, Clinician-Administered PTSD Scale; IES, Impact of Events Scale; SI-PTSD, Structured Interview for PTSD; PSS-SR, PTSD Symptom Scale—Self Report version; IES-R, Impact of Events Scale—Revised. Effect sizes are Hedges's unbiased *g* based on pretreatment and posttreatment comparisons only. Negative effect sizes indicate that the EMDR group was more symptomatic than the comparison group. *Results:* > indicates that first treatment had lower mean scores than second treatment, and < indicates the opposite; *ns*, nonsignificant.

[a]Complete group effect size computed based on Cohen's *d* provided by the primary author.

[b]Complete group only, but overall analysis of covariance was nonsignificant.

[c]Results the same for both ITT and complete groups.

[d]Data provided by primary author.

[e]EMDR group significantly worse on CAPS total at baseline. [f]Three additional treatment sessions offered, if needed, following the posttreatment assessment.

More recently, many studies followed the recommendations of the previous EMDR review. For example, van der Kolk and colleagues (2007) conducted the first psychosocial and pharmacological direct comparison study of PTSD. In this study, 88 male and female participants with PTSD as a result of various traumas were randomly assigned to EMDR, fluoxetine, or pill placebo for eight weekly treatment sessions. Participants with child-onset traumas had significantly more PTSD symptoms at baseline. Seventy-six participants completed treatment without significant differences in dropout rates between treatment conditions. Reliable and valid measures were administered at pretreatment, posttreatment, and 6-month follow-up by blind evaluators who received extensive training and ongoing supervision. Treatment manuals were provided for both active treatment conditions, and fidelity checks were completed on over 10% of the EMDR sessions by an EMDR expert. An omnibus analysis of covariance (ANCOVA) revealed that all three conditions reduced symptoms of PTSD and depression at posttreatment and follow-up. In direct comparison analyses, EMDR was significantly superior to pill placebo for the completer sample at posttreatment. EMDR was also significantly better than fluoxetine at 6-month follow-up for PTSD symptoms, percent asymptomatic, and depression for both the completer and intent-to-treat (ITT) sample. Secondary analyses revealed that within the EMDR condition, individuals with adult-onset traumas responded significantly better to treatment than those with child-onset index events.

A second well-controlled study was conducted by Taylor and colleagues (2003), who randomly assigned 60 participants with PTSD to eight weekly sessions of EMDR, exposure therapy, or relaxation. Forty-five participants completed treatment. Exposure therapy included four imaginal sessions followed by four *in vivo* sessions. Assessments were completed by blind assessors at pretreatment, 1-month posttreatment, and 3-month follow-up. Treatment integrity was rated for 59% of the sessions; 28% were also rated by experts in the procedure. Raters evaluated treatment-nonspecific components, treatment-specific, and nonprotocol interventions. All three treatments reduced PTSD symptoms, guilt, anger, and depression at posttreatment and follow-up. Exposure therapy produced a greater percentage of participants with clinically significant change and greater reductions in reexperiencing and avoidance symptoms.

In a similarly methodologically sound clinical trial, Rothbaum, Astin, and Marsteller (2005) randomly assigned 74 female rape survivors with PTSD to EMDR, PE, or a wait-list control ($N = 20$ completers per group). Treatment sessions comprised nine sessions, twice weekly. The EMDR protocol was modified to be more consistent with PE and included information gathering, psychoeducation, treatment rationale, and preparation. Blind assessments were completed at pretreatment and 1-week posttreatment, and at 6-month follow-up. Treatment integrity, adherence, and competence ratings were completed for 25% of the treatment sessions by experts in each condition. No information was provided on nonprotocol elements or reliability of the treatment integrity checks. Both treatments produced clinically and statistically significant improvements on PTSD symptoms, depression, anxiety, and dissociation. Both EMDR and PE demonstrated better end-state functioning (based on the Clinician-Administered PTSD Scale [CAPS], the Beck Depression Inventory [BDI], and State–Trait Anxiety Inventory—State Anxiety [STAI-S]) than wait-list at posttreatment. PE demonstrated better end-state functioning than EMDR at 6-month follow-up, although the EMDR group had significantly higher scores on several measures at baseline. EMDR was significantly better than PE on dissociation at posttreatment only.

Other studies also provided support for the efficacy of EMDR. Power and colleagues (2002) randomly assigned 105 Scottish primary care patients with PTSD to EMDR ($N = 39$), exposure plus cognitive restructuring (EXP+CR) ($N = 37$) or a wait list ($N = 29$). Participants in each treatment condition received up to 10 sessions. Blind assessors completed assessments at pre- and posttreatment. A 15-month follow-up CAPS assessment was conducted by therapists not blind to condition. Although the authors stated that treatment integrity was maintained, no details were provided. Participants in EMDR had an average of 4.2 sessions, whereas EXP+CR participants had 6.4 sessions. Findings indicated that both treatment groups improved significantly and equally better than the wait list on total scores of the PTSD measures, with 60% of EMDR compared to 50% of EXP+CR participants achieving clinically significant change in PTSD symptoms.

In another study, Lee, Gavriel, Drummond, Richards, and Greenwald (2002) randomly assigned 24 participants with PTSD to seven sessions of EMDR or stress inoculation training plus PE (SIT+PE). Over half of this sample was involved in litigation. Treatment fidelity was assessed by experts in each treatment, and both received acceptable fidelity ratings. EMDR and SIT+PE were found to be equally efficacious on global measures of PTSD at posttreatment, with 83% of EMDR participants and 75% of those in SIT+PE no longer meeting criteria for PTSD. EMDR led to greater reductions in intrusion symptoms at posttreatment and performed significantly better on all measures at 3-month follow-up. Clinically significant improvement was found in 67% of participants in each treatment condition at posttreatment and in 92% of EMDR and 50% of SIT+PE participants at follow-up.

Two additional studies compared EMDR to PE or other exposure-based procedures, but each suffered significant methodological weaknesses. Ironson, Freund, Strauss, and Williams (2002) examined the efficacy, tolerability, and maintenance of EMDR versus PE for 22 randomly assigned participants. Treatment in both groups comprised three preparatory sessions (one of which was the baseline assessment), up to three active treatment sessions, and *in vivo* homework. Treatment integrity was not assessed. Seven out of 10 EMDR participants met criteria for "improved" (i.e., 70% reduction in PTSD symptoms) after three active treatment sessions, compared to 2 out of 12 participants in PE. Remaining participants were offered three additional active treatment sessions. Due to dropout, follow-up analyses were completed on six PE and six EMDR participants. At posttreatment and 3-month follow-up, both treatments were equally effective in reducing symptoms of PTSD and depression.

Rogers and colleagues (1999) treated 12 Vietnam War veterans in a group format, with one session of EMDR or exposure. No differences were found in amount of exposure received or overall patient rating of the treatment. Greater within-session SUDs decreases were found for the EMDR group. Posttreatment results on the Impact of Events Scale (IES) indicated that participants in both groups improved significantly, but the amount of symptom reduction was small (7 points and 2 points, respectively, on the IES). See Table 11.1 for an analysis of effect sizes across the investigations presented here.

In summary, these seven studies suggest that EMDR is an efficacious treatment for PTSD. The recent comparisons of EMDR to PE indicate that EMDR appears to be roughly as effective as PE. These conclusions are also noted in other major reviews conducted by the Veterans Administration/Department of Defense (2003), National Institute for Clinical Excellence (NICE; 2005), and the Australian Centre for Posttraumatic Mental Health (ACPMH; 2007). The lack of support for EMDR by the Institute of Medicine (2008) is the exception.

Future research comparing EMDR and exposure therapy could enhance and improve the literature by including better measures of treatment fidelity, such as treatment integrity (essential components implemented as intended), competence, and treatment differentiation (ensuring no contamination from the other condition). Fidelity should be assessed by multiple, independent raters who rate both treatments. Reporting symptom severity from each of the clusters of PTSD would more precisely address mechanisms and site of action. Finally, additional studies are needed by investigators with no obvious stake in the superiority of EMDR, PE, or any additional compared intervention. Where this is not possible, the investigator's(s') allegiance to one treatment or the other might be assessed and/or declared. This is a concern with no easy solution except multisite investigations, with specific assessments for both site and technique allegiance, and the use of novice therapists whose competence meets specific criteria would assist in meeting this objective.

Dismantling Studies

Numerous studies demonstrate that eye movements do not significantly contribute to the efficacy of EMDR (for a comprehensive review, see Chemtob et al., 2000). In a meta-analysis, Davidson and Parker (2001) examined whether eye movements or any alternating movement is a necessary component of EMDR. The authors concluded that the published data do not support an incremental benefit of eye movements or other alternating movements on treatment outcome.

Despite this conclusion, several studies have continued to examine the impact of eye movements and other forms of stimulation in reducing emotional memories. Specifically, in a recent pilot study, the effects of three different types of auditory and kinesthetic stimulation (intermittent alternating, intermittent simultaneous bilateral, and continuous bilateral) were compared in 20 individuals with single-event PTSD (Servan-Schreiber, Schooler, Dew, Carter, & Bartone, 2006). All three forms of stimulation resulted in a significant reduction in SUDs scores during three EMDR sessions, and the alternating stimulation led to faster reductions when new target memories were utilized.

One other study utilized a clinical sample (Elofsson, von Schèele, Theorell, & Söndergaard, in press) of 13 male refugees with PTSD and found reduced physiological arousal with EMDR treatment. However, a control or alternative treatment condition was not utilized, making conclusions about the incremental contribution of eye movements equivocal. The remaining studies examining the impact of various forms of stimulation have utilized either nonclinical samples of college students (Andrade, Kavanagh, & Baddeley, 1997; Barrowcliff, Gray, Freeman, & MacCulloch, 2004; Barrowcliff, Gray, MacCulloch, Freeman, & MacCulloch, 2003; Christman, Garvey, Propper, & Phaneuf, 2003; Kavanagh, Freese, Andrade, & May, 2001; Sharpley, Montgomery, & Scalzo, 1996; van den Hout, Muris, Salemink, & Kindt, 2001) or those with a history of trauma exposure only, without a PTSD diagnosis (Kuiken, Bears, Miall, & Smith, 2001–2002; Wilson, Silver, Covi, & Foster, 1996). Given the previous dismantling studies related to eye movements and various other forms of stimulation, and the recent lack of well-controlled clinical studies focused on this issue, the best provisional conclusion so far is that the bilateral stimulation component of EMDR does not incrementally influence treatment outcome.

One additional dismantling study assessed the contribution of the cognitive elements of EMDR (Cusack & Spates, 1999). Thirty-eight randomly assigned participants received up to three 90-minute sessions of standard EMDR or a similar protocol without the cognitive components (EMD; i.e., positive cognition, VoC, and installation with the positive cognition). Blind assessment of PTSD symptoms was conducted at posttreatment and at 1- and 2-month follow-up. Treatment integrity was assessed for a random sample of sessions. Eleven participants dropped out of the study (7 in EMD and 4 in EMDR) and displayed significantly higher scores on several measures. The final sample included 27 subjects (13 in EMD and 14 in EMDR). Both conditions produced significant improvements from pre- to posttreatment, with no differences between the treatments. These improvements were maintained at follow-up. Because this is the only study in the literature addressing the cognitive components of the EMDR protocol, additional studies are needed to determine its contribution to treatment efficacy.

Follow-Up Investigation

Marcus, Marquis, and Sakai (2004) provided 3- and 6-month follow-up data on their previous study of the effectiveness of EMDR compared to standard care in an HMO setting (Marcus et al., 1997). Out of 67 participants with PTSD, 44 individuals completed the 3-month follow-up and 36 finished the 6-month follow-up. Treatment gains were maintained at both follow-ups, with EMDR superior to standard care. Depression and state anxiety also improved significantly from the 3- to 6-month follow-up for the EMDR group. Follow-up assessors were not always blind to the treatment condition due to participant disclosure.

Process-Oriented Investigation

Lee, Taylor, and Drummond (2006) investigated empirically whether the content of subjects' responses during EMDR treatment was what might be expected according to the theoretical framework of dual process of attention. This was the first data-based effort to evaluate the mechanisms underlying EMDR effects as proposed by the associated theory. This study drew for comparison purposes upon previous claims in the literature that suggested "reliving" as the putative mechanism underlying traditional exposure therapy. Instead, the conclusion from the Lee and colleagues investigation was that "distancing" better characterized the subjective content of experiences of EMDR-treated subjects during their first treatment session: "Greatest improvement on a measure of PTSD symptoms occurred when the participant processed the trauma in a more detached manner" (p. 97). Unfortunately, the evidence would have been stronger had the investigators made empirical comparisons of subjects treated with traditional exposure and a separate group with EMDR because it is quite possible that exposure-treated subjects might have had similar subjective reactions using the same measurement tool, despite prior theoretical claims. It is worth noting nonetheless that "detached" processing might be a product of explicit instructions utilized in the EMDR protocol to observe passively what is taking place, without judging the experience or process. Referred to as "mindfulness" in contemporary behavior therapy, this feature of treatment is receiving increased attention for its possible contribution to treatment outcome.

Children and Adolescents

In the first edition of the practice guidelines, the recommended rating of EMDR for the treatment of child and adolescent PTSD was Level B–C (Cohen, Berliner, & March, 2000). Evidence supporting EMDR's efficacy in children and adolescents was derived from anecdotal evidence, case reports, and a single randomized, lagged-groups design study comparing EMDR to no treatment (Chemtob, Nakashima, & Carlson, 2002).

Since that time, EMDR has continued to show promise as an efficacious treatment for child and adolescent PTSD. In a well-controlled study meeting six out of Foa and Meadows's (1997) seven "gold standard" criteria, Jabergha-deri, Greenwald, Rubin, Zand, and Dolatabadi (2004) compared EMDR to cognitive-behavioral therapy (CBT) in the treatment of sexually abused Ira-nian girls between the ages of 12 and 13. Fourteen subjects were randomly assigned to up to 12 sessions of either EMDR or CBT. Both treatments had high levels of subject retention. There were no differences between groups on measures of treatment outcome; both evidenced reduction of symptoms. However, EMDR appeared to be more efficient than CBT, with participants requiring fewer sessions and less homework to achieve similar levels of symp-tom reduction.

Several additional studies investigating EMDR in children and adoles-cents were published but did not meet the inclusion criteria of the current review. For example, Oras, Cancela de Ezpeleta, and Ahmad (2004) exam-ined the effectiveness of adding one to six EMDR sessions to the psychody-namic treatment of 13 refugee boys and girls, between the ages of 8 and 16, diagnosed with PTSD. Participants showed improvement on measures of posttraumatic symptoms and global functioning, but there was not a con-trol or comparison condition. Likewise, Jarero, Artigas, and Hartung (2006) describe an uncontrolled examination of a group variant of EMDR applied to child and adolescent survivors of a flood. Participants showed improvement on a measure of trauma-related symptoms. Fernandez, Gallinari, and Loren-zetti (2003) evaluated a school-based EMDR intervention for children who had witnessed a plane crash. However, there was no control or comparison condition, and no standard measure of PTSD symptoms was used. In a ran-domized, controlled investigation, Rubin and colleagues (2001) compared EMDR to treatment as usual (TAU) in a child guidance center. However, this investigation did not specifically target PTSD; therefore, no standard mea-sure of PTSD was included.

Finally, Soberman, Greenwald, and Rule (2002), compared three sessions of EMDR administered within the context of residential or day treatment to TAU for 29 boys, ages 10–16, with conduct problems. This investigation techni-cally did not meet the criteria for inclusion because it did not specifically target PTSD. Rather, it targeted acting-out behaviors in children, while testing the hypothesis that many of these behavior problems are trauma-related. Indeed, 31% of the sample had a diagnosis of PTSD, and all participants were admin-istered measures to assess PTSD symptoms. Compared to the control group, the treatment group showed significantly more improvement on a measure of problem behaviors at 2-month follow-up. Although the outcomes on PTSD measures were nonsignificant, there were trends toward greater improvement for participants receiving EMDR versus the control condition on one measure at posttreatment and on a second measure at 2-month follow-up. A number of methodological weaknesses may have affected the results, including lack of blind assessment for some of the outcome measures, lack of procedures to assess treatment adherence, potential contamination of the independent variable, and administration of the treatment by a single therapist.

In summary, although these findings on children treated with EMDR do not raise the intervention to the status of front-line child trauma treatment enjoyed by CBT, they are optimistic developments that lay the groundwork for future studies. Future studies should clarify whether the difference in efficiency in the Jaberghaderi and colleagues (2004) study is a methodological artifact or represents a true advantage over CBT. Finally, there is clear recognition that both assessment and treatment of PTSD must take into account developmental factors. Future studies should examine the effects of such modifications on the efficacy of the intervention, as well as other developmentally sensitive modifications that might potentially enhance outcomes.

Meta-Analytic Studies of EMDR and Effect Sizes

We identified meta-analyses using an electronic search of PsycINFO and MEDLINE, using key words "EMDR," "Eye movement desensitization and reprocessing," and "PTSD and meta-analyses." We then manually reviewed meta-analyses and non-meta-analytic reviews for additional studies. Articles included must have performed a meta-analysis of EMDR treatment for PTSD. In addition to EMDR, meta-analyses may have included other forms of treatment for PTSD. Both published and unpublished studies were included. Eight studies met criteria (six published and two unpublished); the author of one unpublished study could not be located; thus, seven studies were included in our review (see Table 11.2).

Characteristics of Meta-Analyses Reviewed

Two of the seven studies were meta-analyses of EMDR treatment for PTSD. The remaining five studies were meta-analyses of PTSD treatments including EMDR. The latter allowed for comparisons of the effects of EMDR to other therapeutic approaches. The average number of studies reviewed in a meta-analysis was 26 (range, 7–61). Only two of the seven meta-analyses included unpublished studies (i.e., Sherman, 1998; Van Etten & Taylor, 1998). Meta-analyses reviewed studies published as early as 1980 and through the year 2005. Four meta-analyses presented some form of quality scoring (i.e., Sack, Lempa, & Lamprecht, 2001; Seidler & Wagner, 2006; Van Etten & Taylor, 1998; Waller, Spates, & Mulick, 2000). Two studies reported observer-rated and self-reported measures of effect sizes separately (Van Etten & Taylor, 1998; Waller et al., 2000), whereas others calculated composites and did not differentiate measures by type.

Some variability was observed in inclusion criteria regarding diagnostic status, random assignment, and measures. Two meta-analyses only included

Text continues on page 297

TABLE 11.2. Characteristics of Meta-Analyses Reviewed

		Methods					Results			
Study	Search strategy	Sample size (no. of studies included)	Selection criteria	Validity assessment	Trial flow[a]	Study characteristics	Quanitative data synthesis	Effect size	Conclusions	Peer review
Seidler & Wagner (2006)	Databases	7	1989–2005; EMDR based on Shapiro's (1995) standard protocol; DSM-IV diagnosis of PTSD; random assignment; age 18+; means and SDs, percentage improvement rates, or statistical values reported; one or more valid and reliable instrument used	Quality scoring (via "gold standards" proposed by Foa and Meadows, 1997) reported for each study	Yes. Number of exclusions and reasons.	Treatment type, treatment fidelity, number of sessions, sample size, admission criteria, independent evaluators	Effect sizes of CBT with exposure versus EMDR (global EMDR symptomatology, depression)	Global symptoms: Post–post $d = 0.28$ Follow-up/ follow-up: $d = 0.13$ Depression: Post–post $d = 0.40$ Follow-up/ follow-up $d = 0.12$	No evidence of superiority of one treatment over the other.	Yes
Waller, Spates, & Mulick (2000)	Databases, handsearching	20	English language, 1988–2000; published; used either exposure-based treatment or EMDR; RCT; data available to calculate effect size; "portion" of the sample met diagnostic criteria for PTSD	Quality scoring via Foa and Meadows (1997) "gold standards" reported for each study	Not discussed.	Treatment type	Effect sizes (observer-rated and self-report measures); posttreatment and follow-up. "Gold standard" comparison of exposure and EMDR studies	Pre–post standard measures EMDR: $d = 1.16$ Exposure: $d = 0.98$	Exposure and EMDR have comparable effects.	No

(continued)

293

TABLE 11.2. *(continued)*

	Methods					Results				Peer review
Study	Search strategy	Sample size (no. of studies included)	Selection criteria	Validity assessment	Trial flow[a]	Study characteristics	Quantitative data synthesis	Effect size	Conclusions	
Van Etten & Taylor (1998)	Databases, handsearching, conference proceedings, secondary sources, contacts with PTSD researchers	61	English, 1984–1996; PTSD diagnosis; 5+ points; published; sufficient information to calculated effect sizes; outcome on at least 1 of 4 commonly used variables	Studies coded by treatment length, controlled vs. uncontrolled, and therapist training	Yes, in text. Number of exclusions and reasons.	Treatment type	Effect size (observer-rated and self-report); analyses accounting for file drawer problem	Pre-post total severity of symptoms self-report/ observer EMDR: $d = 1.24$ $d = 0.69$ Behavior therapy: $d = 1.27$ $d = 1.89$ Drug therapy: $d = 0.69$ $d = 1.05$	Exposure and EMDR are equally effective, and comparable to drugs, but lower dropout. No differential dropout for exposure and EMDR.	Yes
Sherman (1998)	Database and hand searching	17	PTSD psychotherapies; no years; published and unpublished; "clinical trials"; comparison group, inferential statistics; objective	None	Not discussed.	Sample size, trauma type, treatment groups	Effect size (composite of all measures used in each study, weighted equally)	Overall effect of all exposure-based treatments across measures $d = 0.52$ ($r = .25$)	Exposure-based treatments (including EMDR) are effective. No reliable differences across treatment modalities.	Yes

294

Study	Source	N	Inclusion criteria	Quality rating	Exclusions	Moderators	Effect sizes	Mean effect sizes	Conclusion	
Davidson & Parker (2001)	Databases, handsearching	34	measures of outcome; threshold PTSD criteria met by patients. Published studies; 1997–March 2000; random assignment, sufficient info for effect size calculation; treatment condition not confounded with therapist	None	Yes, in text. Number of exclusions and reasons.	Trauma type	Effect sizes (posttreatment only)	Mean effect sizes for outcome measures EMDR (pre–post): r = .63 EMDR/ EMDR without eye movements: r = .10	EMDR is effective, no incremental benefit of eye movements.	Yes
Sack, Lempa, & Lamprecht (2001)	Databases	17	Published studies only; EMDR only; 5+ patients treated with EMDR; follow-up or both; standardized measures; controlled design, follow-up, or both; standardized measures	Quality scoring via Foa and Meadows (1997) "gold standards" reported for each study and incorporated into analyses	Yes, in text. Number of exclusions and reasons.	Sample size, trauma type	Effect sizes by quality rating (low, medium, and high)	Mean pre–post effect sizes for EMDR Low-quality studies: d = 0.43 Medium-quality studies: d = 1.20 High-quality studies: d = 1.76	EMDR is effective. No evidence for differential efficacy from medication and psychotherapy interventions.	Yes

(continued)

295

TABLE 11.2. *(continued)*

	Methods					Results				
Study	Search strategy	Sample size (no. of studies included)	Selection criteria	Validity assessment	Trial flow[a]	Study characteristics	Quantitative data synthesis	Effect size	Conclusions	Peer review
Bradley, Greene, Russ, Dutra, & Westen (2005)	Databases, handsearching	26	PTSD psychotherapies; published 1980–2003; adult patients excluded unpublished studies; randomized controlled trials, > 10 patients/ condition; Control or comparison conditions, validated measures, reported in English	None	Not discussed.	Sample size, trauma type, outcome, intervention type	Effect size, completion rates, improvement rates, posttreatment symptoms, long-term follow-up	PTSD symptom changes (pre–post; treatment versus wait list control, treatment versus supportive control) Exposure $d = 1.57$, 1.26, .84 EMDR $d = 1.43$, 1.25, .75	No differential efficacy of exposure and EMDR. Both better than no treatment.	Yes

[a]Number of studies excluded from meta-analyses and reasons for excluding, along with frequencies.

trials that recruited patients who met DSM-III-R or -IV criteria for PTSD (i.e., Seidler & Wagner, 2006; Van Etten & Taylor, 1998), whereas two included trials in which most or all patients met criteria for PTSD (i.e., Sherman, 1998; Waller et al., 2000). One meta-analysis did not have inclusion criteria regarding diagnosis, but diagnostic status was a quality criterion (i.e., Sack et al., 2001), and another included only studies that used standardized diagnostic measures but did not explicitly state inclusion criteria relevant to diagnostic status. Finally, one study did not specifically mention inclusion criteria relevant to diagnostic status (i.e., Davidson & Parker, 2001).

Three meta-analyses only included studies that used random assignment (Bradley, Greene, Russ, Dutra, & Westen, 2005; Seidler & Wagner, 2006; Waller et al., 2000) and another did the same but made one exception (Davidson & Parker, 2001). One meta-analysis included both randomized and nonrandomized designs, but random assignment was a quality scoring criterion for which they adjusted in the analyses (i.e., Sack et al., 2001). Two studies included only controlled trials but did not specifically state that random assignment was an inclusion criterion (i.e., Sherman, 1998; Van Etten & Taylor, 1998).

Five meta-analyses included only studies that employed standardized or validated measures of PTSD symptoms (i.e., Bradley et al., 2005; Sack et al., 2001; Seidler & Wagner, 2006; Van Etten & Taylor, 1998; Waller et al., 2000), whereas one included studies that employed objective measures of outcome (i.e., Sherman, 1998) and another did not state inclusion criteria relevant to measures (i.e., Davidson & Parker, 2001).

Results

EFFECT OF EMDR ON PTSD

In spite of some variability in the characteristics of meta-analyses, all concluded that EMDR is an effective treatment for PTSD. The four meta-analyses that reviewed studies comparing EMDR to a control condition found large mean effect sizes (Cohen's $d = 0.8$; i.e., Bradley et al., 2005; Davidson & Parker, 2001; Sack et al., 2001; Van Etten & Taylor, 1998). Sack and colleagues (2001) showed that studies with higher methodological quality produced the largest effect sizes, and that low effect sizes were only evident in studies with serious methodological problems. One meta-analysis determined that studies with therapists trained at the EMDR Institute did not produce better outcomes than those with therapists not trained at the EMDR Institute (Davidson & Parker, 2001).

DIFFERENTIAL EFFICACY FOR EMDR AND EXPOSURE TREATMENT

Four meta-analyses reviewed studies that compared the efficacy of EMDR and exposure therapies, and none found differential efficacy at posttreatment

(Davidson & Parker, 2001; Seidler & Wagner, 2006; Waller et al., 2000) or follow-up (Seidler & Wagner, 2006; Van Etten & Taylor, 1998; Waller et al., 2000). One exception was an investigation that found exposure therapy superior to EMDR at posttreatment on observer-rated (but not self-report) scales (Van Etten & Taylor, 1998); however, that effect diminished by follow-up.

ADDED VALUE OF EYE MOVEMENTS

One meta-analysis addressed whether eye movements or any alternating movement is a necessary component of EMDR (Davidson & Parker, 2001). The authors conclude that the published data do not support an incremental benefit of eye movements or other alternating movements on single- or composite outcome measures.

Summary

A review of seven meta-analyses revealed that EMDR is an effective treatment for PTSD, and equally effective as exposure-based therapies. Large effect sizes were reported across all meta-analyses reviewed, suggesting that EMDR is a potent treatment for PTSD. No evidence exists based on these investigations to support the use of eye movements or any other alternating movements in EMDR; thus, EMDR could be delivered in a more parsimonious manner without detracting from efficacy. Stated otherwise, the intervention is quite robust in its effects, even without the saccadic eye movement or alternating stimulation feature. Future RCTs should assess proposed mechanisms of action to elucidate further whether EMDR and exposure-based therapies operate via the same or different mechanisms. By doing so we might learn what elements of both approaches are essential and beneficial, and might lead to newer, more integrated, efficient, and parsimonious models of treatment. Seidler and Wagner (2006) also recommend that future research address which patients are most likely to benefit from one treatment approach or the other.

Efficacy Rating

Based on this review of seven new controlled efficacy/effectiveness studies of EMDR and seven new meta-analytic investigations of this technique, we assigned EMDR for treatment of adult PTSD an AHCPR rating of Level A. Studies have continued to improve in quality and relative importance of research focus. To be sure, continued research is warranted, as is continued methodological improvement in that research. However, in our view, these caveats are appropriate for all techniques addressing trauma treatment (i.e., sample size increases, improvements in fidelity and integrity ratings, and additional comparisons that further clarify the question of which patients benefit most). With regard to the application of EMDR to children, we assign an AHCPR rating of Level B. Clearly, the direction in the examination of EMDR for children has been a greater emphasis on RCTs, but the area still suffers from a lack of quantity and replication of such investigations. As the number and quality of these studies improve, meta-analytic investigations will also assist the move to a higher classification.

Summary and Recommendations

Questions for Future Research

Authors in the previous update recommended several lines of investigation that would clarify the standing of EMDR as a front-line intervention for PTSD. Since that time, many of these recommendations have been attempted. Specifically, as shown in this review, comparisons to other trauma-focused treatments, modestly larger sample sizes, treatment efficiency, evaluation of efficacy in children with PTSD, and patient comfort or tolerance have all been targets of investigation. Yet not reflected in the literature is attention to patient characteristics that predict improvement and very large, field-based trials utilizing the large voluminous pool of trained therapists. We believe these remain important research directions, and their accomplishment would advance the reliability of our knowledge of this intervention. In light of the current update, we have several additional recommendations, which include the following.

Dismantling Research Strategies
Targeting Process and Outcome

One of the beneficial effects of the recent adoption of dismantling strategies (Borkovec & Castonguay, 1998) across the field of psychotherapy research is that they provide a window into the most parsimonious accounting of treatment effects as they relate to steps in a treatment procedure. All things being equal, when minimal elements achieve the identical outcomes as more elaborate features of a treatment protocol, it is likely that that minimal features account for the observed outcomes. Absent further evidence on incremental utility, this calls into question the essentiality of the additional elements. This dismantling strategy has been aptly applied in areas outside of PTSD treatment as well, including treatment of depression (Jacobson et al., 1996), panic disorder (Öst, Thulin, & Ramnerö, 2004), and specific phobia (Koch, Spates, & Himle, 2004). In all instances, leading hypotheses regarding required procedural features were challenged by results. Our current recommendation supports continued dismantling studies with this intervention, as well as others targeting PTSD, so as to identify essential empirically supported components of therapy packages. As for EMDR, we suggest that priority attention include the role of *in vivo* homework assignments, journaling as a supplement to core treatment, and additional attention to the role of the highly visible cognitive elements of the protocol. As a result of the application of this research strategy, constructive research designs (Borkovec & Castonguay, 1998) could then be deployed to package those elements of treatments that have empirical support, so that the most powerful interventions emerge based on scientific research. In our view the field is positioned to gain from this approach given the present state of knowledge.

Comparative Efficiency of EMDR

Recent investigations have attempted to examine the comparative efficiency of EMDR and PE in trauma treatment. Results suggest the possibility that the dosed exposure, along with postexposure "mindfulness" features comprising EMDR, might confer advantages over conventional prolonged exposure to trauma memories. However this hypothesis requires substantially more research to test its validity. In some ways the treatment of panic disorder has similarly benefited from this approach entailing a specific focus on interoceptive sources of distress immediately following specific arousal induction procedures (Barlow, 2002).

Combination with Trauma-Focused Medication Treatments

Since the original development and dissemination of EMDR, several medications have been approved by the U.S. Food and Drug Administration (FDA) for specific application to this disorder; thus, many patients seen in practice are either already taking these medications or may initiate a trial during EMDR treatment. Equally as important as understanding the individual efficacy of these interventions is understanding of the empirical basis for combined efficacy because their joint use is a likely reality in practice. The overall findings on combined use of medications and efficacious psychological interventions is a complex one and depends on the disorder treated, as well as the nature of the interactions between the two types of interventions. It should not be assumed that "more is better"; instead, this assumption bears empirical investigation.

Research on Tolerability and Acceptability

Finally, we recommend that "implementation research" (Sanders & Haines, 2006) place emphasis on examining client acceptability of treatment in an effort to elucidate further which treatment is more suited to which type of client. The repeated finding of high dropout rates with PTSD treatment (see Foa & Rothbaum, 1998; Zayfert, Becker, & Gillock, 2002; Zayfert & Black,

2000), necessitates that we understand the role of patient and therapist toler-ability and acceptability as they affect efficacious interventions.

References

Andrade, J., Kavanagh, D., & Baddeley, A. (1997). Eye-movements and visual imagery: A working memory approach to the treatment of post-traumatic stress disorder. *British Journal of Clinical Psychology, 36,* 209–223.

Australian Centre for Posttraumatic Mental Health. (2007). *Australian guidelines for the treatment of adults with acute stress disorder and posttraumatic stress disorder.* Melbourne: Author.

Barlow, D. H. (2002). *Anxiety and its disorders: The nature and treatment of anxiety and panic* (2nd ed.). New York: Guilford Press.

Barrowcliff, A. L., Gray, N. S., Freeman, T. C. A., & MacCulloch, M. J. (2004). Eye-movements reduce the vividness, emotional valence and electrodermal arousal associated with negative autobiographical memories. *Journal of Forensic Psychiatry and Psychology, 15,* 325–345.

Barrowcliff, A. L., Gray, N. S., MacCulloch, S., Freeman, T. C. A., & MacCulloch, M. J. (2003). Horizontal rhythmical eye movements consistently diminish the arousal provoked by auditory stimuli. *British Journal of Clinical Psychology, 42,* 289–302.

Borkovec, T. D., & Castonguay, L. G. (1998). What is the scientific meaning of "empiri-cally supported therapy"? *Journal of Consulting and Clinical Psychology, 66,* 136–142.

Bradley, R., Greene, J., Russ, E., Dutra, L., & Westen, D. (2005). A multidimensional meta-analysis of psychotherapy for PTSD. *American Journal of Psychiatry, 162,* 214–227.

Carlson, J. G., Chemtob, C. M., Rusnak, K., Hedlund, N. L., & Muraoka, M. Y. (1998). Eye movement desensitization and reprocessing (EMD/R) treatment for combat-related posttraumatic stress disorder. *Journal of Traumatic Stress, 11,* 3–24.

Chemtob, C. M., Nakashima, J., & Carlson, J. G. (2002). Brief treatment for elemen-tary school children with disaster-related posttraumatic stress disorder: A field study. *Journal of Clinical Psychology, 58,* 99–112.

Chemtob, C. M., Tolin, D. F., van der Kolk, B. A., & Pitman, R. K. (2000). Eye move-ment desensitization and reprocessing. In E. B. Foa, T. M. Keane, & M. J. Fried-man (Eds.), *Effective treatments for PTSD: Practice guidelines from the International Society for Traumatic Stress Studies* (pp. 139–154). New York: Guilford Press.

Christman, S. D., Garvey, K. J., Propper, R. E., & Phaneuf, K. A. (2003). Bilateral eye movements enhance the retrieval of episodic memories. *Neuropsychology, 17,* 221–229.

Cohen, J. A., Berliner, L., & March, J. S. (2000). Treatment of children and adoles-cents. In E. B. Foa, T. M. Keane, & M. J. Friedman (Eds.), *Effective treatments for PTSD: Practice guidelines from the International Society for Traumatic Stress Studies* (pp. 106–138, 330–332). New York: Guilford Press.

Cusack, K., & Spates, C. R. (1999). The cognitive dismantling of eye movement desen-sitization and reprocessing (EMDR) treatment of posttraumatic stress disorder (PTSD). *Journal of Anxiety Disorders, 13,* 87–99.

Davidson, P. R., & Parker, K. C. H. (2001). Eye movement desensitization and reprocessing (EMDR): A meta-analysis. *Journal of Consulting and Clinical Psychology, 69,* 305–316.

Devilly, G. J., Spence, S. H., & Rapee, R. M. (1998). Statistical and reliable change with eye movement desensitization and reprocessing: Treating trauma with a veteran population. *Behavior Therapy, 29,* 435–455.

Elofsson, U. O. E., von Schèele, B., Theorell, T., & Söndergaard, H. P. (2008). Physiological correlates of eye movement desensitization and reprocessing. *Journal of Anxiety Disorders, 22,* 622–634.

Fernandez, I., Gallinari, E., & Lorenzetti, A. (2004). A school-based eye movement desensitization and reprocessing intervention for children who witnessed the Pirelli Building airplane crash in Milan, Italy. *Journal of Brief Therapy, 2*(2), 129–136.

Foa, E. B., Keane, T. M., & Friedman, M. J. (Eds.). (2000). *Effective treatments for PTSD: Practice guidelines from the International Society for Traumatic Stress Studies.* New York: Guilford Press.

Foa, E. B., & Meadows, E. A. (1997). Psychosocial treatments for posttraumatic stress disorder: A critical review. *Annual Review of Psychology, 48,* 449–480.

Foa, E. B., & Rothbaum, B. O. (1998). *Treating the trauma of rape: Cognitive-behavioral therapy for PTSD.* New York: Guilford Press.

Herbert, J. D., & Mueser, K. T. (1992). Eye movement desensitization: A critique of the evidence. *Journal of Behavior Therapy and Experimental Psychiatry, 23,* 169–174.

Institute of Medicine of the National Academies, Committee on Treatment of Posttraumatic Stress Disorder, Board on Population Health and Public Health Practice. (2008). *Treatment of posttraumatic stress disorder: An assessment of the evidence.* Washington, DC: National Academies Press.

Ironson, G., Freud, B., Strauss, J. L., & Williams, J. (2002). Comparison of two treatments for traumatic stress: A community-based study of EMDR and prolonged exposure. *Journal of Clinical Psychology, 58,* 113–128.

Jaberghaderi, N., Greenwald, R., Rubin, A., Zand, S. O., & Dolatabadi, S. (2004). A comparison of CBT and EMDR for sexually abused Iranian girls. *Clinical Psychology and Psychotherapy, 11,* 358–368.

Jacobson, N. S., Dobson, K. S., Truax, P. A., Addis, M. E., Koerner, K., Gollan, J. K., et al. (1996). A component analysis of cognitive-behavioral treatment for depression. *Journal of Consulting and Clinical Psychology, 64,* 295–304.

Jarero, I., Artigas, L., & Hartung, J. (2006). EMDR integrative group treatment protocol: A postdisaster trauma intervention for children and adults. *Traumatology, 12*(2), 121–129.

Kavanagh, D. J., Freese, S., Andrade, J., & May, J. (2001). Effects of visuospatial tasks on desensitization to emotive memories. *British Journal of Clinical Psychology, 40,* 267–280.

Koch, E. I., Spates, C. R., & Himle, J. A. (2004). Comparison of behavioral and cognitive behavioral one-session exposure treatments for small animal phobias. *Behaviour Research and Therapy, 42,* 1483–1504.

Kuiken, D., Bears, M., Miall, D., & Smith, L. (2001–2002). Eye movement desensitization reprocessing facilitates attentional orienting. *Imagination, Cognition and Personality, 21,* 3–20.

Lee, C., Gavriel, H., Drummond, P., Richards, J., & Greenwald, R. (2002). Treatment of PTSD: Stress inoculation training with prolonged exposure compared to EMDR. *Journal of Clinical Psychology, 58,* 1071–1089.

Lee, C., Taylor, G., & Drummond, P. (2006). The active ingredient in EMDR: Is it tra-ditional exposure or dual focus of attention? *Clinical Psychology and Psychotherapy, 13*, 97–107.

Marcus, S. V., Marquis, P., & Sakai, C. (1997). Controlled study of treatment of PTSD using EMDR in an HMO setting. *Psychotherapy: Theory, Research, Practice and Train-ing, 34*, 307–315.

Marcus, S. V., Marquis, P., & Sakai, C. (2004). Three- and 6-month follow-up of EMDR treatment of PTSD in an HMO setting. *International Journal of Stress Management, 11*, 195–208.

National Institute for Clinical Excellence. (2005). *Posttraumatic stress disorder: The man-agement of PTSD in adults and children in primary and secondary care.* London: Royal College of Psychiatrists.

Oras, R., Cancela de Ezpeleta, S., & Ahmad, A. (2004). Treatment of traumatized refugee children with eye movement desensitization and reprocessing in a psy-chodynamic context. *Nordic Journal of Psychiatry, 58*, 199–203.

Öst, L.-G., Thulin, U., & Ramnerö, J. (2004). Cognitive behavior therapy vs. exposure *in vivo* in the treatment of panic disorder with agrophobia. *Behaviour Research and Therapy, 42*, 1105–1127.

Pitman, R., Orr, S., Altman, B., Longpre, R., Poire, R., & Macklin, M. (1996). Emo-tional processing during eye movement desensitization and reprocessing therapy of Vietnam veterans with chronic posttraumatic stress disorder. *Comprehensive Psychiatry, 37*, 419–429.

Power, K., McGoldrick, T., Brown, K., Buchanan, R., Sharp, D., Swanson, V., et al. (2002). A controlled comparison of eye movement desensitization and repro-cessing versus exposure plus cognitive restructuring versus waiting list in the treatment of posttraumatic stress disorder. *Clinical Psychology and Psychotherapy, 9*, 299–318.

Renfrey, G., & Spates, C. R. (1995). Eye movement desensitization: A partial disman-tling study. *Journal of Behavior Therapy and Experimental Psychiatry, 25*, 231–239.

Rogers, S., Silver, S. M., Goss, J., Obenchain, J., Willis, A., & Whitney, R. L. (1999). A single session, group study of exposure and eye movement desensitization and reprocessing in treating posttraumatic stress disorder among Vietnam War vet-erans: Preliminary data. *Journal of Anxiety Disorders, 13*, 119–130.

Rothbaum, B. O., Astin, M. C., & Marsteller, F. (2005). Prolonged exposure versus eye movement desensitization and reprocessing (EMDR) for PTSD rape victims. *Journal of Traumatic Stress, 18*, 607–616.

Rubin, A., Bischofshausen, S., Conroy-Moore, K., Dennis, B., Hastie, M., Melnick, L., et al. (2001). The effectiveness of EMDR in a child guidance center. *Research on Social Work Practice, 11*(4), 435–457.

Sack, M., Lempa, W., & Lamprecht, F. (2001). Study quality and effect sizes: A meta-analysis of EMDR-treatment for posttraumatic stress disorder. *Psychotherapie Psy-chosomatik Medizinische Psychologie, 51*(9–10), 350–355.

Sanders, D., & Haines, A. (2006). Implementation research is needed to achieve inter-national health goals. *Public Library of Science: Medicine, 3*, 719–722.

Seidler, G. H., & Wagner, F. E. (2006). Comparing the efficacy of EMDR and trauma-focused cognitive behavioral therapy in the treatment of PTSD: A meta-analytic study. *Psychological Medicine, 6*, 1–8.

Servan-Schreiber, D., Schooler, J., Dew, M. A., Carter, C., & Bartone, P. (2006). Eye movement desensitization and reprocessing for posttraumatic stress disorder: A pilot blinded, randomized study of stimulation type. *Psychotherapy and Psychoso-matics, 75,* 290–297.

Shapiro, F. (1989a). Efficacy of the eye movement desensitization procedure in the treatment of traumatic memories. *Journal of Traumatic Stress Studies, 2,* 199–223.

Shapiro, F. (1989b). Eye movement desensitization: A new treatment for post-traumatic stress disorder. *Journal of Behavior Therapy and Experimental Psychiatry, 20,* 211–217.

Shapiro, F. (1995). *Eye movement desensitization and reprocessing (EMDR): Basic principles, protocols, and procedures.* New York: Guilford Press.

Shapiro, F., & Maxfield, L. (2002). Eye movement desensitization and reprocessing (EMDR): Information processing in the treatment of trauma. *Journal of Clinical Psychology, 58,* 933–946.

Sharpley, C. F., Montgomery, I. M., & Scalzo, L. A. (1996). Comparative efficacy of EMDR and alternative procedures in reducing the vividness of mental images. *Scandinavian Journal of Behaviour Therapy, 25,* 37–42.

Sherman, J. J. (1998). Effects of psychotherapeutic treatments for PTSD: A meta-analysis of controlled clinical trials. *Journal of Traumatic Stress, 11,* 413–435.

Soberman, G. B., Greenwald, R., & Rule, D. L. (2002). A controlled study of eye move-ment desensitization and reprocessing (EMDR) for boys with conduct problems. *Journal of Aggression, Maltreatment and Trauma, 6*(1), 217–236.

Taylor, S., Thordarson, D. S., Maxfield, L., Fedoroff, I. C., Lovell, K., & Ogrodniczuk, J. (2003). Comparative efficacy, speed, and adverse effects of three PTSD treat-ments: Exposure therapy, EMDR, and relaxation training. *Journal of Consulting and Clinical Psychology, 71,* 330–338.

Tinker, R. H., & Wilson, S. A. (1999). *Through the eyes of a child: EMDR with children.* New York: Norton.

van den Hout, M., Muris, P., Salemink, E., & Kindt, M. (2001). Autobiographical memories become less vivid and emotional after eye movements. *British Journal of Clinical Psychology, 40,* 121–130.

van der Kolk, B. A., Spinazzola, J., Blaustein, M. E., Hopper, J. W., Hopper, E. K., Korn, D. L., et al. (2007). A randomized clinical trial of eye movement desensitization and reprocessing (EMDR), fluoxetine, and pill placebo in the treatment of post-traumatic stress disorder: Treatment effects and long-term maintenance. *Journal of Clinical Psychiatry, 68,* 37–46.

Van Etten, M. L., & Taylor, S. (1998). Comparative efficacy of treatments for post-traumatic stress disorder: A meta-analysis. *Clinical Psychology and Psychotherapy, 5,* 126–144.

Vaughn, K., Armstrong, M. S., Gold, R., O'Connor, N., Jenneke, W., & Tarrier, N. (1994). A trial of eye movement desensitization compared to image habituation training and applied muscle relaxation in post-traumatic stress disorder. *Journal of Behavior Therapy and Experimental Psychiatry, 25,* 283–291.

Veteran Administration/Department of Defense Clinical Practice Guideline Work-ing Group. (2003). *Management of post-traumatic stress.* Washington, DC: Veter-ans Health Administration, Department of Veterans Affairs and Health Affairs, Department of Defense.

Waller, S., Spates, C. R., & Mulick, P. (2000). *A meta-analysis of leading psychological interventions for PTSD: The effect of selected moderator variables.* Paper presented at the 3rd International Conference of Traumatic Stress, Melbourne, Australia.

Wilson, D. L., Silver, S. M., Covi, W. G., & Foster, S. (1996). Eye movement desensitization and reprocessing: Effectiveness and autonomic correlates. *Journal of Behavior Therapy and Experimental Psychiatry, 27,* 219–229.

Zayfert, C., Becker, C. B., & Gillock, K. L. (2002). Managing obstacles to the utilization of exposure therapy with PTSD patients. In L. VandeCreek & T. L. Jackson (Eds.), *Innovations in clinical practice: A source book* (Vol. 20, pp. 201–222). Sarasota, FL: Professional Resource Press.

Zayfert, C., & Black, C. (2000). Implementation of empirically supported treatment for PTSD: Obstacles and innovations. *Behavior Therapist, 23,* 161–168.

CHAPTER 12

Group Therapy

M. Tracie Shea, Meghan McDevitt-Murphy,
David J. Ready, and Paula P. Schnurr

Group therapy is one of the most common treatment modalities for post-traumatic stress disorder (PTSD). This chapter provides an updated critical review of research on group approaches. Following an initial overview of the use of groups to treat PTSD, we present a summary of the theoretical rationales, strategies, and techniques of different types of group approaches and a review of findings from empirical studies.

Theoretical Context

Group approaches to PTSD vary on several dimensions, including goals and objectives, theoretical rationales and strategies, structure of the group (open or closed), frequency and length of sessions, and duration of treatment. The rationale for the use of a group modality also may vary. Groups are sometimes used because they are thought to be superior to individual treatments for individuals with trauma, although to date there is no empirical support for this belief. Groups may be used efficiently to apply to multiple patients some of the same therapeutic strategies used in individual treatment. For example, most cognitive-behavioral groups teach coping or other types of skills (e.g., assertion training, anxiety management), saving therapist time by treating multiple individuals simultaneously. In other cases, the group format is itself critical to the presumed therapeutic factors, as in process-oriented groups characterized by a focus on interactions among group members as a basis for learning and therapeutic change. In either type of group, this modality offers important advantages to survivors of trauma, in whom estrangement, isolation, and alienation are often prominent. An important shared theoretical principle underlying groups for PTSD is that because of their interpersonal nature, groups can serve as excellent environments to restore a sense of safety, trust, self-esteem, and intimacy with other people (Allen & Bloom, 1994). Participation in a group can decrease the sense of isolation and alienation for patients with PTSD as they come to feel that others can understand them, and experience support in their efforts to recover from trauma related symptoms. This experience can contribute to the reestablishment of trust and a sense of connection with others.

An important broad distinction among group treatment approaches is the emphasis on reintegration of the traumatic experience as key to the change process. Trauma-focused groups assume integration of the traumatic memory on an affective, cognitive, and/or physiological level as the mechanism to reduce symptoms and modify the meaning of the trauma for the individual. Present-focused approaches, in contrast, use the group to decrease patients' isolation and increase their sense of competence, thus improving adaptation and functioning.

A focus on trauma may or may not be present in any of the various theoretical modalities characterizing group approaches to PTSD, with the exception of supportive therapy groups, which tend to avoid direct focus on trauma material. For example, psychodynamic groups that include a focus on trauma similar to that in cognitive-behavioral approaches aim to help the individual to reconstruct the trauma and to integrate disassociated affect and cognitions. The difference lies in both the conceptualization of the processes involved in successful integration (e.g., making unconscious aspects conscious vs. habituation, extinction, or cognitive reconstruction) and the strategies used to address the traumatic experiences.

Among groups focused on the present, there is considerable overlap among those described as psychodynamic, interpersonal, and process oriented. Gaining insight into maladaptive interpersonal patterns, and how these patterns are related to the experience of trauma, is important to all of these approaches. A shared theoretical assumption for such groups emphasizes the social nature—hence, the social effects—of trauma. It follows that central to treatment of PTSD is the need to address the individual's relationship to others. Many of these groups incorporate the principles of group therapy described by Yalom (1995), for whom interpersonal interaction is the core of therapeutic change in group therapy. The focus on here-and-now interactions within the group provides an experiential basis for interpersonal learning and change, or what some refer to as a "corrective emotional experience." For trauma survivors, the development or reestablishment of trust is critical to this corrective experience. Interpersonal psychotherapy (IPT), originally developed as an individual therapy for depression (Klerman, Weiss-

man, Rounsaville, & Chevron, 1984), was adapted for delivery in a group format for PTSD (Krupnick, Green, Miranda, Stockton, & Mete, in press). The
theoretical basis for the IPT model is that symptoms occur in an interpersonal context: Symptoms may cause or accentuate interpersonal problems,
may be the result of interpersonal problems, or both; regardless of the direction of causality, treatment needs to address interpersonal functioning. In
addition to the usual IPT themes of relationship disputes, social deficits, role
transitions, and relationship losses, group IPT for PTSD emphasizes relationship behaviors that decrease social support or lead to further exploitation or
abuse, and how these patterns are related to PTSD symptoms.

Most groups contain elements of support. For groups defined as "supportive," the theoretical rationale is based on the role of emotional support
and empathy in enhancing adaptive defenses and increasing a sense of mastery, self-esteem, and connection with others. Such groups may be indicated
when traumatic memories are too intrusive and the ability of the individual
to cope with strong affect is limited or currently fragile. A group environment
of nonjudgmental acceptance provides a sense of safety and comfort, thus
helping to contain the distressing affect. The acceptance and support may
also enhance trust, reducing the sense of isolation common among those
with PTSD.

Group approaches described as "cognitive-behavioral" typically focus on
behavioral skills training, cognitive restructuring, trauma exposure, or some
combination of these. The theoretical underpinnings of these approaches
are similar to those underlying individual therapies for PTSD. For example,
the use of prolonged imaginal exposure, based on principles of classical
and operant conditioning, is hypothesized to reduce trauma-related anxiety
through desensitization to reminders. It also reduces avoidance responses
that have been motivated by fear, and reinforced by fear reduction. The use
of exposure is also theorized to facilitate change in maladaptive thoughts
and beliefs surrounding the trauma, by allowing them to come into clearer
focus and to be challenged. These may include inflated perceptions of danger, developed through generalization, or inaccurate perceptions of responsibility for the trauma. The use of the group, in principle, may enhance
cognitive restructuring by incorporating feedback from others with similar
experiences.

Description of Techniques

A wide range of techniques is used in groups for PTSD, within and across
theoretical modalities. Strategies designed to establish a sense of safety,
increase trust, and develop group cohesion are common to most groups. The
following is a brief description of strategies and techniques used in the group
approaches covered.

Psychodynamic, Interpersonal, and Process Groups

Although the studies included in this broad group incorporate a range of strategies and techniques, a key characteristic common to all is the emphasis on techniques facilitating insight-based learning and change. As noted earlier, an explicit focus on trauma may or may not be present in these groups. When trauma is a focus of the group, these approaches differ from cognitive-behavioral approaches in strategies used to elicit the traumatic material. In psychodynamic groups, the trauma material arises in a less structured manner than in cognitive-behavioral trauma-focused groups. Trauma material may arise overtly or covertly. Group members are encouraged to describe and to reconstruct their experiences, to experience the affect associated with the trauma, and to modify the negative views of self that developed. Psychodynamic approaches emphasize increasing awareness of unconscious fears and maladaptive patterns that have arisen as a result of an interaction between a patient's childhood and his or her traumatic experiences. The aim is to bring the traumatic memories into conscious awareness as an integrated narrative. There is an emphasis on understanding the meaning of the trauma symptoms, how the trauma has influenced concepts of self and others, and becoming aware of how unconsciously driven patterns of behavior stem from the trauma. The group focus may shift back and forth from the past to the present in the process of making connections and gaining insight into how current difficulties may be linked to the trauma.

"Process" groups typically maintain focus on the immediate present. Attention is directed to group members' here-and-now experiences as they relate to experiencing trauma symptoms and to their interaction with one another in the group. Therapists help group members increase awareness of their own feelings as they occur and express their needs, or fears, as they occur (Classen, Koopman, Nevill-Manning, & Spiegel, 2001). Feedback among members allows individuals to learn how others perceive them and to modify faulty assumptions about themselves and others. The IPT group model (Krupnick et al., in press) helps group members to identify their specific relationship difficulties in terms of the four problem areas of relationship disputes, social deficits, role transitions, and relationship losses. Group members are helped to identify patterns and behaviors that prevent them from receiving social support, or that repeatedly increase risk by making them vulnerable to exploitation from others. The final phase of the group facilitates mourning relative to the loss of the group and to prior relationship losses and disappointments.

Supportive Groups

The aim of groups described as "supportive" is to enhance daily functioning by providing a safe and supportive atmosphere in which participants can begin to let down their guard, increase trust and connection with others, feel accepted and validated, and develop an increased sense of mastery over their problems through the feedback and support of the group members. Whereas most groups contain some elements of such support, the heart of this type of group is the encouragement of interpersonal connections, through the giving and receiving of emotional support and feedback. The focus is on current life issues rather than traumatic experiences. Therapeutic strategies include normalizing the symptoms and experiences of group members, facilitating interactions among group members, increasing group cohesion, encouraging and reinforcing adaptive behaviors, and enhancing a sense of mastery and competence among individuals. Support groups are often used with patients whose PTSD symptoms are judged as not severe enough to justify intensive treatment, or who are considered too fragile, due to severe comorbid conditions, to tolerate a trauma-focused therapy.

Cognitive-Behavioral Group Therapy

The other broad category of group approaches is cognitive-behavioral, including skills training and exposure techniques—singly or in combination. Strategies range from education about the symptoms of PTSD to exposure sessions in which the patient is expected to describe repeatedly the details of his or her traumatic experiences within the group. Most cognitive-behavioral groups include training in skills to manage and reduce symptoms of PTSD, particularly anxiety and arousal. These include relaxation training; grounding techniques; identification and modification of maladaptive thoughts and beliefs; and/or use of role playing, rehearsal, and assertion training to enhance interpersonal functioning. The most comprehensive cognitive-behavioral group approaches for PTSD have been used in veteran samples, and generally incorporate imaginal exposure and cognitive restructuring, in addition to skills training and other components (e.g., Foy, Ruzek, Glynn, Riney, & Gusman, 1997; Ready et al., 2008). For example, trauma-focused group therapy for combat-related PTSD (TFGT) includes three phases. The introductory phase includes education about PTSD, teaching and reinforcing basic coping skills, helping members get to know each other, and preparing members for the work on traumatic memories. The second phase begins with identification of a trauma scene for each member that will be the focus of the reexperiencing and repeated, systematic imaginal exposure to key aspects of the trauma memories. One-third of all sessions are devoted to individualized focus work. Group members are also required to listen to audiotapes of their scenes as homework to increase the dosage of exposure. Exposure sessions include identifying and challenging cognitive distortions. A final phase emphasizes relapse prevention planning and identifying and reviewing coping strategies for predictable high-risk situations.

Method of Collecting Data

Our search for relevant studies began with a review of studies included in the earlier version of this chapter (Foy et al., 2000). Searches for additional articles used the Published International Literature on Traumatic Stress (PILOTS) database from the National Center for PTSD website, and the PsycINFO database maintained by the American Psychological Association. Search terms included "Trauma," "PTSD," "group," "treatment," and "therapy." Searches focused on the years from 1998 to present. Additionally, we used the Social Science Citation Index and the Science Citation Index to locate articles citing the version of this chapter in the previous edition, in an effort to locate additional treatment outcome studies. We also contacted investigators known to be conducting studies of group therapy approaches for possible additions to published material. We included studies that targeted populations with trauma, assessed symptoms of PTSD at pre- and posttreatment, and had at least 10 participants in the group therapy condition being studied. Given the still relatively small number of controlled studies, we did not require that studies include only participants meeting criteria for PTSD. We excluded studies that combined multiple interventions in addition to group therapy, obscuring the effect of group treatment itself.

Literature Review

These criteria resulted in a total of 22 studies (Tables 12.1 and 12.2), including seven randomized and six nonrandomized trials comparing at least one active group to a comparison or control condition (Table 12.1), and nine studies reporting on pre- to posttreatment change for a single treatment (Table 12.2). The most common type of control condition (10 of 13 studies) involved no treatment—primarily wait-list or assessment controls. The most common treatment orientation of the groups studied was cognitive-behavioral—14 of the 22 studies. Psychodynamic or IPT approaches were the focus of four studies. Three studies investigated groups we have labeled insight-oriented: one described as psychoeducational/insight oriented, and two that examined a feminist model of group therapy. Three studies included supportive therapy group conditions.

In terms of types of trauma studied, interpersonal (primarily sexual) abuse was the most common (15 studies), followed by combat veteran samples (five studies). Five studies focused on PTSD with a comorbid disorder—either substance use disorders (four studies) or panic disorder (one study).

Text continues on page 318

TABLE 12.1. Studies with Control or Comparison Groups

Study [AHCPR level]	Target population[a]	Number/length of sessions	Treatment(s); control[b]	Major findings	Between-group effect sizes	Within-group effect sizes
Randomized studies						
Classen, Koopman, Nevill-Manning, & Spiegel (2001); Speigel, Classen, Thurston, & Butler (2004) [B]	55 females with PTSD; childhood sexual abuse	24 1.5-hr sessions	*Psychodynamic* 24 trauma focused (TF) 19 present focused (PF) [33 wait-list [WL] control][c]	Treatment groups (combined) showed significantly more improvement in dissociation, sexual abuse trauma index, and interpersonal problems than WL. No different than WL when groups were analyzed separately.	*Trauma Symptom Checklist–40 (TSC-40)* **All Ss with data** PF vs. TF 0.04 TF vs. WL 0.23 PF vs. WL 0.19 Combined vs. WL 0.26	*TSC-40* **Intent to treat** PF 0.16 TF 0.26 WL 0.20
Falsetti, Resnick, Davis, & Gallagher (2001); Falsetti, Resnick, & Davis (2005) [B]	22 females with PTSD and panic disorder; diverse traumas	12 weekly 1.5-hr sessions	*Cognitive-behavioral* 12 multichannel exposure therapy (MCET) [15 WL control][c]	Significant reduction in PTSD found in treatment group relative to WL.	*MPSS* **Completers** MCET vs. WL 0.94* (*based on *F* value)	Insufficient data
Krakow et al. (2000, 2001) [A]	168 females with PTSD; most with childhood abuse	Two 3-hr sessions, and one 1-hr session over 5 wk	*Cognitive-behavioral* 88 imagery rehearsal therapy (IRT) 80 WL control	Significantly more improvement in nightmares, sleep, and PTSD for IRT compared to WL; improvements maintained at 6 mo.	*Clinician-Administered PTSD Scale (CAPS)* **Intent to treat** IRT vs. WL 0.72 *PTSD Symptom Scale (PSS)* IRT vs. WL 0.72	*CAPS* **Intent to treat** IRT 1.54 WL 0.43 *PSS* IRT 1.06 WL 0.27
Krupnick, Green, Miranda, & Stockton (in press) [A]	48 females with PTSD; interpersonal trauma history (e.g., assault, abuse, and molestation)	16 2-hr sessions, with 3–5 group members	32 *Interpersonal therapy* (IPT) 16 WL control	PTSD, depression, and interpersonal functioning improved significantly more in IPT group than in WL.	*CAPS* **Intent to treat** IPT vs. WL 0.70	*CAPS* **Intent to treat** IPT 1.15 WL 0.26

Study	Sample	Dosage	Treatment	Results	Measure	Measure
Schnurr et al. (2003) [A]	360 male veterans with PTSD	30 weekly + 5 monthly booster 1.5- to 2-hr exposure sessions	*Cognitive-behavioral* 162 trauma-focused group therapy (TFGT) 165 present-centered group therapy (PCGT)	Significant pre- to posttest improvements in PTSD for both treatment groups, but no overall differences between therapy groups. Improvements maintained at 12 mo.	*CAPS* **TFGT vs. PCGT** **Intent to treat** Unadjusted 0.11 Adjusted[d] 0.09 **Completers** Unadjusted 0.15 Adjusted[d] 0.11	*CAPS* **TFGT** **Intent to treat** Unadjusted 0.31 Adjusted[d] 0.25 PCGT Unadjusted 0.27 Adjusted[d] 0.21 **Completers** Unadjusted 0.27 Adjusted[d] 0.20 PCGT Unadjusted 0.21 Adjusted[d] 0.14
Stalker & Fry (1999) [A]	77 females; childhood sexual abuse	10 sessions, 1.5-hr group, 50 min for individual sessions	*Insight-oriented* Feminist model 24 group treatment 28 individual treatment All participants had 10-wk waiting period prior to treatment	No differences in outcome for group compared to individual therapy. Significant pre- to posttest improvements in PTSD, distress, and Global Assessment Scale (GAS) for group and individual treatment. All improvement maintained at 6 mo except GAS.	*TSC-40* **Completers** Group vs. individual 0.10* *Posttraumatic Stress Scale (PTSS)* Group vs. individual 0.07* (*based on F value)	Insufficient data
Zlotnick et al. (1997) [A]	48 females with PTSD; childhood sexual abuse	Weekly 2-hr sessions over 15 wk plus treatment as usual (TAU; individual psychotherapy + medication)	*Cognitive-behavioral* 16 affect management (AM) 17 WL control	AM group reported significantly fewer symptoms of dissociation and PTSD than did WL.	*Davidson Trauma Scale (DTS)* **Completers** AM vs. WL 0.83	*DTS* **Completers** AM 0.72 WL 0.06

(continued)

TABLE 12.1. (continued)

Study [AHCPR level]	Target population[a]	Number/length of sessions	Treatment(s); control[b]	Major findings	Between-group effect sizes	Within-group effect sizes
Nonrandomized studies						
Cloitre & Koenen (2001) [B]	60 females with PTSD; childhood sexual abuse	12 weekly 1.5-hr sessions	34 *Process/interpersonal* 16 in groups with borderline personality disorder (BPD) 18 in groups without BPD 15 WL control	PTSD, anger, and depression significantly reduced in BPD group. No improvements in WL or BPD+ groups (BPD+ showed worsening anger).		*PSS* Within-group effect sizes BPD+ 0.20 BPD− 0.88 WL 0.35
Morgan & Cummings (1999) [B]	89 females, some with PTSD childhood sexual abuse	20 weekly sessions	*Insight-oriented* Feminist empowerment therapy (FET) 40 FET 40 assessment control	Significantly more improvement in treatment group vs. control in depression, social maladjustment, self-blame, and PTSD; maintained at 3-mo follow-up.		*PTSD subscale of Response to Childhood Incest Questionnaire (RCIQ)* FET 0.63 Control 0.00
Resick, Jordan, Girelli, Hunter, & Marhoefer-Dvorak (1988) [B]	43 females; sexual assault	Six 2-hr sessions	*Cognitive-behavioral* 12 stress inoculation (SI) 13 assertion (Assert) 12 supportive psychotherapy (SP) [13 WL control][c]	Significant improvement on fear, depression, anxiety, self-esteem, self-concept, and PTSD. Similar improvement for all treatment groups. No improvement for WL. All improvements maintained at 3 mo.		*Impact of Events Scale (IES) Avoidance* SI 0.57 Assert 0.57 SP 0.29 WL −0.34 *IES Intrusion* SI 0.48

Study	Sample (N[a])	Dose	Treatment conditions (N[b])	Results	Effect sizes
Resick & Schnicke (1992) [B]	41 female rape (childhood or adulthood) survivors with significant PTSD symptoms	12 weekly 1.5-hr sessions	*Cognitive-behavioral* 18 cognitive processing therapy (CPT) 20 WL control	Significant improvements for CPT on PTSD, depression, distress, and social adjustment; improvement maintained at 6 mo. No change for WL from pre- to posttest.	Assert 0.62 SP 0.34 WL 0.13 *Symptom Checklist-90 (SCL-90) PTSD* CPT 0.89 WL 0.02
Saxe & Johnson (1999) [B]	38 female incest survivors entering group 31 WL	20 weekly 2.5-hr sessions	*Supportive* 32 SP 31 WL control	Significantly more improvement for SP than WL in depression, PTSD, distress, and self-concept. Improvements maintained at 6 mo; intrusions significantly improved from posttest to 6 mo.	*IES Avoidance* SP 0.92 WL 0.00 *IES Intrusion* SP 0.28 WL 0.08
Wallis (2002) [B]	83 males and females with childhood abuse/neglect; PTSD not required	12 wk	*Insight-oriented* 64 Psychoeducation/insight 19 WL control	Significant improvement for treatment group on 7 of 10 Trauma Symptom Inventory (TSI) scales. No change in trauma symptoms for control group.	*TSI trauma composite* Treatment 0.71 WL 0.10

[a]N = subjects starting study or treatment.

[b]N = subjects in data analyses.

[c]{} indicates that participants in WL and treatment conditions overlap.

[d]Adjusted for unit of analysis and group intraclass correlation.

TABLE 12.2. Studies without Control or Comparison Conditions

Study [AHCPR level]	Target population[a]	Number/length of sessions	Treatment orientation[b]	Major findings	Within-group effect size[c]
Cook, Walser, Kane, Ruzek, & Woody (2006) [B]	25 veterans with combat PTSD + substance use disorders (SUDs)	25 sessions	*Cognitive-behavioral* 18 Seeking Safety	Significant improvement in PTSD and quality of life.	*PTSD Checklist—Military Version (PCL-M)* 1.18
Creamer, Elliott, Forbes, Biddle, & Hawthorne (2006) [B]	2,223 Vietnam War veterans with PTSD	Predominantly group-based program, plus limited individual therapy sessions; 12 weeks; 6-member cohorts	*Predominantly cognitive-behavioral*	Significant improvements in PTSD, anxiety, depression, and anger at 6 mo; smaller gains through 24 mo follow-up.	*PCL* Pretreatment to: 6 mo 0.59 12 mo 0.70 24 mo 0.85
Donovan, Padin-Rivera, & Kowaliw (2001) [B]	46 male veterans with combat PTSD + SUDs	12 weeks; 10 hrs of group treatment per wk	*Cognitive-behavioral* 35 skills training, trauma processing, peer support	Significant decreases in PTSD and addiction severity; maintained at 6 and 12 mo.	*CAPS* 0.67
Frueh, Turner, Beidel, Mirabella, & Jones (1996) [C]	15 male Vietnam War combat veterans with PTSD	15 individual sessions—education and exposure 14 group sessions—social/rehabilitation 1.5-hr sessions (1–3 per week)	*Cognitive-behavioral* 11 trauma management therapy (TMT)	Significant improvement in locus of control, sexual problems, self-esteem, trauma-related symptoms, and general distress.	*CAPS* 1.09
Hazzard, Rogers, & Angert (1993) [C]	148 females; childhood sexual abuse; no PTSD required	1.5-hr weekly sessions for 1 year	*Process-oriented* 78 process-oriented group therapy	Significant improvements in locus of control, sexual problems, self-esteem, PTSD, and distress.	*TSC-33** 0.44 (*based on 34 subjects with data)

Lubin, Loris, Burt, & Johnson (1998) [C]	33 females with multiple traumas— sexual assault, physical assault, or violent accidents in childhood or adulthood	16 weekly 1.5-hr sessions	Cognitive-behavioral 29 trauma-focused/ psychoeducational group therapy	Significant improvement on three PTSD clusters and depression; improvements sustained at 6-mo follow-up.	CAPS 0.81 IES 0.32
Stauffer & Deblinger (1996) [C]	34 nonoffending mothers of young sexually abused children	11 weekly 2-hr sessions	18 Cognitive-behavioral	Significant improvement in maternal distress and avoidance, and child behavior; maintained at 3-mo follow-up.	IES Avoidance 0.56 Intrusion 0.24
Najavits, Weiss, Shaw, & Muenz (1998) [B]	27 females with PTSD and SUDs; severe trauma history— sexual and physical abuse and "other criminal victimization"	24 1.5-hr sessions (2 times per week)	Cognitive-behavioral 17 Seeking safety	Significant improvement in substance use, PTSD, depression, psychosocial functioning, suicidality; all maintained at 3-mo follow-up.	TSC-40 total 3-mo follow-up 0.56
Zlotnick, Najavits, Rohsenow, & Johnson (2003) [B]	18 incarcerated females with PTSD and SUDs; sexual and physical abuse.	24 1.5-hr sessions (2 times per wk) Plus TAU	Cognitive-behavioral 17 Seeking safety	Significant improvement in PTSD and drug and alcohol use; maintained at 3-mo follow-up.	CAPS 1.28* *Based on t value

[a]N = subjects starting study or treatment.

[b]N = subjects in data analyses.

[c]Within-group effect size only.

Psychodynamic, Interpersonal, Process, and Insight-Oriented Group Therapy

All studies of group treatments described as psychodynamic, interpersonal, or process-oriented focused on samples with sexual assault histories, primarily during childhood. Randomized designs were used in two small-scale studies. Comparison of a trauma-focused group and a present-focused group, both based on psychodynamic principles, showed no differences for either relative to a wait-list control (Spiegel, Classen, Thurston, & Butler, 2004), although, when combined, the groups differed from the control on some non-PTSD measures (Classen et al., 2001). Krupnick and colleagues (in press) found significant effects for an IPT group compared to a wait-list control on PTSD. Cloitre and Koenen (2001) reported significant improvement for an interpersonal/process group compared to a nonrandomized wait-list control, but only for groups that did not have members with borderline personality disorder (BPD).

Six studies investigated insight-oriented or supportive groups. Stalker and Fry (1999) used a randomized design to compare group versus individual delivery of a feminist model of insight-oriented therapy; both conditions showed significant improvement in PTSD and did not differ from each other. The other studies compared group approaches to wait-list or assessment-only controls in nonrandomized designs; all reported significant findings for the group treatment compared to the control. Two studies used supportive groups as comparison conditions to examine the effects of cognitive-behavioral treatments (Resick, Jordan, Girelli, Hutter, & Marhoefer-Dvorak, 1988; Schnurr et al., 2003). In both, there were significant pre–post differences, but within-group effect sizes were small.

Summarizing results from this broad category, findings for groups described as interpersonal are strongest and warrant further study with larger samples. All of the group approaches were associated with positive change, with pre–post effect sizes ranging from small to medium. This is important given that these kinds of groups, providing the benefits of normalization, peer-support, and reframing of symptoms and problems, are the most frequently used type of group therapy treatment for PTSD in clinical settings.

Cognitive-Behavioral Group Therapy Approaches

Fourteen studies examined cognitive-behavioral approaches. Four were randomized; two of these were preliminary or pilot studies. The other randomized studies are notable for their larger sample sizes. Significant effects for imagery rehearsal therapy (IRT), developed to treat PTSD-related nightmares, were found in a study of 168 females with PTSD (Krakow et al., 2001). TFGT was investigated in male veterans of the Vietnam War, in the largest and most rigorous study to date of group therapy for PTSD (Schnurr et al., 2003). TFGT was compared to a present-centered group therapy (PCGT) condition, designed to provide the "nonspecific" but often potent factors of support and interpersonal connection provided by the group format. The primary intention-to-treat (ITT) analyses did not find differences on PTSD or any other outcome measure, and average improvement was modest in both conditions. Dropout during treatment, although higher in TFGT (22.8%) than in PCGT (8.6%), was sufficiently low to conclude that the treatment was tolerable for the majority of participants in the exposure-based condition. Secondary analyses including only those receiving at least 24 sessions of treatment were more favorable for TFGT, with a marginally significant treatment main effect for TFGT and a significant treatment × cohort interaction. TFGT showed significantly better outcome than PCGT for the second and third cohorts (Schnurr et al., 2003).

A naturalistic program evaluation study reported on the outcomes of Australian veterans of the Vietnam War participating in 12-week, group-based PTSD programs (Creamer, Elliott, Forbes, Biddle, & Hawthorne, 2006). Although uncontrolled, this study reflects clinical practice because it is typically conducted in a real-world setting and has the advantage of a very large sample (2,223 male veterans). The predominately group-based cognitive-behavioral approach has components similar to TFGT (Foy et al., 1997), including trauma exposure. Dropout was 3%, and within-treatment effect sizes were moderate to large and continued to increase over follow-up.

The cognitive-behavioral approach called Seeking Safety (Najavits, 2002) shows promise as a group intervention for PTSD complicated by substance abuse or dependence, with three preliminary studies reporting significant improvement for both PTSD symptoms and substance abuse/dependence. Studies comparing this approach with control groups are needed.

In summary, there is significant empirical support for cognitive-behavioral group approaches, in both combat veterans (mean of 0.81 pre- to posttreatment effect size across studies) and in adults with histories of sexual abuse (mean of 0.89 across studies). Within-group effect sizes ranged from small (0.31) to very large (1.54).

Comparisons of Treatment Approaches

Few studies provide direct comparisons of different forms of group therapy. An important question for the treatment of PTSD more broadly is whether treatments focusing on the trauma are more effective for symptoms of PTSD than treatments that do not focus on the trauma. As noted, the largest controlled study to date (Schnurr et al., 2003) did not find evidence for superiority of the trauma-focused group compared to the present-centered supportive group in the primary analyses, although secondary analyses of those with an adequate number of sessions did show an effect for the trauma-focused group. The two other studies comparing two or more types of therapy (Classen et al., 2001; Resick et al., 1988) did not find differences but had small sample sizes, thus limiting statistical power to provide an adequate test.

TABLE 12.3. Within-Group Treatment Effect Sizes by Presence or Absence of Trauma Focus

Groups addressing trauma	Effect size	Groups not addressing trauma	Effect size
Classen et al. (2001)	0.26	Classen et al. (2001)	0.16
Cloitre & Koenen (2001)	0.63	Cook et al. (2006)	1.18
Creamer et al. (2006)	0.59	Krupnick et al. (in press)	1.15
Donovan et al. (2001)	0.67	Najavits et al. (1998)	0.56
Frueh et al. (1996)	1.09	Resick et al. (1988)	0.60[a]
Hazzard et al. (1993)	0.44	Resick et al. (1988)	0.32[a]
Krakow et al. (2001)	1.54	Schnurr et al. (2003)	0.27
Lubin et al. (1998)	0.81	Wallis (2002)	0.71
Morgan & Cummings (1999)	0.63	Zlotnick et al. (1997)	0.72
Resick et al. (1988)	0.53[a]	Zlotnick et al. (2003)	1.28
Resick & Schnicke (1992)	0.89		
Saxe & Johnson (1999)	0.60[a]		
Schnurr et al. (2003)	0.31		
Stauffer & Deblinger, 1996	0.40*		

[a]Mean of Impact of Event Intrusion and Avoidance scales.

To address this question using the results from the literature more broadly, we summarized the pre- to posttreatment effect sizes from the treatment conditions that addressed trauma as part of the group work, and from those that did not focus on trauma (Table 12.3). The average effect size for the two groups of studies is nearly identical (0.69 and 0.70, respectively). Thus, there is currently little evidence that groups focusing on trauma provide superior outcome to those that do not. This question, however, has only been addressed by one controlled study with a sufficiently large sample size to detect differences (Schnurr et al., 2003). It also remains possible that trauma-focused groups may provide superior outcomes for certain types of patients, but as we discuss below, there has been little study of this question.

Summary and Recommendations

The empirical literature on group treatment for PTSD has grown since the first edition of this book, published in 2000. Fifteen additional studies met our criteria for inclusion; among these are six additional randomized studies. The study by Schnurr and colleagues (2003) represents a major advance in terms of sample size and overall methodological rigor. However, five of the seven randomized studies had small sample sizes, and most used wait-list controls. Overall, the research shows that treatment with group therapy is associated with improvement in symptoms of PTSD, with pre- to posttreatment effect sizes ranging from small to large. The amount of change exceeded that of wait-list controls for most studies of interpersonal, process-oriented, and cognitive-behavioral approaches, but not for the single study using a psycho-dynamic approach. Whether the improvement found is due to the strategies used by the different types of group therapy remains unknown. The only ran-domized study with adequate statistical power and an active control condition (Schnurr et al., 2003) did not find a significant advantage for the treatment under investigation (TFGT) compared to a present-focused supportive group therapy in the primary analyses. The fact that the secondary analyses, includ-ing those with at least 24 sessions, showed significant differences suggests that trauma-focused groups may be more effective than present-centered groups for participants who receive an adequate "dose" of treatment, and/or for cer-tain types of patients. There is little evidence, unfortunately, to guide deci-sions regarding the latter.

An important concern is that most studies of group treatments failed to use analytic methods that account for clustering of observations within groups. With the exception of a few studies (Creamer et al., 2006; Ready et al., 2008; Schnurr et al., 2003) the typical approach is to treat the individual par-ticipant as the unit of analysis. This is an unwarranted assumption because individuals in group therapy are part of a shared therapy environment and likely influence other participants' symptoms. A recent analysis (Baldwin, Murray, & Shadish, 2005) examined findings from 33 studies of treatments on the American Psychological Association's list of evidence-based group treatment, all with statistically significant effects, as published. Correcting the degrees of freedom resulted in the loss of statistical significance for over 30% of the studies, and correction for group clustering by varying the intraclass correlation resulted in a loss of statistical significance for additional studies. It is likely that the true effects for group treatment for PTSD are more mod-est than reported. On the other hand, the use of methodologically rigorous controlled studies of group treatments precludes the kind of careful selection of group members that can take place in clinical settings, which could under-estimate the effects if such selection does in fact improve the group process and outcome.

Little is known about factors that may moderate or mediate outcome in group therapy of any type because few studies have addressed such factors. An exception is a study (Cloitre & Koenen, 2001) that compared the effects of a process/interpersonal group for women with childhood sexual abuse by the presence or absence of one or more individuals with BPD in any given group. Groups without BPD members showed a large within-treatment effect size (0.88), in contrast to the effect size (0.20) for the groups including at least one member with BPD. Interestingly, the poorer outcomes were explained not simply by less change among those with BPD, but by less change in the groups with a BPD member, which suggests that having one or more BPD members significantly alters the group process. This finding has potentially important implications for selecting group members for process-oriented groups for individuals with PTSD. Individuals with an additional diagnosis of

BPD may do better in more structured group approaches emphasizing skills training, such as dialectical behavior therapy (Linehan, 1993).

Foy and colleagues (2000) summarized the factors identified in the literature as important considerations for group therapy in general, and for trauma versus supportive groups more specifically. Many of the contraindications for group therapy (e.g., active psychosis, limited cognitive capacity, and current suicidal or homicidal risk) are typically exclusion criteria for studies of group treatments. A key feature commonly thought to be important for successful trauma-focused group treatment is the ability to tolerate high anxiety or other strong affects. Although this makes clinical sense, there is no clear method of assessing this feature, and studies of trauma-focused groups have neither made this a requirement nor examined it as a predictor of outcome. A related issue is the possibility of negative effects for some individuals in trauma-focused groups as a result of vicarious traumatization. Despite an absence of published evidence of such negative effects, this question warrants investigation. Furthermore, it is possible that some types of trauma populations are more vulnerable than others to such effects. Also unaddressed in the empirical literature is the question of the importance of homogeneity of groups in terms of type of trauma. This question is most relevant to trauma-focused groups.

In terms of mechanisms of change, the process of desensitization is presumed to play a central role in facilitating change in trauma-focused cognitive-behavioral groups. A key assumption is that the trauma-related anxiety state, along with physiological arousal, must be reactivated frequently enough for desensitization to occur. Some have questioned the adequacy of exposure procedures in group approaches, specifically, whether the social support developed within the group might minimize the development of the anxiety state (Woodward et al., 1997), and whether the smaller number of personal exposures within a group versus within-individual treatment provides an adequate "dosage" of exposure. An examination of heart rate as an indicator of sympathetic arousal during group exposure therapy for six Vietnam veterans by Woodward and colleagues (1997) indicated that during sessions of their own personal exposure, participants exhibited higher whole-session heart rates, thus demonstrating that arousal does occur within the group context. On the other hand, those not actively engaged in their own exposure showed mild linear declines in heart rate from the beginning to the end of the sessions, suggesting that "vicarious" exposure did not occur.

The minimum number of exposures required for an adequate test of a group-based, trauma-focused treatment is a key question because the number of in-session personal exposures is limited, typically, to no more than two. Exposure sessions in group approaches are typically augmented with repeated exposures outside of the group, using audiotaped recordings, although the number of exposures required outside the group varies. The TFGT condition (Schnurr et al., 2003) required a minimum of eight additional exposures outside of the two exposures in the group. Ready and colleagues (2008) have reported preliminary findings from a trauma-focused group approach called group-based exposure therapy (GBET). GBET is a 16-week outpatient program, similar to TFGT, but with a significantly larger exposure component. Patients make two war trauma presentations within their groups and listen to audiocassette recordings of presentations a minimum of 10 times each. Assuming compliance with out-of-session homework exposures, GBET involves 22 exposures, compared to 10 in TFGT. This approach is shorter term but more intensive in administration, with 3 hours of group therapy per day, twice a week. It also involves larger cohorts (10 vs. 6). Ready and colleagues found large effect sizes on the Clinician-Administered PTSD Scale (CAPS), although a limit is that the assessments were administered by treating clinicians. Self-report PTSD measures showed moderate to large effect sizes. Effects were maintained at 6-month posttreatment (Ready et al., 2008). To date, none of the patients have required psychiatric hospitalization during the exposure phase of GBET, and the overall dropout rate was 3%. A controlled study of GBET is planned.

Further study of the possible benefits of increased number of exposures is important given that the group format is the most frequent mode of delivery of exposure treatment within both the U.S. and Australian Veteran Administration (VA) systems, and the current influx of large numbers of veterans with PTSD from the Iraq War. Data on the comparative effects of individual versus group trauma-focused therapy in this new, less chronic sample of veterans are sorely needed.

A question largely unaddressed in the literature is the comparative efficacy of group versus individual modalities of different therapy approaches. The single study that compared individual and group therapy (Stalker & Fry, 1999) found no differences in outcome. In veteran samples, although there are no direct comparisons, the rates of retention in trauma-focused treatments appear to be better when given in group rather than individual format. Another area in which groups might have an advantage over individual therapy is in outcomes other than PTSD symptoms. The interpersonal interactions and support associated with group approaches could, in principle, provide an advantage in social adjustment and quality-of-life measures compared to individual approaches, but this question has not been tested.

In conclusion, despite advances, there are still relatively few well-designed randomized studies in this area to provide definitive answers to several questions. The research evidence for group therapy for PTSD shows positive change from pre- to posttreatment, and superiority relative to wait-list controls. Cognitive-behavioral approaches remain the most frequently studied. There is no evidence of superiority of one type of group therapy versus another, nor of additional benefits of focusing on trauma, although this question warrants further study. Little is known regarding moderators and mediators of treatment outcome in group therapy for PTSD. Future studies are needed to determine the mechanisms of change in different modalities of group therapy.

References

Allen, S. N., & Bloom, S. L. (1994). Group and family treatment of posttraumatic stress disorder. *Psychiatric Clinics of North America, 17*, 425–437.

Baldwin, S. A., Murray, D. M., & Shadish, W. R. (2005). Empirically supported treatments or Type I errors?: Problems with the analysis of data from group-administered treatments. *Journal of Consulting and Clinical Psychology, 73*, 924–935.

Classen, C., Koopman, C., Nevill-Manning, K., & Spiegel, D. (2001). A preliminary report comparing trauma-focused and present-focused group therapy against a wait-listed condition among childhood sexual abuse survivors. *Journal of Aggression, Maltreatment and Trauma, 4*, 265–288.

Cloitre, M., & Koenen, K. C. (2001). The impact of borderline personality disorder on process group outcome among women with posttraumatic stress disorder related to childhood abuse. *International Journal of Group Psychotherapy, 51*, 379–398.

Cook, J. M., Walser, R. D., Kane, V., Ruzek, J. I., & Woody, G. (2006). Dissemination and feasibility of a cognitive-behavioral treatment for substance use disorders and posttraumatic stress disorder in the veterans administration. *Journal of Psychoactive Drugs, 38*, 89–92.

Creamer, M., Elliott, P., Forbes, D., Biddle, D., & Hawthorne, G. (2006). Treatment for combat-related posttraumatic stress disorder: Two-year follow-up. *Journal of Traumatic Stress, 19*, 675–685.

Donovan, B., Padin-Rivera, E., & Kowaliw, S. (2001). "Transcend": Initial outcomes from a posttraumatic stress disorder/substance abuse treatment program. *Journal of Traumatic Stress, 14*, 757–772.

Falsetti, S. A., Resnick, H. S., & Davis, J. (2005). Multiple channel exposure therapy: Combining cognitive-behavioral therapies for the treatment of posttraumatic stress disorder with panic attacks. *Behavior Modification, 29*, 70–94.

Falsetti, S. A., Resnick, H. S., Davis, J., & Gallagher, N. G. (2001). Treatment of posttraumatic stress disorder with comorbid panic attacks: Combining cognitive processing therapy with panic control treatment techniques. *Group Dynamics: Theory, Research, and Practice, 5*, 252–261.

Foy, D. W., Glynn, S. M., Schnurr, P. P., Jankowski, M. K., Wattenberg, M. S., Weiss, D. S., et al. (2000). Group therapy. In E. B. Foa, T. M. Keane, & M. J. Friedman (Eds.), *Effective treatments for PTSD: Practice guidelines from the International Society for Traumatic Stress Studies* (pp. 155–175). New York: Guilford Press.

Foy, D. W., Ruzek, J. I., Glynn, S. M., Riney, S. A., & Gusman, F. D. (1997). Trauma focused group therapy for combat-related PTSD. *Journal of Clinical Psychology, 3*, 59–73.

Frueh, B. C., Turner, S. M., Beidel, D. C., Mirabella, R. F., & Jones, W. J. (1996). Trauma management therapy: A preliminary evaluation of a multicomponent behavioral treatment for chronic combat-related PTSD. *Behaviour Therapy and Research, 34*, 533–543.

Hazzard, A., Rogers, J., & Angert, L. (1993). Factors affecting group therapy outcome for adult sexual abuse survivors. *International Journal of Group Psychotherapy, 43*(4), 453–468.

Klerman, G. L., Weissman, M. M., Rounsaville, B. J., & Chevron, E. S. (1984). *Interpersonal psychotherapy of depression.* New York: Basic Books.

Krakow, B., Hollifield, M., Johnston, L., Koss, M., Schrader, R., Warner, T. D., et al. (2001). Imagery rehearsal therapy for chronic nightmares in sexual assault survivors with posttraumatic stress disorder. *Journal of the American Medical Association, 286,* 537–545.

Krakow, B., Hollifield, M., Scharader, R., Koss, M., Tandberg, D., Lauriello, J., et al. (2000). A controlled study of imagery rehearsal for chronic nightmares with PTSD: A preliminary report. *Journal of Traumatic Stress, 13,* 589–609.

Krupnick, J. L., Green, B. L., Miranda, J., Stockton, P., & Mete, M. (in press). Group interpersonal therapy for low-income women with PTSD. *Psychotherapy Research.*

Linehan, M. M. (1993). *Cognitive-behavioral treatment of borderline personality disorder.* New York: Guilford Press.

Lubin, H., Loris, M., Burt, J., & Johnson, D. (1998). Efficacy of psychoeducational group therapy in reducing symptoms of posttraumatic stress disorder among multiply traumatized women. *American Journal of Psychiatry, 155*(9), 1172–1177.

Morgan, T., & Cummings, A. (1999). Change experienced during group therapy by female survivors of childhood sexual abuse. *Journal of Consulting and Clinical Psychology, 67*(1), 28–36.

Najavits, L. M. (2002). *Seeking Safety: Cognitive-behavioral therapy for PTSD and substance abuse.* New York: Guilford Press.

Najavits, L. M., Weiss, R. D., Shaw, S. R., & Muenz, L. R. (1998). "Seeking Safety": Outcome of a new cognitive-behavioral psychotherapy for women with posttraumatic stress disorder and substance dependence. *Journal of Traumatic Stress, 11,* 437–456.

Ready, D. J., Thomas, K. R., Worley, V., Backscheider, A. G., Harvey, L. A. C., Baltzell, D., et al. (2008). A field test of group based exposure therapy with 102 veterans with war-related posttraumatic stress disorder. *Journal of Traumatic Stress, 21,* 150–157.

Resick, P., Jordan, C., Girelli, S., Hutter, C., & Marhoefer-Dvorak, S. (1988). A comparative outcome study of behavioral group therapy for sexual assault victims. *Behavior Therapy, 19,* 385–401.

Resick, P., & Schnicke, M. (1992). Cognitive processing therapy for sexual assault victims. *Journal of Consulting and Clinical Psychology, 60*(5), 748–756.

Saxe, B. J., & Johnson, S. M. (1999). An empirical investigation of group treatment for a clinical population of adult female incest survivors. *Journal of Child Sexual Abuse, 8*(1), 67–88.

Schnurr, P. P., Friedman, M. J., Foy, D. W., Shea, M. T., Hsieh, F. Y., Lavori, P. W., et al. (2003). Randomized trial of trauma-focused group therapy for posttraumatic stress disorder. *Archives of General Psychiatry, 60,* 481–488.

Spiegel, D., Classen, C., Thurston, E., & Butler, L. (2004). Trauma-focused versus present-focused models of group therapy for women sexually abused in childhood. In L. J. Koenig, L. S. Doll, A. O'Leary, & W. Pequegnat (Eds.), *From childhood sexual abuse to adult sexual risk: Trauma, revictimization, and intervention* (pp. 251–268). Washington, DC: American Psychological Association.

Stalker, C., & Fry, R. (1999). A comparison of short-term group and individual therapy for sexually abused women. *Canadian Journal of Psychiatry, 44*(2), 168–174.

Stauffer, L., & Deblinger, E. (1996). Cognitive-behavioral groups for nonoffending mothers and their young sexually abused children: A preliminary treatment outcome study. *Child Maltreatment, 1*(1), 65–76.

Wallis, D. A. N. (2002). Reduction of trauma symptoms following group therapy. *Australian and New Zealand Journal of Psychiatry, 36,* 67–74.

Woodward, S. H., Dresher, K. D., Murphy, R. T., Ruzek, J. I., Foy, D. W., Arsenault, N. J., et al. (1997). Heart rate during group flooding therapy for PTSD. *Integrative Physiological and Behavioral Science, 32,* 19–30.

Yalom, I. D. (1995). *The theory and practice of group psychotherapy* (4th ed.). New York: Basic Books.

Zlotnick, C., Najavits, L. M., Rohsenow, D. J., & Johnson, D. M. (2003). A cognitive-behavioral treatment for incarcerated women with substance abuse disorder and posttraumatic stress disorder: Findings from a pilot study. *Journal of Substance Abuse Treatment, 25,* 99–105.

Zlotnick, C., Shea, T., Rosen, K., Simpson, E., Mulrenin, K., Begin, A., et al. (1997). An affect-management group for women with posttraumatic stress disorder and histories of childhood sexual abuse. *Journal of Traumatic Stress, 10*(3), 425–436.

CHAPTER 13

School-Based Treatment for Children and Adolescents

Lisa H. Jaycox, Bradley D. Stein,
and Lisa Amaya-Jackson

Theoretical Context

The field of child traumatic stress has grown substantially over the last decade—with research and policy efforts targeting the impact of trauma in the lives of children well beyond the accommodations made in the diagnostic criteria for posttraumatic stress disorder (PTSD) in DSM-IV (American Psychiatric Association, 1994, 2000). Subsequent development of trauma-focused interventions for children and adolescents has been gaining empirical momentum, with study outcomes targeting not only full-blown PTSD but also the broader presence of symptoms of PTSD, depression, anxiety, disruptive behaviors, and emotional dysregulation. Refinements of these protocols include considerations made for a child developmental framework, a time line guiding whether interventions should ideally be delivered in the acute aftermath of a traumatic event or somewhat later, and an appropriate delivery setting. This chapter focuses on the development and implementation of trauma programs in the school setting. Several lines of recent research support the increased emphasis on developing, evaluating, and delivering trauma-focused programs in schools and include the following:

1. The sheer number of traumatized children attending schools is a public health concern that demands a public health approach to treatment using schools as the base and context in which children function on a daily basis.
2. Trauma affects learning and academic performance, making school the logical environment in which to address these issues, while also utilizing the school environment to facilitate healing of other aspects of traumatic consequence.
3. High-profile, catastrophic traumatic events happening to children in schools have mandated a mental health response at the school level. Early studies in this area led to the recognition that many of these children had been exposed to multiple traumatic events and traumatic stress levels rather than to a single school crisis incident.

This chapter briefly highlights the context for treating child traumatic stress in school settings, reviews the literature supporting treatment approaches in schools, offers a description of techniques used, and identifies empirical support for the reviewed school-based treatment or intervention programs for child traumatic stress.

Child Traumatic Stress and Its Impact

Exposure to trauma—as a witness or as a victim—is a large problem for youth in the United States. Particularly noteworthy is exposure to community and home interpersonal violence (including child abuse and neglect). In fact, pubic health officials have declared that interpersonal violence is one of the most significant public health issues globally (Koop & Lundberg, 1992; Krug, Dahlberg, Mercy, Zwi, & Lozano, 2002; U.S. Public Health Service, 2000). Other forms of trauma—sudden death of a loved one, acute or chronic medical illness, and vehicular and other accidents—also have a significant impact on youth. War, terrorism, and large-scale natural disasters have highlighted the issues of trauma exposure and loss around the globe, with a growing recognition of the impact of these horrors on children.

Trauma often leaves lingering mental health problems that interfere with key developmental and functional outcomes. Trauma exposure may precipitate PTSD, anxiety and depressive symptoms, and aggressive and delinquent behaviors (American Academy of Child and Adolescent Psychiatry, 1998). Traumatic life experiences, particularly interpersonal ones, have important public health implications because they increase the risk of serious health problems (Sachs-Ericsson, Plant, Blazer, & Arnow, 2005); high-risk behaviors, such as alcohol and substance use (Back et al., 2000; DeBellis, 2002), teen pregnancy (Anda et al., 2002); and suicidal ideation and suicidal behavior (Ullman & Brecklin, 2002; Ystgaard, Hestetun, Loeb, & Mehlum, 2004). Trauma exposure affects school functioning (Garbarino, Dubrow, Kostelny, & Pardo, 1992; Hurt, Malmud, Brodsky, & Giannetta, 2001; Saigh, Mroueh, & Bremner, 1997; Schwab-Stone et al., 1995), and violence exposure is associated with lower grade point average (GPA), more days of school absence (Hurt et al., 2001), and decreased rates of high school graduation (Beers & DeBellis, 2002; Delaney-Black et al., 2002; Grogger, 1997), as well as significant deficits in attention, abstract reasoning, long-term memory for verbal information, and reading ability, and decreased IQ (Beers & DeBellis, 2002). Given the effects of trauma across multiple developmental domains, including a negative effect on successful academic achievement, there is a pressing need to combine mental health and educational efforts to support traumatized children.

In the United States, a disproportionate burden of trauma exposure is borne by low-income and minority children and their families, for whom environmental factors, such as poverty, low median value of housing, and high percentage of adults who dropped out of school, are associated with an increased risk factors for violence exposure and mental health problems (Coulton, Korbin, Su, & Chow, 1995; Garbarino, 1995; Stein, Jaycox, Kataoka, Rhodes, & Vestal, 2003; Straussner & Straussner, 1997). From the perspective of educators, the negative effects of trauma exposure on academic functioning may explain one aspect of the "racial achievement gap," the fact that African American and Latino students trail behind their European American peers in schools and have higher high school dropout rates (Shin, 2005).

Socioeconomically disadvantaged children also have the greatest difficulty accessing mental health services (U.S. Public Health Service, 2000). Uninsured children, and Latino and African American children, are at risk for not receiving specialty mental health care (Bussing, Zima, Perwien, Belin, & Widawski, 1998; Kataoka, Zhang, & Wells, 2002; Zima, Bussing, Yang, & Belin, 2000). Traumatized individuals are also less likely than their nontraumatized counterparts to seek health services (Guterman, Hahm, & Cameron, 2002). Thus, our most vulnerable youth are those least likely ever to receive traditional clinic-based mental health care.

Schools can serve an important role in addressing unmet mental health needs following trauma, beginning with their role in the immediate aftermath of a communitywide disaster or school crisis. In the immediate aftermath of traumatic events, both crisis intervention, which provides emotional support and psychoeducation as the school environment is stabilized and immediate safety concerns are addressed, and psychological first aid, which seeks to calm and reassure the school population once things are stabilized, are commonly used to support students.

Crisis intervention usually follows immediately after a critical incident in a school, such as violence on the school campus or the death of a student or teacher. During this period, the focus is on restoring stability to the school environment, helping highly affected students or teachers function, and ensuring safety and security in the school. Recommendations for such procedures have facilitated a standardized school crisis response across the country (see Dorn & Dorn, 2005; Duda, Shepherd, Dorn, Wong, & Thomas, 2004a, 2004b). These procedures, however, have not been formally evaluated.

Once stability has been restored, early intervention that focuses on support and education may begin. The lack of well-controlled studies supporting the effectiveness of early interventions is largely due to logistical and ethical issues in conducting studies in such situations (National Institute of Mental Health, 2002). However, a few programs implemented in schools have been evaluated (see Chapter 5 by Brymer et al., this volume, on psychological first aid for nonschool crisis intervention). For instance, a naturalistic study of students exposed to the *Jupiter* shipping disaster, who underwent a problem-solving debriefing meeting 10 days postdisaster compared with affected students in another school who did not accept the intervention, found that students in the intervention school reported fewer PTSD symptoms and less fear 5–9 months later (Yule, 1992).

Collectively, these lines of evidence suggest that schools have much potential as a setting in which to intervene for trauma-related behavioral and emotional problems. Delivering mental health services in schools can address key financial and structural barriers that often prevent socioeconomically disadvantaged and minority children from receiving needed services (Garrison, Roy, & Azar, 1999). Schools have long been identified as an ideal entry point for improving access to mental health services for children (Allensworth, Lawson, Nicholson, & Wyche, 1997). In addition to providing access to children who otherwise may not have received services in traditional service settings, use of the school environment where children do their day-to-day "work"— that of learning with the help of trusted authority figures—can facilitate a sense of normality and integration of the work done in treatment with the natural progression of academic and social learning with peers. Group work is more easily facilitated in schools than in clinics by virtue of the number of students of similar age range that is present. Links to how trauma reminders and traumatic symptoms affect day-to-day function and peer relations can often be addressed easily, particularly in a group scenario. This principle of using the natural environment to facilitate recovery is considered critical following mass tragedy and disaster (Amaya-Jackson et al., 2003; Macy, 2003; National Child Traumatic Stress Network, 2006), and should be considered and evaluated as to whether it may be a mediator for treatment outcome for other traumas. Regardless of whether an intervention is designed as an acute or intermediate response to traumatic events, or whether the interventions are schoolwide or represent focused treatment for select children, the positive effect of a trauma-informed school environment does not happen automatically, instead requiring work and nurtured partnership between mental health and school personnel.

Description of Techniques

School interventions can be of several types, including schoolwide, curricular-type interventions, selected or indicated interventions for "at-risk" students, or treatment for children with PTSD that occurs at school. Most of the school programs developed to date are of the second type; therefore, they include some kind of screening or identification process to determine which students might benefit from the intervention.

School intervention programs for trauma or PTSD have incorporated several different kinds of techniques, but the predominant techniques are drawn from cognitive-behavioral therapy (CBT). The core components of CBT can be summarized by the acronym PRACTICE: Parental treatment component, Psychoeducation, Relaxation and stress management skills, Affective expression and modulation skills, Cognitive coping skills, Trauma narrative, *In vivo* desensitization of trauma reminders, Conjoint sessions for parents, and Enhancing safety and future development (Cohen, Mannarino, & Deblinger, 2006). Because most of these techniques lend themselves well to group formats in the school setting, they can be adapted for school use; several such programs have been developed and tested. In addition, some incorporate techniques drawn from psychodynamic theories or crisis intervention models as well (see Lieberman, Ghosh Ippen, & Marans, Chapter 15, and Brymer et al., Chapter 5, this volume). However, several important adjustments to clinic-based CBT are required for successful school interventions.

First, CBT in clinics is usually delivered in individual or conjoint (parent and child) sessions, whereas school-based programs tend to be delivered in group format. Thus, the didactics are presented in a classroom-style format, and exercises and experiential learning are reformatted to include a group of children rather than an individual child. This group formatting does not allow as easily for individual tailoring of the pace and focus of therapy, but it does provide a way for students to learn from their peers, and to gain and utilize peer support in a way that is lacking in individual therapy.

Second, as outlined earlier, school-based interventions may be more feasible and acceptable to some families. Issues related to stigma and barriers to intervention, such as cost, transportation, and time, are at least partially removed in the school setting, enabling children in families who are not yet "ready" to seek specialty care, or who are unable to do so easily, to receive much-needed services.

Third, conjoint parent sessions are rarely feasible in the school setting due to both scheduling issues and the fact that parents are not as engaged in the therapy process as they are in clinic-based therapy. Normally, school programs identify children in need and offer services, whereas parents bring children in for treatment in a clinic setting. Thus, parents are not necessarily "ready" to engage in therapy themselves in a school-based intervention. The advantage of being able to work with children who have not entered the specialty mental health sector may be offset in some cases by the lack of full engagement of parents in services. When the latter is true, considerable effort on the part of treatment providers may be required when parental involvement is necessary. By the same token, youth whose parents are unable or unwilling to engage in treatment are able to access services they would otherwise not receive, and have additional allies in the treatment process that they might not otherwise have had.

Fourth, facilitation of the trauma narrative may be less comprehensive in school-based interventions, which are often briefer than clinic-based interventions. Time and logistical limitations of school-based interventions do not always allow for thorough processing for all relevant traumas, particularly for children who have multiple traumatic events, and students sometimes need to be referred into continuing care for a secondary phase of therapy.

Method of Collecting Data

Because this is a newly developing field, we conducted a formal literature search and augmented it in several ways. For the formal literature, we searched several relevant databases for papers in English period 1986–2006: Cumulative Index to Nursing and Allied Health Literature (CINAHL); Criminal Justice Abstracts; Education Research Information Center (ERIC); National Criminal Justice Reference Service Abstracts; PubMed; PsycINFO; Social Science Abstracts; Social Services Abstracts; and Sociological Abstracts. We included five concepts: (trauma *or* disaster *or* abuse *or* violence); (adolescent *or* child*); (PTSD *or* stress *or* post-traumatic stress *or* posttraumatic stress); (treat* *or* intervention *or* psych* *or* psychotherapy); and (school). This search produced 186 potentially relevant articles that we examined more closely for inclusion. We examined studies and programs presented in review articles that this search discovered as well. Our augmentation of this search by programs listed on the National Child Traumatic Stress Network website, by expert nomination, and through work we conducted in the Gulf States region following the hurricanes of 2005 uncovered some additional programs. This augmentation (snowball technique) uncovered a number of programs that, although under development, are not yet evaluated in the published literature.

We eliminated the following from our review: programs not specifically focused on trauma; those not conducted in regular school settings or as only a small part of a larger community effort or program; programs based on dissertation studies only; clinic treatments offered to schoolchildren but not as a school program per se; and preventive rather than intervention programs. We did not include community-based programs that simply include some school involvement (e.g., a wraparound program that includes school personnel in service consultation). We also do not discuss therapy elements or medication that school-based clinicians might use in their individual treatment of traumatized students. We also excluded from discussion programs described in a single paper, whose evaluation component we could not trace or for which we could find no updates on the Internet as to continued implementation or evaluation efforts.

Literature Review

A large number of programs have been developed with a treatment or intervention focus on reduction of students' trauma-related symptoms that endure beyond the immediate crisis. We focus only on school-specific programs that have a detailed program protocol or manual. We categorize them by the type of trauma they address, although several of them are flexible and can be used for many different types of trauma. We highlight within each category those programs that have been evaluated in published studies. Those studies that are rated as Level A or B in terms of evidence for reduction in PTSD symptoms are presented in Tables 13.1 and 13.2, respectively For the purposes of this chapter, Level A studies are defined as studies employing a randomized controlled design, and Level B studies employ a nonrandomized comparison group design. At present, there are two programs supported by Level A randomized trials, and three with Level B studies with uncontrolled comparison groups. Uncontrolled studies, and ones that do not assess PTSD symptoms directly, are not included in the tables, but they are described in the text. However, we also briefly present other, not yet evaluated programs because many promising approaches in this relatively new area of research have not yet undergone rigorous evaluation.

Programs Addressing Trauma of Many Types or Nonspecific Trauma

Evidence-Based Programs

Three programs have been developed specifically for use in schools and focus on a broad array of traumas: the cognitive-behavioral intervention for trauma in schools (CBITS; Jaycox, 2003); the multimodality trauma treatment (MMTT; Amaya-Jackson et al., 2003; March, Amaya-Jackson, Murray, & Schulte, 1998), and the UCLA Trauma/Grief Program (Goenjian et al., 2005; Saltzman, Steinberg, Layne, Aisenberg, & Pynoos, 2001). All three draw on evidence-based practices in treating trauma, largely cognitive-behavioral techniques, and all three have some empirical support for the reduction of trauma-related symptoms. CBITS has been evaluated in a quasi-experimental design for recent immigrant students ($N = 152$, treatment group; $N = 47$, waitlist control group) and in a randomized controlled trial of sixth and seventh graders ($N = 126$), and students have shown reductions in PTSD symptoms, as well as behavioral problems (Kataoka et al., 2003; Stein, Jaycox, Kataoka, Wong, et al., 2003). MMTT, evaluated with a staggered start date control design, showed decreases in PTSD, depressive, and anxiety symptoms among 14 treated students (March et al., 1998), and these effects have been replicated in subsequent studies (Amaya-Jackson et al., 2003). The UCLA Trauma/Grief Program showed reductions in PTSD and grief symptoms, and improve-

TABLE 13.1. A-Level Studies (Randomized Designs)

Study	Target population[a]	Number/length of sessions	Treatment(s)/control[b]	Major findings	Between-group effect sizes	Within-group effect sizes
Berger et al. (2007)	142 elementary students in Israel exposed to repeated terror attacks	8 weekly, 90-min sessions	*Overcoming the Threat of Terrorism (OTT)* 70 in OTT 64 in no treatment (NT)	In this randomized controlled trial (RCT), OTT participants showed significant reductions of PTSD symptoms, somatic complaints, and generalized and separation anxiety symptoms in 1 and 2 mo compared to NT controls.	*UCLA Reaction Index for DSM-IV* Intent to treat OTT vs. NT: 1.06	OTT: 1.14; NT: 0.04
Stein, Jaycox, Kataoka, Wong, et al. (2003)	126 middle school students in Los Angeles	10 weekly group sessions for 45–60 min; 1–3 individual sessions, 2–4 optional parent sessions, and 1 teacher educational session	*Cognitive-Behavioral Intervention for Trauma in Schools (CBITS)* 54 in CBITS 63 in wait list (WL)	In this RCT, CBITS participants showed significant reductions in PTSD symptoms, depressive symptoms, and parent (but not teacher) reports of behavior problems compared to controls.	*Child PTSD Symptom Scale* Completers CBITS vs. WL: 1.08 (reported by authors)	Unable to calculate

[a]N = subjects starting study or treatment.
[b]N = subjects in data analyses.

334

TABLE 13.2. B-Level Studies (Nonrandomized Control Groups)

Study	Target population[a]	Number/length of sessions	Treatment(s); control[b]	Major findings	Between-group effect sizes	Within-group effect sizes
Goenjian et al. (1997, 2005)	64 early adolescents exposed to the 1988 earthquake in Armenia	16–20 group sessions held weekly, lasting 50 min	*UCLA Trauma/Grief Program* 32 in program 27 in no treatment (NT)	In this quasi-experimental, controlled study, program participants showed significant reductions in PTSD and depression, and improvements in academic performance and classroom behaviors.	PTSD Reaction Index: 1.29 (1997) and 0.69 (2005, 2-year follow-up of population)	1997 1.5 to 3 yr program: 1.13; NT: 0.60 2005 1.5 to 5 yr program: 1.71; NT: 0.55
Kataoka et al. (2003)	113 Spanish-speaking recent immigrant students in Los Angeles	8 group sessions held weekly for 45–60 min; 1–3 individual sessions, 2–4 optional parent sessions, and 1 teacher educational session	*Cognitive-Behavioral Intervention for Trauma in Schools (CBITS)* 67 in CBITS 46 in wait list (WL)	In this quasi-experimental, controlled study, CBITS participants showed significant reductions in PTSD symptoms, depressive symptoms, and parent reports of behavior problems compared to controls.	Child PTSD Symptom Scale: 0.29	CBITS: 0.86; WL: 0.27
Khamis, Macy, & Coignez (2004)	Palestinian children ages 6–16	15 classroom sessions, three times a week over 5 wk	*Classroom-based intervention (CBI)* 380 in CBI 284 in WL	In this large, quasi-experimental field trial, CBI participants showed improved peer relations, communication, and day-to-day psychosocial functioning in West Bank/Gaza schools and camps compared to controls.	Impact of Events Scale (IES): 0.21 (ages 6–11) and 0.07 (ages 12–16)	IES, ages 6–11 CBI: 0.34; WL: 0.20 IES, ages 12–16 CBI: 0.19; WL: 0.08
March et al. (1998)	17 elementary and junior high students following a single-incident stressor	14 group sessions held weekly for 45–60 min and 2 individual sessions	*Multimodality Trauma Treatment (MMTT)* 14 in single-case across-setting design	In this single-case across-setting study, MMTT participants showed significant decreases in PTSD, depressive, and anxiety symptoms.	1.15	Unable to calculate

[a]*N* = subjects starting study or treatment.
[b]*N* = subjects in data analyses.

335

improvements in GPA among 26 participants, but no changes in depressive symptoms between pre- and posttest when adapted for community violence and implemented in Southern California (Layne, Pynoos, & Cardenas, 2001; Saltzman, Pynoos, Layne, Steinberg, & Aisenberg, 2001). Likewise, it demonstrated reductions in PTSD symptoms in two field trials of a brief version of the program following an earthquake in Armenia (Goenjian et al., 1997, 2005). In addition, the program was implemented in postwar Bosnia (Layne, Pynoos, Saltzman, et al., 2001).

These three programs focus on both symptom reduction and skills building (affect regulation and anxiety reduction via specific coping skills), and include some method for processing the traumatic event through imagination, drawing, or construction of a trauma narrative. The CBITS and MMTT programs are implemented with groups of students, whereas the UCLA Trauma/Grief Program is run with individual students or groups. All three programs serve students from late elementary school through early high school, and are being implemented in several school districts in the United States.

Emerging Programs

Several other programs fit into this category, but do not yet have effectiveness data to consider. These include an adaptation of trauma-focused cognitive-behavioral therapy (TF-CBT; Cohen, Deblinger, Mannarino, & Steer, 2004) that has recently been implemented in school settings; the Community Outreach Program—Esperanza (COPE; de Arellano et al., 2005), which integrates the core components of a TF-CBT package with parent–child interaction therapy (Chaffin et al., 2004; Eyberg et al., 2001); and a trauma-focused motivational/CBT/eye movement desensitization and reprocessing (EMDR)–based program for adolescents with conduct problems (Greenwald, 2002). In addition, there are two programs that focus on the whole classroom or school rather than selecting students in need: the School Interaction Project (SIP), with a focus on affect regulation and problem solving (see Jaycox, Morse, Tanielian, & Stein, 2006, for details); and Better Todays, Better Tomorrows for Children's Mental Health (B2-T2; Kirkwood & Stamm, 2004, 2006), which educates school staff to raise awareness about the emotional consequences of trauma rather than intervening directly with students. Neither of these has been evaluated to date.

Programs Addressing Disasters (Natural or Man Made), Terrorism, and War

Evidence-Based Programs

There also have been some notable international efforts in regions affected by disaster or ongoing terrorist threat, five of which have been evaluated. The classroom-based intervention program (CBI; Macy, Bary, & Noam, 2003), a 15-session, classroom-based intervention providing a psychoeducational curriculum for children ages 7–19, is used to address critical needs of children and youth exposed to threat and terror. The themes are (1) information, safety, and control; (2) stabilization, awareness, and self-esteem; (3) survival narrative—thoughts and reactions during danger to the individual and his or her loved ones; (4) survival narrative—resource identification and coping skills; and (5) resource installation and future planning (Macy et al., 2003). Preliminary evaluations in Turkey following an earthquake and in the West Bank/Gaza schools and camps for Palestinian refugees show improvements among children (ages 4–11) and female adolescents (ages 12–16) in a large, randomized controlled field trial of 664 children and adolescents. Improvements were noted on multiple domains, including communication, social support, negotiation skills, use of relaxation as a coping strategy, and, among younger children, decreasing emotional and behavior problems. No improvements were noted among adolescent boys (ages 12–16), however (Khamis, Macy, & Coignez, 2004). An eight-session program for second through sixth graders, Overshadowing the Threat of Terrorism (OTT), has been used and evaluated in Israel (Berger, Pat-Horenczyk, & Gelkopf, 2007). In this randomized controlled trial, 70 children who took part in the intervention showed reduced PTSD, somatic, and anxiety symptoms 2 months after the intervention, as compared to controls. OTT includes coping skills and psychoeducation to help children handle the ongoing threat of terrorism.

Another disaster-related program, the Maile Project, is a four-session psychoeducational program developed for students with lingering PTSD symptoms following Hurricane Iniki in Hawaii. Designed for symptomatic elementary school children, the program, via statewide screening, showed reductions in trauma-related problems among 214 children who underwent either group or individual versions of the program (Chemtob, Nakashima, & Hamada, 2002).

The catastrophic stress intervention (CSI), implemented in the aftermath of Hurricane Hugo in affected South Carolina high schools, comprises group meetings three times each year, for 3 years, focused on understanding stress and coping, increasing social support, and increasing self-efficacy through art. In a quasi-experimental field study, the program was shown to be effective in reducing mental distress during the 2 years following the hurricane but dissipated at later time points (Hardin, Weinrich, Garrison, Addy, & Hardin, 2002). Another program implemented in Turkey following the 1999 earthquake showed positive impact of a teacher-mediated intervention compared to a matched control group (Wolmer, Laor, Dedeoglu, Siev, & Yazgan, 2005).

Emerging Programs

Several other, similar programs have been developed but not yet evaluated: an adaptation of CBI being implemented by Save the Children in the aftermath of Hurricane Katrina called psychosocial structured activities (PSSA; for details, see *www.savethechildren.org* or Jaycox, Morse, et al., 2006); two programs in the development phase called Journey to Resilience and Enhancing Resilience among Students Experiencing Stress (ERASE-S; for details, see Jaycox, Morse, et al., 2006); and three other programs developed for children exposed to war. These programs also have had some positive impact in uncontrolled trials or small pilot studies, including a mind–body skills program for children exposed to war in Kosovo (Gordon, Staples, Blyta, & Bytyqi, 2004); a cognitive-behavioral program for refugees and asylum seekers (Ehntholt, Smith, & Yule, 2005), a trauma healing and peace program for children exposed to war in Croatia (Woodside, Santa Barbara, & Benner, 1999), and three programs implemented for students displaced by Hurricanes Katrina and Rita: Silver Linings, Friends and New Places, and an adaptation of the UCLA Trauma/Grief Program in the wake of Hurricane Katrina (for details, see Jaycox, Morse, et al., 2006). In addition, Healing after Trauma Skills (HATS; Gurwitch & Messenbaugh, 2005) was developed for use in Oklahoma City schools following the Oklahoma City bombing in 1995, and the Resiliency and Skills Building Workshop Series, a five-session curriculum implemented in Health classes in high schools, has been implemented in New York City schools impacted by the attacks on September 11, 2001 (for details, see Jaycox, Morse, et al., 2006).

Evidence-Based Programs Addressing Loss

Most of the trauma programs described earlier have some focus on loss, which is often a part of the traumatic experience, but some school programs have been developed specifically for loss, such as the sudden or violent death of a loved one. Unfortunately, only one program has undergone any evaluation. The Three-Dimensional Grief Program, also known as the School-Based Mourning Project (Sklarew, Krupnick, Ward-Wimmer, & Napoli, 2002), is for school-age children and focuses on the loss of any loved one. It aims to facilitate the grieving process and restore ego-integrity. In a randomized study of 43 treated and 30 control children, participants showed significant improvement on developmental indicators from Draw-a-Person tests, and teachers and parents reported children's increased capacity for empathy and compassion and ability to concentrate, and a decreased tendency to act out aggressive impulses (Skarlew, Krupnick, Ward-Wimmer, & Napoli, 2004; Sklarew et al., 2002), but the data presented do not allow effect size calculation. Three other programs, the Loss and Bereavement Program for Children and Adolescents (L&BP), PeaceZone (Prothrow-Stith et al., 2005), and Rainbows, all focus on loss but have no published evaluations (for details, see *www.rainbows.org* or Jaycox, Morse, et al., 2006).

Programs Addressing Violence

Evidence-Based Programs

In addition to programs like CBITS and MMTT that include children exposed to violence, one evaluated program focused specifically on violence.

Children's well-being groups are offered to those referred by school staff or parents, and focus on reducing behavior problems and improving social competence among elementary students exposed to domestic violence or other adversities at home. Data from an open trial show pre- to posttest improvements on these dimensions (Johnston, 2003).

Emerging Programs

Two other approaches have been developed that operate at the school level, without identifying specific students, but neither has been formally evaluated to date. Safe Harbor (U.S. Department of Justice Office for Victims of Crime, 2003) is a schoolwide program for sixth- to 12th-grade students, and a related program, Relation Abuse Prevention Program (RAPP), is very similar to Safe Harbor but focuses on dating and relationship violence.

Emerging Programs Addressing Complex Trauma

Several programs also have been developed to address complex trauma in schools. "Complex trauma" is defined as experiences of multiple traumatic events within the caregiving system, in place of the safety and stability that is normally provided therein (Cook, Blaustein, Spinazzola, & van der Kolk, 2003). Although students participating in the programs described earlier often have experienced more than one traumatic event, sometimes including complex trauma, these particular programs are designed to deal with personality issues, difficulties with emotion regulation, and impulsive or risky behaviors seen in the aftermath of complex trauma. None of these programs to date has published effectiveness studies in children. Life Skills/Life Stories (Cloitre, Koenen, Cohen, & Han, 2002), a clinical program for women, has been adapted for female high school students with histories of sexual victimization and child abuse. Trauma adaptive recovery group education and therapy for adolescents (TARGET-A; Ford, Mahoney, & Russo, 2001) focuses on body self-regulation, memory, interpersonal problem solving, and stress management. Structured Psychotherapy for Adolescents Responding to Chronic Stress (SPARCS; DeRosa & Pelcovitz, 2008) is for teens of both genders and focuses on coping, relationships, and improving functioning in the present. It comprises 22 group sessions and combines techniques from trauma programs (UCLA Trauma/Grief Program and TARGET-A) and from dialectical behavior therapy for adolescents (Rathus & Miller, 2000).

Summary and Recommendations

As can be seen in this literature review, a great deal of work is being done to bring trauma-focused interventions into schools. Much of this work is international, in war-torn regions, but it also occurs within the United States in response to issues such as natural disasters, terrorism, violence, and loss.

Although intervention development is burgeoning, evaluation of these programs is lagging behind. To date, there are only a handful of studies for which effect sizes have been reported or can be calculated. Of these programs, some report nonsignificant findings, whereas others report large effects. Only two studies to date have used randomized controlled trials, and both (CBITS and OTT) reported moderate to large effects (Berger et al., 2007; Stein, Jaycox, Kataoka, Wong, et al., 2003). Because school-based research can be extremely challenging, particularly when it deals with sensitive issues such as violence and trauma exposure (Jaycox, McCaffrey, et al., 2006), many other studies have relied on quasi-experimental designs. Several of these programs have shown medium effects (e.g., CBI: Khamis et al., 2004; MMTT: March et al., 1998; UCLA Trauma/Grief Program: Goengian et al., 1997, 2005).

In general, cognitive-behavioral programs show positive effects in the school setting, but many other approaches remain untested. Clearly, more research is needed in this area. Worth noting is that most of these programs have been developed and initiated in the school setting, reducing implementation challenges involved in translation from clinic or university settings that are unfamiliar with school-specific needs and barriers. Implementation evaluation and research on intervention use in "real-world settings" have been heralded as critical next steps for the field of mental health effectiveness studies. Noted researchers are challenging the field to make treatments "community-based" instead of university-based, to allow for effectiveness in real-world settings (Chorpita et al., 2002; Weisz, Donenberg, Han, & Weiss, 1995). Increasing integration of the systems issues schools face in total, and the intervention delivery issues schools face specifically, into intervention development and research has clearly begun in the interventions described in this chapter, and will be a critical element in the challenge of broader dissemination and intervention of these and other school-based mental health treatments.

References

Allensworth, D., Lawson, E., Nicholson, L., & Wyche, J. (1997). *Schools and health: Our nation's investment.* Washington, DC: National Academy Press.

Amaya-Jackson, L., Reynolds, V., Murray, M. C., McCarthy, G., Nelson, A., Cherney, M. S., et al. (2003). Cognitive-behavioral treatment for pediatric posttraumatic stress disorder: Protocol and application in school and community settings. *Cognitive and Behavioral Practice, 10*(3), 204–213.

American Academy of Child and Adolescent Psychiatry. (1998). Practice parameters for the diagnosis and treatment of posttraumatic stress disorder in children and adolescents. *Journal of the American Academy of Child and Adolescent Psychiatry, 36*(Suppl.), 4S–26S.

American Psychiatric Association. (1994). *Diagnostic and statistical manual of mental disorders* (4th ed.). Washington, DC: Author.

American Psychiatric Association. (2000). *Diagnostic and statistical manual of mental disorders* (4th ed. text revision). Washington, DC: Author.

Anda, R. F., Chapman, D. P., Felitti, V. J., Edwards, V., Williamson, D. F., Croft, J. B., et al. (2002). Adverse childhood experiences and risk of paternity in teen pregnancy. *Obstetrics and Gynecology, 100*(1), 37–45.

Back, S., Dansky, B., Coffey, S., Saladin, M., Sonne, S., & Brady, K. (2000). Cocaine dependence with and without posttraumatic stress disorder: A comparison of substance abuse, trauma history and psychiatric comorbidity. *American Journal on Addictions, 9*(1), 51–62.

Beers, S., & DeBellis, M. (2002). Neuropsychological function in children with maltreatment-related posttraumatic stress disorder. *American Journal of Psychiatry, 159,* 483–486.

Berger, R., Pat-Horenczyk, R., & Gelkopf, M. (2007). School-based intervention for prevention and treatment of elementary students' terror-related distress in Israel: A quasi-randomized controlled trial. *Journal of Traumatic Stress, 20*(4), 541–552.

Bussing, R., Zima, B. T., Perwien, A. R., Belin, T. R., & Widawski, M. (1998). Children in special education programs: Attention deficit hyperactivity disorder, use of services, and unmet needs. *American Journal of Public Health, 88*(6), 880–886.

Chaffin, M., Silovsky, J. F., Funderburk, B., Valle, L. A., Brestan, E. V., Balachova, T., et al. (2004). Parent–child interaction therapy with physically abusive parents: Efficacy for reducing future abuse reports. *Journal of Consulting and Clinical Psychology, 72*(3), 500–510.

Chemtob, C. M., Nakashima, J. P., & Hamada, R. S. (2002). Psychosocial intervention for postdisaster trauma symptoms in elementary school children: A controlled community field study. *Archives of Pediatrics and Adolescent Medicine, 156*(3), 211–216.

Chorpita, B. F., Yim, L. M., Dorkervoet, J. C., Arensdorf, A., Admundsen, M. J., McGee, C., et al. (2002). Toward large-scale implementation of empirically supported treatments for children: A review and observations by the Hawaii Empirical Basis to Services Task Force. *Clinical Psychology: Science and Practice, 9*(2), 165–190.

Cloitre, M., Koenen, K., Cohen, L. R., & Han, H. (2002). Skills training in affective and interpersonal regulation followed by exposure: A phase-based treatment for PTSD related to childhood abuse. *Journal of Consulting and Clinical Psychology, 70,* 1067–1074.

Cohen, J. A., Deblinger, E., Mannarino, A. P., & Steer, R. A. (2004). A multisite, randomized controlled trial for children with sexual abuse-related PTSD symptoms. *Journal of the American Academy of Child and Adolescent Psychiatry, 43*(4), 393–402.

Cohen, J. A., Mannarino, A. P., & Deblinger, E. (2006). *Treating trauma and traumatic grief in children and adolescents.* New York: Guilford Press.

Cook, A., Blaustein, M., Spinazzola, J., & van der Kolk, B. (2003). *Complex trauma in children and adolescents: National Child Traumatic Stress Network.* Retrieved April 7, 2006, from *www.nctsnet.org/nctsn_assets/pdfs/edu_materials/complextrauma_all.pdf*

Coulton, C. J., Korbin, J. E., Su, M., & Chow, J. (1995). Community level factors and child maltreatment rates. *Child Development, 66*(5), 1262–1276.

de Arellano, M. A., Waldrop, A. E., Deblinger, E., Cohen, J. A., Danielson, C. K., & Mannarino, A. R. (2005). Community outreach program for child victims of traumatic events: A community-based project for underserved populations. *Behavior Modification* [Special issue: Beyond Exposure for Posttraumatic Stress Disorder Symptoms: Broad Spectrum PTSD Treatment Strategies], *29*(1), 130–155.

DeBellis, M. (2002). Developmental traumatology: A contributory mechanism for alcohol and substance use disorders. *Psychoneuroendocrinology, 27*(1–2), 155–170.

Delaney-Black, V., Covington, C., Ondersma, S. J., Nordstrom-Klee, B., Templin, T., Ager, J., et al. (2002). Violence exposure, trauma, and IQ and/or reading deficits among urban children. *Archives of Pediatric and Adolescent Medicine, 156,* 280–285.

DeRosa, R., & Pelcovitz, D. (2008). Group treatment for chronically traumatized adolescents: Igniting SPARCS of change. In J. D. Brom, R. Pat-Horenczyk, & J. Ford (Eds.), *Treating traumatized children: Risk, resilience, and recovery* (pp. 225–239). London: Routledge.

Dorn, M., & Dorn, C. (2005). *Innocent targets: When terrorism comes to school.* Macon, GA: Safe Havens International.

Duda, R., Shepherd, S., Dorn, M., Wong, M., & Thomas, G. (2004a). *Jane's: School safety handbook, second edition.* Coulsdon, UK: Jane's Information Group.

Duda, R., Shepherd, S., Dorn, M., Wong, M., & Thomas, G. (2004b). *Jane's: Teachers' safety guide.* Coulsdon, UK: Jane's Information Group.

Ehntholt, K. A., Smith, P. A., & Yule, W. (2005). School-based cognitive-behavioural therapy group intervention for refugee children who have experienced war-related trauma. *Clinical Child Psychology and Psychiatry, 10*(2), 235–250.

Eyberg, S., Funderburk, B., Hembree-Kigin, T., McNeil, C., Querido, J., & Hood, K. (2001). Parent–child interaction therapy with behavior problem children: One and two year maintenance of treatment effects in the family. *Child and Family Behavior Therapy, 23,* 1–20.

Ford, J., Mahoney, K., & Russo, E. (2001). *TARGET and FREEDOM (for children).* Farmington: University of Connecticut Health Center.

Garbarino, J. (1995). The American war zone: What children can tell us about living with violence. *Journal of Developmental and Behavioral Pediatrics, 16*(6), 431–435.

Garbarino, J., Dubrow, N., Kostelny, K., & Pardo, C. (1992). *Children in danger: Coping with the consequences of community violence.* San Francisco: Jossey-Bass.

Garrison, E. G., Roy, I. S., & Azar, V. (1999). Responding to the mental health needs of Latino children and families through school-based services. *Clinical Psychology Review, 19*(2), 199–219.

Goenjian A. K., Pynoos, R. S., Karayan, I., Minassian, D., Najarian, L. M., Steinberg, A. M., et al. (1997). Outcome of psychotherapy among pre-adolescents after the 1988 earthquake in Armenia. *American Journal of Psychiatry, 154,* 536–542.

Goenjian, A. K., Walling, D., Steinberg, A. M., Karayan, I., Najarian, L. M., & Pynoos, R. S. (2005). A prospective study of posttraumatic stress and depressive reactions among treated and untreated adolescents 5 years after a catastrophic disaster. *American Journal of Psychiatry, 162,* 2302–2308.

Gordon, J. S., Staples, J. K., Blyta, A., & Bytyqi, M. (2004). Treatment of posttraumatic stress disorder in postwar Kosovo high school students using mind–body skills groups: A pilot study. *Journal of Traumatic Stress, 17*(2), 143–147.

Greenwald, R. (2002). Motivation–adaptive skills–trauma resolution (MASTR) therapy for adolescents with conduct problems: An open trial. *Journal of Aggression, Maltreatment and Trauma, 6*(1), 237–261.

Grogger, J. (1997). Local violence and educational attainment. *Journal of Human Resources, 32*(4), 659–682.

Gurwitch, R. H., & Messenbaugh, A. K. (2005). *Healing after trauma skills, 2nd edition.* Retrieved April 7, 2006, from *www.nctsnet.org/nctsn_assets/pdfs/edu_materials/ hats2ndedition.pdf*

Guterman, N. B., Hahm, H. C., & Cameron, M. (2002). Adolescent victimization and subsequent use of mental health counseling services. *Journal of Adolescent Health, 30*(5), 336–345.

Hardin, S. B., Weinrich, M., Garrison, C., Addy, C., & Hardin, T. L. (2002). Effects of a long-term psychosocial nursing intervention on adolescents exposed to catastrophic stress. *Issues in Mental Health Nursing, 23*(6), 537–551.

Hurt, H., Malmud, E., Brodsky, N. L., & Giannetta, J. (2001). Exposure to violence: Psychological and academic correlates in child witnesses. *Archives of Pediatrics and Adolescent Medicine, 155*, 1351–1356.

Jaycox, L. H. (2003). *Cognitive-behavioral intervention for trauma in schools.* Longmont, CO: Sopris West Educational Services.

Jaycox, L. H., McCaffrey, D. F., Ocampo, B. W., Shelley, G. A., Blake, S. M., Peterson, D. J., et al. (2006). Challenges in the evaluation and implementation of school-based prevention and intervention programs on sensitive topics. *American Journal of Evaluation, 27*(3), 320–336.

Jaycox, L. H., Morse, L., Tanielian, T., & Stein, B. D. (2006). *How schools can help students recover from traumatic experiences: A toolkit for supporting long-term recovery.* Santa Monica, CA: RAND Corporation.

Johnston, J. R. (2003). Group interventions for children at risk from family abuse and exposure to violence: A report of a study. *Journal of Emotional Abuse, 3*(3/4), 203–226.

Kataoka, S. H., Stein, B. D., Jaycox, L. H., Wong, M., Escudero, P., Tu, W., et al. (2003). A school-based mental health program for traumatized Latino immigrant children. *Journal of the American Academy of Child and Adolescent Psychiatry, 42*(3), 311–318.

Kataoka, S. H., Zhang, L., & Wells, K. B. (2002). Unmet need for mental health care among U.S. children: Variation by ethnicity and insurance status. *American Journal of Psychiatry, 159*(9), 1548–1555.

Khamis, V., Macy, R., & Coignez, V. (2004). *Impact of the Classroom/Community/Camp-Based Intervention Program on Palestinian children: USAID Report on Palestinian Children.* Available at *http://savethechildren.org/publications/technical-resources/education/CBI.Impact.Evaluation.pdf*

Kirkwood, A. D., & Stamm, B. H. (2004). Confronting stigma: An Idaho community-based social marketing campaign. In K. Robinson (Ed.), *Advances in school-based mental health care: Best practices and program models* (pp. 21–22). Kingston, NJ: Civic Research Institute.

Kirkwood, A. D., & Stamm, B. H. (2006). A social marketing approach to challenging stigma. *Professional Psychology: Research and Practice, 37*(5), 472–476.

Koop, C. E., & Lundberg, G. B. (1992). Violence in America: A public health emergency: Time to bite the bullet back. *Journal of the American Medical Association, 267*, 3075–3076.

Krug, E. G., Dahlberg, L. L., Mercy, J. A., Zwi, A. B., & Lozano, R. (Eds.). (2002). *World report on violence and health.* Geneva: World Health Organization.

Layne, C. M., Pynoos, R. S., & Cardenas, J. (2001). Wounded adolescence: School-based group psychotherapy for adolescents who sustained or witnessed violent injury. In M. Shafii & S. Shafii (Eds.), *School violence: Contributing factors, management, and prevention* (pp. 163–180). Washington, DC: American Psychiatric Press.

Layne, C. M., Pynoos, R. S., Saltzman, W. R., Arslanagic, B., Black, M., Savjak, N., et al. (2001). Trauma/grief-focused group psychotherapy: School-based postwar intervention with traumatized Bosnian adolescents. *Group Dynamics, 5,* 277–290.

Macy, R. D. (2003). Community-based trauma response for youth. *New Directions for Youth Development, 98,* 29–49.

Macy, R. D., Bary, S., & Noam, G. G. (2003). Youth facing threat and terror: Supporting preparedness and resilience. In *New directions for youth development* (pp. 51–79). San Francisco: Jossey-Bass.

March, J. S., Amaya-Jackson, L., Murray, M. C., & Schulte, A. (1998). Cognitive-behavioral psychotherapy for children and adolescents with posttraumatic stress disorder after a single-incident stressor. *Journal of the American Academy of Child and Adolescent Psychiatry, 37*(6), 585–593.

National Child Traumatic Stress Network and National Center for PTSD. (2006). *Psychological first aid: Field operations guide* (2nd ed.). Available online at *www.nctsn. org* and *www.ncptsd.va.gov*

National Institute of Mental Health. (2002). *Mental health and mass violence: Evidence-based early psychological intervention for victims/survivors of mass violence: A workshop to reach consensus on best practices.* Washington, DC: U.S. Government Printing Office.

Prothrow-Stith, D., Chery, T., Oliver, J., Feldman, M., Chery, J., & Shamis, F. (2005). *The PeaceZone: A program for social literacy.* Champaign, IL: Research Press.

Rathus, J. H., & Miller, A. L. (2000). DBT for adolescents: Dialectical dilemmas and secondary treatment targets. *Cognitive and Behavioral Practice, 7,* 425–434.

Sachs-Ericsson, N., Plant, E., Blazer, D., & Arnow, B. (2005). Childhood sexual abuse and physical abuse and the 1-year prevalence of medical problems in the National Comorbidity Survey. *Health Psychology, 24*(1), 32–40.

Saigh, P. A., Mroueh, M., & Bremner, J. D. (1997). Scholastic impairments among traumatized adolescents. *Behaviour Research and Therapy, 35*(5), 429–436.

Saltzman, W. R., Pynoos, R. S., Layne, C. M., Steinberg, A. M., & Aisenberg, E. (2001). Trauma- and grief-focused intervention for adolescents exposed to community violence: Results of a school-based screening and group treatment protocol. *Group Dynamics: Theory, Research, and Practice, 5,* 291–303.

Saltzman, W. R., Steinberg, A. M., Layne, C. M., Aisenberg, E., & Pynoos, R. S. (2001). A developmental approach to school-based treatment of adolescents exposed to trauma and traumatic loss. *Journal of Child and Adolescent Group Therapy, 11*(2/3), 43–56.

Schwab-Stone, M. E., Ayers, T. S., Kasprow, W., Voyce, C., Barone, C., Shriver, T., et al. (1995). No safe haven: A study of violence exposure in an urban community. *Journal of the American Academy of Child and Adolescent Psychiatry, 34*(10), 1343–1352.

Shin, H. B. (2005). *School enrollment–social and economic characteristics of students: October 2003 population characteristics (P20-554).* Washington, DC: U.S. Bureau of the Census.

Sklarew, B., Krupnick, J., Ward-Wimmer, D., & Napoli, C. (2002). The School-Based Mourning Project: A preventive intervention in the cycle of inner-city violence. *Journal of Applied Psychoanalytic Studies, 4*(3), 317–330.

Skarlew, B., Krupnick, J., Ward-Wimmer, D., & Napoli, C. (2004). The School-Based Mourning Project: A preventive intervention in the cycle of inner-city violence. In B. Sklarew, S. Twemlow, & S. Wilkinson (Eds.), *Analysts in the trenches: Streets, schools, war zones* (pp. 196–210). Hillsdale, NJ: Analytic Press.

Stein, B. D., Jaycox, L. H., Kataoka, S., Rhodes, H. J., & Vestal, K. D. (2003). Prevalence of child and adolescent exposure to community violence. *Clinical Child and Family Psychology Review, 6*(4), 247–264.

Stein, B. D., Jaycox, L. H., Kataoka, S. H., Wong, M., Tu, W., Elliott, M. N., et al. (2003). A mental health intervention for schoolchildren exposed to violence: A randomized controlled trial. *Journal of the American Medical Association, 290*(5), 603–611.

Straussner, J. H., & Straussner, S. L. (1997). Impact of community school violence on children. In N. K. Phillips & S. L. A. Straussner (Eds.), *Children in the urban environment: Linking social policy and clinical practice* (pp. 61–77). Springfield, IL: Thomas.

Ullman, S., & Brecklin, L. (2002). Sexual assault history and suicidal behavior in a national sample of women. *Suicide and Life-Threatening Behavior, 32*(2), 117–130.

U.S. Department of Justice Office for Victims of Crime. (2003, January). *Safe Harbor: A school-based victim assistance/violence prevention program.* Washington, DC: Author.

U.S. Public Health Service. (2000). *Report of the Surgeon General's Conference on Children's Mental Health: A National Action Agenda.* Washington, DC: U.S. Department of Health and Human Services.

Weisz, J. R., Donenberg, G. R., Han, S. S., & Weiss, B. (1995). Bridging the gap between laboratory and clinic in child and adolescent psychotherapy. *Journal of Consulting and Clinical Psychology, 63*(5), 688–701.

Wolmer, L., Laor, N., Dedeoglu, C., Siev, J., & Yazgan, Y. (2005). Teacher-mediated intervention after disaster: A controlled three-year follow-up of children's functioning. *Journal of Child Psychology and Psychiatry, 46*(11), 1161–1168.

Woodside, D., Santa Barbara, J., & Benner, D. G. (1999). Psychological trauma and social healing in Croatia. *Medicine, Conflict, and Survival, 15*(4), 355–367.

Ystgaard, M., Hestetun, I., Loeb, M., & Mehlum, L. (2004). Is there a specific relationship between childhood sexual abuse and physical abuse and repeated suicidal behavior? *Child Abuse and Neglect, 28*(8), 863–875.

Yule, W. (1992). Post-traumatic stress disorder in child survivors of shipping disasters: The sinking of the *Jupiter. Psychotherapy and Psychosomatics, 57*(4), 200–205.

Zima, B. T., Bussing, R., Yang, X., & Belin, T. R. (2000). Help-seeking steps and service use among children in foster care. *Journal of Behavioral Health Services and Research, 27,* 271–285.

CHAPTER 14

Psychodynamic Therapy for Adults

Harold S. Kudler, Janice L. Krupnick,
Arthur S. Blank Jr., Judith L. Herman,
and Mardi J. Horowitz

Theoretical Context

Psychodynamic therapy for posttraumatic symptomatology has been evolving for over a century. Its principles and practices can facilitate treatment across a broad range of approaches, psychodynamic and otherwise. In our experience, psychodynamic formulations provide an invaluable guide through the maze of pretraumatic personality dispositions, peritraumatic experiences, and posttraumatic symptoms and syndromes that so often complicate the aftermath of overwhelming events.

In *Studies on Hysteria*, Joseph Breuer and Sigmund Freud (1895/1955) proposed that mental disorders may be rooted in psychological trauma. This was a radical notion given the contemporary belief that psychiatric patients suffered mainly from biological defects. Janet had already developed an effective psychotherapy for trauma survivors (1886, 1889/1973), but his approach was founded on a belief that his patients' brains were too degenerate to integrate traumatic memories properly. Breuer and Freud held that a psychological trauma could, in itself, be pathogenic.

Breuer, who wrote the first case history in the *Studies*, used hypnosis to probe for, identify, and remove traumatic memories. Under hypnosis, his patient recalled links between each of her symptoms and specific traumatic events that had preceded them. When she remembered the trauma while reexperiencing the emotions associated with it ("abreaction"), the symptom would disappear. By repeating the process for each of his patient's symptoms, Breuer eventually brought her to health. This cathartic treatment was the first method of analyzing the psyche.

Although Freud began by employing Breuer's method, he distrusted hypnosis. Following a patient's advice (Frau Emmy in the *Studies*), Freud invited his patients to speak as candidly as possible about their symptoms and to follow their own thoughts from there ("free association"). He listened actively to facilitate his patients' ability to understand and accept their experiences, along with the internal struggles which they had engendered. Freud hypothesized that hysterical patients "repress" awareness of traumatic memories as a "defense" against them and their implications. Repressed memories are not forgotten; they are actively maintained outside of consciousness.

Freud conceived of the interplay between what was conscious and unconscious as a dynamic give and take between defense (an "ego," or *myself* component of the psyche) and what was being defended against (confined to the "id," or *not me*, component). In this formulation, psychic balance is maintained by a "compromise" that partially expresses the repressed trauma and its associations (including its affective component) in the form of a symptom.

Case Example

A man presented with complaints of a recurrent nightmare in which a local hotel collapsed. The nightmare interfered with his sleep and tortured his waking thoughts. He could not understand why he kept dreaming about something that had never happened. In taking a history, his therapist discovered that the patient, who had been a medic during the first Gulf War, had been responsible for pulling bodies out of a barracks that had received a direct missile hit. The patient had never associated the dream about his hometown with his horrific war memories. He generally avoided his war memories in his waking thoughts. Although the man was reluctant to believe the therapist's interpretation that his dream might be an acceptable expression of an unacceptable memory, he never had the nightmare again.

Psychic balance comes at a price. To the extent that the patient represses, he or she distorts reality. The patient retreats into a life founded on a wish of how the world should be. Ideally, a survivor learns to cope with the residua of trauma and achieve a new psychic balance, but if the patient reaches a stalemate, symptoms may grow so severe or so numerous that they become incapacitating. At such times, "psychodynamic psychotherapy" may be indicated.

Like Breuer, Freud originally thought of traumatic memories as foreign objects festering in the psyche: One simply needed to pluck them out, and health would ensue. Over time, he realized that analysis of defenses was as important as analysis of repressed material. Thus, Freud replaced the idea of catharsis with the concept of "working through," which requires thorough, iterative exploration of the dynamic processes involved in symptom formation. From the psychodynamic perspective, a posttraumatic symptom is not a simple defect: It is an adaptive attempt to manage the trauma.

The external world may or may not be a meaningful place (this is a question for philosophy and theology), but mental life is inextricably caught up in meaning making. Psychodynamic psychotherapy elicits and explicates meanings to make unconscious meanings conscious. The patient's progressive understanding of his or her own premises and operating principles provides him or her with an opportunity to cope more effectively. The concept of symptoms as compromises whose meaning must be understood and worked through is a fundamental proposition that distinguishes psychodynamic psychotherapy from the theories and treatments that preceded it.

Another distinguishing proposition of psychodynamic psychotherapy is the concept of "transference." When a patient enters into a working relationship with a therapist, some of the patient's responses reflect a realistic appraisal of the therapist and a practical alliance in the service of successful treatment. Yet, as Freud and subsequent clinicians observed, in each therapeutic relationship there also develops a very different class of attitudes toward the therapist that primarily repeat the patient's important past relationships in a manner inappropriate to the current situation (Greenson, 1967). When Freud first encountered transference, he considered it an interference (or "resistance") and tried to overcome it through appeals to reason or by the weight of his authority. Over time he realized that, like hysterical symptoms (and dreams), transference is a compromise expression of psychic life. Through mutual effort to understand the transference, patient and therapist gain a clearer view of the underpinnings of the problem that brought them together.

Modern psychoanalytic technique is designed to precipitate transference. Frequent meetings promote an intense relationship. The couch and the therapist's *neutrality* and relative anonymity combine to provide a *blank screen* upon which transference can be *projected*. Psychoanalysis has become the "analysis of the transference."

All psychodynamic psychotherapies are informed by the transference, but there is a differential in the way that transference is dealt with across the spectrum of therapies. For example, in *supportive psychotherapy* the therapist rarely brings unobjectionable positive transference to the patient's attention, but consistently confronts the irrationality in negative transference reactions as early as possible to keep the treatment from derailing. In contrast, in formal psychoanalysis, both positive and negative transference are generally allowed to evolve to the point of being well defined and quite palpable in the patient's behavior and conscious awareness. Interpretations and the patient's working through of this fully formed transference then become the focus and driving force of treatment. This emphasis on interpretation of the transference distinguishes formal psychoanalysis from other psychodynamic psychotherapies.

Forging a therapeutic relationship with a patient is always demanding. It is still more complex when the patient is a trauma survivor (see, e.g., Courtois, 1999; De Wind, 1984). In working closely with a survivor, a therapist must contend with his or her own personal responses to what the patient has been through and to those demands that the patient makes upon the therapist. This can evoke powerful *countertransference* reactions. "Countertransference" has been variously defined but, for the purposes of this chapter, it refers to therapist responses (thoughts, feelings, interventions, etc.) that more closely express the therapist's personal issues than they reflect a rational, clinically appropriate response to the patient. At such times, it is the therapist who may for a time lose track of reality. Even therapists who do not think of themselves as psychodynamically oriented tend to pay close attention to countertransference and its possible corollary of "compassion fatigue" (Figley, 1995).

Many valuable articles and texts have been written on the importance of countertransference in treating trauma survivors (Danieli, 1984; Davies & Frawley, 1994; Haley, 1974; Pearlman & Saakvitne, 1995; Wilson & Lindy, 1994). It is generally agreed that therapists should guard against acting on countertransference but, being human, they often discover their countertransferential responses precisely because they have become enmeshed in these thoughts, feelings, and/or enactments. Many therapists seek personal psychodynamic psychotherapy to achieve greater awareness of their personal countertransference tendencies. Although it is important to minimize acting out of countertransference, it is neither possible nor even preferable to eradicate personal responses to patients. No one can be useful to a patient about whom he or she has no feelings at all, and repression of such feelings only creates blind spots. Learning to acknowledge and to work with countertransference helps the therapist understand what is going on in the therapy.

The relationship between patient and psychotherapist cannot be reduced to transference and countertransference. Patient and therapist also take part in a *real relationship* that is relatively free from distortions and central to their *therapeutic alliance* (Greenson, 1967). Loewald (1960) suggested that the patient–therapist relationship is itself the critical therapeutic factor in psychoanalysis. As Bruch pointed out, "[Psychodynamic] psychotherapy rests on the assumption that problems with an origin in damaging and confusing early experiences are capable of correction through a new and different intimate personal relationship" (1974, p. 19). A distorted sense of self and others can be reworked in the context of that new relationship. The interpersonal aspects of psychotherapy are no less important in psychodynamic work with trauma survivors. The patient–therapist relationship complements the use of other interventions in the therapeutic action of psychodynamic psychotherapy. As Solomon and Johnson (2002) point out, "The success of any PTSD [posttraumatic stress disorder] treatment depends upon establishing and maintaining a therapeutic context of sufficient safety and trust for positive emotional change to occur" (p. 959).

The psychoanalytic concept of trauma continues to evolve. Early in his clinical work, Freud found that every hysterical patient he treated, male or female, reported a history of sexual abuse (Freud, 1896/1962). Because Freud at first presumed that children do not have sexual feelings, he concluded that molestation prematurely and traumatically awakened their sexuality. He later abandoned this "seduction theory" on the grounds that (1) not all hysterical patients had been seduced, and (2) children do, indeed, have sexual feelings (Freud, 1905/1953). Throughout his career, Freud held to the concept that some mental health problems stem from sexual abuse during childhood, but he also came to believe that psychological problems could arise from dynamic conflict between sexual impulses and personal or social inhibitions (Freud, 1925/1959; Gay, 1988). At that point in his career, Freud took a hiatus from trauma theory to address more general questions about psychological development.

Freud's attention was drawn back to the problem of psychological trauma by the many psychological casualties among veterans of World War I. In *Beyond the Pleasure Principle* (1920/1955), Freud defined "psychological trauma" as the result of a breach in a psychic "stimulus barrier."

Like Janet (van der Hart, Brown, & van der Kolk, 1989), Freud understood survivors' intrusive and avoidant symptoms (later core elements of PTSD) as a biphasic attempt to cope with trauma. Freud speculated that survivors repeat these memories in the hope of mastering them. He revised his theory of dreams to include a special class of posttraumatic dreams rooted in this "repetition compulsion." He also hypothesized that although all living things have an inherent instinct for self-preservation, they also strive to nullify any and all noxious stimulation, internal or external, even if it means giving up life entirely ("death instinct").

One of Freud's colleagues, Abram Kardiner, treated hundreds of combat veterans in World War I and published his findings early in World War II (1941). Kardiner accepted Freud's premises about psychological trauma but emphasized the interplay between psychological and biological factors in what he termed the "physioneurosis" of combat survivors. The two world wars forced many clinicians and theorists (Fairbairn, 1943b; Ferenczi, Abraham, Simmel, & Jones, 1921; Greenson, 1949/1978; Grinker & Speigel, 1945; Kardiner & Spiegel, 1947; Lidz, 1946; Lindemann, 1944; Rivers, 1918) to ponder psychodynamic models and to forge therapeutic interventions. Abreactive models, employing amytal and hypnosis (well described by Sargant & Slater [1969] and dramatically chronicled by John Huston [1948] in his documentary film *Let There Be Light*) were combined with supportive and psychoeducational interventions in highly effective treatments of what was then called "combat fatigue." This successful application of psychoanalytic theory spurred worldwide interest in psychoanalysis in the postwar years.

World War II also demanded that therapists confront the effects of massive psychic trauma on noncombatants. Studies on survivors of the Holocaust (Krystal, 1968) and of Hiroshima (Lifton, 1967) demonstrated that overwhelming events could numb basic human capacities and result in a kind of "death in life." Krystal (1988) went on to develop an information-processing model of psychological trauma, which included the idea that overwhelming events can disable the psyche's ability to utilize anxiety as a signal for the mobilization of defense. Once this system is disrupted, anxiety and other affects fail to serve psychic needs. Affects may become muted, overwhelming, or inappropriate. One possible outcome is "alexithymia" (a profound disconnection between words and feelings).

Another psychodynamic information-processing model was then suggested by Horowitz (1973, 2001). The reason for his reformulation was a series of clinical, experimental, and field studies that showed a phasic variation in states of mind in the dimensions of memory, emotion, and cognition. He empirically validated the centrality of intrusive thinking and also its seeming opposite: avoidance of relevant ideation and numbing of emotional responses. Horowitz utilized models of schematic change such as those that take place in mourning to explicate adjustment and posttraumatic disorders. These he described in terms of pretraumatic beliefs about self and others that then take on new meaning in the wake of horrendous events.

Concern about identity issues during and after trauma was also central to Kohut's *self psychology* theory, which has also been applied to the problem of psychological trauma (Ulman & Brothers, 1988). A stable sense of self (and the regulatory systems that maintain it) is refined in the course of normal narcissistic development, but it can be disrupted or even shattered by experiences that threaten the very relevance of the self.

Object relations theory, which seeks to understand how intrapsychic functions and structures develop in the context of interpersonal experiences, offers valuable insights into how shattered personal assumptions, relationships, and social contracts can lead to psychopathology. D. W. Winnicott's (1965) description of the "holding environment," which enables children to overcome fears of physical and psychological annihilation as they move toward greater autonomy, provides valuable clues as to how adults maintain or fail to maintain psychic balance in the face of trauma. Kudler (1991) has suggested that Winnicott's holding environment essentially creates Freud's stimulus barrier.

Fairbairn (1943a) conceived of trauma as releasing repressed, internalized relationships with so-called "bad objects." When a hated and feared object (e.g., a frustrating parent) is also recognized by the child as essential for survival, the psyche may become flooded with anxiety. Traumatic events can revivify early experiences and identifications with such objects by disrupting an achieved balance of autonomy and aggression. Treatment focuses on restoring that balance.

Many commentators have depicted psychoanalysis as being more concerned with intrapsychic reality than with the effects of real external events. The work of Shengold (1989, 1991), Terr (1979), Lindy (1985), and a host of others demonstrates the clinical relevance and conceptual power that psychoanalytic perspectives bring to the problem of psychological trauma. Kudler (2007), in response to the wide-ranging public health implications of post-deployment mental health problems faced by new combat veterans and their families, points out that these problems are better understood and addressed within the adaptational, dimensional context of psychodynamic principles than in the descriptive, categorical terms that typify the prevailing medical model of PTSD. The treatment of this profoundly human problem requires understanding and intervention at the level of human nature. Psychodynamic psychotherapy approaches PTSD by way of the mind. As such, it offers a unique perspective on psychological trauma.

Description of Techniques

Psychoanalytic theory continues to evolve and has given rise to a broad array of techniques referred to as "psychodynamic psychotherapies." These are grounded in psychoanalytic concepts of defense, conflict, symptoms as meaningful representations, conscious and unconscious levels of mental activity, transference, countertransference, and the therapeutic relationship. Techniques can vary greatly with regard to how these concepts are applied.

In *formal psychoanalysis*, patient and therapist meet four to five times per week over the course of 2–7 years (or more). Treatment is directed at personality disturbances of long standing as may be evoked by a combination of temperament, character, and early childhood deprivations and traumas, which might include uncompensated losses and physical or sexual abuse. Adults and children are treated. Whereas adults are expected to interact with the analyst through free association of ideas on the couch, children generally bring intrapsychic material into analysis through play. Although analysts vary in their degree of activity, they strive to remain equidistant between polarities of conflict and proadaptational in their responses to the patient. As Anna Freud (1966) pointed out, this means that the analyst avoids siding with any one aspect of the patient's intrapsychic contents, structure, or function (be it wish, defense, or demand to adhere to social standards). The analyst's only investment is in the patient's progress toward autonomy and health.

Progress in psychoanalysis stems from growth in the patient's understanding of his or her own premises, strategies, perceptions, and responses to the external environment. This is accomplished in the context of a strong *working alliance* with a trustworthy and considerate analyst, and a shared commitment to honesty and openness. The patient follows the *fundamental rule* of saying whatever is on his or her mind, no matter how irrelevant, noxious, or banal that thought might appear. The analysis follows these associations and explores dreams, symptomatic acts, transference, and countertransference to explicate the complex network of ideas, memories, wishes, fears, and constitutional givens that comprise the psyche of this unique person. Another way to think of psychoanalysis is as a constant sifting and sorting of what is true and what is fantasy in the patient's assessment of him- or herself and his or her world. The therapist employs observations, confrontations, and interpretations to test hypotheses with the patient. It is important to emphasize that the therapist is simply a facilitator in this process. Ultimately, the patient analyzes him- or herself.

In *psychodynamic psychotherapy*, meetings may be held once or twice weekly, or even less often. Patient and therapist face one another without benefit of the couch. While therapists tend to be more active (make more comments, be more emotionally available in the hour), they may still strive for neutrality vis-à-vis the patient's conscious and unconscious concerns. The process may or may not center on the interpretation of transference. There may be more emphasis on here-and-now issues as opposed to the developmental and historical issues plumbed in formal psychoanalysis. Consistent, positive relational experiences with the therapist may enhance self-esteem and challenge erroneous interpersonal expectations.

Psychodynamic psychotherapy is a composite of supportive and expressive methods that may enlarge the patient's understanding of unconscious issues in the context of a strong therapeutic alliance. Goals include improved self-understanding and greater "ego strength" (intrapsychic integrity and capacity to cope).

In the now considerable body of work describing psychodynamic psychotherapy for survivors of trauma (e.g., see Briere, 1996; Chu, 1998; Lindy, 1986, 1996; McCann & Pearlman, 1990; Ochberg, 1988; Parson, 1984; Roth & Batson, 1997; van der Kolk, McFarlane, & Weisaeth, 1996), psychoanalytic roots are not always explicit. The boundaries between these treatments and the cognitive-behavioral therapies are sometimes blurred. A variety of interventions may be applied at different phases of treatment. The broad range of psychodynamic techniques acknowledges the variety of survivor populations, the specific needs of individual patients, and the particular treatment goals established by different clinicians. Theories and findings may or may not be generalizable across survivor populations.

Mann (1973) pointed out that patients in long-term therapy often make significant gains as they approach termination. He hypothesized that impending separation from the therapist impels this final spurt of progress. This led him to develop a *brief psychodynamic therapy* (12 sessions) that exploits the factor of separation by emphasizing how few sessions remain. This technique may be particularly useful when issues of separation and loss are prominent in the patient's presentation (as in work with trauma survivors). A number of manualized, brief dynamic therapies have grown around another idea proposed by Mann: Brief therapies work best when the patient presents a problem that can be understood within a single metaphor or theme (as in Luborsky's [1990] "core conflictual relationship theme").

Brief psychodynamic psychotherapies have been developed specifically for the treatment of trauma survivors. Horowitz (1974; Horowitz & Kaltreider, 1979) presented a transference-based, 20-session model (later revised to 12 sessions) that takes into account how a survivor's preexisting personality and defensive style interact with his or her traumatic experience to produce particular conflicts and specific kinds of relationships—including specific therapeutic relationships (see also Horowitz et al., 1984; Horowitz, Marmar, Weiss, DeWitt, & Rosenbaum, 1984). Marmar and Freeman (1988) applied Horowitz's ideas in developing a brief treatment method focused on the management of narcissistic regression in the face of trauma. Brom, Kleber, and Defares (1989) employed Horowitz's manualized, brief psychodynamic psychotherapy for PTSD and found it effective in an empirical study.

Horowitz (2003) has updated his manual for the brief psychodynamic treatment of stress response syndromes. His theory of how interacting systems can either precipitate or relieve symptoms, advance coping capacity or diminish it, and, ultimately, reconfigure character structure (Horowitz, 1998) is an example of a multimodal brief approach based on reliable, research-validated strategies.

In Horowitz's (1997) model, a systematic, individualized case formulation (based on psychoanalytic concepts of how defense and unconscious information processing affect mood and behavioral patterns) informs the therapist when to use behavioral techniques for guided desensitization (to achieve shock mastery), cognitive techniques (to modify dysfunctional conscious beliefs and plan possible futures), and/or supportive and expressive dynamic techniques (to modify defensive resistances to processing of stressful events). The therapist employs this model to guide changes in how the patient's emotions are regulated and to facilitate identity reschematization and affiliation reformation.

Supportive psychotherapy is often characterized as being less expressive than other forms of psychodynamic psychotherapy. Therapists are generally more active in their interventions and less likely to interpret than to "support" the patient's defenses by bolstering self-esteem and allying with those coping strategies that the patient has already found useful. The focus is less on uncovering unconscious conflicts than on restoring intrapsychic equilibrium. Problems are managed in the here and now rather than through extended elaborations of development and intrapsychic structure. Although the therapist is less likely to make transference interpretations, interventions are nonetheless informed by a psychodynamic understanding of the patient's problems and relationship patterns (including transference and countertransference issues), and by an appreciation of how supportive interventions affect the intrapsychic balance (Werman, 1984).

Interpersonal psychotherapy (IPT) is a time-limited, manualized treatment in which the therapist takes an exploratory stance and focuses interventions on the patient's outside relationships rather than on transference. Although IPT was developed for the treatment of individuals with major depression (Klerman, Weissman, Rounsaville, & Chevron, 1984), it has been adapted for use in anxiety disorders, including PTSD (Krupnick, Green, & Miranda, 1998). IPT targets impairment in relationships. Because interpersonal trauma can lead to PTSD, and PTSD itself is associated with impaired interpersonal function, an approach that helps survivors find new ways to understand and behave in relationships holds great promise.

Although this chapter focuses on the techniques described earlier, many other therapeutic techniques, including group, family, and cognitive psychotherapies, have also derived from psychodynamic concepts. Many group and family therapies remain well within the bounds of psychodynamic psychotherapy, whereas others do not. Cognitive theory, which emphasizes the role of unconscious schemas in the production of symptoms, has blossomed into several forms of therapy that, although "officially" separate from psychodynamic therapy, bear many similarities to it (the assumption of unconscious levels of process, the effects of past experience on current behaviors, the importance of a strong therapeutic alliance, and the centrality of reworking maladaptive patterns of response in order to alleviate suffering and open the path for further growth among others).

Psychodynamic systems of case formulation and methods of intervention often influence therapists who otherwise distance themselves from psychoanalysis. Such clinicians often pay careful attention to unconscious meanings, symbolic acts, and the concepts of transference and countertransference. As Marshall, Yehuda, and Bone (2000) point out, "Confronting the traumatic memory, experiencing the associated affects within a supportive relationship, and thereby processing the traumatic experience may be the common mechanism of efficacy across trauma therapies" (p. 350).

Method of Collecting Data

We obtained the literature on psychodynamic psychotherapy of PTSD from searches using MEDLINE, PsycINFO, Published International Literature on Traumatic Stress (PILOTS), *Title Key Word and Author Index to Psychoanalytic Journals, 1920–1986* (Mosher, 1987), papers furnished by members of the Working Group, review of most books that include chapters on PTSD treatment published since 1980, review of all issues of the *Journal of Traumatic Stress*, and review of references in published articles and chapters. Items chosen bear directly on theory, technique, and outcome.

The psychodynamic literature is particularly rich in case reports. There is ongoing debate over the relative value of the case report compared to the randomized, double-blind, controlled studies typical of pharmacological research. Our position is that each is a legitimate form of scholarship, and neither is suited for application in every field of research. Case reports are valuable because they extract clinical material from a particular case, or a small series of cases, to inform theory and practice. Case studies neither provide ultimate tests for psychodynamic hypotheses nor define the limits of psychopathology, theory, or technique. They do, however, provide the groundwork for hypotheses that can be tested empirically.

This task force has set standards by which research is to be judged. These favor designs that involve many individuals and tightly controlled variables. This is not the optimal lens for studying psychodynamic psychotherapy. As Fonagy, Target, Cottrell, Phillips, and Kurtz (2002) point out, "From the clinician's standpoint, research of almost any sort, but particularly outcome research, has profound intrinsic limitations" (p. 371). To conform to the other position papers in this series, this section concentrates on the relatively few studies of this nature in the psychodynamic literature. Note that each of these studies involves brief psychodynamic psychotherapy. Their findings may not be generalizable to formal psychoanalysis, to long-term psychodynamic psychotherapy, or to supportive psychotherapy. Although most psychodynamic case reports receive low scores in the classification of Level of Evidence chosen by the Agency for Health Care Policy and Research (AHCPR) Guidelines Committee, it must be emphasized that the psychodynamic literature is an essential part of the scientific effort to understand the human impact of psychological trauma.

Literature Review

Empirical Studies

Horowitz and colleagues conducted several empirical studies (Horowitz, 1995; Horowitz et al., 1993, 1994) testing the hypothesis that survivors of traumatic events experience heightened intrusive *and* avoidant symptoms related to traumatic memories and themes. These studies employed a manualized, brief psychodynamic psychotherapy. Horowitz holds that this biphasic response generates intense conflict as the survivor attempts to integrate traumatic memories while defending against external and internal dangers. Horowitz and colleagues found that when a conflictual topic (one linked to the traumatic event) emerges in a psychodynamic session, it is accompanied by intrusions and avoidances, emotionality, fragmentation of important ideas, verbal and nonverbal warding-off behaviors, and stifling of facial emotional expression (Horowitz et al., 1993 [AHCPR Level D]; 1994 [AHCPR Level C]). Recognition of these responses can cue patient and therapist to the emergence of traumatic themes in therapy and better enable them to process this material. Such recognition may also help patients become aware of inadequate or even pathological attempts at coping that have interfered with their working through a posttraumatic problem. These findings are pertinent to all psychodynamic approaches.

Brom and colleagues (1989) constructed a controlled outcome study on the efficacy of three modes of therapy: trauma desensitization, hypnotherapy, and a brief psychodynamic therapy (based on Horowitz's model and involving Horowitz's direct assistance in supervising therapists). The outcome objective was to see which therapy most reduced PTSD symptoms of intrusion and avoidance. The 112 subjects diagnosed with PTSD were randomly assigned to one of the three therapies or to a wait-list control group. Therapists had over 10 years of experience in their respective methods. Each therapist was supervised by a recognized expert in the specific treatment. The mean length of treatment in each setting was 15 sessions (desensitization), 14.4 sessions (hypnotherapy), and 18.8 sessions (psychodynamic therapy). The authors concluded that "the treatments do benefit some in comparison with a control group and using stringent methodological techniques but they do not benefit everyone, the effects are not always substantial, and the differences between the therapies are small" (p. 610). Although the psychodynamic treatment involved the most sessions and showed the least improvement in terms of intrusive symptoms on initial scores, follow-up data indicated that subjects in the psychodynamic treatment group showed greater improvement during the posttermination phase than did subjects in the other two therapies. This finding of an accruing posttreatment improvement, similar to that noted by Horowitz, Marmar, Weiss, Kaltreider, and Wilner (1986), suggests that psychodynamic therapy mobilizes coping mechanisms that continue to strengthen following termination. The Brom and colleagues (1989) findings are most relevant to brief psychodynamic psychotherapy but may be generalizable to longer-term psychodynamic treatments (effect size = 1.14, AHCPR Level A).

Clinical Studies

Bleiberg and Markowitz (2005) conducted an open trial of brief (14 week) interpersonal psychotherapy (IPT) with 14 subjects with chronic PTSD recruited by referral and advertisement. At termination, 12 of the 13 subjects who completed treatment no longer met criteria for PTSD on the Clinician-Administered PTSD Scale (CAPS). Effect sizes for symptom reduction on measures of reexperiencing, avoidance, and hyperarousal ranged from 1.7 to 2.1. Ongoing follow-up of these subjects is planned to measure whether these gains are maintained posttreatment. A treatment manual developed in this study will be used for future randomized controlled trials (AHCPR Level B).

Talbot and her colleagues (2005) also conducted an open trial of brief (16 session) IPT for 25 depressed women with childhood sexual abuse histories, treated in a community mental health center. Ten women completed treatment, and 15 completed eight or more sessions. Significant improvements in depression and general mental health functioning were reported. However, despite the fact that over half the subjects were diagnosed with PTSD at the outset, changes in PTSD were not measured (AHCPR Level B).

Similarly, Price, Hilsenroth, Callahan, Petrectic-Jackson, and Bonge (2004) conducted an open trial of psychodynamic psychotherapy with a cohort of 14 patients with childhood sexual abuse histories, seen at a university-based outpatient clinic. Mean treatment length was 26 sessions. Twelve patients completed treatment. Symptom improvement measured by the Symptom Checklist-90 (SCL-90) and other self-reports showed effect sizes ranging from 0.66 to 0.98; clinician ratings of improvement in Global Assessment of

Functioning (GAF) showed an effect size of 1.51. However, no measure of PTSD symptoms was included in the test battery (AHCPR Level B).

Lindy (1988) reported outcomes in a clinical series of 37 combat veterans of the Vietnam War, each of whom met DSM-III criteria for PTSD. Treatment involved a psychodynamic psychotherapy engaging traumatic war memories. The treatment rationale was to help subjects learn to deal with traumatic memories rather than repress them. Treatment objectives looked beyond symptom reduction. The ultimate goal was intrapsychic change. Treatment was manualized and included three phases: opening, working through, and termination. Working alliance, transference, and countertransference factors were monitored. The average number of sessions was 56. For the 23 subjects who completed treatment, significant changes were noted on clinical ratings by independent clinicians and on global ratings by patients and therapists. Significant differences were also noted on self-report measures including the SCL-90, the Impact of Events Scale (IES), and the Cincinnati Stress Response Schedule. Intrusive phenomena, feelings of alienation and depression, and associated features of hostility and substance abuse were most notably changed. Although clinical ratings at the end of treatment indicated that patients were still not at "normal" levels, subjects showed increased capacity to trust and to manage traumatic stress precipitated in an interview. They also seemed to have moved from a state of psychic numbing to an appreciation of being alive. They experienced a greater sense of personal integrity and dignity with regard to their own experiences as combat soldiers. There was less estrangement and more investment in adult roles and socially constructive activities. Each subject also expressed a greater sense of continuity with the person he or she had been before the war (AHCPR Level B).

Weiss and Marmar (1993) described a 12-session psychodynamic treatment for adult survivors of single traumatic events. They employed a treatment manual and reported on results in work with over 200 patients. They did not employ systematic outcome measures. The thrust of their article is that this method is "teachable." This finding is most relevant to brief psychodynamic psychotherapy, but it may be generalizable to longer-term psychodynamic treatments (AHCPR Level C).

Roth and Batson (1997) conducted a systematic evaluation of a yearlong psychodynamic treatment of six adult female childhood incest survivors with PTSD. Markers of improvement in the areas represented by PTSD and other psychiatric diagnoses, trauma themes, and complex PTSD symptoms demonstrated significant clinical change. The therapeutic effects for trauma themes occurred in survivors' processing of the traumatic origins of their fear, shame, alienation, and rage (AHCPR Level B).

Numerous clinical studies were neither controlled nor strict in their choice of outcome measures but are sufficiently compelling to warrant the use of psychodynamic psychotherapy and the application of psychodynamic approaches to survivors of traumatic events (AHCPR Level C). These include Herman's (1992) description of her work with trauma survivors, most of whom were adult women who had survived childhood rape or incest. Treatment involved a combination of expressive and supportive psychodynamic psychotherapy techniques that sequentially emphasized issues of safety, remembrance/ mourning, and reconnection in the context of a strong, positive relationship with a trusted therapist. Shengold (1989, 1991) advocated strongly for formal psychoanalysis of adult survivors of childhood sexual trauma, many of whom evidenced severe character pathology. He suggests that a child may respond to sexual abuse by isolating and compartmentalizing feelings, thoughts, and identifications. Murderous rage may represent the greatest burden for such patients. These feelings must be carefully confronted and interpreted, so that what has been held apart can be reintegrated.

De Wind (1971) presented salutary results in the treatment of 23 Holocaust survivors by formal psychoanalysis. Success seemed to depend on the patient's ability to mourn lost love objects and to tolerate his or her own aggression. In addition to better management of posttraumatic symptoms, patients were also reported to have achieved a deeper sense of integration and meaning.

Rose (1991) described successful experience with psychodynamic psychotherapy in a series (number unspecified) of adult female patients who had been raped. The treatment emphasized confrontation and management of intense rage. Rose found that patients improved in terms of their posttraumatic symptoms and, in some cases, seemed to make progress in dealing with preexisting conflicts. The findings of these studies are limited to the populations and techniques peculiar to each report, but they are potentially generalizable to other psychodynamic psychotherapies.

Single- or small-series case reports, starting with Breuer and Freud's *Studies on Hysteria* (1895/1955), comprise the bulk of evidence for the efficacy of psychodynamic treatment of trauma survivors. These are, at best, AHCPR Level D evidence (based on long-standing and widespread clinical practice that has not been subjected to empirical tests in PTSD). For example, Goldschmidt (1986) reported a positive outcome with an adult patient who, as a 4-year-old child, witnessed the suicide of his parents (who also attempted to poison him). The treatment comprised a 20-session, brief psychodynamic psychotherapy, in which the therapist identified and interpreted elements of the traumatic situation that were being relived in the therapy setting. The patient improved in terms of his ability to mourn. He also was able to curtail his previously frequent reenactments of the trauma (including urges to hurt himself, extreme avoidance, and marked anxiety). The patient went on to begin formal psychoanalysis. Krupnick (1997) reported a single case study demonstrating the efficacy of brief (12 sessions) psychodynamic psychotherapy for PTSD. The treatment was largely of a supportive nature, but transference interpretations were also offered. The therapist attempted to help the patient "reestablish a sense of coherence and meaning" (p. 77). Treatment was meant to alleviate PTSD symptoms, but it also focused on helping the patient move forward in her life without guilt. By accepting her rage and aggressive feelings, the patient became able to integrate a more mature sense of self. Taken together, these reports document that psychoanalysis and psychodynamic psychotherapy have demonstrated effectiveness in the treatment of trauma survivors.

Recommendations

When considering a patient for a psychodynamic psychotherapy, be it formal psychoanalysis, psychodynamic psychotherapy, brief psychodynamic psychotherapy, or supportive psychotherapy, one should evaluate certain patient attributes. Initially, therapist and patient team up to review the patient's goals. Is the patient focused on immediate symptom reduction and "getting on with life," or is he or she seeking a broader understanding of his or her reactions, life history, goals, and options? What has his or her experience been with other treatments? What practical considerations (financial factors, available time, career pressures) pertain to the therapy? By the end of the evaluation (which might require anywhere from one to five or more sessions), the therapist should be able to offer the patient a concise statement of the problem and general recommendations for treatment.

Given that a diagnosis of PTSD does not lead to a fixed prescription for treatment, there can be no substitute for a thoughtful, individualized case formulation (Horowitz, 1997, 2005). The psychodynamic approach focuses on factors that distinguish each person as an individual (as opposed to the descriptive approach of the DSM diagnostic system, which groups patients by features they share in common). From a psychodynamic perspective, the traumatic event is not the sole cause of the conflicts, painful distress, and symptoms often encountered in survivors. Formulation has to consider biopsychosocial interactions, premorbid dispositions, comorbidities, developmental and family history, and quality and quantity of social support, among other factors. Initial formulation is partial at best. Constant reformulation is necessary as more information is gained and treatment progresses.

The final choice of treatment modality is best made collaboratively. Certain guidelines may be helpful in making this decision. Gabbard (2005) lists the indications for highly expressive psychodynamic psychotherapy (including formal psychoanalysis) as follows: (1) a strong motivation to understand oneself; (2) suffering that interferes with life to such an extent that it becomes an incentive for the patient to endure the rigors of treatment; (3) the ability not only to regress and give up control of feelings and thoughts but also to regain control quickly and reflect on that regression (regression in the service of the ego; Greenson, 1967); (4) tolerance for frustration; (5) a capacity for insight and for understanding oneself in psychological terms ("psychological mindedness"); (6) intact reality testing; (7) meaningful and enduring object relations; (8) reasonably good impulse control; and (9) ability to sustain a job (Bachrach & Leaff, 1978) (p. 114). Gabbard also emphasizes the patient's ability to form a strong, trusting relationship with the therapist. Luborsky, Crits-Christoph, Mintz, and Auerbach (1988) add that a good outcome is more likely when there is a positive relationship between therapist and patient at the outset of treatment.

Patients with PTSD may lack one or more of the attributes listed earlier because of the following tendencies: avoidance of traumatic material; fears of being overwhelmed by feelings, thoughts, and images; decreased tolerance for frustration; impaired ability to begin or sustain relationships; weakened impulse control; and difficulty sustaining employment. As Courtois's (1999) review of current trauma-focused models of psychodynamic psychotherapy indicates, vulnerabilities of these kinds can often be addressed by phase-oriented treatments that incorporate multiple techniques and emphasize pacing of the work to the individual's needs and capacities. If methods are use to increase self-observational capacity, some patients who are not initially psychologically minded can learn to increase self-governance by thinking through a problem instead of acting precipitously. In a study of a two-phase treatment for childhood abuse survivors with PTSD, in which the initial phase focused explicitly on fostering the therapeutic alliance, Cloitre, Stoval-McClough, Miranda, and Chemtob (2004) demonstrated that the strength of the therapeutic alliance reliably predicts improvement in PTSD symptoms.

Another key indicator for expressive psychodynamic psychotherapy derived from clinical wisdom is the patient's ability to stand back from his or her own position and see him- or herself objectively. This capacity, referred to as an "observing ego," is generally believed to strengthen in the course of treatment and is sometimes used to gauge the patient's readiness to terminate. The combination of a strong observing ego and reasonable self-understanding may equip an individual to maintain or even improve his or her psychic balance, without ongoing assistance from a therapist.

The following characteristics would indicate the need for a more supportive psychodynamic psychotherapy: long-standing ego weakness; acute life crisis; poor tolerance for anxiety and/or frustration; poor capacity for insight; poor reality testing; severely impaired object relations; limited impulse control; low intelligence or organic cognitive dysfunction (including significant traumatic brain injury); difficulty with self-observation; and tenuous ability to form a therapeutic alliance (Gabbard, 2005).

The next issue to resolve is whether the therapy should be long term or brief. The choice depends to some extent on practical considerations. Third-party payers and the patient's financial resources may be critical factors. The choice also depends on the agreed-upon goals of treatment and the patient's capacities. Brief therapy demands that the patient be able to form a trusting relationship quickly with the therapist. The patient and therapist must also be able to agree on a clear focus for the work. Brief psychodynamic therapy is not "less therapy." It is a technically refined, highly focused, psychotherapeutic approach that is indicated when patient and therapist are in close agreement about the nature of the problem and the mode of intervention. It requires a patient with quick intelligence, a high degree of trust, a strong ability to toler-ate harsh feelings, and a well-developed ability to think about him- or herself with clarity and perspective.

Although the studies by Brom and colleagues (1989) and Horowitz and colleagues (1986) suggest that brief therapy can continue to have a salutary effect long after treatment ends, it is also true that brief therapy is most clearly indicated when the problem itself is focal. Many patients who have experienced traumatic events have problems that are much less focal. The concept of "complex PTSD" (Herman, 1992; Pelcovitz et al., 1997) is based on an understanding that trauma experienced during earlier developmen-tal periods has strong implications for later development. For many such survivors, the posttraumatic state combines PTSD symptoms with more gen-eral difficulties in regulation of affect, impulsivity, dissociative tendencies, damaging perceptions of self and others, somatization, and alterations in systems of meaning. McCann and Pearlman (1990) and Roth and Batson (1997) have detailed the disruptions in central beliefs and self-image that underlie the psychology of the adult survivor of childhood trauma. McCann and Pearlman note, for example, that transference and countertransfer-ence issues are consequently harsh and powerful, and specify difficulties in the areas of safety, trust/dependency, esteem, and independence. Davies and Frawley (1994) have described the defensive use of dissociation, in which the adult survivor of childhood incest expresses traumatic material while simultaneously warding off traumatic memories, affects, and fanta-sies. McCann and Pearlman summarize research suggesting that survivors of childhood trauma may be particularly vulnerable to later victimization, and may be at increased risk for PTSD secondary to traumas experienced later in life.

Because traumatic experiences and certain personality disorders predis-pose individuals to emotional instability, a period of supportive therapy may be indicated to help a patient avoid out-of-control states of mind and develop self-observational and self-governance skills that better equip him or her to participate in more intense, expressive modes of therapy. This preparatory phase helps the patient achieve greater mastery of emotional and cognitive responses, and develop a more solid therapeutic alliance as a foundation for the expressive work to follow.

Danieli (1989) has suggested that group treatment may be indicated in work with Holocaust survivors and their children. Homogeneous groups of first- or second-generation survivors or mixed, intergenerational groups can create a contemporary "family" that helps members reaffirm their iden-tity and rework their relationships with others. Mobilization of internalized and trauma-tainted object relationships within the group may provide sorely needed opportunities for mourning and progression. Danieli's recommen-dations are echoed by those of Shay (1994), who stressed the importance of the *communalization* of war experience through the sharing of narrative within groups of combat veterans. The reader is referred to Cohen, Mannarino, Deblinger, and Berliner (Chapter 8, this volume) for a more complete discussion of group treatment.

The contraindications to psychodynamic modes of therapy comprise largely the opposites of those indications listed previously. An inability to form a therapeutic alliance, a lack of psychological mindedness, a limited observing ego, impaired reality testing, and inability to tolerate strong emotions are important contraindications to expressive modes of therapy. The patient may simply be unable to contain the issues expected to arise in the course of treatment.

Countertransference to trauma survivors can be profound; significant countertransference on the part of the therapist can serve as a relative contraindication to undertaking or continuing a therapy. Appropriate training, continuous self-reflection, collegial support, consultation, ongoing supervision, and personal psychotherapy can each play a role in helping a therapist maintain his or her therapeutic stance in the course of work with trauma survivors.

Areas Requiring Further Exploration

Psychodynamic researchers have had significant problems employing conventional research paradigms to evaluate their work. Some of the studies cited earlier (especially the work by Brom et al. [1989], Horowitz [2005], Lindy [1996], and Luborsky [1990]) point the way toward making this paradigmatic leap. It is essential that psychodynamic psychotherapists find ways to state their propositions as testable hypotheses. Research would be enriched by more case reports and large-scale studies that describe treatment effects among different populations of survivors. Historical reviews are needed to retrace the evolution of key theoretical concepts, so that they may be reconsidered and, in some cases, redefined. The new *Psychodynamic Diagnostic Manual* (PDM Task Force, 2006) of the Alliance of Psychoanalytic Organizations and the new Empirical Studies of Psychoanalytic Treatments, Process, and Concepts section of the American Psychoanalytic Association (2007) website (*www.apsa.org/research/empiricalstudiesinpsychoanalysis/tabid/449/default.aspx*) represent new and potentially valuable efforts to systematize and extend psychodynamic research. As Gabbard (2006) points out, "The recent emphasis on more naturalistic effectiveness trials may be particularly applicable to the assessment of psychotherapies" (p. 182). Interdisciplinary efforts are needed to bring psychodynamic perspectives in closer contact with neuroscience and genomics, as well as with developmental, cognitive, and behavioral approaches in psychology. Finally, and perhaps most important, competition among rivals must be reformulated as collaboration among colleagues (Kudler, 1989). This Guidelines Project is a good step in that direction.

Summary

Psychodynamic treatment seeks to reengage normal mechanisms of adaptation by addressing what is unconscious and, in tolerable doses, making it conscious. The psychological meaning of a traumatic event is progressively understood within the context of the survivor's unique history, constitution, and aspirations. This includes collaborative sifting and sorting through wishes, fantasies, fears, and defenses stirred up by the event. Transference and countertransference are universal phenomena that should be recognized by therapists, but that may or may not be explicitly addressed depending on treatment modality and therapist judgment. Psychodynamic treatment requires insight and courage, and is best approached in a therapeutic relationship that emphasizes safety and honesty. The therapist–patient relationship is itself a crucial factor in the patient's response. The wide range and broad public health implications of posttraumatic responses are best understood and addressed within the adaptational, dimensional context of psychodynamic principles rather than the descriptive, categorical terms that typify the prevailing medical model of PTSD. Psychodynamic psychotherapy approaches PTSD by way of the mind. As such, it offers a unique and useful clinical tool.

Acknowledgments

We wish to acknowledge the members of the Working Group on Psychodynamic Psychotherapy for PTSD, including Nanette Auerhahn, Ronald Batson, Elizabeth Brett, Danny Brom, Richard Gartner, Nancy Hartevelt Kobrin, Dori Laub, Elana Newman, Laurie Pearlman, Susan Roth, Bessel van der Kolk, and Lars Weisaeth. We also thank reviewers Matthew Friedman, Patricia Resick, Susan Roth, and Terry Keane for their efforts on behalf of this project.

References

American Psychoanalytic Association. (2007). *Empirical studies of psychoanalytic treatments, process, and concepts.* Retrieved July 14, 2007, from *www.apsa.org/research/empiricalstudiesinpsychoanalysis/tabid/449/default.aspx*

Bachrach, H. M., & Leaff, L. A. (1978). "Analyzability": A systematic review of the clinical and quantitative literature. *Journal of the American Psychoanalytic Association, 26,* 881–920.

Bleiberg, K. L., & Markowitz, J. C. (2005). A pilot study of interpersonal psychotherapy for posttraumatic stress disorder. *American Journal of Psychiatry, 162,* 181–183.

Breuer, J., & Freud, S. (1955). *Studies on hysteria.* In J. Strachey (Ed. & Trans.), *The standard edition of the complete psychological works of Sigmund Freud* (Vol. 2, pp. 1–335). London: Hogarth Press. (Original work published 1895)

Briere, J. (1996). *Therapy for adults molested as children: Beyond survival* (2nd ed.). New York: Springer.

Brom, D., Kleber, R. J., & Defares, P. B. (1989). Brief psychotherapy for posttraumatic stress disorders. *Journal of Consulting and Clinical Psychology, 57*, 607–612.

Bruch, H. (1974). *Learning psychotherapy: Rationale and ground rules.* Cambridge, MA: Harvard University Press.

Chu, J. A. (1998). *Rebuilding shattered lives: The responsible treatment of complex posttraumatic and dissociative disorders.* New York: Wiley.

Cloitre, M. , Stovall-McClough, K. D., Miranda, R., & Chemtob, C. (2004). Therapeutic alliance, negative mood regulation, and treatment outcome in child-abuse-related posttraumatic stress disorder. *Journal of Consulting and Clinical Psychology, 72*, 411–416.

Courtois, C. A. (1999). *Recollections of sexual abuse: Treatment principles and guidelines.* New York: Norton.

Danieli, Y. (1984). Psychotherapists' participation in the conspiracy of silence about the Holocaust. *Psychoanalytic Psychology, 1*, 23–42.

Danieli, Y. (1989). Mourning in survivors and children of survivors of the Nazi Holocaust: The role of group and community modalities. In D. R. Dietrich & P. C. Shabad (Eds.), *The problem of loss and mourning: Psychoanalytic perspectives* (pp. 427–460). Madison, CT: International Universities Press.

Davies, J. M., & Frawley, M. G. (1994). *Treating the adult survivor of childhood sexual abuse: A psychoanalytic perspective.* New York: Basic Books.

De Wind, E. (1971). Psychotherapy after traumatization caused by persecution. In H. Krystal & W. G. Niederland (Eds.), *Psychic traumatization* (pp. 93–114). Boston: Little, Brown.

De Wind, E. (1984). Some implications of former massive traumatization upon the actual analytic process. *International Journal of Psychoanalysis, 65*, 273–281.

Fairbairn, W. R. D. (1943a). The repression and return of bad objects (with special reference to the "war neuroses"). In W. R. D. Fairbairn (Ed.), *Psychoanalytic studies of the personality* (pp. 59–81). London: Tavistock.

Fairbairn, W. R. D. (1943b). The war neuroses—their nature and significance. In W. R. D. Fairbairn (Ed.), *Psychoanalytic studies of the personality* (pp. 256–288). London: Tavistock.

Ferenczi, S., Abraham, K., Simmel, E., & Jones, E. (1921). *Psycho-analysis and the war neuroses.* New York: International Psycho-Analytical Press.

Figley, C. R. (Ed.). (1995). *Compassion fatigue: Coping with secondary traumatic stress disorder in those who treat the traumatized.* New York: Brunner/Mazel.

Fonagy, P., Target, M., Cottrell, D., Phillips, J., & Kurtz, Z. (2002). *What works for whom?: A critical review of treatments for children and adolescents.* New York: Guilford Press.

Freud, A. (1966). The ego and the mechanisms of defense. In *The writings of Anna Freud* (Vol. 2, pp. 1–191). New York: International Universities Press. (Original work published 1936)

Freud, S. (1953). Three essays on the theory of sexuality. In J. Strachey (Ed. & Trans.), *The standard edition of the complete psychological works of Sigmund Freud* (Vol. 7, pp. 123–245). London: Hogarth Press. (Original work published 1905)

Freud, S. (1955). Beyond the pleasure principle. In J. Strachey (Ed. & Trans.), *The standard edition of the complete psychological works of Sigmund Freud* (Vol. 18, pp. 1–64). London: Hogarth Press. (Original work published 1920)

Freud, S. (1959). An autobiographical study. In J. Strachey (Ed. & Trans.), *The standard edition of the complete psychological works of Sigmund Freud* (Vol. 20, pp. 1–74). London: Hogarth Press. (Original work published 1925)

Freud, S. (1962). The aetiology of hysteria. In J. Strachey (Ed. & Trans.), *The standard edition of the complete psychological works of Sigmund Freud* (Vol. 3, pp. 187–221). London: Hogarth Press. (Original work published 1896)

Gabbard, G. O. (2005). *Psychodynamic psychiatry in clinical practice: Fourth edition.* Washington, DC: American Psychiatric Press.

Gabbard, G. O. (2006). Psychotherapy in the *Journal*: What's missing? [Editorial]. *American Journal of Psychiatry, 163*, 182–183.

Gay, P. (1988). *Freud: A life for our time.* New York: Norton.

Goldschmidt, O. (1986). A contribution to the subject of psychic trauma based on the course of a psychoanalytic short therapy. *International Review of Psycho-Analysis, 13*, 181–199.

Greenson, R. R. (1967). *The technique and practice of psychoanalysis.* New York: International Universities Press.

Greenson, R. R. (1978). The psychology of apathy. In *Explorations in psychoanalysis* (pp. 17–30). New York: International Universities Press. (Original work published 1949)

Grinker, R., & Spiegel, J. (1945). *Men under stress.* New York: McGraw-Hill.

Haley, S. (1974). When the patient reports atrocities. *Archives of General Psychiatry, 30*, 191–196.

Herman, J. (1992). *Trauma and recovery.* New York: Basic Books.

Horowitz, M. J. (1973). Phase-oriented treatment of stress response syndromes. *American Journal of Psychotherapy, 27*(4), 506–515.

Horowitz, M. J. (1974). Stress response syndromes: Character style and dynamic psychotherapy. *Archives of General Psychiatry, 31*, 768–781.

Horowitz, M. J. (1995). Defensive control of states and person schemas. In T. Shapiro & R. N. Emde (Eds.), *Research in psychoanalysis: Process, development, outcome* (pp. 67–89). Madison, CT: International Universities Press.

Horowitz, M. J. (1997). *Formulation as a basis for planning psychotherapy.* Washington, DC: American Psychiatric Press.

Horowitz, M. J. (1998). *Cognitive psychodynamics: From conflict to character.* New York: Wiley.

Horowitz, M. J. (2001). *Stress response syndromes* (4th ed.). Northvale, NJ: Aronson.

Horowitz, M. J. (2003). *Treatment of stress response syndromes.* Arlington, VA: American Psychiatric Publishing.

Horowitz, M. J. (2005). *Understanding psychotherapy change: A practical guide to configurational analysis.* Washington, DC: American Psychological Association Press.

Horowitz, M. J., & Kaltreider, N. (1979). Brief therapy of the stress response syndrome. *Psychiatric Clinics of North America, 2*, 365–377.

Horowitz, M. J., Marmar, C., Krupnick, J., Wilner, N., Kaltreider, N., & Wallerstein, R. (1984a). *Personality styles and brief psychotherapy.* New York: Basic Books.

Horowitz, M. J., Marmar, C., Weiss, D. S., DeWitt, K., & Rosenbaum, R. (1984b). Brief therapy of bereavement reactions: The relation of process to outcome. *Archives of General Psychiatry, 41*, 438–448.

Horowitz, M. J., Marmar, C., Weiss, D., Kaltreider, N., & Wilner, N. (1986). Comprehensive analysis of change after brief dynamic psychotherapy. *American Journal of Psychiatry, 143*, 582–589.

Horowitz, M. J., Milbrath, C., Jordan, D., Stinson, C., Ewert, M., Redington, D., et al. (1994). Expressive and defensive behavior during discourse on unresolved topics: A single case study. *Journal of Personality, 62*, 527–563.

Horowitz, M. J., Stinson, C., Curtis, D., Ewert, M., Redington, D., Singer, J. L., et al. (1993). Topics and signs: Defensive control of emotional expression. *Journal of Consulting and Clinical Psychology, 61*, 421–430.

Huston, J. (1948). *Let there be light* (PMF5019). Washington, DC: Film Production of the U. S. Army.

Janet, P. (1886). Les actes inconscients et la mémoire pendant le somnambulism [Unconscious acts and memory under somnambulism]. *Revue Philosophique, 25*(1), 238–279.

Janet, P. (1973). *L'automatisme psychologique* [Psychological automatism]. Paris: Société Pierre Janet. (Original work published 1889)

Kardiner, A. (1941). *The traumatic neuroses of war.* New York: Hoeber.

Kardiner, A., & Spiegel, H. (1947). *War stress and neurotic illness.* New York: Hoeber.

Klerman, G. L., Weissman, M. M., Rounsaville, B. J., & Chevron, E. (1984). *Interpersonal psychotherapy of depression.* New York: Basic Books.

Krupnick, J. (1997). Brief psychodynamic treatment of PTSD. *Journal of Clinical Psychology, 3*, 75–89.

Krupnick, J. L., Green, B. L., & Miranda, J. (1998, June). *Group interpersonal psychotherapy for the treatment of PTSD following interpersonal trauma.* Paper presented at the annual meeting of the Society for Psychotherapy Research, Snowbird, UT.

Krystal, H. (Ed.). (1968). *Massive psychic trauma.* New York: International Universities Press.

Krystal, H. (1988). *Integration and self-healing.* Hillsdale, NJ: Analytic Press.

Kudler, H. (1989). The tension between psychoanalysis and neuroscience: A perspective on dream theory in psychiatry. *Psychoanalysis and Contemporary Thought, 12*, 599–617.

Kudler, H. (1991). What is psychological trauma? *National Center for Post-Traumatic Stress Disorder Clinical Newsletter, 2*, 8.

Kudler, H. (2007). The need for psychodynamic principles in outreach to new combat veterans and their families. *Journal of the American Academy of Psychoanalysis and Dynamic Psychiatry, 35*(1), 39–50.

Lidz, T. (1946). Nightmares and the combat neurosis. *Psychiatry, 3*, 37–49.

Lifton, R. J. (1967). *Death in life: Survivors of Hiroshima.* New York: Random House.

Lindemann, E. (1944). Symptomatology and management of acute grief. *American Journal of Psychiatry, 101*, 141–146.

Lindy, J. (1985). The trauma membrane and other clinical concepts derived from psychotherapeutic work with survivors of natural disasters. *Psychiatric Annals, 15*, 153–160.

Lindy, J. (1986). An outline for the psychoanalytic psychotherapy of post-traumatic stress disorder. In C. Figley (Ed.), *Trauma and its wake* (Vol. II, pp. 195–212). New York: Plenum Press.

Lindy, J. (1988). *Vietnam: A casebook.* New York: Brunner/Mazel.

Lindy, J. D. (1996). Psychoanalytic psychotherapy of posttraumatic stress disorder: The nature of the therapeutic relationship. In B. A. van der Kolk, A. C. McFarlane, & L. Weisaeth (Eds.), *Traumatic stress: The effects of overwhelming experiences on mind, body, and society* (pp. 525–536). New York: Guilford Press.

Loewald, H. W. (1960). On the therapeutic action of psychoanalysis. *International Journal of Psychoanalysis, 41*, 16–33.

Luborsky, L. (1990). A guide to the CCRT method. In L. Luborsky & P. Crits-

Christoph (Eds.), *Understanding transference: The core conflictual relationship theme method* (pp. 15–36). New York: Basic Books.

Luborsky, L., Crits-Christoph, P., Mintz, J., & Auerbach, A. (1988). *Who will benefit from psychotherapy?: Predicting therapeutic outcomes.* New York: Basic Books.

Mann, J. (1973). *Time-limited psychotherapy.* Cambridge, MA: Harvard University Press.

Marmar, C., & Freeman, M. (1988). Brief dynamic psychotherapy of post-traumatic stress disorders: Management of narcissistic regression. *Journal of Traumatic Stress, 1,* 323–337.

Marshall, R. D., Yehuda, R., & Bone, S. (2000). Trauma-focused psychodynamic psychotherapy. In A. Y. Shalev, R. Yehuda, & A. C. McFarlane (Eds.), *International handbook of human response to trauma* (pp. 347–361). New York: Kluwer Academic/Plenum Press.

McCann, I. L., & Pearlman, L. A. (1990). *Psychological trauma and the adult survivor: Theory, therapy, and transformation.* New York: Brunner/Mazel.

Mosher, P. W. (Ed.). (1987). *Title key word and author index to psychoanalytic journals, 1920–1986.* New York: American Psychoanalytic Association.

Ochberg, F. M. (Ed.). (1988). *Post-traumatic therapy and victims of violence.* New York: Brunner/Mazel.

Parson, E. R. (1984). The reparation of the self: Clinical and theoretical dimensions in the treatment of Vietnam combat veterans. *Journal of Contemporary Psychotherapy, 14*(1), 4–56.

PDM Task Force. (2006). *Psychodynamic diagnostic manual.* Silver Spring, MD: Alliance of Psychoanalytic Organizations.

Pearlman, L. A., & Saakvitne, K. W. (1995). *Trauma and the therapist: Countertransference and vicarious traumatization in psychotherapy with incest survivors.* New York: Norton.

Pelcovitz, D., van der Kolk, B., Roth, S., Mandel, F. S., Kaplan, S., & Resik, P. A. (1997). Development of a criteria set and a Structured Interview for Disorders of Extreme Stress (SIDES). *Journal of Traumatic Stress, 10,* 3–17.

Price, J. L., Hilsenroth, M., Callahan, K. L., Petrectic-Jackson, P. A., & Bonge, D. (2004). A pilot study of psychodynamic psychotherapy for adult survivors of childhood sexual abuse. *Clinical Psychology and Psychotherapy, 11,* 378–391.

Rivers, W. H. R. (1918, February). An address on the repression of war experience. *Lancet,* pp. 173–177.

Rose, D. (1991). A model for psychodynamic psychotherapy with the rape victim. *Psychotherapy, 28,* 85–95.

Roth, S., & Batson, R. (1997). *Naming the shadows: A new approach to individual and group psychotherapy for adult survivors of childhood incest.* New York: Free Press.

Sargant, W., & Slater, E. (1969). *An introduction to physical methods of treatment in psychiatry* (4th ed.). Edinburgh, UK: Livingstone.

Shay, J. (1994). *Achilles in Vietnam: Combat trauma and the undoing of character.* New York: Atheneum/Macmillan.

Shengold, L. (1989). *Soul murder: The effects of childhood abuse and deprivation.* New Haven, CT: Yale University Press.

Shengold, L. (1991). *"Father, don't you see I'm burning?": Reflections on sex, narcissism, symbolism, and murder.* New Haven, CT: Yale University Press.

Solomon, S. D., & Johnson, D. M. (2002). Psychosocial treatment of posttraumatic stress disorder: A practice-friendly review of outcome research. *Journal of Clinical Psychology, 58*, 947–959.

Talbot, N. L., Conwell, Y., O'Hara, M. W., Stuart, S., Ward, E. A., Gamble, S. A., et al. (2005). Interpersonal psychotherapy for depressed women with sexual abuse histories. *Journal of Nervous and Mental Disease, 193*, 847–850.

Terr, L. (1979). Children of Chowchilla. *Psychoanalytic Study of the Child, 34*, 547–623.

Ulman, R., & Brothers, D. (1988). *The shattered self: Psychoanalytic study of trauma.* Hillsdale, NJ: Analytic Press.

van der Hart, O., Brown, P., & van der Kolk, B. A. (1989). Pierre Janet's treatment of posttraumatic stress. *Journal of Traumatic Stress, 2*, 379–395.

van der Kolk, B. A., McFarlane, A. C., & Weisaeth, L. (Eds.). (1996). *Traumatic stress: The effect of overwhelming experience on mind, body and society.* New York: Guilford Press.

Weiss, D., & Marmar, C. (1993). Teaching time-limited dynamic psychotherapy for posttraumatic stress disorder and pathological grief. *Psychotherapy, 30*, 587–591.

Werman, D. S. (1984). *The practice of supportive psychotherapy.* New York: Brunner/Mazel.

Wilson, J. P., & Lindy, J. D. (Eds.). (1994). *Countertransference in the treatment of PTSD.* New York: Guilford Press.

Winnicott, D. W. (1965). *The maturational processes and the facilitating environment: Studies in the theory of emotional development.* London: Hogarth Press.

CHAPTER 15

Psychodynamic Therapy for Child Trauma

Alicia F. Lieberman, Chandra Ghosh Ippen,
and Steven Marans

Theoretical Context

From the earliest days of psychoanalysis, Sigmund Freud put trauma at the center of his theories about emotional disturbances, tracing their origin to the lasting repercussions of traumatic experiences on personality development. This central premise remained a constant amid Freud's many revisions of his ideas, and the characteristics of traumatic phenomena that he elucidated remain the subject of clinical and research focus to this day. The basic features of the traumatic moment include the following elements: (1) Unpredictable and immediate danger to life and personal integrity elicits high levels of terror and helplessness that overwhelm the individual's ability to anticipate and cope; (2) a convergence between the impact of external dangers and "internal dangers" or anxieties that become salient at different stages of development; and (3) a potential for enduring impact on personality structure of the protective/defensive mechanisms mobilized in response to trauma (Freud, 1926/1959, 1940/1964).

Freud attributed the impact of trauma to the interaction between two sets of factors: the objective features of the event, and the individual characteristics of the person experiencing it, including constitutional makeup, developmental stage, and prior history. He also stressed the pivotal role of "helplessness," defined as the dual inability to tolerate the overwhelming affective responses to the situation and to take effective protective action to

370

cope with it. The helpless response to overwhelming danger is the key feature that distinguishes the traumatic experience from anxiety. Unlike the collapse of coping mechanisms that characterizes the traumatic response, anxiety serves as a signal for preparation and action whose aim is to avoid or decrease the threat of the perceived danger. In developing attachment theory, Bowlby (1969/1982, 1980) adapted Freud's concept of the mother as the child's "protective shield" against unbearable levels of stimulation, framing the maternal role in the context of ethological principles, and highlighting attachment as a biologically determined emotional bond with the mother that promotes species survival and psychological security in situations of uncertainty and danger. Clinical experience and empirical research in the subsequent decades have repeatedly demonstrated the soundness of many of Freud's and Bowlby's basic formulations, which continue to influence trauma treatment for children and adults across different theoretical orientations (Cohen, Mannarino, & Deblinger, 2006; Horowitz, 2003; Putnam, 1997; Pynoos, Steinberg, & Piacentini, 1999).

Children's developmental stage plays a major role in their response to trauma, and must inform and guide the course of treatment. Young children are deeply affected by their parents' or primary caregivers' presence and response to the traumatic event because they are primarily dependent on the parents for protection and have a self-referential understanding of causality, whereas older children and adolescents tend to be more responsive to the specific characteristics of the traumatic event (Berkowitz & Marans, 2006; Laor et al., 1997). Children of all ages tend to compensate for their increased sense of vulnerability and helplessness following trauma with a range of symptoms that aim to reestablish a sense of greater control. These defensive efforts may include avoidant and phobic behaviors, oppositional behavior, revenge fantasies, somatic complaints, increased arousal, separation anxiety, aggression, and other protective maneuvers (Marans, 1996; Marans & Adelman, 1997; Pynoos et al., 1999). Underlying these situational traumatic responses are the four normative anxieties that unfold in succession in the course of development: fear of abandonment, fear of losing the parent's love, fear of body damage (referred to in classic psychoanalysis as "castration fear"), and fear of superego condemnation (Freud, 1926/1959). These internal dangers, labeled by Brenner (1976) as the "four calamities," because they pervade the child's emotional life with the anticipation of catastrophe, converge with external dangers to shape the individual child's specific responses to trauma (Marans, 2005; Pynoos, Steinberg, & Wraith, 1995).

Description of Techniques

The psychodynamic treatment of child trauma is guided by the therapist's understanding of the child's inner life in the context of the child's daily life and history. The psychodynamic psychotherapist focuses on the specific meanings the child gives to the traumatic event based on his or her constitutional, developmental, and environmental circumstances and history. Parents and/or other significant adults are engaged as allies in treatment to reestablish psychological safety and the reassuring routines that are essential to recovery.

The ultimate goal of psychodynamic psychotherapies is to promote personality coherence and healthy development rather than to alleviate symptom severity alone. In work with younger children, free play during the session is viewed as the most developmentally appropriate entry point into the child's experience. Toys and other materials are provided, with the goal of promoting imaginative play and organized narratives that often lead to the child's reenactment of the traumatic events or to the expression, in displacement, of the key ingredients that constituted the most frightening aspects of the convergence of internal and external dangers. The therapist closely follows the child's enactments to help describe what happened and to put feelings into words to promote narrative coherence and cognitive mastery of overwhelming emotional reactions. Interventions also focus on the child's fantasies or cognitive misunderstandings about his or her own role in precipitating the traumatic event or its consequences to correct misconceptions and promote reality testing. In keeping with Freud's famous dictum, "Where id was, there shall ego be," the therapist strives to help the child replace destructive emotions and self-damaging fantasies of revenge with prosocial, constructive images and behaviors that restore a sense of internal safety and trust in the self and others.

With infants, toddlers, and preschoolers, the parent or primary caregiver is customarily engaged as a partner in treatment, whether through collateral sessions or through the parent's physical presence during the sessions. Relationship-based psychotherapies address situations in which the parents are either the perpetrators of the trauma or fail to support the child's healthy development. In infant–parent psychotherapy (IPP; Fraiberg, 1980; Lieberman, Silverman, & Pawl, 2000), toddler–parent psychotherapy (TPP; Lieberman, 1992), and preschool–parent psychotherapy (PPP; Toth, Maughan, Manly, Spagnola, & Cicchetti, 2002), the focus of the intervention is on the relationship itself, to address negative parental attributions to the child and correct mutual traumatic expectations between the parent(s) and the child. Although these treatments are geared to the specific demands of the child's age and developmental needs, all relationship-based approaches share an emphasis on translating the parent's and the child's experiences to each other as a vehicle to enhanced emotional reciprocity. For this reason, Lieberman (2004) advocates use of the term "child–parent psychotherapy" (CPP) as an umbrella concept.

Consideration of individual characteristics, developmental context, history, and current environment are equally important in work with older children and adolescents. The adolescent's thrust toward autonomy and mastery, and away from perceived dependent relationships, may pose particular challenges to the treatment of trauma. Psychotherapeutic intervention with traumatized adolescents may require a psychoeducational introduction that aims to (1) mobilize more mature cognitive capacities; (2) explain symptomatology; (3) identify traumatic reminders; (4) clarify environmental factors that may complicate recovery, such as interactions that promote developmental regression; and (5) make explicit the ways that overwhelming fear and helplessness of the traumatic situation run counter to age-appropriate strivings for a sense of agency and self-competence. The relatively unstructured nature of the interviews that follow may promote a return of the locus of control and greater comfort, encouraging self-observation and reflection to distinguish between both the real and psychological origins of the dangers, and the past and current nature of the threat.

Method of Collecting Data

We conducted a series of literature searches using PsycINFO and Published International Literature on Traumatic Stress (PILOTS). A preliminary search for the key words "(psychodynamic or psychoanalytic), treatment, randomized and (child or children or adolescents)" revealed only three studies, none of which was specific to the treatment of traumatized children. This result was surprising because it failed to identify several well-known studies involving psychodynamic treatment. We hypothesized that psychodynamic child trauma clinical researchers may be less likely than practitioners of other psychotherapy approaches to "brand" their work because they tend to use an integrative developmental psychopathology framework that incorporates dynamic, relational, attachment-oriented, cognitive, behavioral, and cultural considerations (Lieberman & Van Horn, 2005). This integrative approach is consistent with the overarching goal of promoting healthy development rather than symptom reduction alone.

Given the sparse results of the initial search, we broadened terms to include the following key words: "(treatment or randomized) and (child or children or adolescents) and (psychodynamic or psychoanalytic or play therapy or dyadic or relational or individual psychotherapy or infant–parent psychotherapy or toddler–parent psychotherapy or preschool–parent psychotherapy or child–parent psychotherapy)." We included treatment studies based on attachment theory because of the psychoanalytic origins of this approach (Bowlby, 1969/1982). We identified additional articles through consultation with colleagues in the field. To be included, the authors needed to identify their treatment as psychodynamic, psychoanalytic, or attachment-based, either in the published article or when contacted. Integrative treatments that targeted the attachment relationship but also included parent training or other cognitive-behavioral methods were not included.

Literature Review

Case Studies

In a series of clinical case studies, Gaensbauer and colleagues (e.g., Gaensbauer & Sands, 1979) described the disruptive impact of trauma in infancy and early childhood on the parent–child relationship. Gaensbauer and Siegel (1995) proposed that including the caregiver in the young child's treatment provides for the child a safe therapeutic environment that allows toleration of feelings associated with the trauma. The caregiver's presence during the sessions may serve to clarify how the child's play is related to the traumatic event, and may correct negative parental attributions to the child by linking the child's problem behavior to the anxiety generated by the trauma rather than to the child's intrinsic negative characteristics. In addition, the caregiver's supportive presence may allow the child to work through feelings of anger and mistrust, and help repair the parent's role as a protector. Parental collaboration is also necessary to develop a plan to manage symptoms that may become temporarily more intense with therapy. When children display symptoms of dissociation, parental involvement in treatment is used to address maladaptive parent–child interactions that may serve to reinforce dissociative states and impede the development of an integrated self (Silberg, 2004).

The effectiveness of psychodynamic and/or relationship-based approaches is supported by numerous case studies that document the course of such treatments for children with single-incident (e.g., Gaensbauer, 1994) and complex, chronic traumas (e.g., Osofsky, Cohen, & Drell, 1995). Other case studies detail how relationship-based interventions can be conducted with trauma-exposed mothers and their young children to reduce the likelihood of an intergenerational transmission of the negative consequences of trauma exposure (Arons, 2005; Mayers, 2005; Schechter, Kaminer, Grienenberger, & Amat, 2003). Space considerations prevent an extensive description of all the case studies, which describe treatments following exposure to a range of traumas, including dog attacks (Gaensbauer, 1994), invasive medical procedures (Gaensbauer, 2000), sexual abuse (Grubbs, 1994; Silberg, 2004), witnessing the murder of a parent (Gaensbauer, Chatoor, Drell, Siegel, & Zeanah, 1995; Marans & Adelman, 1997; Osofsky et al., 1995), and chronic traumas, including domestic violence, physical abuse, neglect, and suspected sexual abuse (Childs & Timberlake, 1995). These case studies demonstrate how psychodynamically oriented play therapy can help young children process experiences that occurred during preverbal periods and as they are developing language skills (Gaensbauer, 1995).

Pretest to Posttest Comparisons

The literature search did not identify any psychodynamic or relationship-based pre- to posttest trials with specific samples of trauma-exposed children.

Randomized Trials

We present each randomized trial using a standardized format to enable comparisons among dynamically oriented treatments, as well as with trauma-informed treatments based in other theoretical orientations. Table 15.1 presents a synopsis of the randomized trials conducted to date.

Relationship-Based Interventions

A key premise of psychodynamic relationship-based psychotherapy is that conflicts originating in the parents' relational history can affect the current relationship with their child through distorted representations and lack of attunement (Fraiberg, Adelson, & Shapiro, 1975). The goal of treatment is to support and strengthen the parent–child relationship as a vehicle to long-term healthy child development. Targets of the intervention include mothers' and children's maladaptive representations of themselves and each other, and interactions and behaviors that interfere with children's mental health. With trauma-exposed samples, these treatments incorporate a focus on trauma experienced by the parent, the child, or both. Over the course of treatment, parent and child are guided in creating a joint narrative of the traumatic event to identify and address traumatic triggers that generate dysregulated behaviors and reinforce mutual traumatic expectations between parent and child, and to place the traumatic experience as an anomalous occurrence within the overall context of satisfying interpersonal relationships, developmentally appropriate activities and goals, and safe and predictable daily routines. Sessions include the parent(s) and the child, and are conducted in the home or a clinic playroom. Individual parent or child sessions may be added as needed.

Four randomized trials support the efficacy of relationship-based therapies with trauma-exposed children. In addition, two randomized trials demonstrate the efficacy of relationship-based interventions with other at-risk groups. These studies are described below.

CPP FOR CHILDREN EXPOSED TO DOMESTIC VIOLENCE

Sample Characteristics. Lieberman, Van Horn, and Ghosh Ippen (2005) conducted a randomized controlled trial of CPP for children who had witnessed domestic violence. Mother–child dyads were randomized to either CPP ($N = 42$) or case management plus community referrals for psychotherapy ($N = 33$). The study involved 36 boys and 39 girls, ages 3–5 ($M = 4.06$; $SD = 0.82$), exposed to domestic violence in addition to other traumas: physical abuse (49%); community violence (46.7%), and sexual abuse (14.4%). Children were from a variety of ethnic backgrounds: 37% mixed ethnicity (predominantly Latino/white), 28% Latino, 14.5% African American, 10.5% white, 7% Asian, and 2% other ethnicity. On average, mothers had experienced 12.36

TABLE 15.1. Studies Based on Randomized Trials

Study	Target population[a]	Number/length of sessions	Treatment(s); control[b]	Major findings	Between-group effect sizes	Within-group effect sizes
Lieberman et al. (2005)	39 females and 36 males ages 3–5 with exposure to domestic violence	50 weekly 1-hr sessions	42 child-parent psychotherapy (CPP) 33 community and case management (CT-CM)	Significantly greater improvements in child traumatic stress and maternal avoidance for CPP relative to comparison.	CPP vs. CT-CM *DC: 0–3 TSD* **Intent to treat:** 0.43 **Completers:** 0.69 *CAPS Avoidance* **Intent to treat:** 0.48 **Completers:** 0.50	*DC: 0–3 TSD* **Intent to treat** CPP: 0.76 CT-CM: 0.09 **Completers** CPP: 1.13 CT-CM: 0.10 *CAPS Avoidance* **Intent to treat** CPP: 0.73 CT-CM: 0.25 **Completers** CPP: 0.99 CT-CM: 0.31
Trowell et al. (2002)	71 sexually abused girls ages 6–14	Individual: Up to 30 sessions, 50 min each Group: Up to 18 sessions	35 individual therapy (IT) 36 group therapy (GT)	IT girls showed significantly greater reductions in PTSD symptoms at 1- and 2-yr assessment points.	Orvaschel's 1989 PTSD Scale IT vs. GT **Completers** Baseline—1st yr follow-up Reexperiencing: 0.60 Avoidance: 0.66 Baseline—2nd yr follow-up Reexperiencing: 0.79 Avoidance: 0.36 Baseline to study exit Reexperiencing: 0.65 Avoidance: 0.60	Insufficient data

Note. DC: 0–3 TSD, Structured Interview for Diagnostic Classification of Mental Health and Development Disorders of Infancy and Early Childhood for Clinicians—Traumatic Stress Disorder Section; CAPS, Clinician-Administered PTSD Scale.

[a]N = subjects starting study.
[b]N = subjects in data analyses.

stressful life events. Mean monthly income was $1,817 ($SD$ = $1,460); 23% received public assistance, and 41% had incomes below the federal poverty level.

Treatment. CPP was conducted over 50 weeks by master's- and PhD-level clinicians. Fidelity was monitored through intensive weekly supervision and case conferences. Comparison group mothers received monthly case management and were connected to community clinics; 73% of mothers and 55% of children received individual psychotherapy.

Attrition and Attendance. The attrition rate was 14.3% in the CPP group and 12% in the comparison group, with no significant group differences. CPP participants on average attended 32.09 sessions (SD = 15.20). Among those who received individual psychotherapy in the comparison group, 50% of mothers and 65% of children attended more than 20 sessions.

Assessment. Children and mothers were assessed at intake, midtreatment, posttreatment, and at 6-month posttreatment. Children were assessed using the Child Behavior Checklist (CBCL; Achenbach, 1991; Achenbach & Edelbrock, 1983) and the Structured Interview for Diagnostic Classification Manual for Mental Health and Development Disorders of Infancy and Early Childhood for Clinicians (DC: 0–3; Scheeringa, Zeanah, Drell, & Larrieu, 1995). Parents were assessed using the Symptom Checklist-90—Revised (SCL-90-R; Derogatis, 1994) and the Clinician-Administered PTSD Scale (CAPS; Blake et al., 1990).

Outcomes. At posttreatment, CPP children showed significantly greater reductions in total behavior problems (Cohen's d = 0.24) and traumatic stress symptoms (d = 0.64). CPP mothers showed significantly greater reductions in avoidant symptomatology (d = 0.50). Results from the 6-month follow-up showed that improvements in children's behavior problems (d = 0.41) and in maternal symptoms (d = 0.38) continued after treatment ended (Lieberman, Ghosh Ippen, & Van Horn, 2006).

PPP FOR MALTREATED CHILDREN

Toth and colleagues (2002) examined the efficacy of two interventions—a psychoeducation model and an attachment-informed intervention—to alter preschoolers' mental representations of their mothers and themselves. Maltreated preschoolers are likely to have negative models of relationships and to generalize them to others. These negative representations may form the basis for children's future relationship expectations.

Sample Characteristics. Randomized assignment of 112 maltreated preschoolers was to PPP (N = 31), psychoeducation home visitation (PHV; N = 48), or community standard (CS; $N = 33$). Abuse types included physical abuse, sexual abuse, emotional maltreatment, and neglect, with 60% of children experiencing more than one form of maltreatment. The design included a nonmaltreated, low-income comparison group (NC: $N = 43$). The final sample included 68 boys and 54 girls (PPP: $N = 23$; PHV: $N = 34$; CS: $N = 30$; NC: $N = 35$) age 4 years at intake ($M = 48.18$ months, $SD = 6.88$). Specific information regarding child ethnicity was not provided, but 76.2% were ethnic minorities. Average group income ranged from $16,700 to $19,930.

Treatment. PPP and PHV were provided over a 12-month period by master's-level therapists. Both treatments are manualized, and fidelity was monitored through weekly supervision. PPP was described earlier. PHV involved social support, psychoeducation, and cognitive-behavioral techniques to reduce risk factors and increase protective factors for child maltreatment. PHV children also participated in a 10-month, full-day preschool program, in which they were taught school readiness and relationship skills. In the CS group, 13% of children and 23% of mothers received individual psychotherapy. Mothers also participated in family or marital counseling (3%), support group or day treatment (10%), and parenting services (17%).

Attrition and Attendance. The attrition rate was as follows: PPP (19.4%); PHV (25%); CS (9%); NC (11.6%). There were no differences in demographic characteristics among dropped and retained participants, and number of sessions and duration of treatment were comparable for PPP and PHV. On average, PPP dyads received 11.63 months of treatment ($SD = 3.13$) and attended approximately 32.39 sessions ($SD = 12.42$). PHV dyads received 13.32 months of treatment ($SD = 6.56$) and on average attended 31.09 sessions ($SD = 14.30$). For CS families, treatment averaged 9.3 months for children and 5.8 months for mothers.

Assessment. Children were assessed at intake, posttreatment, and at 1 and 3 years' postintervention. Children's attributions were measured with the MacArthur Story-Stem Battery (MSSB) and coded for adaptive maternal representations; maladaptive maternal representations; global relationship expectations; and positive, negative, and false self-representations (Bretherton, Oppenheim, Buchsbaum, Emde, & the MacArthur Narrative Group, 1990).

Outcomes. PPP was more effective in improving representations of self and caregivers. The authors did not report effect sizes, but means and standard deviations provided in the article were used to calculate effect size (Cohen, 1988). For maladaptive maternal attributions, there was a significant group × time interaction, with the PPP group showing the greatest decline (PPP vs. PHV: Cohen's $d = 0.38$; PPP vs. CS: $d = 0.53$). For negative self-representations, the PPP children showed significant declines (PPP vs. PHV: $d = 0.64$.; PPP vs. CS: $d = 0.53$). There was also a significant treatment effect for relationship expectations, with PPP children showing the largest increase (PPP vs. PHV: $d = 0.69$; PPP vs. CS: $d = 0.68$). These findings highlight the importance of a relationship-focused model for changing internal working models.

IPP FOR MALTREATED CHILDREN

Cicchetti and colleagues (2006) examined the relative efficacy of a relationship-based versus a behavioral intervention in changing maltreated children's attachment classification.

Sample Characteristics. Through a review of Child Protective Services (CPS) records, 1-year-old infants ($M = 13.31$ months; $SD = 0.81$ months) were classified as maltreated or living in maltreating families and randomly assigned to IPP ($N = 53$), psychoeducational parenting intervention (PPI; $N = 49$), or community standard (CS; $N = 35$). A fourth group of 52 NC infants was also recruited. Fifty-three percent of the infants were girls; the majority of mothers (74.1%) were ethnic minorities, and the average annual family income was $17,151.

Treatment. IPP and PPI involved 1 year of weekly home visitation by master's-level therapists. Both treatments were manualized, and fidelity was monitored through weekly supervision. IPP was described earlier. The PPI intervention included didactic training in child development, parenting skills, coping strategies for managing stress, and assistance in developing social support networks. Details on services received by the CS group were not provided.

Attrition and Attendance. Although intensive recruitment strategies were used, the initial dropout rate was high: 39.6% of IPP and 51% of PPI mothers initially randomized could not be engaged. The authors noted that these rates may reflect the fact that families were not seeking treatment. Those who dropped out did not differ from those who engaged in terms of demographic or other variables. Following engagement, the overall attrition rate was 21.7%, with the greatest attrition in the CS group (42.9%) and no significant differences between IPP and PPI groups. The length of intervention and average number of sessions conducted were comparable for both groups (IPP: 46.4 weeks and 21.56 sessions; PPI: 49.4 weeks and 25.38 sessions).

Assessment. Assessments were conducted at intake and at follow-up, when the children were approximately 26 months old. Mothers and infants participated in the Strange Situation procedure, which enabled coding of infants' primary attachment classification.

Outcomes. Contrary to the authors' hypothesis, both treatments had similar efficacy in terms of altering children's attachment classifications and were significantly more effective that the CS. The rate of secure attachment changed from 3.1 to 60.7% for the IPP group and from 0.0 to 54.5% for the PPI group. In contrast, the CS group's rate of secure attachment was similar at intake (32.7%) and exit (38.6%). The NC group also did not show an increase in secure attachment over time. The authors reported effect sizes, *h*, for contrasts with the CS group of 1.51 and 1.41 for the IPP and PPI groups, respectively. Similar results were found with respect to disorganized attachment. Results were maintained for intent-to-treat (ITT) analyses.

ATTACHMENT AND BIOBEHAVIORAL CATCH-UP IN A MALTREATED SAMPLE

Dozier and colleagues (2006; Dozier, Brohawn, Lindhiem, Perkins, & Peloso, in press) examined the preliminary effectiveness of Attachment and Biobehavioral Catch-Up (ABC), an attachment-based intervention for young maltreated children in foster care.

Sample Characteristics. Sixty children ages 3.6 to 39.4 months, half boys and half girls, participated. Ethnicity was African American (63%), white (32%), or biracial (5%). Children and their foster parents were randomly assigned to ABC or to an educational intervention. Data were also gathered from 104 non-foster-care children. Dozier and colleagues (in press) included an overlapping sample of 46 of these children.

Treatment. ABC is a relationship-based intervention that seeks to reduce children's affect dysregulation by improving the child–caregiver relationship. Caregivers learn to reinterpret the child's alienating behaviors, to process their own issues that interfere with their ability to provide nurturing care, and to create an environment that nurtures the child's regulatory capabilities. The educational intervention, Developmental Education for Families (DEF), targets cognitive development, including language development. Both interventions were conducted through 10 individual, home-based sessions with the foster parents. Therapists were professional social workers or psychologists, with a minimum of 5 years clinical experience. ABC and DEF are manualized, and fidelity to the manual was monitored with videotapes of sessions.

Attrition and Attendance. Data on attrition and attendance were not reported.

Assessment. Children and caregivers were assessed at intake and 1 month after the end of treatment. Salivary cortisol samples were collected by caregivers over a 2-day period. Caregivers also completed the Parent Daily Report (PDR; Chamberlain & Reid, 1987) and a Parent Attachment Diary to track infant reactions following distress. Child reactions were coded for secure behavior (proximity seeking/contact maintenance and successful calming by the caregiver), avoidance, or resistance.

Outcomes. At posttreatment, ABC children showed lower cortisol values than DEF children. DEF children had higher cortisol than the comparison group, but ABC children did not. When distressed, ABC children showed significantly less avoidance than DEF children.

RELATIONSHIP-BASED INTERVENTIONS WITH OTHER AT-RISK SAMPLES

Four additional published studies support the efficacy of relationship-based models with at-risk samples, including anxiously attached dyads (Lieberman, Weston, & Pawl, 1991) and children of depressed mothers (Cicchetti, Rogosch, & Toth, 2000; Cicchetti, Toth, & Rogosch, 1999; Toth, Rogosch, Cicchetti, & Manly, 2006). These studies are not described here because they do not focus specifically on traumatized children. However, they are significant because they demonstrate that a child–parent focus is efficacious with diverse samples, including low-income, Spanish-speaking dyads (Lieberman et al., 1991), and that this approach has a beneficial effect on important outcomes that are not usually the focus of treatment outcome research, such as children's cognitive functioning and attachment security (Cicchetti et al., 1999, 2000, 2006; Toth et al., 2006).

SUMMARY OF RELATIONSHIP-BASED TREATMENTS

The research detailed here provides support for the use of relationship-based treatments for young children with documented maltreatment histories or exposure to domestic violence. Children and their mothers in these studies appear to have experienced multiple types of interpersonal traumas. This is noteworthy because few trauma-focused interventions exist for working with individuals with complex or chronic traumas. Importantly, four of the randomized trials involved predominantly ethnic/minority samples, including Spanish-speaking dyads, suggesting that a relationship-based approach has ecological validity for different cultural groups. Domains of improvement across studies include child and parent symptomatology; children's attributions of parents, themselves, and relationships; parent–child relationships; attachment classification; and physiological changes.

Individual Psychoanalytic Treatment for Sexual Abuse

Sample Characteristics. Trowell and colleagues (2002) examined the relative efficacy of a psychoanalytically based individual therapy ($N = 35$) and a psychoeducation-based group treatment ($N = 36$) with a group of 71 sexually abused girls, ages 6–14 ($M = 10$; $SD = 2.2$). Ethnicity included 63% white, 11%

black Caribbean, 10% mixed, 5% Chinese, 6% Mediterranean origin, and 3% unknown.

Treatment. Individual therapy included up to 30 weekly sessions of brief, focused, psychoanalytic treatment occurring over three phases: (1) engagement; (2) focus on issues relevant to that participant; and (3) separation, ending, and reworking key topics. Children were given play materials, and therapists ensured that topics listed in a manual were raised (no reference was provided for the manual). They completed checklists to ensure fidelity. Caregivers met independently with social workers approximately every 2 weeks. Group treatment comprised up to 18 sessions, including psychotherapeutic or psychoeducational components. Caregivers were seen either individually or in caregiver groups. The authors report that although there were differences in the number of sessions, the "length of each session was such that the face-to-face contact time was approximately the same" (Trowell et al., 2002, p. 235).

Attrition and Attendance. The mean percentage of attended sessions was 88% for individual and group treatment. Examining both groups, 97% received treatment as allocated.

Assessment. Children and caregivers were assessed at pretest, 1-year, and 2-year follow-up. Assessment instruments included the Schedule for Affective Disorders and Schizophrenia for School-Age Children (K-SADS; Chambers et al., 1985), the Kiddie Global Assessment Scale (K-GAS; Chambers et al., 1985), and Orvaschel's 1989 PTSD Scale, which is an extension of the K-SADS (Orvaschel, 1989). Data were not available for all participants; some girls declined assessment because they did not wish to think about their traumatic experiences. At the first follow-up, 83% of the individual therapy and 81% of the group therapy participants completed assessment measures. At the 2-year follow-up, 80% of the individual therapy and 72% of the group therapy participants were assessed.

Outcomes. Although the authors initially hypothesized greater effects for group treatment, the results favor the psychoanalytically based individual treatment. Girls in this group showed significantly greater reductions in PTSD symptoms at 1- and 2-year assessment points. For reexperiencing, the authors report a between-group effect size of 0.60 from baseline to 1-year follow-up, and 0.79 from baseline to 2-year follow-up. For persistent avoidance, effect size was 0.66 from baseline to 1-year follow-up, and 0.36 from baseline to 2-year follow-up. There were no significant group differences with regard to K-GAS impairment scores or PTSD arousal. Both groups declined significantly. These findings provide initial support for the use of psychoanalytic therapy for the treatment of child sexual abuse.

Summary and Recommendations

There is growing evidence of the effectiveness and efficacy of psychodynamic approaches in the treatment of traumatized children. This is a promising trend toward painting a more complete picture of the empirical support that exists for different forms of psychotherapy for traumatized children. Paradoxically, the pervasive influence of Freud's ideas on the evolution of approaches to psychotherapy generally, and trauma treatment in particular, makes it difficult to circumscribe the boundaries of what constitutes psychodynamic treatment, an observation also made by Kudler, Krupnick, Blank, Herman, and Horowitz (Chapter 14, this volume). The challenge is compounded by the many shared characteristics of different approaches to psychotherapy, which is defined as "an interpersonal process designed to bring about modifications of *feelings, cognitions, attitudes* and *behavior* which have proved troublesome to the person seeking help from a trained professional" (Strupp, 1978, p. 3, emphasis added). Cognitive, behavioral, and interpersonal psychotherapies routinely incorporate therapeutic elements that are central components of psychodynamic approaches, such as attention to the quality of the client–therapist relationship and sustained focus on identification of traumatic triggers of maladaptive affective states, pathogenic interpersonal attributions, and obstacles to therapeutic progress. Reciprocally, psychodynamic psychotherapies utilize therapeutic strategies derived from cognitive, behavioral, and interpersonal approaches to promote safety in everyday life, maintain predictable routines that uphold continuity in the sense of self, and encourage engagement with developmentally appropriate goals and activities. The overlap between modern cognitive-behavioral approaches and psychoanalysis has been explicated by Roth and Fonagy (2005), who highlight as specific commonalities the premise of irrational cognitive processes and the concepts of helplessness, discrepancy between perceived self and ideal self, self-destructiveness of negative cognitions, and avoidance of painful cognitions (p. 8), and go on to observe that "there is much that is 'borrowed' from different orientations by all practitioners" (p. 15).

Roth and Fonagy (2005) describe the complexities of defining what constitute empirically supported therapies (ESTs), pointing out that lack of empirical evidence is not equivalent to lack of effectiveness/efficacy. They also stress the potential mistakes of equating ESTs with best practice. Many currently available ESTs are cognitive-behavioral therapies because psychodynamic treatments do not have a quantitative research tradition that enables their practitioners to undertake randomized controlled trials readily. This is the case, in part, because the relatively unstructured, individually driven approach of psychodynamic treatment leaves many practitioners generally distrustful of manualized treatments that are intended to be implemented in standardized fashion across different clinical research participants. In addition, the goals of psychodynamic treatment involve broader changes in character structure and relationship patterns that often cannot be measured as succinctly or readily as circumscribed symptom with instruments that are currently available. In spite of these obstacles to empirical documentation, a substantial body of evidence demonstrates the effectiveness of psychodynamic treatment with adults (Roth & Fonagy, 2005). This review gives reason for optimism that there is momentum toward gathering similar empirical evidence supporting the psychodynamic treatment of traumatized children as well.

References

Achenbach, T. M. (1991). *Manual for the Child Behavior Checklist 4-18 and 1991 Profile.* Burlington: University of Vermont Department of Psychiatry

Achenbach, T. M., & Edelbrock, C. S. (1983). *Manual for the Child Behavior Checklist and Revised Child Behavioral Profile.* Burlington: University of Vermont Department of Psychiatry.

Arons, J. (2005). "In a black hole": The (negative) space between longing and dread: Home-based psychotherapy with a traumatized mother and her infant son. *Psychoanalytic Study of the Child, 60,* 101–127.

Berkowitz, S. J., & Marans, S. (2006). Crisis intervention: Secondary prevention for children exposed to violence. In M. M. Feerick & G. B. Silverman (Eds.), *Children exposed to violence* (pp. 137–158). Baltimore: Brookes.

Blake, D. D., Weathers, F., Nagy, L., Kaloupek, D. G., Klauminzer, G., Charney, D., et al. (1990). Clinician-Administered PTSD Scale. *Behavior Therapist, 18,* 12–14.

Bowlby, J. (1980). *Attachment and loss.* New York: Basic Books.

Bowlby, J. (1982). *Attachment and loss: Vol. I. Attachment.* New York: Basic Books. (Original work published 1969)

Brenner, C. (1976). *Psychoanalytic technique and psychic conflict.* New York: International University Press.

Bretherton, I., Oppenheim, D., Buchsbaum, H., Emde, R. N., & the MacArthur Narrative Group. (1990). *MacArthur Story-Stem Battery.* Unpublished manual.

Chamberlain, P., & Reid, J. B. (1987). Parent observation and report of child symptoms. *Behavioral Assessment, 9,* 97–109.

Chambers, W. J., Puig-Antich, J., Hirsch, M., Paez, P., Ambrosini, P., Tabrizi, M. A., et al. (1985). The assessment of affective disorders in children and adolescents by semi-structured interview. *Archives of General Psychiatry, 42,* 697–702.

Childs, L. S., & Timberlake, E. M. (1995). Assessing clinical progress: A case study of Daryl. *Child and Adolescent Social Work Journal, 12,* 289–315.

Cicchetti, D., Rogosch, F. A., & Toth, S. L. (2000). The efficacy of toddler–parent psychotherapy for fostering cognitive development in offspring of depressed mothers. *Journal of Abnormal Child Psychology, 28,* 135–148.

Cicchetti, D., Rogosch, F. A., & Toth, S. L. (2006). Fostering secure attachment in infants in maltreating families through preventive interventions. *Development and Psychopathology, 18,* 623–650.

Cicchetti, D., Toth, S. L., & Rogosch, F. A. (1999). The efficacy of toddler–parent psychotherapy to increase attachment security in offspring of depressed mothers. *Attachment and Human Development, 1,* 34–66.

Cohen, J. (1988). *Statistical power analysis for the behavioral sciences* (2nd ed.). Hillsdale, NJ: Erlbaum.

Cohen, J. A., Mannarino, A. P., & Deblinger, E. (2006). *Treating trauma and traumatic grief in children and adolescents.* New York: Guilford Press.

Derogatis, L. R. (1994). *Symptom Checklist-90-R: Administration, scoring, and procedures manual.* Minneapolis, MN: National Computer Systems.

Dozier, M., Brohawn, D., Lindhiem, O., Perkins, E., & Peloso, E. (in press). Effects of a foster parent training program on children's attachment behaviors: Preliminary evidence from a randomized clinical trial. *Child and Adolescent Social Work Journal.*

Dozier, M., Peloso, E., Lindhiem, O., Gordon, M. K., Manni, M., Sepulveda, S., et al. (2006). Preliminary evidence from a randomized clinical trial: Intervention effects on foster children's behavioral and biological regulation. *Journal of Social Issues, 62,* 767–785.

Fraiberg, S. (1980). *Clinical studies in infant mental health.* New York: Basic Books.

Fraiberg, S., Adelson, E., & Shapiro, V. (1975). Ghosts in the nursery: A psychoanalytic approach to impaired infant–mother relationships. *Journal of the American Academy of Child Psychiatry, 14,* 387–421.

Freud, S. (1959). Inhibitions, symptoms and anxiety. In J. Strachey (Ed. & Trans.), *The standard edition of the complete psychological works of Sigmund Freud* (Vol. 20). London: Hogarth Press. (Original work published 1925–1926)

Freud, S. (1964). An outline of psychoanalysis. In J. Strachey (Ed. & Trans.), *The standard edition of the complete psychological work of Sigmund Freud* (Vol. 23). London: Hogarth Press. (Original work published 1940)

Gaensbauer, T. J. (1994). Therapeutic work with a traumatized toddler. *Psychoanalytic Study of the Child, 49,* 412–433.

Gaensbauer, T. J. (1995). Trauma in the preverbal period: Symptoms, memories, and developmental impact. *Psychoanalytic Study of the Child, 50,* 122–149.

Gaensbauer, T. J. (2000). Psychotherapeutic treatment of traumatized infants and toddlers: A case report. *Clinical Child Psychology and Psychiatry, 5,* 373–385.

Gaensbauer, T. J., Chatoor, I., Drell, M., Siegel, D., & Zeanah, C. H. (1995). Traumatic loss in a one-year-old girl. *Journal of the American Academy of Child and Adolescent Psychiatry, 34,* 520–528.

Gaensbauer, T. J., & Sands, K. (1979). Distorted affective communications in abused/ neglected infants and their potential impact on caretakers. *Journal of the American Academy of Child and Adolescent Psychiatry, 18,* 236–250.

Gaensbauer, T. J., & Siegel, C. H. (1995). Therapeutic approaches to posttraumatic stress disorder in infants and toddlers. *Infant Mental Health Journal, 16,* 292–305.

Grubbs, G. A. (1994). An abused child's use of sandplay in the healing process. *Clinical Social Work Journal, 22,* 193–209.

Horowitz, M. J. (2003). *Treatment of stress response syndromes.* Washington, DC: American Psychiatric Association.

Laor, N., Wolmer, I., Mayesl, L. C., Gershon, A., Weizman, R., & Cohen, D. J. (1997). Israeli preschoolers under SCUDs: A thirty-month follow up. *Journal of the American Academy of Child and Adolescent Psychiatry, 36,* 349–356.

Lieberman, A. F. (1992). Infant–parent psychotherapy with toddlers. *Development and Psychopathology, 4* 559–574.

Lieberman, A. F. (2004). Traumatic stress and quality of attachment: Reality and

internalization in disorders of infant mental health. *Infant Mental Health Journal,*
   25, 336–351.

Lieberman, A. F., Ghosh Ippen, C., & van Horn, P. (2006). Child–parent psychotherapy: 6-month follow-up of a randomized controlled trial. *Journal of the American*
   Academy of Child and Adolescent Psychiatry, 45, 913–918.

Lieberman, A. F., Silverman, R., & Pawl, J. H. (2000). Infant–parent psychotherapy:
   Core concepts and current approaches. In C. H. Zeanah (Ed.), *Handbook of infant*
   mental health (2nd ed., pp. 472–484). New York: Guilford Press.

Lieberman, A. F., & van Horn, P. (2005). *Don't hit my mommy: A manual for child–parent*
   psychotherapy with young witnesses of family violence. Washington, DC: Zero-to-Three
   Press.

Lieberman, A. F., van Horn, P. J., & Ghosh Ippen, C. (2005). Toward evidence-based
   treatment: Child–parent psychotherapy with preschoolers exposed to marital
   violence. *Journal of the American Academy of Child and Adolescent Psychiatry, 44,*
   1241–1248.

Lieberman, A. F., Weston, D. R., & Pawl, J. H. (1991). Preventive intervention and outcome with anxiously attached dyads. *Child Development, 62,* 199–209.

Marans, S. (1996). Psychoanalysis on the beat: Children, police, and urban trauma.
   Psychoanalytic Study of the Child, 51, 522–541.

Marans, S. (2005). When we all need someone to lean on. *International Journal of*
   Group Psychotherapy [Special issue: Children and Adolescents in the Aftermath
   of 9/11: Group Approaches towards Healing Trauma and Building Resilence],
   55(3), 443–454.

Marans, S., & Adelman, A. (1997). Experiencing violence in a developmental context.
   In J. D. Osofsky (Ed.), *Children in a violent society* (pp. 202–222). New York: Guilford Press.

Mayers, H. A. (2005). Treatment of a traumatized adolescent mother and her two-
   year-old son. *Clinical Social Work Journal, 33,* 419–431.

Orvaschel, H. (1989). *Kiddie SADS-E Section: Designed to assess PTSD.* Philadelphia:
   Medical College of Pennsylvania.

Osofsky, J. D., Cohen, G., & Drell, M. (1995). The effects of trauma on young children:
   A case of 2-year old twins. *International Journal of Psycho-Analysis, 76,* 595–607.

Putnam, F. W. (1997). *Dissociation in children and adolescents: A developmental perspective.*
   New York: Guilford Press.

Pynoos, R., Steinberg, A. M., & Piacentini, J. C. (1999). A developmental psychopathology model of childhood traumatic stress and intersection with anxiety disorders. *Biological Psychiatry, 46,* 1542–1554.

Pynoos, R. S., Steinberg, A. M., & Wraith, R. (1995). A developmental model of childhood traumatic stress. In D. Cicchetti & D. J. Cohen (Eds.), *Developmental psycho-*
   pathology: Vol. 2. Risk, disorder, and adaptation (pp. 72–95). Oxford, UK: Wiley.

Roth, A., & Fonagy, P. (2005). *What works for whom?: A critical review of psychotherapy*
   research (2nd ed.). New York: Guilford Press.

Schechter, D. S., Kaminer, T., Grienenberger, J. F., & Amat, J. (2003). Fits and starts:
   A mother–infant case study involving intergenerational violent trauma and pseu-
   doseizures across three generations. *Infant Mental Health Journal, 24,* 510–528.

Scheeringa, M. S., Zeanah, C. H., Drell, M. J., & Larrieu, J. A. (1995). Two approaches
   to the diagnosis of posttraumatic stress disorder in infancy and early childhood.
   Journal of the American Academy of Child and Adolescent Psychiatry, 34, 191–200.

Silberg, J. L. (2004). The treatment of dissociation in sexually abused children from a family attachment perspective. *Psychotherapy: Theory, Research, Practice and Training, 41*, 487–495.

Strupp, H. H. (1978). Psychotherapy research and practice: An overview. In A. E. Bergin & S. L. Garfield (Eds.), *Handbook of psychotherapy and behavior change* (2nd ed., pp. 3–22). New York: Wiley.

Toth, S. L., Maughan, A., Manly, J. T., Spagnola, M., & Cicchetti, D. (2002). The relative efficacy of two interventions in altering maltreated preschool children's representational models: Implications for attachment theory. *Developmental Psychopathology, 14*, 877–908.

Toth, S. L., Rogosch, F. A., Cicchetti, D., & Manly, J. T. (2006). The efficacy of toddler–parent psychotherapy to reorganize attachment in young offspring of mothers with major depressive disorder: A randomized trial. *Journal of Consulting and Clinical Psychology, 74*(6), 1006–1016.

Trowell, J., Kolvin, I., Weeramanthri, T., Sadowski, H., Berelowitz, M., Glasser, D., et al. (2002). Psychotherapy for sexually abused girls: Psychopathological outcome findings and patterns. *British Journal of Psychiatry, 180*, 234–247.

CHAPTER 16

Psychosocial Rehabilitation

Shirley M. Glynn, Charles Drebing, and Walter Penk

The world has changed since publication of the first psychosocial rehabilitation clinical practice guidelines for posttraumatic stress disorder (PTSD) (Penk & Flannery, 2000). On the positive side, the growth of the recovery movement is providing more hope and optimism for persons with psychiatric disorders (President's New Freedom Commission on Mental Health, 2003). A critical tenet of the recovery movement is that those meeting criteria for mental disorders should get needed support for the greatest quality of life possible, even if they continue to experience symptoms. Consistent with the recovery movement, growing access to Internet and other resources enables trauma survivors to assume greater personal control over their own learning and care (e.g., Bandura, 2006). On the negative side, social well-being and quality of life are declining as dangers in living increase (Diener & Tov, 2007).

These changes are leading clinicians to broaden approaches for treating PTSD beyond symptom reduction toward enhancement of social and occupational functioning. This chapter builds upon psychosocial rehabilitation techniques already demonstrated as effective for mental disorders in general and examines whether such interventions are beneficial when treating PTSD, either as adjunctive and supplemental services or as primary rehabilitation. We conclude that although benefits of psychosocial rehabilitation still need to be substantiated, we clinicians can proceed with confidence to develop and to use such techniques as we await confirmatory findings from randomized clinical trials currently underway and nearing completion.

September 11, 2001,
and a War against Terrorists and Terrorism

On September 11, 2001, terrorists piloted planes into the World Trade Center in New York City. These attacks destroyed a commercial center, killed more than 3,000 people, and forever disturbed the sense of personal safety into which millions had been lulled. Reactions were swift. The United States launched a War on Terrorism and Terrorists, overthrowing a Taliban government in Afghanistan and deposing a harsh dictator in Iraq. There quickly followed, in response, *jihads* and other attacks against civilians, with suicide bombings in countries from Indonesia and Malaysia to Spain and England. At the same time, genocides in Africa expanded in the 21st century to Somalia and Ethiopia. The historical strife between Israel and terrorist groups continued. A clash between Christian and Islamic religions, started in the ninth century but suspended by the 17th century, may now be resuming in the 21st century, at least by Islamic extremists.

The War on Terrorism is a conflict fought among civilians in places where they work, in homes where they live, in malls where they shop, in resorts where they seek rest and relaxation, in schools where they seek to advance themselves, and in churches and mosques where they worship and seek spiritual comfort. Terrorism and the War on Terrorism now magnify the numbers of persons exposed to trauma. This proliferation of traumatized individuals amplifies the need for effective interventions to assuage symptoms associated with trauma; many of these treatments are outlined in this volume. Although they are often effective, access can be a problem because there are not enough monies and therapists to provide for all.

DSM-IV-TR Adds Psychosocial Factors
to PTSD Diagnostic Criteria

With the populations of traumatized individuals increasing and far exceeding the number of trained therapist, it is also important to note that the diagnostic criteria of PTSD itself have also changed. Before 2000, PTSD criteria were limited to symptoms of cognitive appraisal, emotional reactivity, and emotion-driven behaviors to avoid reminders of trauma. In 2000, PTSD diagnostic criteria were expanded to include Criterion F, specifically, "The disturbance causes clinically significant distress or impairment in social, occupational, or other important areas of functioning" (American Psychiatric Association, 2000, p. 468). With the diagnostic formulation of PTSD currently including criteria that require attention to social and occupational dimensions of adjustment, clinicians now must expand the scope of their treatments beyond symptom reduction to include assessment and treatments for interferences in family, social, and work interactions when they are not improved by focalized treatment of symptoms of Criteria B–D. Criterion F not only marks a significant expansion of what clinicians must assess about PTSD but also highlights their need to attend to the psychosocial adjustment of persons presenting with PTSD. Toward this end, psychosocial rehabilitation and self-help techniques have been designed and are beginning to produce positive results (Hirai & Clum, 2005). As a consequence, psychosocial rehabilitation strategies, once considered as adjunctive or supplemental, also might now be considered primary, if they address trauma-related dysfunction.

Before DSM-IV-TR paradigmatically shifted the criteria of PTSD from symptoms *within the skin* of the traumatized (remembrances of the trauma, fears arising from reminders, startle responses, flashbacks, etc.) to include symptoms *outside the skin* (i.e., interferences in family, work, and community functioning), treatments were thought of as two basic types. Fenichel (1945) long ago classified and called these two approaches as "the quieting-down method" and the "stormy" method. Quieting-down methods comprise "take it easy" approaches, such as removing the person from traumatizing situations, providing rest, medicating, hospitalizing, and so forth—any approach that withdraws the person from traumatic situations and/or remind him or her about trauma. Stormy methods include the cathartic blend of teaching a person to relax while simultaneously reexposing him or her to other-induced or self-engendered reminders of trauma, which, when combined with relaxation techniques, reduce negative emotions associated with recalling trauma. Stormy methods are those that reexpose the person to memories and/or simulations of the trauma, induce catharsis, and reduce emotional reactivity: By encouraging the person to talk about and otherwise reexperience the trauma, therapists hope that such emotion-focused treatments decrease patients' emotional avoidance of trauma and modify emotion-driven behaviors (e.g., Moses & Barlow, 2006).

To both quieting-down and stormy methods (described in considerable detail in preceding chapters) we now must add methods that strengthen survivors' instrumental and social role functioning. These approaches go beyond those and range from medication, which involves reducing vulnerabilities to stress, and exposure or cognitive processing therapy, which involves increasing abilities to cope with or eliminate symptoms, to psychosocial rehabilitation—that is, taking responsibility for managing one's trauma and symptoms associated with it, taking charge of one's own life, improving personal relationships, and reinforcing a sense of purpose and accomplishment in living (e.g., Anthony, 1993; Drake, Becker, Bond, & Mueser, 2003; Liberman, 1992). Bandura (2006) has described such approaches as the "primacy of human agency" in self-directing one's recovery.

Recovery Models:
New Freedom Commission on Mental Health

Recognition of the importance of real-world functioning in recovery from psychiatric illness is mirrored in the recommendations of a Presidential

Task Force (President's New Freedom Commission on Mental Health, 2003), designed to begin transformation of mental health services delivery from a disease model to a rehabilitation model of recovery. "Recovery" means that clinicians and those receiving their services (i.e., "consumers")[1] participate in rehabilitation processes designed to ensure that patients live, work, learn, and participate fully in their communities. The emphasis goes beyond the remission of patients' psychiatric symptoms to surviving in the community and being trained to live fulfilling and productive lives. The recovery model, as promulgated in the New Freedom Commission, promotes living with a sense of mastery, competence, and hope, even if the person still experiences symptoms. Learned helplessness, a characteristic of PTSD, is assuaged by psychosocial techniques designed to decrease social stigma, social misattributions, and social avoidance after trauma and other stresses. Optimism, positive psychology, and successful problem-solving skills are emphasized. Consumer-directed care is a key tenet of the model. Treatments based on a recovery model must be consumer- and family-centered, fostering the ability to cope successfully with life's challenges and build resilience to withstand subsequent stresses and trauma. Psychosocial rehabilitation strategies are uniquely qualified to meet these directives.

Treatment Models Shift from Medical to Public Health Models

In light of both recognition of the increasing prevalence of traumatic events and the importance of attending to the broad potential spectrum of negative psychosocial sequelae, it is not surprising that PTSD treatment models have expanded from concerns and practices derived exclusively from the medical models to those incorporating public health concepts. Some refer to this change as a contrast between "compensation" and "capitalization" treatment models, in which "compensation" refers to therapies that remedy weaknesses, and "capitalization" is defined by therapies that elicit and draw on strengths (e.g., Snow, 1991). Kudler, Straits-Troster, and Jones (2006), for example, have summarized the current transition from a medical to a recovery model in the Veterans Health Administration (VHA) in their writings about the status of VHA care of veterans of the OIF/OEF Era (Occupation Iraqi Freedom and Occupation Enduring Freedom): More than 500,000 OIF/OEF veterans are eligible for VHA care; of these, nearly 150,000 already have sought VHA medical services, with the three most common problems being mental health, musculoskeletal, and dental care. The most common mental health problems thus far are nondependent use of drugs (38%), depressive disorder (30%), and PTSD (15%). Although many OIF/OEF veterans are already seeking treatment for mental health problems, most traumatized veterans stay away from services that might assuage symptoms. Reasons for avoiding treatment may be implicit in PTSD, a disorder in which the structure of the symptom complex is to cope by avoiding reminders of trauma. When surveyed for explanations, non-treatment-seeking respondents list reasons such as treatment is a sign of weakness; the fear that others might perceive that they cannot do their jobs and, as a consequence, that they will lose their employment; and anticipating that their colleagues will lose confidence in their leadership. Only one-third of those judged to need treatment actually receive interventions that help (Hoge et al., 2004; Hoge, Auchterlonie, & Milliken, 2006).

The disparity between mental health need and use has not gone unnoticed by the Department of Defense (DoD) and the VHA. Both agencies now actively provide interventions that are consistent with a public health model, incorporating outreach and recovery (President's New Freedom Commission on Mental Health, 2003). Goals of public health model treatment and rehabilitation approaches are to help combatants and their families retain a healthy balance in everyday living despite multiple stressors arising from military deployment. The public health model differs notably from a medical model, in which PTSD is diagnosed as disease and healers take full responsibility to prescribe a cure (Kudler et al., 2006). Kudler and colleagues' (2006) public health model posits that interventions must be driven by the psychosocial needs of the veteran and his or her family, and that services must find their way to the combatant rather than waiting for those with PTSD to find their way to the right mix of services. The public health model directly increases access to services and reduces stigma for those traumatized in war. It also emphasizes helping patients to strengthen functioning.

Another example of the public health model for PTSD is the Battlemind training program (*www.battlemind.org*), developed by the Walter Reed Army Institute of Research (*carlcastro@us.army.mil*). This form of the public health model, as distinguished from the medical model, is based on participant *training* rather than *treatment*. This training emphasizes adaptive change, resilience, and the capacity for growth. Participation in Battlemind is a self-directed process. Soldiers becoming civilians are trained to revise their mindsets about thoughts and behaviors that worked in war zones to the mindsets that they need to live, work, and enjoy life as civilians. Battlemind separates thinking that was useful on the battlefield from the kind of thinking needed to succeed in civilian adjustment across a number of critical domains: buddies versus withdrawal (teaching people how not to be alone), accountability versus control (relinquishing control), targeted versus inappropriate aggression (controlling instead of expressing anger), tactical awareness versus hypervigilance, lethally armed versus unarmed, emotional control versus anger or detachment, mission versus secretiveness, individual responsibility versus guilt, nondefensive driving versus aggressive driving, and discipline and ordering versus conflict.

Kudler and his colleagues (2006) are creating civilian analogues to Battlemind, similar to what Kudler calls "Reset training" for combatants returning from the war zone. "Reset" is the military metaphor of rechecking and upgrading one's equipment after battle, in this case, one's mind. Reset training focuses on changing mindsets by eliminating behaviors that worked for survival in combat and remastering behaviors that are positive and adaptive for civilian survival. Thoughts and behaviors in resetting mindsets include caring and sharing at home: rebalancing control issues with spouses, overcoming emotional withdrawal, dealing with hypervigilance and startle; getting back to sleep; reconnecting with kids; avoiding the stigma; involving the family in treatment; and so forth.

Reset training is comparable to the psychosocial rehabilitation approaches reviewed in this chapter, arising from a similar self-directed, self-regulating, self-reflecting approach to developing management of one's own symptoms. The implications are that, as a society increasingly vulnerable to experiences of trauma, we must learn how to train ourselves and others for the aftermath of life-threatening experiences that most of us will experience in our lifetimes.

The VA and DoD
Add Recovery Rehabilitation to PTSD Treatment

Another change that signifies the growing prominence of psychosocial rehabilitation in PTSD is reflected in the recent (VA, 2004) publication of the second edition of PTSD clinical practice guidelines by the VA in collaboration with the DoD. Whereas the original 1997 VA guidelines for the management of persons with major depressive disorder, substance abuse, and PTSD contained neither algorithms nor descriptions of psychosocial rehabilitation techniques, the 2004 revision contains descriptions and evaluations of psychosocial rehabilitation techniques, such as patient education, supported housing, marital/family skills training, social skills training, vocational rehabilitation, and case management. These techniques are identical to those presented by Penk and Flannery (2000) in their clinical review of promising but still-to-be-validated psychosocial rehabilitation interventions. The VA/DoD recommends that clinicians use a checklist systematically to determine whether problems exist in any of these areas, and offer services if needs are identified. Since 2002, some randomized clinical trials of psychosocial rehabilitation strategies for PTSD have been completed, and reports are beginning to appear in the peer-reviewed literature. Likewise, many studies were done well before 2002, using samples likely to have been exposed to multiple traumas, which refers in this instance to studies of not only VA patients but also of seriously mentally ill patients in whom PTSD is underdiagnosed as a co-occurring disorder (Brady, Rierdan, Penk, Meschede, & Losardo, 2003).

Although absent in the VA's 1997 clinical practice guidelines, the presence of psychosocial rehabilitation in the 2004 VA/DoD best practices heralds a sea change in thinking about PTSD interventions. Psychosocial rehabilitation at the least merits status on the periphery of empirically based services to be recommended in treatment planning for PTSD. If and when more randomized clinical trials are performed, and if patients with PTSD turn out to attain greater, more significant treatment gains than those from placebo and other treatments, then the adjunctive forms of psychosocial rehabilitation currently on the periphery may start to shift to the center as primary treatments.

Theoretical Context

Tests of the benefits of psychosocial rehabilitation interventions for PTSD are few in number, and most have been driven by practice, and not by theory. Heuristic frames of reference, however, are available from many theorists to guide tests of the efficacy and effectiveness of psychosocial rehabilitation (e.g., Bandura, 2006; Moses & Barlow, 2006). One relevant theory for testing benefits of psychosocial rehabilitation is the "agentic" theory of human development, adaptation, and change advanced by Albert Bandura. The core belief that is the foundation of human agency is Bandura's concept of self-efficacy. "Self-efficacy"—the extent to which people believe that they can produce desired effects by their actions—is a key resource in personal development and change. Measures of self-efficacy are widely used in testing hypotheses about the benefits of treatment for PTSD. Degrees of self-efficacy influence properties of human agency—intentionality, forethought, self-reactiveness, and self-reflectiveness. Bandura's theoretical approach conceptualizes the person as a contributor to his or her life circumstances and not merely as a product; the person is a proactive agent in adjustment, not just an onlooker. Self-efficacy is found to be influenced negatively by trauma (Bandura, 1973). Effective treatments are found to increase self-efficacy positively (Bandura, 1997). Psychosocial rehabilitation techniques, designed to improve the capacity of people to regain mastery over their environment, seem well-suited to increasing self-efficacy and reducing PTSD symptoms. As Bandura has written, "Much of psychology is concerned with discovering principles about how to structure environmental conditions to promote given personal and social outcomes and with the psychosocial mechanisms throughout which the environmental influences produce their effects" (Bandura, 2006, p. 169). Theories such as Bandura's (2006) psychology of human agency provide a rich array of testable hypotheses about the benefits of psychosocial rehabilitation techniques for the treatment of PTSD.

Description of Techniques

In the first edition of this book, seven types of psychosocial rehabilitation techniques were described as beneficial for treating many mental disorders, although systematic application of these interventions to PTSD was just beginning. We have added an eighth technique, supported education, in this edition. Manualized treatment approaches, described in greater detail below, have been written for all eight techniques, and many are in the process of being field-tested for efficacy and effectiveness for PTSD:

1. *Patient education techniques.* Training comprises educating trauma survivors about symptoms associated with trauma and traumatic loss, possible consequences of trauma exposure, ways of coping with feelings and behaviors associated with trauma, processes of recovery, and treatments for trauma.

2. *Supported education.* Many trauma survivors want to enter new professions and find that they need more education to do so. For these individuals, participation in supported education programs, can be critical. These programs help individuals to navigate school regulations while assisting them to access disability services that can help them compensate for difficulties in attention, memory, and concentration.

3. *Self-care and independent living skills.* These techniques build upon a history of successful studies among persons with serious mental disorders, demonstrating that persons can be taught to improve their skills in taking care of their physical and mental health, and can be taught skills to live independently at home and in the least restrictive environments of their choice.

4. *Supported housing services.* Particularly for trauma survivors who have become homeless, training is needed to recover skills in learning to live in and maintain their own households. Even among those with PTSD already living independently, the ability to maintain an independent household can be challenging. Training techniques have been developed to improve efficiency in maintaining a household.

5. *Supported family services.* Treatment techniques have been developed to address marital and family discord arising from trauma. Psychosocial rehabilitation techniques are centered mainly on educating families to understand and to learn how to support the traumatized family member. Families are taught techniques in how to be supportive and to help traumatized persons make adaptation transitions to posttrauma experiences.

6. *Social skills training.* Training to reduce social isolation associated with mental disorders has been found to be effective, particularly with serious mental disorders. Social isolation is one of several primary symptoms of PTSD. Available resources include training manuals designed to identify problems with avoiding social contacts and to substitute coping skills to increase social interactions.

7. *Supported employment.* Loss of mastery of the environment, another of the primary symptoms of PTSD, results in high rates of unemployment and underemployment. Treatment manuals have been written to support efforts to regain and to maintain employment, and to advance at work.

8. *Case management.* Persons who are traumatized are at times unable to development treatment plans for recovery and feel overwhelmed by fragmented mental health agencies, where treatments are separated into many different forms across settings. Case management provides experts support

and to coach traumatized persons through a maze of services needed for recovery.

Literature Review

To update the literature review presented in the Penk and Flannery (2000) chapter on psychosocial rehabilitation in the previous edition of this volume, the authors used typical variants of the labels for each of these interventions (e.g., "family therapy," "family treatment," "couple therapy," and "marital therapy") and "PTSD" and "posttraumatic stress disorder" in searches for intervention investigations in the PsycLIT, Published International Literature on Traumatic Stress (PILOTS), and MEDLINE databases from 1998 to 2007. Randomized controlled trials, naturalistic studies, and case studies all were examined for relevance. There have been relatively few randomized controlled PTSD trials conducted in the eight specified psychosocial domains. Where information from PTSD-specific programs is lacking, descriptions of the programs, as utilized with other psychiatric illnesses, are provided in the review.

Patient Education Interventions

A great deal has been written in the past 7 years about psychoeducational interventions for persons with PTSD or those who are at risk for developing PTSD due to trauma exposure. Several factors make the emerging literature difficult to negotiate. First, the term "education" is used in a variety of ways, sometimes referring to traditional models of information transfer, but also including interactive models that may be more commonly described as "individual" or "group psychotherapy." Second, whereas there are studies that focus on educational interventions alone, many examine educational interventions as part of larger interventions that include different forms of psychotherapies and other rehabilitation services (Kubany, Hill, & Owens, 2003; Mosig, 2006; Rosenberg, Mueser, Jankowski, & Salyers, 2004). In these studies, it is difficult to determine the efficacy of the educational element of the intervention. Third, a growing number of clinical trials of forms of psychotherapy use psychoeducational interventions as the comparison condition (Trowell et al., 2002; Mosig, 2006). Although some valuable information can be gleaned from these studies, the design necessarily limits what can be said about the efficacy of the educational intervention.

In the past 7 years, more than 30 empirical studies examining psychoeducational interventions for victims of trauma and PTSD have been identified in the literature search. Of those, three randomized clinical trials of interventions that were primarily educational in nature were identified. Naturalistic studies and case studies are supplemented by papers discussing content and/or strategies for educational interventions. The interventions described in this growing literature vary widely in the target population for the intervention, the content and format for the intervention, and the outcome variables examined. For example, the literature includes studies of educational interventions applied to individuals diagnosed with PTSD (David, Simpson, & Cotton, 2006; Fujimoto, 2002), individuals at risk for PTSD due to trauma (Fries, 2003; Rauch, Hembree, & Foa, 2001; Turpin, Downs, & Mason, 2005), and large population groups that may include trauma victims (Howard & Goelitz, 2004; Lukens, 2004; Souza & Sloot, 2003). Interventions have been administered to trauma victims of all ages (Glodich, 2000; Trowell et al., 2002; Turpin et al., 2005), as well as to individuals in the social support network of the person with PTSD, including parents (Kataoka et al., 2003), significant others (Morris, 2004), caregivers (Peckham, Howlett, & Corbett, 2007), teachers (Kataoka et al., 2003), and children (Stephens, McDonald, & Jouriles, 2000).

Specialty interventions have been developed for a variety of traumatic experiences, including military personnel exposed to combat-related trauma (Lubin & Johnson, 2000), military sexual trauma (David et al., 2006), rape (Bryant-Davis, 2004), domestic violence (Kubany et al., 2003), violent crime (Jaycox, Marshall, & Schell, 2004), child abuse (Fujimoto, 2002), and traumatic events such as the attacks of September 11, 2001 (Howard & Goelitz, 2004; Lukens, 2004; Underwood & Kalafat, 2002). Specialty interventions have been developed for unique populations, including traumatized adults who also have comorbid serious mental illness (SMI) (Rosenberg et al., 2004), comorbid substance dependence (Back, Dansky, Carroll, & Foa, 2001), comorbid intellectual disabilities (Peckham et al., 2007), or are members of particular target groups, such as immigrants (Kataoka et al., 2003) or children living in homeless shelters (Stephens et al., 2000).

Psychoeducational interventions can be delivered in a wide variety of formats, as reflected in the use of group and individual meetings, as well as theater (Souza & Sloot, 2003), film (Bryant-Davis, 2004), radio (Hamdani, 2003), self-help books (Flannery, 1992), and online websites (Lange et al., 2003). The interventions described in the literature range widely in length, from a single session up to 21 sessions (Osterman, Barbiaz, & Johnson, 2001). The physical settings for the interventions also vary widely, including jails and prisons (McMackin, Leisen, Sattler, Krinsley, & Riggs, 2002), schools (Kataoka et al., 2003; Mabalango, 2003), workplaces (Barsky-Carrow, 2000), psychiatric inpatient programs (Pratt et al., 2005), medical inpatient programs (Jaycox et al., 2004), and refugee resettlement programs. Finally, the content delivered by these interventions also varies and includes the symptoms of PTSD (Jagodic & Kontac, 2002), the range of reactions to trauma (Glodich, 2000; Underwood & Kalafat, 2002), the different types of available treatments (Back et al., 2001), symptom management and self-regulation (Glodich, 2001), stress and stress management techniques (Fries, 2003), problem solving (Glodich, 2001), assertiveness and self-advocacy (Wald, Taylor, & Scamvourgeras, 2004), empathy (Glodich, 2001), and avoidance of retraumatization.

Randomized Trials of Educational Interventions for PTSD

Turpin and colleagues (2005) evaluated the effectiveness of providing self-help information about trauma and trauma reactions to adults exposed to automobile accidents that involved traumatic injury. One hundred forty-two adults were randomized to two conditions: (1) an experimental group given self-help information ($N = 75$) and (2) a control group not given any material ($N = 67$). PTSD symptoms, anxiety, and depression were assessed 2 weeks post trauma exposure, and again at 3 and 6 months. Both groups showed significant improvement on all three outcome variables from the initial evaluation to the 6-month follow-up, but no significant treatment effect was identified.

Glodich (2000) conducted a randomized trial of an 8-week psychoeducational group designed for adolescents who had been exposed to violence and abuse. Forty-seven adolescents between ages 14 and 18 were randomly assigned to participate in the group or to a wait-list condition. Results indicate that the intervention group did show evidence of a significant increase in knowledge about trauma and its effects. There was also evidence of statistically significant improvements in adaptive attitudes toward risk-taking behavior, but no significant treatment effect was found for measures of PTSD symptoms.

Lange and colleagues (2003) examined the effectiveness of an Internet-based intervention combining psychoeducation and an interactive written therapy intervention for adults with a history of trauma, along with symptoms of PTSD. Participants were randomly assigned to participate in the online intervention ($N = 69$) or to a wait-list control group ($N = 32$). The treatment group showed significantly greater improvement than the wait-listed group on a range of outcome measures, including measures of PTSD symptoms, depression, anxiety, somatization, and sleep problems. The authors concluded that this "Interapy" intervention effectively reduced trauma-related symptomatology.

As can be seen in Table 16.1, effect sizes for interventions using education alone to address PTSD symptoms are not significant. The Interapy intervention has a greater impact. The studies suggest that education has important benefits other than symptom reduction, including increased knowledge and potential change in high-risk behavior.

Clinical Issues Regarding Psychoeducational Interventions and PTSD

Besides the psychoeducational interventions evaluated earlier, there is a wide range of educational opportunities to help the trauma victim recover an active and productive lifestyle. After gaining a clear sense of the clinical and rehabilitative needs of the client, the clinician typically considers arranging for education for the following: diagnosis and nature of PTSD; treatment options, including medication, talking therapies, and rehabilitation treatment options; treatment expectations and importance of compliance;

socialization programs (social skills training); integrated substance abuse/ dual-diagnosis treatments; and vocational rehabilitation services (e.g., transitional or supported employment). Psychoeducational offerings that are less specific to PTSD treatment but may be important for some clients include physical health education and promotion, such as smoking cessation, stress management, drug use, health, and relapse (Marlatt & Gordon, 1985; Nowinsky, Baker, & Carroll, 1994); sexually transmitted diseases (Cates & Graham, 1993); smoking cessation (American Psychiatric Association, 1996); and diet and exercise (Byrne, Brown, Voorberg, & Schofield, 1994).

Layperson Educational Materials

Self-help manuals for PTSD are commonly available, including *"I Can't Get Over It": A Handbook for Trauma Survivors* (Matsakis, 1996), *The Courage to Heal: A Guide for Women Survivors of Child Abuse* (Bass & Davis, 1988), *Post-Traumatic Stress Disorder: The Victim's Guide to Healing and Recovery* (Flannery, 1992), and Flannery's (1998) peer-help program for health care staff assaulted by their patients. There is also a self-help book for teenage children of persons who have been traumatized: *Finding My Way* (Sherman & Sherman, 2005). Clients and clinicians report that such self-help materials are useful.

Supported Education

In contrast to psychoeducational interventions, "supported education" is a term that refers to rehabilitation services in which the consumer is supported in entering and completing a formal education program, typically in a community setting, such as a high school, college, or graduate school (Anthony, 1992). Many adults who qualify for support by state or local rehabilitation services may be provided funding to enter a vocational or specialized education program. In contrast, supported education is a model of service that focuses more on providing the personal support that many adults with PTSD may need, whether or not they receive financial support. As in supported employment and supported housing, the emphasis in supported education is on the provision of individualized services that allow the person to be successful in the education process.

There are fairly limited empirical data regarding this model, and the existing literature is dominated by descriptions of programs across a broad spectrum of psychiatric disorders, although not specific to PTSD. For example, Isenwater, Lanham, and Thornhill (2002) described the College Link Program, a typical supported employment program located in London. Data are provided on 16 participants who completed the program. Positive outcomes were noted relative to baseline evaluations, including increased self-esteem, improved social functioning, and enhanced confidence and independence. Ratzlaff, McDiarmid, Marty, and Rapp (2006) described a specialized supported educational program in which adults with mental illness were trained

TABLE 16.1. Educational Interventions

Study and treatment	Population	N	Comparison groups	Duration of trial	Main outcome measure	Within-group effect size		Between-group effect size		Results
						ITT	Completer	ITT	Completer	
Turpin et al. (2005): provision of psychoeducation materials	142 adults exposed to trauma	75	Received self-help materials	26 weeks	Posttraumatic Diagnostic Scale (PDS)	0.12		0.03		Treatment effects were not significant.
		67	Received no materials			0.06				
Lange et al. (2003): Interapy	101 adults self-identified as "traumatized" and seeking assistance through the Internet	69	Combination of psychoeducation and 10-session interactive written therapy protocol	5 weeks	Impact of Event, Intrusion scale		1.08		1.20	Treatment was associated with a significant reduction in Intrusion and Avoidance scale scores.
		32	Placed on a wait list		Avoidance scale		−0.24			
		69	Combination of psychoeducation and 10-session interactive written therapy protocol	5 weeks	Impact of Event, Intrusion scale		1.04		1.48	
		32	Placed on a wait list		Avoidance scale		−0.6			

Study	Sample	Group	N	Duration	Measure			Outcome
Glodich (2000): Psychoeducation	47 adolescents with self-reported exposure to trauma	8-week psychoeducation group	23	8 weeks	Impact of Event, Intrusion scale	0.41	0.02	Treatment was not associated with a significant change in Intrusion scale scores.
		Placed on a wait list	24			0.49		
		8-week psychoeducation group	23	8 weeks	Avoidance scale	0.34	0.23	Treatment was not associated with a significant change in Avoidance scale scores.
		Placed on a wait list	24			0.15		
		8-week psychoeducation group	23	8 weeks	Hyperarousal scale	0.07	0.12	Treatment was not associated with a significant change in Hyperarousal scale scores.
		Placed on a wait list	24			0.47		
Glynn et al. (1999): behavioral family therapy (BFT)	Vietnam War combat veterans	Exposure + BFT	17	9 + 22 weeks	Composite PTSD-positive symptom factor	0.71	Exp + BFT vs. WL: 0.65	Both treatment groups significantly different from control; no difference between treatment groups.
		Exposure (Exp) alone	12	9 weeks		0.29	Exp vs. WL: 0.85	
		Wait list (WL)	13	9 weeks		−0.08	Exp + BFT vs. Exp: 0.07	
		Exposure + BFT	17	9 + 22 weeks	Composite PTSD-negative symptom factor	0.82	Exp + BFT vs. WL: 0.45	Treatment effects were not significant.
		Exp alone	12	9 weeks		0.68	Exp vs. WL: 0.76	
		WL	13	9 weeks		0.21	Exp + BFT vs. Exp: −0.20	

Note. ITT, intention to treat.

to be consumer-providers of mental health services. Students completed a 15-week process that included both classroom and internship experiences, along with support in the form of a "mentorship." Outcome data on 84 graduates were reported, with significant increases noted on measures of hope, self-esteem, and "recovery stage." Collins, Mowbray, and Bybee (2000) randomly assigned 397 participants to one of three formats for supported education: group support, classroom support, or individual support. All three were shown to have a positive impact on educational enrollment and vocational education, whereas different models appeared to have particular benefits in terms of academic self-efficacy, empowerment, and motivation.

Although the literature evaluating supported education is modest in size and does not include studies that specifically address PTSD, the evidence provides some support for the use of supported education with adults with mental illness. A clinician will want to access supported education services and programs in the community when he or she has an appropriate client; that is, when the clinician and the client have examined the client's interests and goals, and have determined that the client wants to pursue an educational goal and is "ready" to pursue that goal in terms having the resources to do so. Supported education services vary in what they offer, so careful discussion should take place before the referral is made to ensure that what is offered fully supports the needs of the client returning to school (Mowbray, Gutierrez, Bellamy, & Szilvagyi, 2003).

Self-Care, Independent Living Skills, and Empowerment Techniques

Concepts and measures of self-care and independent skills trainings are expanding as clinicians and consumers learn more about the many proficiencies that must be mastered by persons with mental disorders to survive successfully in the community. The need for self-care and independent living skills, along with empowerment training, is being identified as essential for many classes of potential trauma victims, such as older adults, and for many women survivors of domestic violence who must learn to live independently after leaving spouses who batter (e.g., Gorde, Helfrich, & Finlayson, 2005).

Assessment of independent living skills needed to survive in the community is proliferating (e.g., Lyons, 2003; Rempfer, Brown, Hamera, & Cromwell, 2003; Rempfer, Hildenbrand, Parker, & Brown, 2003). Reviews of tests and manuals, including techniques centering on trauma and its comorbidities, have been summarized in a recent report from the American Psychological Association/Committee for the Advancement of Professional Practice (APA/CAPP) Task Force on Serious Mental Illness and Severe Emotional Disturbance, available from *www.apa.org/practice/grid.html*. Manual-based techniques are now available in the self-care/independent skills domains of health, leisure, cooking, home management, transportation, shopping, and money management, building upon the pioneering work of Ayllon and Azrin

(1968) and Liberman and colleagues (1993). Self-care and independent living skills training are essential ingredients in the VA inpatient and outpatient services and appear prominently in the VA clinical practice guidelines for PTSD.

No formal randomized trials on self-care, independent living skills, and empowerment approaches have as yet been tested for clients with PTSD, although such work is underway. Whereas self-care and independent skills training have proven effective in studies of patients with schizophrenia and other serious mental disorders (e.g., Lehman et al., 2002), evidence from these studies is sufficiently positive that one may readily conclude that what has been beneficial for veterans with serious mental disorders is highly likely to have positive effects for persons meeting criteria for a primary diagnosis of PTSD. Clinicians are encouraged to assess clients' health, social, and familial lifestyles, their capacities to continue living on their own and with their families, then, when deficiencies are noted, to link clients to appropriate skills development training.

Supported Housing Techniques

During the course of treatment, the client with PTSD and the clinician may determine that the client has a problem with housing that significantly affects rehabilitation. Rehabilitation services that focus on housing problems take a variety of forms, most of which have not been empirically evaluated. The model of services that is most commonly cited as a best practice and as having an evidence base is supported housing (Rog, 2006). Although there is some variety in how this model is employed (Felce, Lowe, & Jones, 2002; Rog, 2006) the term "supported housing" typically refers to a model of services in which the client is provided immediate access to independent housing that is fully integrated into the community, along with ongoing support in that living situation. The model was developed in contrast to more traditional models that typically use a graduated sequence of housing options through which the client is supposed to progress. Unfortunately, there is evidence that a large portion of clients in these continuum models do not graduate to independent housing, but are caught cycling through the initial levels of the continuum (Tsemberis & Asmussen, 1999; Tsemberis & Eisenberg, 2000).

Supported housing emphasizes immediate access as a means to ensure that clients reach independent housing and to give the rehabilitation process a greater degree of stability, if only in the dimension of where the person lives. Many traditional housing models also rely heavily on "congregate housing," in which homeless adults with mental illness are housed together or in sites that are separate from standard community housing, such as housing facilities on hospital grounds and near homeless shelters. The supported housing model seeks to integrate clients fully into the community by using housing options that are spread throughout general residential areas, and that do not pool clients together in large concentrations. This element reflects the reality that clients prefer to live in integrated settings, and that the end goal of the rehabilitation process is full participation in the community. The supported housing model also includes clinical support that typically takes the form of assertive community treatment services that maintain ongoing contact with clients, providing treatment in the home to support clients' efforts to remain independent.

Although there have been no specific empirical studies of supported housing for adults with PTSD, a small but growing quasi-experimental literature evaluates supported housing for the larger group of adults with mental illness. Mares, Kasprow, and Rosenheck (2004) compared housing outcomes for veterans placed in supported housing in 18 VA sites with those of individuals participating in prior residential treatment. After correcting for case–mix variables and program variables, no differences were found between the two groups with respect to housing outcomes. It should be noted that treatment fidelity varied significantly across supported housing sites. Tsemberis and Eisenberg (2000) compared housing outcomes for 242 participants in the Pathways to Housing program, with 1,600 persons participating in housing service continua. The results indicate that after 5 years of participation, 88% of the Pathway to Housing participants were still housed compared to 47% of participants in traditional housing service continua. The advantage for Pathways to Housing was maintained even after controlling for case–mix factors. Culhane, Metraux, and Hadley (2002) compared homeless adults who participated in supported housing with those who did not participate in any housing services. They found that supported housing participants were housed at more than twice the rate of the comparison group (69 vs. 30%). After reviewing a range of experimental and quasi-experimental evaluations, Rog (2006) concluded that with respect to the supported housing model, a limited number of studies have evaluated the model, but that those studies do provide a moderate level of support.

A range of other types of housing services, most of which have not been well examined empirically, have received some attention in the form or program descriptions, pilot studies, and archival studies that use administrative data. This growing literature on the wider range of housing services does suggest that particularly those services that provide case management and linkages to specialized clinical services are more effective than the standard solutions for homelessness—either "single-room occupancy" (e.g., providing a room but not other forms of rehabilitation or case management) or "warehousing" in shelters without other forms of support (e.g., Goldfinger et al., 1999). Forms of housing considered more effective are those in which clinical services are integrated or treating staff make an effort to foster community living (e.g., Goldfinger et al., 1999; McHugo et al., 2004). Naturalistic studies at VA Connecticut continue to provide empirical support for the essential role of clinical services integrated into housing interventions in the treatment of persons with PTSD and other disorders (e.g., Rossman, Sridharan, & Buck, 1998).

Other types of housing problems are common and may need clinical support to resolve. Clients may have significant problems securing safe, quality, affordable, stable housing, or they may have adequate housing that is not satisfactory for other reasons. Because housing problems typically have a major impact on the success of other treatment efforts, it is important the housing issues be dealt with proactively, typically with coordination and/or referral to rehabilitation specialists. Many housing interventions involve referring the client to other specialists for purposes of solving homelessness. Such referrals tend to fragment rehabilitation and decrease opportunities to integrate homelessness services with other forms of rehabilitation. Supported housing outcomes may be enhanced if clients and clinicians integrate PTSD treatment with housing and other rehabilitation services. Furthermore, treating the frequently co-occurring problem of substance use should also be integrated into supported housing interventions when homelessness is associated with PTSD (e.g., Goldfinger et al., 1999).

Family Interventions

Prominent PTSD symptoms include feelings of detachment or estrangement from others, restricted range of affect, and irritability or outbursts of anger. In light of how these symptoms may affect close personal relationships, it is not surprising that family stress and dysfunction often accompanies PTSD. This association has been studied most frequently in the families of combat veterans with PTSD, in which higher rates of relationship stress (Carroll, Rueger, Foy, & Donahoe, 1985; Roberts et al., 1982), violence (Beckham, Feldman, Kirby, Hertzberg, & Moore, 1997; Marshall, Panuzio, & Taft, 2005), and separation and divorce (Prigerson, Maciejewski, & Rosenheck, 2002) are reported. Partners of combat veterans with PTSD are also more likely to report psychological distress and burden (Beckham, Lytle, & Feldman, 1996; Galovski & Lyons, 2004; Manguno-Mire et al., 2007). Riggs, Byrne, Weathers, and Litz (1998) have noted that emotional numbing may be particularly deleterious to a relationship. Children of combat veterans with PTSD also suffer (Jordan et al., 1992). Also, a smaller body of literature indicates that family members of adult sexual assault survivors may be very distressed and express negative attitudes to the survivors (Ahrens & Campbell, 2000). High rates of family stress have been related to poor treatment outcomes across a mixed-trauma sample with PTSD (Tarrier, Sommerfield, & Pilgrim, 1999).

In spite of (or perhaps because of) the difficulties that PTSD may impose on relationships, it is not surprising that two large meta-analyses of predictors of PTSD outcomes have found a significant association between posttrauma social support and lower symptom levels across a range of traumatic events (Brewin, Andrews, & Valentine, 2000; Ozer, Best, Lipsey, & Weiss, 2003). The importance of social support in recovery from trauma has also been demonstrated in combat veterans (King, King, Foy, Keane, & Fairbank, 1999). However, data suggest that both veterans (Keane, Scott, Chavoya, Lamparski, & Fairbank, 1985) and nonveterans (Regehr, Hill, Knott, & Sault, 2003) with PTSD may experience a diminution of perceived social support after the trauma that may be mediated by PTSD symptoms (Lui, Glynn, & Shetty, 2008).

Family Skills Training Approaches to Dealing with Psychiatric Illnesses and/or Relationship Distress

Clinicians have articulated how PTSD symptoms may affect relationships and how conjoint treatment may be especially appropriate for PTSD (Glynn, 2008; Riggs, 2000; Sherman et al., 2005). They have also noted an interest in both individual and family therapy among partners of persons with PTSD, although rates of participation in therapy are low (Galovski & Lyons, 2004; Sherman et al., 2005). Many descriptions of family-based interventions for PTSD are available (Beckerman, 2004; Johnson, Feldman, & Lubin, 1995; Marrs, 1984; Rabin & Nardi, 1991; Sherman, 2006), but data supporting their use are scant (Riggs, 2000).

In considering potential rehabilitation resources for treating PTSD and its concomitant social dysfunction in a family context, two sets of scientific data appear relevant: the literature on family psychoeducational approaches to serious and persisting psychiatric illnesses, and the literature on behavioral marital therapy for couple distress. Consistent with a psychiatric rehabilitation focus, these interventions share an emphasis on behaviorally oriented communication and problem-solving training to manage problems in daily living, as well as illness management issues. Participants typically practice skills in session, then are encouraged to complete out-of-session assignments to strengthen their use.

Despite their similarities, the literatures on family psychoeducational approaches to psychiatric conditions and on utilizing behavioral marital therapy for couple distress also differ in significant ways. For example, family psychoeducation is appropriate for any family relationship and has been used in both families of origin and romantic relationships. Thus, it can easily accommodate hierarchical family relationships. Furthermore, the treatment typically involves formal acknowledgment that a specific family member has a vulnerability to a psychiatric disorder, and that recovery is facilitated when family members learn to accommodate for this disability (Glynn, Cohen, Dixon, & Niv, 2006). Behavioral marital therapy typically views participant relationships as more egalitarian, and often includes other behavioral strategies (e.g., contingency contracting, behavioral exchange) designed to strengthen the dyadic relation (Shadish & Baldwin, 2005). Although the psychiatric diagnosis of a specific participant may be acknowledged, there is a greater emphasis on viewing this disorder in a systemic context.

Both family psychoeducation and behavioral marital therapy have been found to be effective interventions in treatment of other psychiatric disorders. For example, meta-analyses of family interventions in schizophrenia have provided extensive evidence for the efficacy of such treatments. Using relapse and rehospitalization as outcomes, a meta-analysis of 25 treatment studies published between 1977 and 1997 concluded that family participation in treatment reduced relapse rates by 20% (Pitschel-Walz, Leucht, Bäuml, Kissling, & Engel, 2001). Study durations ranged from 2 weeks to 4 years and were primarily psychoeducational models. The effect size (ES) comparing family intervention to treatment as usual (TAU) was 0.20 (confidence interval [CI]: 0.14–0.27), indicating superior outcomes in the family condition. Another meta-analysis of 18 randomized controlled trials of family interventions (Pilling et al., 2002), with a minimum duration of 6 weeks, reported even stronger findings than those established by the Pitschel-Walz and colleagues (2001) study. Family interventions conferred greater benefits than all other treatments combined (ES = 0.63; CI: 0.46–0.86) or standard care alone (ES = 0.37; CI: 0.23–0.59) in regard to relapse within 1 year.

Similarly, the benefits of participation in behavioral marital therapy are well established. In a recent meta-analysis of 30 randomized controlled trials published since 1988, Shadish and Baldwin (2005) found an ES of 0.585 (CI; 431–737) with regard to reducing martial distress. Behavioral marital therapy has been found to be an effective treatment of depression (Halford, Bouma, Kelly, & Young, 1999) and substance use disorders (Epstein & McCrady, 1998; O'Farrell & Fals-Stewart, 2003), which often co-occur with PTSD.

The empirical literature on tests of family-based skills training interventions that target adults with PTSD is limited to a randomized trial of a variant of family psychoeducation (Glynn et al., 1999) and a pre- and posttreatment study of cognitive-behavioral couple treatment, a variant of behavioral marital therapy (Monson, Schnurr, Stevens, & Guthrie, 2004). Glynn and associates (1999) randomized 42 combat veterans with PTSD and a key family member to individual exposure therapy, individual exposure therapy and behavioral family therapy, or a wait-list control group. Both of the active treatment groups improved with regard to PTSD positive symptoms (reexperiencing, and hyperarousal) compared to the control group, but the addition of the family treatment conferred no additional statistically significant benefits. Possible explanations for this null effect include small sample size, greater relative dropout in the family therapy condition, and a treatment ceiling effect during a specific time period. In the Monson and colleagues (2004) trial, participation in cognitive-behavioral couple treatment was associated with improvements in PTSD symptoms in seven combat veterans with PTSD; the partners also reported improved relationship satisfaction at posttreatment. Comparison of these two trials might indicate that behavior marital therapy is a more effective treatment than behavioral family therapy for chronic PTSD, but the lack of a randomized control group in the Monson et al. trial limits conclusions that can be drawn.

The rationale for tests of family interventions for PTSD is strong, but the database for their efficacy is weak. It seems clear that here the primary need is for further tests of interventions for PTSD. Work is especially needed in three areas: (1) brief interventions that specifically target difficulties with treatment engagement on both the survivor's and the relative's part; (2) tests to compare the relative advantages of a family psychoeducation and a behavioral couple therapy approach to intervention for PTSD; and (3) more work with nonveteran samples of survivors to understand the issues these families confront, as well as the interventions that might be most helpful for them.

Social Skills Training

Many people with serious psychiatric disabilities exhibit deficits in measurable skills that are necessary to interact effectively with others. These deficits may occur at a micro level (e.g., poor eye contact, long speech latency) or at a more macro level (e.g., poor grooming, refusal to participate in conversations). With the rise of the behavioral treatment movement in the 1960s, clinicians began to apply learning principles to remediate these deficits in persons with serious and persisting psychiatric illnesses (Bellack, Mueser, Gingerich, & Agresta, 2004). Techniques such as modeling, coaching, chaining, prompting, extinction, providing positive reinforcement, and ensuring multiple practice opportunities are all aspects of an effective social skills training program. Forty years later, cumulative data in this area indicate that specific social skills can be taught to patients in the clinic, and that careful application of learning principles can increase likelihood of generalization of these skills to the community, which often can then improve patients' overall instrumental role functioning (Bellack et al., 2004). However, these skills training programs appear to have relatively little impact on core psychiatric symptoms (e.g., hallucinations, delusions, manic behavior, sadness) not targeted by the training.

The application of socials skills training approaches to the treatment of PTSD has been very limited in spite of its utility in other disorders. In part, this lack of application of social skills techniques likely reflects the belief that core PTSD symptoms (e.g., flashbacks, distressing dreams, numbing, sleep disturbances) are not skills deficits. However, it can certainly be argued that some PTSD symptoms (e.g., avoidance of reminders of the trauma, feelings of detachment or estrangement from others, a restricted range of affect, and irritability or outbursts of anger) might be reflected in observable social skills deficits that could profitably be targeted in behavioral interventions.

Social Skills Training in PTSD

There are no published trials of circumscribed social skills interventions in PTSD. However, a few investigators have included a specific social skills training component as part of a more comprehensive treatment program, typically including exposure therapy, with promising results. For example, Frueh and colleagues (Frueh, Turner, Beidel, Mirabella, & Jones, 1996; Turner, Beidel, & Frueh, 2005) reported on the development of a 29-session, multicomponent behavioral treatment for chronic combat-related PTSD called "trauma management therapy." In addition to education, exposure, and attention to personal topics, the treatment includes four sessions of interpersonal skills training and four sessions of anger management training (which can be understood as a variant of social skills training). Pre- to posttreatment data across the entire 17-week program demonstrate that participation was associated with significant reductions in sleep difficulties, nightmares, and flashbacks, as well as more involvement in social activities (Frueh et al., 1996). It is impossible to know, of course, which components of the program were responsible for the benefits. Similarly, Cloitre, Koenen, Cohen, and Han (2002) developed a treatment (STAIR—skills training in affective and interpersonal regulation) that includes an initial phase of skills training in affect and interpersonal regulation, followed by a subsequent phase of prolonged exposure for PTSD related to childhood abuse. Compared to a wait-list control, participation in the two-phase treatment was associated with improvements in affect regulation and interpersonal problems, as well as PTSD symptoms. However, without a dismantling design, it is impossible to discern the unique benefits of the social skills training.

The place of social skills training programs in treatment for PTSD is still not clear. Dismantling studies designed to examine the specific components of the treatment we described earlier, or smaller trials that just look at the impact of social skills training, especially on the "negative" symptoms of PTSD, are needed.

Vocational Rehabilitation Techniques

The interrelationship of work and PTSD is bidirectional. Traumatization and the development of psychological difficulties such as PTSD can result in subsequent work difficulties and/or unemployment (Ainspan, 2008). Furthermore, some occupations (e.g., nurse, first responder) associated with higher rates of traumatic exposure have higher prevalence of PTSD. In view of the relation between employment and PTSD, it is somewhat surprising that there is very little empirical work on the topic.

The Impact of PTSD on Work Functioning

Early studies focused on the impact of PTSD on subsequent work performance among Vietnam War combat veterans. A consistent finding was that most veterans made good employment adjustment after their discharge from the service, unless they had significant psychological or physical problems related to their military experience (Iversen et al., 2005; Savoca & Rosenheck, 2000). In combat veterans, PTSD has been related to a higher likelihood of unemployment and lower earnings among workers. Similarly, more severe PTSD symptoms in combat veterans have been associated with fewer hours worked (Magruder et al., 2004; Smith, Schnurr, & Rosenheck, 2005) and/ or performance problems at work (Solomon, 1989). In light of the fact that many veterans receive compensation for PTSD, it is perhaps not surprising that Johnson, Fontana, Lubin, Corn, and Rosenheck (2004), in their 6-year follow-up of participants of their intensive inpatient program for combat-related PTSD, reported that veterans' self-ratings indicated improvement in all areas of functioning except employment. Employment difficulties associated with PTSD may be chronic, at least in the subsample of individuals who receive some kind of compensation or disability payment for the disorder.

It is notable that the deleterious impact of trauma on employment is not limited to combat veterans. Surveys of other trauma survivors have documented similar negative outcomes. For example, Michaels and colleagues (2000), in a sample of 247 adults admitted to a level one trauma unit, found that poor work outcomes at 12 months were related to both physical problems and psychological distress, as reflected on the Brief Symptom Inventory (BSI) Depression score (Derogatis, 1993) and the civilian form of the Mississippi Scale for PTSD (Lauterbach, Vrana, King, & King, 1997) at 1 year posttrauma. Matthews (2005) reported that among a sample of injured automobile accident survivors who were employed at the time of their accident, those with PTSD at follow-up (a mean 8.6 months after the event) were significantly less likely than those without PTSD to return to work (with PTSD, 58%; without PTSD, 89%). Although the PTSD-positive group reported more pain, the groups did not differ in injury severity or physical functioning capacity. Intriguingly, the PTSD-positive group also reported greater extrinsic motivation to work. In a random-digit dialing study of community residents, Breslau, Lucia, and Davis (1985) found that a lifetime diagnosis of PTSD was predictive of time lost from work during the 30-day period when the participant was "most upset" about the experience.

The deleterious impact of personal exposure to the events of September 11, 2001, has been well documented (e.g., DeLisi et al., 2003). In addition to the trauma suffered, many individuals had their work lives disrupted (destruction of work site, loss of job), and this vocational interruption may have rendered them even more vulnerable to poor outcomes. In one random-digit dialing study in the New York metropolitan area approximately 6 months after the incident, predictors of persisting PTSD were assessed. Job loss as a result of the catastrophe emerged as a significant independent predictor of PTSD at 6 months, whether or not the individual was again employed at follow-up (Galea et al., 2003).

Overall, the results outlined here suggest that both military and civilian trauma can have a significant negative impact on work life. This dysfunction can be seen both in the short term and even years after the traumatic event. Some individuals never return to work.

The Impact of Work on PTSD Prevalence

Stress and/or injuries at work can, of course, result in the development of PTSD. MacDonald, Colotla, Flamer, and Karlinsky (2003) examined 44 workers whose claims were accepted for workers' compensation in the absence of documented physical injuries, and found that the majority (82%) had experienced direct exposure to a traumatic event, whereas the rest witnessed such an event. Over half (54%) had been proximal to an armed robbery. Across the entire sample, only 43% returned to their previous job with the same employer.

Some occupations, such as first responder to accidents or other life-endangering events, are more likely to result in exposure to trauma and have an increased prevalence of PTSD (Wilhelm, Kovess, Rios-Seidel, & Finch, 2004). For example, a report by the Centers for Disease Control and Prevention (CDC; 2006) found that police officers and firefighters who had exposure to Hurricane Katrina reported high levels of physical injuries and psychological strain. Nineteen percent of the police officers and 22% of the firefighters surveyed met diagnostic criteria for PTSD according to the PTSD Checklist (PCL) (Weathers, Litz, Herman, Huska, & Keane, 1993) approximately 3 months after the hurricane; depression rates as assessed by the Center for Epidemiologic Studies Depression Scale (CES-D; Breslau et al., 1985) were also high.

It is notable that baseline levels of PTSD and depression are often not assessed in these employment studies, and these levels might be high. For example, Regehr and colleagues (2003) compared the traumatic exposure levels, depression, and PTSD severity of new firefighter recruits and experienced firefighters. Compared to the seasoned firefighters, the new recruits reported significantly less exposure to multiple casualties, the death of a child, or witnessing violence against others, but they did not differ in the amount of violence directed toward themselves or exposure to near-death situations. Nevertheless, the seasoned firefighters had significantly higher scores on the Impact of Events scale (IES) (Horowitz, Wilner, & Alvarez, 1979) and on the Beck Depression Inventory (BDI) (Beck, Ward, Mendelson, Mock, & Erbaugh, 1961), suggesting that the development of untoward psychological outcomes may be heightened by cumulative exposure to trauma.

The psychological cost of work-related exposure to the events of September 11, 2001, is becoming more apparent. Immediate exposure to the site of the traumatic events, not surprisingly, has been associated with negative outcomes. For example, an open-ended survey of transportation and construction workers (truck drivers, heavy equipment operators, laborers, and carpenters) who worked rescue and cleanup at the World Trade Towers site reported high levels of depression, substance use, and posttraumatic stress (Johnson et al., 2005). Even those with primarily vicarious exposure to the catastrophe could be negatively affected. In a large-scale mail survey of American Airlines flight attendants approximately 10 months after the event, 18.2% of the respondents reported symptoms on the PCL (Weathers et al., 1993) consistent with a likely diagnosis of PTSD (Lating, Sherman, Everly, Lowry, & Peragine, 2004).

Taken together, these studies indicate that PTSD in the workplace may be a common problem. Furthermore, members of some occupations may be particularly at risk due to cumulative exposure to traumatic events. Greater attention to this topic is clearly needed.

Psychiatric Rehabilitation Strategies to Reduce Work Dysfunction in Persons with PTSD

In light of the previous discussion highlighting the negative interaction of work and PTSD, it is discouraging that so little attention has been paid to designing and evaluating strategies to improve vocational functioning in trauma survivors. Furthermore, what little data there are suggest that interventions tested to date are not particularly effective. For example, Nhiwatiwa (2003) evaluated a brief psychoeducational intervention to assist with nurses' feelings about patient assaults. Unfortunately, nurses randomized to the educational condition reported more distress than the control (no intervention) condition at 3 months.

In a larger-scale naturalistic effort, Rosenheck, Stolar, and Fontana (2000) examined the outcomes of veterans with chronic combat-related PTSD who participated in the compensated (on-site, sheltered) work therapy program while they were in inpatient or residential treatment programs (they could continue with the work program postdischarge). A sophisticated statistical model to match work therapy participants with similar nonparticipants was implemented, and outcomes at 4-month follow-up were assessed. Participation in the work therapy program was not associated with greater improvement on any of outcome domains, including PTSD symptoms, violence, substance use, medical problems, or community employment. Although this was not a randomized trial, the results of this investigation do little to reassure survivors or policymakers that the most widely available type of vocational services in the VA will lead to improvements in job status.

Over the past 15 years, manualized psychiatric rehabilitation strategies, such as supported employment (Bond, 2004), have been implemented for unemployed persons with serious and persisting psychiatric illnesses, many of them involving psychosis, with promising results (Cook & Razzano, 2000). Bond (2004) noted the following key elements of supported employment for persons with serious and persisting psychiatric illnesses: (1) services focused on securing competitive employment (not sheltered or transitional); (2) eligibility for the service based on consumer preference (rather than judgment of "work readiness" by others); (3) rapid job search (rather than extensive prevocational assessment or participation in "work preparation" programs); (4) integration of rehabilitation and mental health treatment; (5) attention to consumer preferences in directing the job search; and (6) unlimited, individualized support.

In the five randomized controlled trials comparing supported employment to conventional vocational rehabilitation services among persons with serious and persisting psychiatric illnesses over an 18- to 24-month period, 51% of the participants receiving supported employment obtained a competitive job versus 18% of those in the comparison groups (weighted mean ES = 0.79; Twamley, Jeste, & Lehman, 2003). There is a published supported employment fidelity scale, programs rated with greater adherence to supported employment manuals appeared to have better outcomes (Becker, Smith, Tanzman, Drake, & Tremblay, 2001). A basic supported employment manual is now available as one of the Substance Abuse and Mental Health Services Administration (SAMHSA) evidence-based toolkits (*www.mentalhealth.samhsa.gov/cmhs/communitysupport/toolkits/employment/*). The VA is now sponsoring a major national effort to expand the availability of supported employment to veterans with psychiatric disorders (Resnick & Rosenheck, 2007).

Although supported employment is the most validated approach for vocational rehabilitation in psychiatric illnesses, there are no published trials on its use in individuals with a primary diagnosis of PTSD, although Smith and colleagues (2005) recommended that the intervention be tested with veterans with PTSD (see also Penk, Drebing, & Schutt, 2002). Mueser, Essock, Haines, Wolfe, and Xie (2004) reported that comorbid PTSD reduced the effectiveness of supported employment in a sample of community-residing persons with serious and persisting psychiatric illnesses, randomized to receive supported employment.

In considering how supported employment might be used with persons with PTSD, the following issues might be fruitfully addressed. First, because many individuals with PTSD already have a job, the primary work would be to help them resolve situations that interfere with job maintenance, including conflicts with others that might result from DSM-IV PTSD Criterion D irritability symptoms or performance issues related to avoidance of anxiety-provoking activities or places consistent with the DSM-IV Criterion C avoidance symptoms. The clinician could easily do much of this work "behind the scenes," using behavioral rehearsal and education in his or her office, which may be preferable for consumers who have not disclosed that they are having any psychiatric difficulties at work. Second, a test of supported employment among trauma survivors who are no longer employed seems warranted.

Case Management

Case management for PTSD has not been tested for efficacy using randomized clinical trials. However, clinical case studies and observations, surveys, personal accounts, and naturalistic studies using pre- and postcase management techniques provide compelling evidence favoring this approach. It is no longer a question of whether case management works; rather, the question is, which form of case management works for which individuals? The clinical literature favors the form of intensive case management in which case managers introduce control over contingencies in managing increases in preferred behaviors and decreases in behaviors considered nonproductive (e.g., Rosenheck, 2004; Rosenheck et al., 2000).

Six elements of case management for traumatized persons are as follows:

1. The case manager is assigned to work with a client who has been traumatized.
2. The case manager conducts a needs assessment designed to capture PTSD symptoms.
3. The case manager and client develop action steps to address the trauma-related problems for which treatment has been sought.
4. The case manager and client together assess client and community resources to reduce trauma symptoms.
5. The case manager monitors client progress in achieving agreed-upon goals in reducing trauma symptoms.
6. The case manager links the client to needed services with service providers who work on behalf of the client (e.g., Drake, Yovetich, Bebout, Harris, & McHugo, 1997).

Contemporary approaches emphasize the importance of case managers' control of contingencies to increase desired outcomes (Sorenson et al., 2005).

Two model programs developed in the VA, build upon assertive community treatment approaches pioneered long ago by Test and Stein, and further developed for local and state mental health agencies in a variety of locales (Test, 1999). The first, for persons with serious mental illness (many with co-occurring PTSD), was developed by Neale, Rosenheck, and their colleagues at the VA in Connecticut (e.g., Neale & Rosenheck, 2000). The other, a care management program developed and tested for its effectiveness among clients seen in primary care and medical and surgical units at the VA in Connecticut, was developed by Noel, Rogers, Vogel, and Rohrbaugh (2004) and Noel, Vogel, Erdos, Cornwall, and Levin (2004). Neale and Rosenheck developed clinical practice guidelines for mental health intensive case management (MHICM), and more than 90 MHICMs are now operational in VAs across the nation, involving more than 5,000 veterans, many with PTSD diagnoses. VA MHICM guidelines are distinguished by a required outcome evaluation system analyzed by the New England Program Evaluation Center (*www.nepec. org*). Annual reports demonstrate benefits for veterans with serious mental disorders, many with co-occurring PTSD diagnoses. Favorable outcomes are reported for reducing inpatient hospitalization, satisfaction with services, improvements in social and occupational role functioning, and decreases in psychiatric symptoms and alcohol/drug abuse.

Checklist to Guide Selection of Rehabilitation Techniques

Use of each of these rehabilitation techniques is predicated on a thorough assessment of the trauma survivor, with careful attention to each of the eight domains of functioning. Figure 16.1 provides a guideline to help the clinician determine which services are most appropriate for which survivors.

Clinicians working with individuals with PTSD are encouraged to assess each of the following domains frequently, typically through interview, and refer individuals for psychosocial rehabilitation services as warranted.

1. **Patient education techniques.** Clinicians should attend to whether clients have a clear understanding of their disorder, especially emphasizing comprehension regarding mutable factors associated with better and worse outcomes. Clients lacking appropriate information can be provided with written materials, videos, and Web-based self-study resources. Clients are encouraged to initiate and to continue personal studies about trauma and its residuals, using portals such as the VA My HealtheVet program (*www.myhealth.va.gov/mhvportal/anonymous. portal?_nfpb=true&_nfto=false&_pageLabel=mhvHome*), and/or information form the National Center for PTSD (*www ncptsd.va.gov*).
2. **Supported education.** Many clients with PTSD often wish to return to school to improve their vocational prospects. These clients often benefit from referrals to supported education program, which can help them not only to navigate school regulations but also access disability services that can compensate for difficulties in attention, memory, and concentration.
3. **Self-care and independent living skills training.** Clinicians refer clients for training in self-care and independent living skills in cases where impairments and interferences in functioning are noted (cf. VA/DoD psychosocial rehabilitation module: *www.oqp.med.va.gov/cpg/cpg.htm*). This includes the following:
   - **Client health education services.** Health education services are recommended in situations where clients engage in high-risk behaviors (e.g., addictions) and are uninformed about proactive health consequences needed in PTSD (e.g., Najavits, 2002).
   - **Services to ensure safety.** Client and clinician take steps to ensure client safety (e.g., Najavits, 2002).
4. **Supported housing services.** Clients who are homeless and/or are not living in safe, stable, affordable housing are referred to housing placement services (see the VA/DoD psychosocial rehabilitation modules for determining needs).
5. **Family psychoeducation services.** As and when needed, family psychoeducation services are recommended to ensure family support and knowledge about PTSD and associated disorders subsequent to trauma (e.g., Glynn et al., 1999).
6. **Social skills training.** To address social isolation associated with PTSD, clients in need are referred to social skills training and other forms of rehabilitation to increase appropriate socialization. Participation in peer-counseling services such as the VA Vet-to-Vet program can also be invaluable. When available, clients are encouraged to establish links with support groups to facilitate home and community adjustment of persons recovering from PTSD and related disorders.
7. **Supported employment.** Unemployed clients who meet criteria for PTSD are encouraged to seek job counseling and job placement services.
8. **Intensive case management.** The care or case manager should be designated when and were appropriate to remove barriers and improve access to requisite treatment and rehabilitation services, and to continue follow-up to ensure that PTSD symptoms are addressed, and home and community adjustment improves.

FIGURE 16.1. Psychosocial rehabilitation services assessment checklist for PTSD.

Summary and Recommendations

We conclude from reviewing the literature on psychosocial rehabilitation that considerable progress has been made in developing both measures and manualized interventions for persons who have been traumatized. Randomized clinical trials are beginning to be published in peer-reviewed journals for the psychosocial rehabilitation domains first specified for PTSD in 2000 by Penk and Flannery. The VA is investing in funding randomized clinical trials for PTSD veterans for types of psychosocial rehabilitation such as vocational rehabilitation, social skills training, family services, physical health, and independent living skills. Based on pilot studies used to justify such investments, results are likely to yield positive findings, further justifying these approaches to treating PTSD. Although psychosocial rehabilitation is promising for those who have been traumatized, clinicians fielding such techniques face many barriers before applications proliferate. One major problem is funding. Despite benefits, third-party payors often do not reimburse for psychosocial rehabilitation. As a consequence, techniques proven to be effective are not likely to be as widely practiced as emerging evidence suggests that they merit.

Our central conclusions are as follows:

1. More randomized clinical trials are needed for each of the eight listed domains of psychosocial rehabilitation listed earlier.
2. Comparisons between psychosocial rehabilitation techniques and other forms of treatment for PTSD are needed.
3. Cost analyses need to be conducted.
4. Strategies need to be generated for reimbursement for psychosocial rehabilitation.
5. Criteria for levels of care within each type of psychosocial rehabilitation need to be developed in terms of who needs such services, degree of frequency and intensity needed for such services, when such services should terminate, and when such services should again be prescribed, if relapse occurs. A PTSD-equivalent to the training grid developed by the American Psychological Association needs to be developed for psychosocial rehabilitation.
6. Functional measures need to be developed for determining when to refer patients with PTSD to services provided for each type of psychosocial rehabilitation.

We conclude, in summary, that each of the eight categories of psychosocial rehabilitation listed represents a modality in its own right. Each already has been demonstrated to be effective for mental disorders in general. Now, a growing literature suggests that these approaches may benefit PTSD. Each of the eight categories can be, and in some instances already has been, specifically and uniquely structured to address problems associated with PTSD. Clinicians and mental health researchers must devise and develop techniques by which each category of psychosocial rehabilitation can become trauma-focused. Staff delivering such services must learn from trauma specialists how to deliver such trauma-focused services. Those receiving the services must learn principles of coping with trauma, so that they are able to direct the course of their self-care. We believe that results from empirical evaluations of psychosocial rehabilitation interventions will document their benefit for this population as more and more of the randomized clinical trials currently underway are completed and published.

Note

1. We use the terms "patient," "client," and "consumer" interchangeably in the rest of the chapter.

References

Ahrens, C. E., & Campbell, R. (2000). Assisting rape victims as they recover from rape: The impact on friends. *Journal of Interpersonal Violence, 15*(9), 959–986.

Ainspan, N. D. (2008). Finding employment as a veteran with a disability. In N. D. Ainspan & W. E. Penk (Eds.), *Returning wars' wounded, injured, and ill: A reference handbook* (pp. 102–138). Westport, CT: Praeger

American Psychiatric Association. (1996). Practice guidelines for the treatment of patients with nicotine dependence. *American Journal of Psychiatry, 153*(Suppl. 10), 1–31.

American Psychiatric Association. (2000). *Diagnostic and statistical manual of mental disorders* (4th ed., text revision). Washington, DC: Author.

Anthony, W. A. (1992). Psychiatric rehabilitation: Key issues and future policy. *Health Aff (Millwood), 11*(3), 164–171.

Anthony, W. A. (1993). Recovery from mental illness: The guiding vision of the mental health service system in the 1990s. *Psychosocial Rehabilitation Journal, 16*, 11–23.

Association, A. P. (1996). Practice guidelines for the treatment of patients with nicotine dependence. *American Journal of Psychiatry, 153*(10, Suppl.), 1–31.

Ayllon, T., & Azrin, N. H. (1968). *The token economy.* New York: Appleton-Century-Crofts.

Back, S. E., Dansky, B. S., Carroll, K. M., & Foa, E. B. (2001). Exposure therapy in the treatment of PTSD among cocaine-dependent individuals: Description of procedures. *Journal of Substance Abuse Treatment, 21*(1), 35–45.

Bandura, A. (1973). *Aggression: A social learning analysis.* Englewood Cliffs, NJ: Prentice-Hall.

Bandura, A. (1997). *Self-efficacy: The exercise of control.* New York: Freeman.

Bandura, A. (2006). Toward a psychology of human agency. *Perspectives on Psychological Science, 1*, 164–180.

Barsky-Carrow, B. M. (2000). Using study circles in the workplace as an educational method of facilitating readjustment after a traumatic life experience. *Dissertation Abstracts International A: Humanities and Social Sciences, 60*(7-A), 2321.

Bass, E., & Davis, L. (1988). *The courage to heal: A guide for women survivors of child abuse.* New York: Harper & Row.

Beck, A. T., Ward, C. H., Mendelson, M., Mock, J., & Erbaugh, J. (1961). An inventory for measuring depression. *Archives of General Psychiatry, 4*, 561–571.

Becker, D. R., Smith, J., Tanzman, B., Drake, R. E., & Tremblay, T. (2001). Fidelity of supported employment programs and employment outcomes. *Psychiatric Services, 52*(6), 834–836.

Beckerman, N. L. (2004). The impact of post-traumatic stress disorder on couples: A theoretical framework for assessment and intervention. *Family Process, 31*(3), 129–144.

Beckham, J. C., Feldman, M. E., Kirby, A. C., Hertzberg, M. A., & Moore, S. D. (1997). Interpersonal violence and its correlates in Vietnam veterans with chronic post-traumatic stress disorder. *Journal of Clinical Psychology, 53*(8), 859–869.

Beckham, J. C., Lytle, B. L., & Feldman, M. E. (1996). Caregiver burden in partners of Vietnam War veterans with posttraumatic stress disorder. *Journal of Consulting and Clinical Psychology, 64*(5), 1068–1072.

Bellack, A. S., Mueser, K. T., Gingerich, S., & Agresta, J. (2004). *Social skills training for schizophrenia: A step-by-step guide* (2nd ed.). New York: Guilford Press.

Bond, G. R. (2004). Supported employment: Evidence for an evidence-based practice. *Psychiatric Rehabilitation Journal, 27*(4), 345–359.

Brady, S., Rierdan, J., Penk, W., Meschede, T., & Losardo, M. (2003). Post-traumatic stress disorder in civilians with serious mental illness. *Journal of Trauma and Dissociation, 4*, 77–90.

Breslau, N., Lucia, V. C., & Davis, G. C. (1985). Partial PTSD versus full PTSD: An empirical examination of associated impairment. *Psychological Medicine, 34*(7), 1205–1214.

Brewin, C. R., Andrews, B., & Valentine, J. D. (2000). Meta-analysis of risk factors for posttraumatic stress disorder in trauma-exposed adults. *Journal of Consulting and Clinical Psychology, 68*(5), 748–766.

Bryant-Davis, T. (2004). Rape is . . . : A medical review for sexual assault psychoeducation. *Trauma, Violence and Abuse, 5*(2), 194–195.

Byrne, C., Brown, B., Voorberg, N., & Schofield, R. (1994). Wellness education for individuals with chronic mental illness living in the community. *Issues in Mental Health Nursing, 15*(3), 239–252.

Carroll, E. M., Rueger, D. B., Foy, D. W., & Donahoe, C. P., Jr. (1985). Vietnam combat veterans with posttraumatic stress disorder: Analysis of marital and cohabitating adjustment. *Journal of Traumatic Stress, 15*(3), 205–212.

Cates, J. A., & Graham, L. L. (1993). HIV and serious mental illness: Reducing the risk. *Community Mental Health Journal, 29*(1), 35–47.

Centers for Disease Control and Prevention. (2006). Health hazard evaluation of police officers and firefighters after hurricane Katrina—New Orleans, Louisiana, October 17–28 and November 30–December 5, 2005. *Mortality and Morbidity Weekly, 55*(16), 456–458.

Cloitre, M., Koenen, K. C., Cohen, L. R., & Han, H. (2002). Skills training in affective and interpersonal regulation followed by exposure: A phase-based treatment for PTSD related to childhood abuse. *Journal of Consulting and Clinical Psychology, 70*(5), 1067–1074.

Collins, M. E., Mowbray, C. T., & Bybee, D. (2000). Characteristics predicting successful outcomes of participants with severe mental illness in supported education. *Psychiatric Services, 51*(6), 774–780.

Cook, J. A., & Razzano, L. (2000). Vocational rehabilitation for persons with schizophrenia: Recent research and implications for practice. *Schizophrenia Bulletin, 26,* 87–103.

Culhane, D. P., Metraux, S., & Hadley, T. (2002). Public service reductions associated with placement of homeless persons with severe mental illness in supportive housing. *Housing Policy Debate, 13*(1), 107–163.

David, W. S., Simpson, T. L., & Cotton, A. J. (2006). Taking charge: A pilot curriculum of self-defense and personal safety training for veterans with PTSD because of military sexual trauma. *Journal of Interpersonal Violence, 21*(4), 555–565.

DeLisi, L. E., Maurizio, A., Yost, M., Papparozzi, C. F., Fulchino, C., Katz, C. L., et al. (2003). A survey of New Yorkers after the September 11, 2001, terrorist attacks. *American Journal of Psychiatry, 160*(4), 780–783.

Derogatis, L. R. (1993). *Brief Symptom Inventory (BSI): Administration, scoring, and procedures manual* (3rd ed.). Minneapolis, MN: National Computer Systems.

Diener, E., & Tov, W. (2007). Culture and subjective well-being. In S. Kitayama & D. Cohen (Eds.), *Handbook of cultural psychology* (pp. 691–713). New York: Guilford Press.

Drake, R. E., Becker, D. R., Bond, G. R., & Mueser, K. T. (2003). A process analysis of integrated and non-integrated approaches to supported employment. *Journal of Vocational Rehabilitation, 18*(1), 51–58.

Drake, R. E., Yovetrich, N. A., Bebout, R. R., Harris, M., & McHugo, G. J. (1997). Integrated treatment for dually diagnosed homeless adults. *Journal of Nervous and Mental Disorders, 185*(5), 298–305.

Epstein, E. E., & McCrady, B. S. (1998). Behavioral couples treatment of alcohol and drug use disorders: Current status and innovations. *Clinical Psychology Review, 18*(6), 689–711.

Felce, D., Lowe, K., & Jones, E. (2002). Association between the provision characteristics and operation of supported employment services and resident outcomes. *Journal of Applied Research in Intellectual Disabilities, 15*(4), 404–418.

Fenichel, O. (1945). *The psychoanalytic theory of neurosis.* New York: Norton.

Flannery, R. B. (1992). *Post-traumatic stress disorder: The victim's guide to healing and recovery.* New York: Crossroads.

Flannery, R. B. (1998). *The Assaulted Staff Action program (ASAP): Coping with the psychological aftermath of violence.* Ellicott City, MD: Chevron.

Fries, E. (2003). Steps towards empowerment for community healing. *Intervention: International Journal of Mental Health, Psychosocial Work and Cooperation in Areas of Armed Conflict, 1*(2), 40–46.

Frueh, B. C., Turner, S. M., Beidel, D. C., Mirabella, R. F., & Jones, W. J. (1996). Trauma management therapy: A preliminary evaluation of multicomponent behavioral treatment for chronic combat-related PTSD. *Behaviour Research and Therapy, 34*(7), 533–543.

Fujimoto, K. L. (2002). Evaluating the effectiveness of a group treatment program: Integrating traumatic stress disorder and childhood trauma literature. *Dissertation Abstracts International B: The Sciences and Engineering, 3799.*

Galea, S., Vlahov, D., Resnick, H., Ahern, J., Susser, E., Gold, J., et al. (2003). Trends of probable post-traumatic stress disorder in New York City after the September 11 terrorist attacks. *American Journal of Epidemiology, 158*(6), 514–524.

Galovski, T., & Lyons, J. A. (2004). Psychological sequelae of combat violence: A review of the impact of PTSD on the veteran's family and possible interventions. *Aggression and Violent Behavior, 9,* 477–501.

Glodich, A. (2000). Psychoeducational groups for adolescents exposed to violence and abuse: The effectiveness of increasing knowledge of trauma to avert reenactment and risk-taking behaviors. *Dissertation Abstracts International A: Humanities and Social Sciences*, 3527.

Glodich, A. (2001). Protocol for a trauma-based psychoeducational group intervention to decrease risk-taking, reenactment, and further violence exposure: Application to the public high school setting. *Journal of Child and Adolescent Group Therapy*, *11*(2–3), 87–107.

Glynn, S. M., Cohen, A. N., Dixon, L. B., & Niv, N. (2006). The potential impact of the recovery movement on family interventions for schizophrenia: Opportunities and obstacles. *Schizophrenia Bulletin*, *32*(3), 451–463.

Glynn, S. M., Eth, S., Randolph, E. T., Foy, D. W., Urbaitis, M., Boxer, L., et al. (1999). A test of behavioral family therapy to augment exposure for combat-related posttraumatic stress disorder. *Journal of Consulting and Clinical Psychology*, *67*(2), 243–251.

Goldfinger, S. M., Schutt, R. K., Tolomiczenko, G. S., Seidman, L., Penk, W. E., Turner, W., et al. (1999). Housing placement and subsequent days homeless among formerly homeless adults with mental illness. *Psychiatric Services*, *50*(5), 674–679.

Gorde, M. W., Helfrich, C. A., & Finlayson, M. L. (2005). Trauma symptoms and life skills needs of domestic violence victims. *Journal of Interpersonal Violence*, *19*, 691–708.

Halford, W. K., Bouma, R., Kelly, A., & Young, R. (1999). Individual psychopathology and marital distress: Analyzing the association and implications for therapy. *Behavior Modification*, *23*(2), 179–216.

Hamdani, N. (2003). Psycho-education through radio. *Intervention: International Journal of Mental Health, Psychosocial Work and Counselling in Areas of Armed Conflict*, *1*(2), 47–49.

Hirai, M., & Clum, G. A. (2005). An Internet-based self-change program for traumatic event related fear, distress, and maladaptive coping. *Journal of Traumatic Stress*, *18*(6), 631–636.

Hoge, C. W., Auchterlonie, J. L., & Milliken, C. S. (2006). Mental health problems, use of mental health services, and attrition from military service after returning from deployment to Iraq or Afghanistan. *Journal of the American Medical Association*, *295*(9), 1023–1032.

Hoge, C. W., Castro, C. A., Messer, S. C., McGurk, D., Cotting, D. I., & Koffman, R. L. (2004). Combat duty in Iraq and Afghanistan, mental health problems, and barriers to care. *New England Journal of Medicine*, *351*(1), 13–22.

Horowitz, M., Wilner, N., & Alvarez, W. (1979). Impact of Event Scale: A measure of subjective stress. *Psychosomatic Medicine*, *41*(3), 209–218.

Howard, J. M., & Goelitz, A. (2004). Psychoeducation as a response to community disaster. *Brief Treatment and Crisis Intervention*, *4*(1), 1–10.

Isenwater, W., Lanham, W., & Thornhill, H. (2002). The College Link Program: Evaluation of a supported education initiative in Great Britain. *Psychosocial Rehabilitation Journal*, *26*(1), 43–50.

Iversen, A., Nikolaou, V., Greenberg, N., Unwin, C., Hull, L., Hotopf, M., et al. (2005). What happens to British veterans when they leave the armed forces? *European Journal of Public Health*, *15*(2), 175–184.

Jagodic, G. K., & Kontac, K. (2002). Normalization: A key to childrens' recovery. In

W. N. Zubenko & J. A. Capozzoli (Eds.), *Children and disasters: A practical guide to healing and recovery* (pp. 159–171). London: Oxford University Press.

Jaycox, L. H., Marshall, G. N., & Schell, T. (2004). Use of mental health services by men injured through community violence. *Psychiatric Services, 55*(4), 415–420.

Johnson, D. R., Feldman, S., & Lubin, H. (1995). Critical interaction therapy: Couples therapy in combat-related posttraumatic stress disorder. *Family Process, 34*(4), 401–412.

Johnson, D. R., Fontana, A., Lubin, H., Corn, B., & Rosenheck, R. (2004). Long-term course of treatment-seeking Vietnam veterans with posttraumatic stress disorder: Mortality, clinical condition, and life satisfaction. *Journal of Nervous and Mental Disease, 192*(1), 35–41.

Johnson, S. B., Langlieb, A. M., Teret, S. P., Gross, R., Schwab, M., Massa, J., et al. (2005). Rethinking first response: Effects of the clean up and recovery effort on workers at the World Trade Center disaster site. *Journal of Occupational and Environmental Medicine, 47*(4), 386–391.

Jordan, B. K., Marmar, C. R., Fairbank, J. A., Schlenger, W. E., Kulka, R. A., Hough, R. L., et al. (1992). Problems in families of male Vietnam veterans with posttraumatic stress disorder. *Journal of Consulting and Clinical Psychology, 60*(6), 916–926.

Kataoka, S. H., Stein, B. D., Jaycox, L. H., Wong, M., Escudero, P., Tu, W., et al. (2003). A school-based mental health program for traumatized Latino immigrant children. *Journal of the American Academy of Child and Adolescent Psychiatry, 42*(3), 311–318.

Keane, T. M., Scott, W. O., Chavoya, G. A., Lamparski, D. M., & Fairbank, J. A. (1985). Social support in veterans with posttraumatic stress disorder: A comparative analysis. *Journal of Consulting and Clinical Psychology, 53*(1), 95–102.

King, D. W., King, L. A., Foy, D. W., Keane, T. M., & Fairbank, J. A. (1999). Posttraumatic stress disorder in a national sample of female and male Vietnam veterans: Risk factors, war-zone stressors, and resilience–recovery variables. *Journal of Abnormal Psychology, 108*(1), 164–170.

Kubany, E. S., Hill, E. E., & Owens, J. A. (2003). Cognitive trauma therapy for battered women with PTSD: Preliminary findings. *Journal of Traumatic Stress, 16*(1), 81–91.

Kudler, H., Straits-Troster, K., & Jones, E. (2006). *Strategies in the service of new combat veterans.* Paper presented at the VISN 17 PTSD Conference, Audie Murphy Memorial VA Hospital, San Antonio, TX. Available from *howard.kudler@med. va.gov*

Lange, A., Rietkijk, D., Hudcovicova, M., van de Ven, J. P., Schrieken, B., & Emmelkamp, P. M. G. (2003). Interapy: A controlled randomized trial of the standardized treatment of posttraumatic stress through the Internet. *Journal of Consulting and Clinical Psychology, 71*(5), 901–909.

Lating, J. M., Sherman, M. F., Everly, G. S., Jr., Lowry, J. L., & Peragine, T. F. (2004). PTSD reactions and functioning of American Airlines flight attendants in the wake of September 11. *Journal of Nervous and Mental Disease, 192*(6), 435–441.

Lauterbach, D., Vrana, S., King, D. W., & King, L. A. (1997). Psychometric properties of the Mississippi PTSD Scale. *Journal of Traumatic Stress, 10*(3), 499–513.

Lehman, A. F., Goldberg, R. W., Dixon, L. B., McNary, S., Postrado, L., Hackman, A., et al. (2002). Improving employment outcomes for persons with severe mental illness. *Archives of General Psychiatry, 59*, 165–172.

Liberman, R. (1992). *Handbook of psychiatric rehabilitation*. Boston: Allyn & Bacon.

Liberman, R. P., Wallace, C. J., Blackwell, G. A., Eckman, T. A., Vaccaro, T. V., & Kuehnel, T. G. (1993). *Innovations in skills training: The UCLA social and independent living skills modules*. Camarillo, CA: Psychiatric Rehabilitation Consultants.

Lubin, H., & Johnson, D. R. (2000). Interactive psychoeducational group therapy in the treatment of authority problems in combat-related posttraumatic stress disorder. *International Journal of Group Psychotherapy, 50*(3), 277–289.

Lui, A., Glynn, S. M., & Shetty, V. (2008). *The interplay of perceived social support and posttraumatic psychological distress following orofacial injury*. Manuscript submitted for publication.

Lukens, E. P. (2004). Building resiliency and cultural collaboration post September 11th: A group model of brief integrative psychoeducation for diverse communities. *Traumatology, 10*(2), 107–129.

Lyons, J. S. (2003). *Young adult needs and strengths assessment*. Evanston, IL: Buddin Praed Foundation.

Mabalango, M. A. G. (2003). A quasi-experimental study of a school-based psychoeducational group for traumatized school-aged children and their parent/caregivers. *Dissertation Abstracts International A: Humanities and Social Sciences, 64*(4), 1409.

MacDonald, H. A., Colotla, V., Flamer, S., & Karlinsky, H. (2003). Posttraumatic stress disorder (PTSD) in the workplace: A descriptive study of workers experiencing PTSD resulting from work injury. *Journal of Occupational Rehabilitation, 13*(2), 63–77.

Magruder, K. M., Frueh, B. C., Knapp, R. G., Johnson, M. R., Vaughan, J. A., III, Carson, T. C., et al. (2004). PTSD symptoms, demographic characteristics, and functional status among veterans treated in VA primary care clinics. *Journal of Traumatic Stress, 17*(4), 293–301.

Mares, A. S., Kasprow, W. J., & Rosenheck, R. (2004). Outcomes of supported housing for homeless veterans with psychiatric and substance abuse problems. *Mental Health Services Research, 6*(4), 199–211.

Marlatt, G. A., & Gordon, J. F. (1985). *Relapse prevention: Maintenance strategies in the treatment of addictive behaviors*. New York: Guilford Press.

Marrs, R. (1984). Why the pain won't stop and what the family can do to help. In S. Breznitz (Ed.), *The denial of stress* (pp. 85–101). New York: International Universities Press.

Marshall, A., Panuzio, J., & Taft, C. T. (2005). Intimate partner violence among military veterans and active duty servicemen. *Clinical Psychology Review, 25*, 882–896.

Matsakis, A. (1996). *"I can't get over it": A handbook for trauma survivors*. Oakland, CA: New Harbinger Press.

Matthews, L. R. (2005). Work potential of road accident survivors with posttraumatic stress disorder. *Behaviour Research and Therapy, 43*(4), 475–483.

McHugo, G. J., Bebout, R. R., Harris, M., Cleghorn, S., Herring, G., Xie, H., et al. (2004). A randomized controlled trial of integrated versus parallel housing services for homeless adults with severe mental illness. *Schizophrenia Bulletin, 30*(4), 969–982.

McMackin, R. A., Leisen, M. B., Sattler, L., Krinsley, K., & Riggs, D. S. (2002). Preliminary development of trauma-focused treatment groups for incarcerated juvenile offenders. In R. Greenwald (Ed.), *Trauma and juvenile delinquency: Theory, research, and interventions* (pp. 175–199). New York: Haworth Maltreatment and Trauma Press/Haworth Press.

Michaels, A. J., Michaels, C. E., Smith, J. S., Moon, C. H., Peterson, C., & Long, W. B. (2000). Outcome from injury: General health, work status, and satisfaction 12 months after trauma. *Journal of Trauma, 48*(5), 841–848.

Monson, C. M., Schnurr, P. P., Stevens, S. P., & Guthrie, K. A. (2004). Cognitive-behavioral couple's treatment for posttraumatic stress disorder: Initial findings. *Journal of Traumatic Stress, 17*(4), 341–344.

Morris, A. S. (2004). Analysis of the impact of PTSD group psychoeducational skills training with spouses and significant others of trauma survivors. *Dissertation Abstracts International B: The Sciences and Engineering, 65*(2), 1034.

Moses, E. B., & Barlow, D. H. (2006). A new unified treatment for emotional disorders. *Current Directions in Psychological Science, 15*, 146–150.

Mosig, A. (2006). The impact of exposure therapy and didactic intervention on reduction of somatic symptoms in posttraumatic stress disorder. *Dissertation Abstracts International B: The Sciences and Engineering, 67*(4), 2235.

Mowbray, C. T., Gutierrez, L. M., Bellamy, C. D., & Szilvagyi, S. (2003). Replication of psychosocial rehabilitation program: A case study analysis of supported education. *Journal of Community Psychology, 31*(5), 437–457.

Mueser, K. T., Essock, S. M., Haines, M., Wolfe, R., & Xie, H. (2004). Posttraumatic stress disorder, supported employment, and outcomes in people with severe mental illness. *CNS Spectrums, 9*(12), 913–925

Najavits, L. M. (2002). Seeking safety: A new psychotherapy for PTSD and substance abuse. In P. Ouimette & P. Brown (Eds.), *Trauma and substance abuse: Causes, consequences, and treatments for co-morbid disorders* (pp. 228–248). Washington, DC: American Psychological Association.

Neale, M. S., & Rosenheck, R. A. (2000). Therapeutic limit setting in assertive community treatment programs. *Psychiatric Services, 51*, 499–505.

Nhiwatiwa, F. G. (2003). The effects of single session education in reducing symptoms of distress following patient assault in nurses working in medium secure settings. *Journal of Psychiatry and Mental Health Nursing, 10*(5), 561–568.

Noel, H. L., Rogers, C., Vogel, D. C., & Rohrbaugh, R. M. (2004). Linking case management, healthy outcomes, and resource use across the continuum. *Care Management, 10*, 21–32.

Noel, H. L., Vogel, D. C., Erdos, J. J., Cornwall, D., & Levin, F. (2004). Home telehealth reduces health care costs. *Telemedicine Journal and E-Health, 10*, 170–183.

Nowinsky, J., Baker, S., & Carroll, K. M. (1994). *Twelve-step facilitation therapy manual* (Vol. 1, NIAA Project MATCH Monograph, NIH Publication No. 94-3722). Washington, DC: U.S. Government Printing Office.

O'Farrell, T. J., & Fals-Stewart, W. (2003). Alcohol abuse. *Journal of Marital and Family Therapy, 29*(1), 121–146.

Osterman, J. E., Barbiaz, J., & Johnson, P. (2001). Emergency interventions for rape victims. *Psychiatric Services, 52*(6), 733–734.

Ozer, E., Best, S., Lipsey, T., & Weiss, D. (2003). Predictors of posttraumatic stress disorder and symptoms in adults: A meta-analysis. *Psychological Bulletin, 129*(1), 52–72.

Peckham, N. G., Howlett, S., & Corbett, A. (2007). Evaluating a survivors group pilot for women with significant intellectual disabilities who have been sexually abused. *Journal of Applied Research in Intellectual Disabilities, 20*(4), 308–322.

Penk, W., Dreving, C., & Schutt, R. (2002). PTSD in the workplace. In J. C. Thomas & M. Hersen (Eds.), *Handbook of mental health in the workplace* (pp. 215–248). Thousand Oaks, CA: Sage.

Penk, W., & Flannery, R. B., Jr. (2000). Psychosocial rehabilitation. In E. B. Foa, T. M. Keane, & M. J. Friedman (Eds.), *Effective treatments for PTSD: Practice guidelines from the International Society of Traumatic Stress Studies* (pp. 224–246). New York: Guilford Press.

Pilling, S., Bebbington, P., Kuipers, E., Garety, P., Geddes, J., Orbach, G., et al. (2002). Psychological treatments in schizophrenia: I. Meta-analysis of family intervention and cognitive behaviour therapy. *Psychological Medicine, 32*, 763–782.

Pitschel-Walz, G., Leucht, S., Bäuml, J., Kissling, W., & Engel, R. R. (2001). The effect of family interventions on relapse and rehospitalization in schizophrenia: A meta-analysis. *Schizophrenia Bulletin, 27*, 73–92.

Pratt, S. I., Rosenberg, S., Mueser, K. T., Brancato, J., Salyers, M. P., Jankowski, M. K., et al. (2005). Evaluation of a PTSD psychoeducational program for psychiatric inpatients. *Journal of Mental Health, 14*(2), 121–127.

President's New Freedom Commission on Mental Health. (2003). *Achieving the promise: Transforming mental health care in America: Final report* (DHHS Publication No. SMA-03-3832). Rockville, MD: Substance Abuse and Mental Health Services Administration.

Prigerson, H. G., Maciejewski, P. K., & Rosenheck, R. A. (2002). Population attributable fractions of psychiatric disorders and behavioral outcomes associated with combat exposure among U.S. men. *American Journal of Public Health, 92*(1), 59–63.

Rabin, C., & Nardi, C. (1991). Treating posttraumatic stress disorder couples: A psychoeducational program. *Community Mental Health Journal, 27*(3), 209–224.

Ratzlaff, S., McDiarmid, D., Marty, D., & Rapp, C. (2006). The Kansas Consumer as Provider Program: Measuring the effects of a supplemental education initiative. *Psychiatric Rehabilitation Journal, 29*(3), 174–182.

Rauch, S. A. A., Hembree, E. A., & Foa, E. B. (2001). Acute psychosocial preventive interventions for posttraumatic stress disorder. *Advances in Mind–Body Medicine, 17*(3), 187–190.

Regehr, C., Hill, J., Knott, T., & Sault, B. (2003). Social support, self-efficacy and trauma in new recruits and experienced firefighters. *Stress and Health, 19*, 189–193.

Rempfer, M., Brown, C., Hamera, E., & Cromwell, R. (2003). The relations between cognition and the independent living skill of shopping in people with schizophrenia. *Psychiatric Research, 117*, 103–112.

Rempfer, M., Hildenbrand, W., Parker, K., & Brown, C. (2003). An interdisciplinary approach to environmental intervention: Ecology of human performance. In L. Letts, P. Rigby, & D. Steward (Eds.), *Using environment to enable occupational performance* (pp. 119–136). Thorofare, NJ: Slack.

Riggs, D. S. (2000). Marital and family therapy. In E. B. Foa, T. M. Keane, & M. J. Friedman (Eds.), *Effective treatments for PTSD: Practice guidelines from the International Society for Traumatic Stress Studies* (pp. 280–301). New York: Guilford Press.

Riggs, D. S., Byrne, C. A., Weathers, F. W., & Litz, B. T. (1998). The quality of the intimate relationships of male Vietnam veterans: Problems associated with posttraumatic stress disorder. *Journal of Trauma and Stress, 11*(1), 87–101.

Roberts, W. R., Penk, W. E., Gearing, M. L., Robinowitz, R., Dolan, M. P., & Patterson, E. T. (1982). Interpersonal problems of Vietnam combat veterans with symptoms of posttraumatic stress disorder. *Journal of Abnormal Psychology, 91*(6), 444–450.

Rog, D. J. (2006). The evidence on supported housing. *Psychiatric Rehabilitation Journal, 29*(3), 334–344.

Rosenberg, S., Mueser, K. T., Jankowski, M. K., & Salyers, M. P. (2004). Cognitive-behavioral treatment of PTSD in severe mental illness: Results of a pilot study. *American Journal of Psychiatric Rehabilitation, 7*(2), 171–186.

Rosenheck, R., Stolar, M., & Fontana, A. (2000). Outcomes monitoring and the testing of new psychiatric treatments: Work therapy in the treatment of chronic post-traumatic stress disorder. *Health Services Research, 35*, 133–151.

Rosenheck, R. A. (2004). *Mental and substance use health services for veterans: Experiences with performance evaluation in the Department of Veterans Affairs.* Washington, DC: Institute of Medicine Committee on Crossing the Quality Chasm.

Rossman, S., Sridharan, S., & Buck, J. (1998). The impact of the opportunity to succeed program on employment success. *National Institute of Justice Journal, 1*, 14–20.

Savoca, E., & Rosenheck, R. (2000). The civilian labor market experiences of Vietnam-era veterans: The influence of psychiatric disorders. *Journal of Mental Health Policy and Economics, 3*(4), 199–207.

Shadish, W. R., & Baldwin, S. A. (2005). Effects of behavioral marital therapy: A meta-analysis of randomized controlled trials. *Journal of Consulting and Clinical Psychology, 73*(1), 6–14.

Sherman, M. D. (2006). Updates and five-year evaluation of the S.A.F.E. Program: A family psychoeducational program for serious mental illness. *Community Mental Health Journal, 42*(2), 213–219.

Sherman, M. D., & Sherman, D. M. (2005). *Finding my way: A teen's guide to living with a parent who has experienced trauma.* Edina, MN: Beavers Pond Press.

Sherman, M. D., Sautter, F., Lyons, J. A., Manguno-Mire, G. M., Han, X., Perry, D., et al. (2005). Mental health needs of cohabitating partners of Vietnam veterans with combat-related PTSD. *Psychiatric Services, 56*(9), 1150–1152.

Smith, M. W., Schnurr, P. P., & Rosenheck, R. A. (2005). Employment outcomes and PTSD symptom severity. *Mental Health Service Research, 7*(2), 89–101.

Snow, R. (1991). Aptitude–treatment interaction as a framework for research on individual differences in psychotherapy. *Journal of Consulting and Clinical Psychology, 59*, 205–216.

Solomon, Z. (1989). PTSD and social functioning: A three year prospective study. *Social Psychiatry and Psychiatric Epidemiology, 24*(3), 127–133.

Sorenson, J. L., Masson, C. L., Delucchi, K., Sporer, K., Bartnett, P. G., Mitsuishi, F., et al. (2005). Randomized trial of drug abuse treatment-linkage strategies. *Journal of Consulting and Clinical Psychology, 73*, 1026–1035.

Souza, R., & Sloot, M. (2003). Folk theatre improves psychosocial work in Kashmir. *Intervention: International Journal of Mental Health, Psychosocial Work and Counselling in Areas of Armed Conflict, 1*(3), 57–61.

Stephens, N., McDonald, R., & Jouriles, E. N. (2000). Helping children who reside at shelters for battered women: Lessons learned. *Journal of Aggression, Maltreatment and Trauma, 3*(1), 147–160.

Tarrier, N., Sommerfield, C., & Pilgrim, H. (1999). Relatives' expressed emotion (EE) and PTSD treatment outcome. *Psychology Medicine, 29*(4), 801–811.

Test, M. A. (1999). The strength's model: Case management with people suffering from severe and persistent mental illness. *Psychiatric Services, 50,* 1502–1503.

Trowell, J., Kolvin, I., Weeramanthri, T., Sadowski, H., Berelowitz, M., & Glasser, D. (2002). Psychotherapy for sexually abused girls: Psychopathological outcome findings and patterns of change. *British Journal of Psychiatry, 180*(3), 234–247.

Tsemberis, S., & Asmussen, S. (1999). From streets to homes: The Pathways to Housing Consumer Preference Supported Housing Model. *Alcoholism Treatment Quarterly, 17*(1–2), 113–131.

Tsemberis, S., & Eisenberg, R. F. (2000). Pathways to Housing: Supported housing for street-dwelling homeless individuals with psychiatric disabilities. *Psychiatric Services, 51*(4), 487–493.

Turner, S. M., Beidel, D. C., & Frueh, B. C. (2005). Multicomponent behavioral treatment for chronic combat-related posttraumatic stress disorder: Trauma management therapy. *Behavior Modification, 29*(1), 39–69.

Turpin, G., Downs, M., & Mason, S. (2005). Effectiveness of providing self-help information following acute traumatic injury: Randomized controlled trial. *British Journal of Psychiatry, 187*(1), 76–82.

Twamley, E. W., Jeste, D. V., & Lehman, A. F. (2003). Vocational rehabilitation in schizophrenia and other psychotic disorders: A literature review and meta-analysis of randomized controlled trials. *Journal of Nervous and Mental Disease, 191*(8), 515–523.

Underwood, M. M., & Kalafat, J. (2002). Crisis intervention in a new context: New Jersey post-September 11, 2001. *Brief Treatment and Crisis Intervention, 2*(1), 75–83.

Veterans Health Administration. (2004). *VA/DoD Clinical Practice Guidelines for the management of PTSD.* Washington, DC: National VA Clinical Practice Guidelines Committee. Available online from *www.oqp.med.va.gov/cpg/cpg.htm*

Wald, J., Taylor, S., & Scamvourgeras, A. (2004). Cognitive behavioral and neuropsychiatric treatment of post-traumatic conversion disorder: A case study. *Cognitive Behaviour Therapy, 33*(1), 12–20.

Weathers, F., Litz, B., Herman, D., Huska, J., & Keane, T. (1993, October). *The PTSD Checklist (PCL): Reliability, validity, and diagnostic utility.* Paper presented at the annual convention of the International Society of Traumatic Stress Studies, San Antonio, TX.

Wilhelm, K., Kovess, V., Rios-Seidel, C., & Finch, A. (2004). Work and mental health. *Social Psychiatry and Psychiatric Epidemiology, 39*(11), 866–873.

CHAPTER 17

Hypnosis

Etzel Cardeña, José R. Maldonado, Onno van der Hart,
and David Spiegel

Theoretical Context

Definitions

Hypnotic phenomena have been described for centuries, but the systematic development of clinical and research hypnosis did not emerge until the 19th century (Ellenberger, 1970). In the specific context of posttraumatic symptomatology, hypnotic techniques have been used for the psychological treatment of "shell shock," "battle fatigue," traumatic neuroses, and their more recent incarnations: posttraumatic stress disorder (PTSD), acute stress disorder (ASD), and dissociative disorders (e.g., Brende, 1985; Cardeña, Butler, & Spiegel, 2003; Spiegel & Spiegel, 1987). In this section, we review hypnosis and related constructs, relate them to dissociation and to posttraumatic symptomatology, and provide a rationale for the use of hypnosis in the treatment of PTSD.

It clarifies matters to distinguish among "hypnosis" as a specific procedure; "hypnotic phenomena" as behavior and experience occurring in the context of the hypnotic procedure; "hypnotic-like phenomena" as similar phenomena to those occurring within hypnosis but occurring in other contexts; and "hypnotizability," "hypnotic susceptibility," or "hypnotic responsiveness" as the ability to respond to a series of suggestions within a formal hypnotic procedure.

"Hypnosis" was defined by Division 30 of the American Psychological Association as "a procedure during which a health professional or researcher suggests that a client, patient, or subject experience changes in sensations, perceptions, thought, or behavior. The hypnotic context is generally established by an induction procedure" (Kirsch, 1994, p. 143). Hypnotic procedures can bring about a state of attentive focal concentration, with a relative suspension of peripheral awareness and heightened sensitivity to suggestions (Spiegel, 1994; Spiegel & Cardeña, 1990). Labeling of the situation as hypnotic and instructions to focus on the hypnotist's suggestions for relaxation, alertness, or a perceptual event, such as a metronome ticking, are common ingredients of hypnotic inductions. The induction procedure can be more or less formal. Despite claims to the contrary, there is no evidence that "indirect" suggestions and lack of a hypnosis context are more effective than direct suggestions and labeling the context as hypnosis (Matthews, Bennett, Bean, & Gallagher, 1985).

Hypnotic inductions typically involve communications to disregard extraneous concerns and to concentrate on the behaviors and experiences proposed by the hypnotist or that occur spontaneously. The induction for the Harvard Group Scale of Hypnotic Susceptibility (HGSHS; Shor & Orne, 1962) serves as a good illustration of a common approach. Its initial stage includes establishing rapport and briefly explaining the nature of the hypnotic procedure (e.g., that it is based on suggestions, and that the hypnotic experience may not be that different from other experiences encountered in everyday life). A more formal procedure follows, in which the individual is told that he or she will become more relaxed and hypnotized as he or she attends to suggestions to relax the muscles of the whole body and to close the eyes. Afterward, the hypnotist counts from 1 to 20 to "deepen" the hypnotic experience, although such techniques are more a continuation of the hypnotic induction at a level determined by the subject's hypnotizability. The following stage comprises giving specific suggestions to alter sensations, behavior, and cognition. The HGSHS and other relaxation-based inductions are often lengthy, but briefer procedures, such as the induction for the Hypnotic Induction Profile (HIP; Spiegel & Spiegel, 1987), require less than a minute. The HIP involves having the individual roll his or her eyes upward, then slowly closing the eyelids while taking a deep breath, exhaling and relaxing, and experiencing floating sensations (Spiegel & Spiegel, 1987).

Although hypnotic inductions commonly entail suggestions for relaxation, suggestions for activity and alertness are equally effective. In that modality, the hypnotist emphasizes mental alertness and has the participant engage in a physical activity, such as riding a stationary bike or moving his or her hand (Cardeña, Alarcón, Capafons, & Bayot, 1998). Use of procedures emphasizing mental alertness and physical activity may be a method of choice for individuals who easily fall asleep, are hypotensive or depressed, or just prefer activity and alertness over relaxation.

With respect to the clinical use of hypnosis, Division 30's definition stated,

> Hypnosis is not a type of therapy, like psychoanalysis or behavior therapy. Instead, it is a procedure that can be used to facilitate therapy. . . . Clinical hyp-

nosis should be used only by properly trained and credentialed health care professionals . . . who have also been trained in the clinical use of hypnosis and are working within the areas of their professional expertise. (Kirsch, 1994, p. 143)

"Hypnotic phenomena" are behavioral, cognitive, and experiential alterations that either emerge or are enhanced by a hypnotic induction. A number of studies have described the following common alterations among "hypnotized" individuals: (1) a sense of compulsion or enhanced suggestibility; (2) a diminution in reflective awareness, related to absorption in the suggested experiences; and (3) various unusual experiences, including body image alterations, altered sense of time, and dissociative experiences, such as feeling detached from oneself or the environment (cf. Cardeña, 2005; Cardeña & Spiegel, 1991). Because some people are not susceptible to hypnotic procedures or may actively resist suggestions, there is no guarantee that a hypnotic procedure will evoke hypnotic phenomena in any particular individual.

"Hypnotic-like phenomena" may occur spontaneously or follow nonhypnotic events, especially among highly hypnotizable individuals, and include behaviors and experiences similar to those found in a hypnotic setting (e.g., perceptual alterations, enhanced suggestibility, and narrow and continuous attentional focus) but encountered in different contexts. As we describe later, a number of acute and chronic traumatic reactions share similarities with those induced during formal hypnosis. Hypnotic-like phenomena can occur in the absence of a hypnotic context, especially with highly hypnotizable individuals or during traumatic situations.

Finally, "hypnotizability, hypnotic susceptibility, or responsiveness" refers to the robust finding of valid and reliable individual differences in response to hypnotic suggestions. With standardized induction and suggestion procedures, about 25% of individuals show substantial to very high hypnotizability, roughly 50% have moderate hypnotizability, and 25% have very low or no susceptibility (Hilgard, 1965). Furthermore, highly hypnotizable individuals are prone to have hypnotic-like experiences, independent of the context (Spiegel & Spiegel, 1987; Tellegen & Atkinson, 1974), and hypnotizability correlates positively with reports of spontaneous and unusual events, including paranormal experiences and a tendency to blur the distinction between different states of consciousness (e.g., Cardeña, Lynn, & Krippner, 2000; Pekala, Kumar, & Marcano, 1995).

Hypnotic responsiveness varies throughout the life cycle. Individuals are more highly hypnotizable during their late childhood years, with a peak in hypnotic capacity around the age of 12. This is followed by a moderate decline, with stabilization later in adulthood (Hilgard, 1965). Hypnotizability does not seem to change much during the adult years. A test–retest study found a strong correlation (.71) between testing conducted during undergraduate years and that taking place 25 years later (Piccione, Hilgard, & Zimbardo, 1989).

Hypnosis, Dissociation, and Posttraumatic Phenomena

Several pioneers of modern psychopathology (e.g., Pierre Janet, Josef Breuer and Sigmund Freud, Morton Prince) studied the triad of hypnosis–dissociation–trauma and developed theories to account for their relationship (Breuer & Freud, 1895/1982; Janet, 1889/1973; van der Hart & Horst, 1989; van der Kolk & van der Hart, 1989). Spiegel and Cardeña (1991) have suggested that trauma may be seen as the process of being made into an object, or being the victim of someone else's rage, organized aggression, or nature's indifference. The helplessness engendered by traumatic experiences may create sudden challenges to normal ways of processing perception, cognition, affect, and relationships (Maldonado & Spiegel, 1994). Experimental and survey data suggest that traumatic and stressful events indeed produce a narrow focus of attention, with a consequent disregard of peripheral information (Cardeña & Spiegel, 1993; Christianson & Loftus, 1987; Classen, Koopman, Hales, & Spiegel, 1998; Koopman, Classen, & Spiegel, 1996), and these attentional processes are similar to those manifested during hypnosis (Cardeña & Spiegel, 1991; Nijenhuis & van der Hart, 1999).

This narrowing of attention, especially if maintained for more than a few moments, is associated with alterations in consciousness, including dissociative phenomena. As a descriptive construct, "dissociation" has been defined as an alteration in consciousness characterized by an experiential disconnection or disengagement from the self and/or the environment (Cardeña, 1994). More theoretically, it was defined as "a structured separation of mental processes . . . that are ordinarily integrated" (Spiegel & Cardeña, 1991, p. 367). Dissociative phenomena include alterations in the sense or perception of self and the environment, the sense of agency or will, memory, and identity (Butler, Duran, Jasiukaitis, Koopman, & Spiegel, 1996; Cardeña, 1997). However, some authors regard alterations in consciousness not as dissociative in nature but as related symptoms (e.g., van der Hart, Nijenhuis, & Steele, 2006). Recently, the concept of somatoform dissociation has stressed dissociative somatic symptomatology, such as lack of sensations or motor control (Nijenhuis, Spinhoven, Van Dyck, van der Hart, & Vanderlinden, 1996).

Since the time of Janet (1889/1973), dissociation has been strongly associated with traumatic events. During, or shortly after, a traumatic event, a high percentage of individuals experience dissociative alterations, including experiential (or passive) detachment, and alterations in memory and perception (e.g., Cardeña & Spiegel, 1993; Foa & Hearst-Ikeda, 1996; Spiegel & Cardeña, 1991). A number of these changes have been described in the hypnosis literature, including alterations in the sense of time, a narrow focus of attention, experiential detachment, and slowing down of responses (Cardeña, 1995). Similarly, Nash (1992, p. 150) remarked that "the description given by patients of some pathological [including, we would add, posttraumatic] states often resembles the report of normal subjects describing their experience during hypnosis."

Furthermore, there is evidence that dissociation at the time of trauma, or following it, is a significant predictor of later PTSD, an issue addressed by the inclusion of the diagnosis of ASD, which includes dissociative symptoms as definitional components, into the DSM-IV (e.g., Bremner et al., 1992; Classen et al., 1998; Koopman et al., 1996; Marmar et al., 1994; Ozer, Best, & Lipsey, 2003; Shalev, Peri, Canetti, & Schreiber, 1996). Although pervasive amnesia after single episodes of trauma is not common (e.g., Cardeña, Grieger, Staab, Fullerton, & Ursano, 1997), other forms of dissociation may be present. Van der Hart and colleagues have formulated a model distinguishing between several levels of dissociation of the personality, with "primary dissociation" referring to an undue division of the personality between one dissociative part dedicated to daily living and the other part fixated in trauma and threat; "secondary dissociation" comprising a daily living part and more than one trauma-fixated part; and "tertiary dissociation" comprising more than one of both types of dissociative parts (e.g., Nijenhuis & van der Hart, 1999; van der Hart et al., 2006).

Trauma victims are not only more prone to experience spontaneous episodes of dissociation or even to induce them deliberately as defenses, but for a long time individuals with posttraumatic symptomatology also have been observed to be highly hypnotizable (e.g., Ross, 1941), an observation for which Gill and Brenman (1961) found some informal mathematical support. Recent systematic studies have confirmed these clinical observations. Masked and nonmasked studies with standardized hypnotizability scales have corroborated that individuals with posttraumatic symptoms, or full ASD and PTSD, tend to score high in hypnotizability scales and are significantly more hypnotizable than most other clinical and nonclinical groups (Bryant, Guthrie, & Moulds, 2001; Cardeña, 1996; Kluft, 1985; Spiegel, Detrick, & Frischholz, 1982; Spiegel, Hunt, & Dondershine 1988; Stutman & Bliss, 1985), have high imagery abilities (Stutman & Bliss, 1985), and may perform especially well on dream-induced and amnesia-type items (Bryant et al., 2001). A longitudinal study suggests that the hypnotizability performance of individuals with PTSD is not always stable and may be related to their PTSD avoidance scores (Bryant, Guthrie, Moulds, Nixon, & Felmingham, 2003). Dissociation, one of the core hypnotic processes (besides absorption, suggestibility, and other alterations of consciousness; Cardeña & Spiegel, 1991), has been related to some forms of avoidance and a failure in processing traumatic information (Foa & Hearst-Ikeda, 1996). However, the relationship between hypnotizability and trauma history in nonclinical groups is equivocal (Putnam & Carlson, 1998). Some studies suggest that a positive correlation between history of trauma and hypnotizability is present only in survivors of repeated rather than isolated instances of trauma (Eisen, Anderson, Cooper, Horton, & Stenzel, 1994). There is also some evidence that chronic dissociation is more likely to occur after repeated rather than single instances of trauma (Terr, 1991).

Rationale for the Use of Hypnotic Techniques in the Treatment of PTSD

Several considerations have led experts to suggest that hypnosis is a useful adjunct to the treatment of PTSD:

1. The high level of hypnotizability observed in many patients with ASD and PTSD can be used purposefully in hypnosis. A meta-analysis found a moderate average correlation ($r = .44$) between hypnotic suggestibility and treatment outcome (Flammer & Bongartz, 2003), although other factors, such as expectancies, may mediate hypnotic responsivity (Schoenberger, Kirsch, Gearan, Montgomery, & Pastyrnak, 1997).

2. Many patients with PTSD have dissociative symptoms (Bremner et al., 1992; Dracu, Riggs, Hearst-Ikeda, Shoyer, & Foa, 1996; Hyer, Albrecht, Poudewyns, Woods, & Brandsma, 1993). In 1920–1921, McDougall remarked that, in the treatment of trauma, "the essential therapeutic step is the relief of the dissociation. . . . Emotional discharge is not necessary to this, though it may play some part in contributing to bring it about" (p. 25). Because hypnosis may induce dissociative experience within a structured and controlled setting, patients can learn specific techniques to modulate and bring under control unbidden and distressing emotions (Benningfield, 1992; Maldonado & Spiegel, 1998; Spiegel & Cardeña, 1990; Valdiserri & Byrne, 1982). Furthermore, dissociative phenomena may be reframed and utilized for therapeutic purposes (Edgette & Edgette, 1995; Phillips, 1993).

3. Hypnotic techniques can be easily integrated into diverse therapeutic approaches, including psychodynamic or cognitive-behavioral therapies, and pharmacotherapy (e.g., Kirsch, 1996; Maldonado, Butler, & Spiegel, 2000; Muraoka, Komiyama, Hosoi, Mine, & Kubo, 1996; Spiegel & Spiegel, 1987). Meta-analyses of research on the use of hypnosis to treat various clinical conditions have shown that hypnosis can have a synergistic effect on therapies with which is used as an adjunct (Kirsch, Capafons, Cardeña, & Amigo, 1999; Kirsch, Montgomery, & Sapirstein, 1995; Smith, Glass, & Miller, 1980). Furthermore, some techniques that have been described recently as "new," such as imagery rescripting (Smucker, Dancu, Foa, & Niederee, 1995) or a focus on inner experience (Watkins, 2008), have been used for more than a century in hypnosis (Crabtree, 1993).

4. Two dominant models in the treatment of PTSD, the psychodynamic and the cognitive-behavioral, emphasize the importance of recollection of the traumatic event, whether in the framework of achieving emotional and cognitive integration or of providing repeated exposure to the traumatic event in the context of enhancing alternative, more adaptive, responses. Both models require recollection of the traumatic event and, as we describe later in detail, hypnosis can facilitate the working through of traumatic memories by giving the patient techniques to pace and control the intensity and associated distress of the traumatic memory. In fact, there is evidence that similar

brain structures become more active during both recall of traumatic events and response to hypnosis (Vermetten & Bremner, 2004).

5. There is evidence that some traumatized individuals have fragmentary, disorganized, or no recall of traumatic events (Brown, Scheflin, & Hammond, 1998). Some patients with PTSD are likely to have experienced dissociative phenomena at the time of trauma, including alterations of memory. This memory impairment can take various forms, including problems encoding new information (Bremner et al., 1993); partial or, more rarely, total amnesia; a decontextualized recall of the event; or impersonal recollection. Hypnosis and traumatic events can produce similar experiences. Thus, for trauma victims who were in a dissociated state at the time of the trauma, use of the structured dissociation of hypnosis may facilitate access to trauma-related memories. The theory of state-dependent memory (Overton, 1978) supports the hypothesis that hypnosis may facilitate the retrieval of memories associated with a state of mind similar to that at the time of the trauma. State-dependent effects may occur, especially when no stronger cues are available (Eich, 1995). Although there is evidence that hypnosis can be helpful in reversing functional amnesia (Kritchevsky, Chang, & Squire, 2004), hypnotic techniques to recall memories needs to be conducted very carefully because hypnosis may enhance the individual's confidence in the reported memory rather than its actual accuracy (Dywan & Bowers, 1983). Length issues prevent us from discussing general topics such as "traumatic transference," and memory and hypnosis, but our discussion of this in the previous edition of this volume (Cardeña, Maldonado, van der Hart, & Spiegel, 2000) remains pertinent. A recent study provides further evidence that favors the use of hypnosis, revealing that misleading questions, but not hypnosis, have a negative effect on memory accuracy (Scoboria, Mazzoni, & Kirsch, 2006). With awareness of the reconstructive nature of memory and of the potential effect of misleading questions or cues on recollection, therapists with solid training should feel comfortable using hypnosis in the treatment of ASD and PTSD whenever it is warranted. The American Society of Clinical Hypnosis has provided guidelines and samples of informed consent forms for hypnosis in memory work that might be of use to clinicians or forensic experts (Hammond et al., 1995).

Description of Techniques

Hypnotic techniques have been used for the treatment of posttraumatic disturbances in various ways for more than a century, including the use of supportive suggestions, uncovering, integrating, or abreacting trauma memories (Brende, 1985; Brown & Fromm, 1986), and even reconstructing past events (as in Janet's substitution of a more benign memory for a traumatic one; van der Hart, Brown, & van der Kolk, 1989; see also Kardiner & Spiegel, 1947).

Trauma treatment, especially for chronic or otherwise complicated post-traumatic conditions, usually follows a phase-oriented model that divides the trauma treatment into phases or stages, each with its own objectives or goals (Brown et al., 1998). Hypnosis can be employed during the three general stages of trauma treatment (first described by Janet; see van der Hart et al., 1989). These stages generally entail (1) establishing the therapeutic relationship and frame, providing short-term relief, and helping to stabilize the patient by making symptoms more manageable and enhancing coping skills; (2) working through and integrating the traumatic events; and (3) furthering integration and self and relational development. Length of treatment likely depends on a number of factors, including (1) the nature of the trauma (e.g., multiple or single events; natural disaster or caused by humans); (2) how soon treatment starts after the traumatic event; (3) the patient's comorbidity, including the degree to which self- and relational schemas are affected; and (4) previous history of chronic abuse or neglect. For posttraumatic conditions following a single, uncomplicated, recent trauma, our clinical experience is that a few sessions may alleviate the symptoms. For chronic or complicated conditions, treatment is more likely to require a number of months or years and entail education on basic skills such as emotional regulation (Gold, 2000). Some clinicians (e.g., Fromm & Nash, 1997) opine that hypnosis usually shortens treatment, and other researchers seem to support this contention (see "Recent Studies").

Treatment Phase 1: Stabilization and Symptom Reduction

During the initial phase, the focus is on stabilizing and alleviating the patient's symptoms, and enhancing self-mastery over symptoms and current concerns and stresses. This initial phase may be revisited even when later phases are being implemented. Hypnotic suggestions can be used to induce relaxation, so that patients can learn to experience a calm and serene state and, through self-hypnosis, maintain this state outside of the consulting room. Specific suggestions can target symptoms associated with PTSD, including anxiety, physical pain, discomfort, and sleep disturbances (e.g., Eichelman, 1985; Jiranek, 1993). Other techniques that may be especially useful at this stage include establishing an imaginal "safe place" (Brown & Fromm, 1986) and using "ego strengthening" procedures (Frederick & McNeal, 1993; Hartland, 1965). Brown and colleagues (1998, p. 480) provide various signs of stabilization in this phase, including skills related to feeling safe, self-soothing, connectedness, alleviation of PTSD symptoms, and so on.

Treatment Phase 2: Treatment of Traumatic Memories

The second phase, after an appropriate therapeutic alliance has been forged and the patient has developed sufficient personal resources to confront dif-

ficult issues without being overwhelmed by them, involves working with traumatic memories. Whether to overcome the avoidance of traumatic memories,
achieve psychological integration (Brown et al., 1998; Spiegel & Cardeña,
1990), or enhance emotional engagement, habituation, and cognitive restructuring (Foa & Meadows, 1997; Jaycox, Foa, & Morral, 1998; Lynn & Cardeña,
2007), authors from diverse perspectives agree on the importance of working with trauma memories. It bears mentioning that since the introduction
of the term "abreaction" by Breuer and Freud (1895/1982), various authors
have borrowed this concept to describe the purpose of trauma treatment.
Although a minority still speaks of "abreactive techniques," a more current
view is that the goal is to integrate the traumatic memories rather than just
to abreact them (van der Hart & Brown, 1992). In terms of van der Hart's
structural model, the goal in treating traumatic memories entails integrating
dis-integrated components of the traumatic memory into a whole, the self-
representational system into a structural whole and, in turn, integrating each
component with the other (van der Hart et al., 2006).

Occasionally the focus may be to make conscious apparently amnesic
material (see Brown et al., 1998). However, in general, during the integration
work of memories it is likely that more detailed or even new and relevant memories will emerge spontaneously. Greater recollection of accurate, meaningful memories after repeated probes has been demonstrated in the laboratory
(Erderlyi, 1994). However, exposing patients to traumatic stimuli or memories
requires careful consideration. There is some evidence that flooding therapy
for PTSD may exacerbate symptoms (Pitman et al., 1991), especially among
perpetrators (Foa & Meadows, 1997). Also, among patients with PTSD in an
intensive, residential treatment, Cardeña observed very enhanced levels of
distress when they were asked repeatedly to recollect traumatic events as part
of research on a manualized treatment. It has also been noted that revisiting
traumatic memories may be counterproductive, unless the patient feels safe
and has enough ego strength to deal with such material (e.g., Peebles, 1989).
Van der Kolk, McFarlane, and van der Hart (1996, p. 436) wrote,

> Only when issues of interpersonal security can be safely negotiated can the
> therapeutic relationship be utilized to hold the patient's psyche together when
> the threat of physical disintegration is re-experienced. . . . Once the traumatic
> experiences have been located in time and place, the person can start making
> distinctions between current life stresses and past trauma, and can decrease the
> impact of the trauma on present experience.

Spiegel (1992) remarked that this process can be facilitated by appropriate attention to transference and countertransference issues related to the
trauma, and that working through issues of trust and mutual acceptance is a
critical part of the psychotherapy of trauma-related symptoms. Patients may
experience the therapist as inflicting trauma rather than treating it, and open

discussion of these feelings is crucial to effective therapy. Hypnotic techniques can help to provide a context in which exposure to traumatic memories can be accomplished in a way that does not overwhelm the patient (Scheff, 1980), although exposure therapy has been successfully conducted without hypnosis (Foa & Meadows, 1997).

As a group, patients with PTSD are highly hypnotizable, so therapists should avoid suggestive or misleading questions or comments when eliciting new information. Questions should neither misinform nor suggest a specific answer. Also, patients need help to control processing of memories, while maintaining a state of comfort and safety. Adequate hypnotic memory retrieval involves the use of techniques that promote physical levels of relaxation and a sense of cognitive and emotional control.

Work with traumatic memories should proceed at a pace that patients can tolerate to avoid retraumatization. Hypnotic techniques should be tailored to a patient's particular needs, with an emphasis on using the occasion to enhance the patients' sense of control over his or her mental and physical state. Many patients fear that if they recall traumatic memories, they will once again lose control and symbolically reenact the helplessness they experienced during the traumatic episode. To some extent this is not an unreasonable fear. Memories can take over the patient's mental life every time he or she experiences a flashback. Hypnosis may allow patients to separate themselves from their memories of events or of their younger selves, as needed (Degun-Mather, 2006). Part of the therapist's role is to help control and structure the retrieval and expression of painful memories and the feelings associated with them. Hypnosis can be used therapeutically to facilitate working through traumatic memories. Traumatic events often produce feelings of helplessness and powerlessness. During the hypnotic process, patients may be given appropriate ego-enhancing suggestions and images to generate experiences of personal power, protection, and competence (e.g., Ebert, 1988). Other techniques, described for patients with dissociation but applicable to PTSD, include "fractionated abreactions," time sense alterations, and trance ratification (Kluft, 1994). We describe here five especially relevant hypnotic techniques: relaxation, projective and restructuring techniques, age regression, and imaginal memory containment.

Relaxation

After the induction of hypnosis, which may itself contain suggestions for relaxation, a deeper level of physical relaxation may easily be achieved by instructing patients to imagine themselves in a place they associate with relaxation and calmness. This might be a place they have been in before or a place they invent in their minds (e.g., floating in a hot tub, pool, or space). Once the desired level of relaxation is achieved, patients are instructed to maintain this state while they are asked to confront emotionally charged traumatic memo-

ries. The objective is to process traumatic memories at a pace they can tolerate, while maintaining the same level of physical and, if possible, emotional
relaxation. Hypnotic techniques may be integrated with systematic desensitization as needed (Wilshire, 1996).

Projective Techniques

Patients may be asked to "project" images, sensations, and thoughts away from
themselves, onto an imaginary screen. Useful images include a movie or computer screen, or the surface of a calm lake, mirror, or blue sky. This technique
seems to facilitate the process of separating memories from physically painful
sensations, if necessary, to minimize the possibility of overwhelming recollections or retraumatization. The screen may allow for the manipulation of the
affect that is mobilized during the retrieval of traumatic memories. Patients
are taught, for instance, to control the intensity of the content by making the
images larger or smaller, or by moving the screen closer or farther away. They
are reminded that, as in a frightening movie, some scenes may be difficult or
even repulsive, but they do not have to reexperience the pain associated with
the traumatic memories or images. The goal of this technique is to increase
patients' sense of control and safety, until they can integrate the information,
sensations, emotions, and so on.

Restructuring

The main goal here is to provide alternative and healthier evaluations of
posttraumatic schemas. A variation of the projective technique calls for
patients to divide the screen in half. While doing this, they are asked to project onto the left side of the screen images of what they need to work on (e.g.,
memories of the trauma), and to picture on the right side something they
did to protect themselves or someone else (Spiegel, 1981, 1992). On occasion, some patients may have difficulty remembering anything good and may
blame themselves inappropriately for not having done enough. The therapist
encourages them to recall anything they might have done to protect themselves and attempts to reinterpret their perception of powerlessness into a
useful survival technique. Fighting back, screaming for help, or just "lying
still" to avoid further injury are examples of common defensive acts. The
idea at this stage is to facilitate the restructuring of traumatic memories to
make them more bearable, while helping the client move from the position
of victim to that of survivor.

The new cognition involves recognizing both the intensity of the threat
and the patient's adaptive response at the time of trauma. At the end, the two
images serve to restructure the memory of the trauma. The image on the left
symbolizes a summary of the trauma itself. The image on the right may help
the patient realize that although indeed victimized, he or she also attempted

to master the situation and displayed courage during a time of overwhelming threat. This process may allow patients to realize that humiliation is only one aspect of the trauma experience. A more radical idea is to imaginally provide an alternative "ending" to a distressing memory, as some hypnosis clinicians have done for a long time (Crabtree, 1993).

Age Regression

In contrast with projective techniques, hypnotically induced regression to an earlier time may not provide patients with the protective advantage of being able to "project" memories away from themselves. Because of this, it may be a more intense experience. In this technique, the therapist suggests that patients, by counting or by some other technique, go back in time in their lives. We have observed that this technique can help patients understand the origin of long forgotten bodily symptoms, such as conversion symptoms and somatic memories. It may even help them recall dissociated memories. Highly hypnotizable individuals are able to use this technique as a form of "role playing" the events, as if they were happening all over again, but with an enhanced sense of control. This may provide a more complete recall of affects and other elements that may have become dissociated from memory of the event. A full recollection may even help to explain some present behaviors, such as a disproportionate response to seemingly benign stressors. Although it may be very difficult to determine to what extent the recalled memory is historically accurate, it is nonetheless useful in making sense of the individual's interpretation of the traumatic event. We should point out that the "regression" that occurs is an imaginal–experiential event, not a literal regression to a younger age (Nash, 1992). Brown and coauthors (1998, p. 353) opine that age regression may bring about significant recovery of accurate memory, if misleading questioning is avoided; in any case, this technique may be very helpful when exploring affect.

Imaginal Memory Containment

With this technique, imagery is used to contain unresolved (parts of) memories until the patient or client is ready for further memory work. An example is an imagined safe, in which the patient places the traumatic memory. The safe is closed and, in the patient's imagination, both patient and therapist use separate keys to lock it. A related, more direct hypnotic approach is to suggest that posthypnotic amnesia for traumatic memories be maintained if the patient's current recollection is too distressing. In general, it is advisable to give permissively formulated suggestions, for example, "Take along from this experience in hypnosis whatever is good to take and for which the time is right, and just leave behind whatever is better left here for the time being" (van der Hart, Boon & van Everdingen, 1990).

Treatment Phase 3: Further Personality Reintegration and Rehabilitation

The third phase of treatment emphasizes maintaining the gains of the two previous phases, achieving a structural integration of the traumatic event into an adaptive sense of the self and the world, and enhancing personal and relational development. Brown and colleagues (1998) proposed that the work in this phase includes stabilizing the previous integration of various psychological processes, developing the self rather than maintaining it crystallized into the trauma, establishing or reestablishing healthy relationships, modulating impulses and emotions, stabilizing psychophysiological responses, and achieving good cognitive restructuring (see also van der Hart et al., 2006). As much as possible, treatment should not deal exclusively with alleviation of pathology, but also with the personal development of the individual. For some patients and therapists, adding a spiritual dimension to treatment may be of great benefit. In this phase, hypnotic techniques are helpful in stabilizing gains outside of the clinic and in proposing alternative forms of coping that the individual can implement on his or her own, for instance, through self-hypnosis. Other techniques, such as age progression, may help to break a hopeless sense of the future by providing a goal to achieve a better, albeit realistic, personal future.

An Eight-Step Model to Treat PTSD

A treatment approach to treat posttraumatic syndromes that details important therapeutic processes that can be easily subsumed under Phases 2 and 3 of the more general phase-oriented treatment was described earlier (Spiegel, 1992; Spiegel & Cardeña, 1990). This approach is designed to help patients recognize and understand factors involved in the development of their symptoms, define one or several particularly frightening memories, learn how to control them, and reintegrate the memories into a more adaptive and healthy sense of self and the world. Of the following eight processes, the first six or seven are particularly indicated for the second treatment phase of trauma therapy (i.e., working through), whereas the last steps (control and congruence) are especially useful for the final treatment phase (i.e., reintegration):

1. *Confrontation* of traumatic memories directly instead of avoiding them, which, paradoxically, may perpetuate them (cf. Foa, Hearst-Ikeda & Perry, 1995; Wegner & Pennebaker, 1993).

2. *Confession* to the therapist of deeds or emotions that may seem embarrassing and at times repugnant. It is also important to help patients distinguish between misplaced guilt and real remorse.

3. *Consolation* from the therapist in a professional manner, lest he or she be perceived as judgmental, as minimizing the pain, or even as reinflicting it.

4. *Conscious experience* of aspects of the memory that the patient may not remember, or that he or she may have experienced in a detached way, but that are necessary to understand fully and move past the traumatic event. A suggestion that allows the patient to remember only the material mentioned during hypnosis that he or she can tolerate at that point can facilitate a gradual and tolerable recall of difficult memories.

5. *Condensation* of crucial aspect of the traumatic experience. The goal of this treatment component is to make the overwhelming aspects of the trauma more manageable by giving them concrete form, while restructuring the experience by joining together previously disparate images.

6. *Concentration* to help contain the effect of the traumatic experience, by having the patient learn to deploy attention voluntarily to that or other events, as appropriate.

7. *Control* over memories to reduce helplessness. Because the most painful aspect of severe trauma can be the absolute sense of helplessness and loss of control over one's body and the course of events, it is important that therapy enhance the patient's sense of control and mastery over those memories.

8. *Congruence* of memories, self-images, and sense of the world, and enhancing the flexibility of cognitive and memory patterns. Use of techniques such as "age progression," in which the patient may create an image of what type of a person he or she aspires to be in the future, can facilitate a new integration between the old and the emerging self. In related terms, Myers (1940) formulated his overall treatment goal with shell-shocked combat soldiers as the reintegration of the traumatic ("emotional") personality state with the "apparently normal" personality state, a similar goal to that of the third treatment phase described earlier. It would also be helpful to encourage a sense of *communal* sharing and support from those close to the patient, as appropriate, within the therapeutic framework.

Method of Collecting Data

The major sources for identifying relevant citations were PsycLIT, MEDLINE, and Published International Literature on Traumatic Stress (PILOTS) databases. We searched these sources using combinations of the following key words: "hypnosis," "hypnotism," "trauma," "PTSD," "ASD," "traumatic neurosis," "shell-shock," and "combat fatigue." We also conducted a library search for relevant books and consulted colleagues in the field. We incorporated references on the related fields of memory and dissociation.

Literature Review

Meta-analyses of studies on the treatment of anxiety, pain, and other conditions show that hypnosis can substantially enhance the effectiveness of psychodynamic and cognitive-behavioral therapies (Kirsch, 1996; Kirsch et al., 1995, 1999; Smith et al., 1980). However, most of the literature on the use of hypnosis for PTSD still entails case studies. The reader should bear in mind the limitations of this method, including a general lack of systematic assessment and a possible bias toward reporting positive rather than negative results. Nonetheless, case reports consistently suggest that hypnosis can be very helpful in the treatment of patients with PTSD. Hypnotic techniques have been reported to be effective for symptoms often associated with PTSD, such as pain (Daly & Wulff, 1987; Jiranek, 1993; Richmond et al., 1996), anxiety (Kirsch et al., 1995), and nightmares (Donatone, 2006; Eichelman, 1985; Kingsbury, 1993). Also, clinical observations suggest that hypnosis can modulate dissociative processes commonly found in patients with PTSD (Benningfield, 1992; Brende & Benedict, 1980; Spiegel, 1981; Spiegel & Cardeña, 1990; van der Hart et al., 1990), although no systematic studies have been conducted to date to evaluate this claim.

A Brief History of the Use of Hypnosis for Posttraumatic Conditions

Use of Hypnosis before and during World War I

Vijselaar and van der Hart (1992) described a very early reference (1813) to Dutch physicians' use of hypnosis to treat traumatic grief. Of the many French therapists using hypnosis around the turn of the century, Pierre Janet, probably more than anybody else, utilized it in the treatment of patients with posttraumatic conditions (e.g., Janet, 1898/1990; cf. van der Hart, Brown, & van der Kolk, 1989). Crocq and De Verbizier (1989) determined through the examination of Janet's major clinical works that approximately half of his patients had been traumatized. Janet described the successful application of hypnotic techniques in symptom reduction, increase of ego strength, and exploration and treatment of traumatic memories. Breuer and Freud (1895/1982) also employed hypnotic techniques to treat some patients who reported traumatic events.

During World War I, although the French prohibited the use of hypnosis in military hospitals (Southard & Fenton, 1919), the American, British, and German armies did not (e.g., Brown, 1919; McDougall, 1926; Myers, 1916, 1940; Nonne, 1915; Simmel, 1919; Smith & Pear, 1917). Myers (1916) described the successful use of hypnosis to alleviate various symptoms of shell-shock, including dissociative amnesia, sensory alterations, and speech disturbances. He later (1940, p. 57) discussed the benefits and limitations of hypnosis for shell-shock:

> [Hypnosis] is a perfectly safe and reliable procedure to adopt, provided that it be only employed for psycho-therapeutic purposes, in particular for mental re-integration or re-synthesis of dissociated or repressed memories, and not merely for the removal of bodily "functional" disorders by suggestion.

In an important discussion in the *British Journal of Psychiatry*, shortly after World War I, Myers (1920–1921), McDougall (1920–1921), and Jung (1921–1922), strongly argued against the use of abreactive techniques. All three agreed instead on the importance of psychological "re-integration" or "re-synthesis."

Rivers (1918) also applied hypnosis occasionally and discussed the importance of having patients experience, not repress, the traumatic events, and of cognitively restructuring the interpretations of the trauma (a process he called "re-education"). Southard and Fenton (1919) presented 589 case studies of shell-shock, including a "comparatively long" (p. 895) series of 27 cases successfully treated with hypnosis. Although they remarked on the "miraculous" cures after hypnosis, they recommended a longer reeducation process for treatment.

Smith and Pear (1917, p. 41) provided keen observations of the objective and subjective components of posttraumatic symptomatology: "In the first place there is the vividness or intensity of the stimulus; in the second, the degree of recency; in the third, the frequency of the stimulus; and in the fourth its relevancy (to the individual's past experience and personality)." They also emphasized the use of hypnosis as an adjunct, concluding that "hypnotic treatment, when used with skill, discretion, and discrimination, has its place in the treatment of shell-shock and similar conditions. . . . Hypnosis alone will be of relative slight use" (p. 40). Hadfield (1944) conducted probably the only systematic study of the use of hypnosis for "shell-shock," through a follow-up with 100 of the 500–600 patients he had treated. He found that 90% of patients treated with "hypno-analysis" were working full time 18 months after discharge. As used in this study, "hypno-analysis" emphasized abreaction of a traumatic memory within a psychoanalytic context. Spanish psychiatrists used hypnosis in the context of war (e.g., Camino Galicia, 1928). One of them, who participated in the Spanish Civil War, wrote that "mild hypnosis" was a useful technique for emotional and imaginative (perhaps highly hypnotizable?) patients (Mira, 1943).

Use of Hypnosis during World War II and the Vietnam War

World War II brought not only a change in terminology, from "shell-shock" to "war neuroses," but also a general shift from the use of hypnosis to pharmacological approaches, such as insulin, ether, sodium amytal and sodium pentothal, to induce sedation and sometimes abreaction. Bleckwenn started using amytal to treat neuropsychiatric disorders in 1930; Lindemann (1932) applied it for psychiatric conditions, and Sargant and Slater (1940) used it for "acute war neuroses" (Naples & Hackett, 1978; Sargant, 1942). Some authors expressed a preference for this procedure over hypnosis (e.g., Gillespie, 1943; Grinker & J. Spiegel, 1945), whereas Kardiner and H. Spiegel (1947) remarked that ordinary therapy, therapy with sedatives, or therapy with hypnosis, had distinct advantages and disadvantages. They concluded that the final integration of the clinical material should occur during the ordinary state of consciousness. In their review of the literature, Brenman and Gill (1947) concluded that narcotherapy was more problematic than hypnotherapy in the induction of catharsis because it induced a "less controllable" state.

During World War II, hypnosis was partly replaced by narcotherapy, although hypnosis remained in use, especially for the treatment of amnesia, fugue, and conversion symptomatology (e.g., Alpern, Carbone, & Brooks, 1946; Fischer, 1943; Kartchner & Korner, 1947; Watkins, 1949). Currently the pendulum seems to have swung again, with a preference for hypnosis over medications in most cases (Putnam, 1992). Perhaps the most thorough description of the foundations and use of hypnosis to treat war neuroses during World War II is that of Watkins (1949) on his experiences at Welsh hospital, where group hypnotic and narcotherapy techniques were also used to enhance motivation and develop insight among patients with various posttraumatic symptoms. Watkins's (1987) "ego therapy" hypnotic approach has been used with posttraumatic patients (e.g., Phillips, 1993). The main concept is that individuals have organized systems of behavior and experience with more or less permeable boundaries, and many of the hypnotic techniques described by Watkins have been very influential in the treatment of combat veterans and other posttraumatic patients. Nonetheless, some aspects of "ego therapy" could be seen as unnecessarily personalizing psychophysiological states, at least among some dissociative patients (cf. International Society for the Study of Dissociation, 1994). Systematic inquiry on this particular approach is clearly warranted.

Kartchner and Korner (1947) reported on hypnotic treatment for approximately one-third of acute patients in a Pacific Island hospital, especially to diminish or clear amnesia, confusion, and other symptoms; to enhance insight; and to help with diagnosis and sedation. They remarked that overall hypnosis was a better procedure than narcotherapy, but that is should be considered an adjunct rather than a comprehensive therapy.

There have been occasional reports of the use of hypnosis to treat Vietnam War veterans with PTSD. Balson and Dempster (1980) described treatment of 15 patients with acute or chronic "war neuroses," comprising an evaluation and therapy preparation phase, treatment, and follow-up and consolidation. The first phase included 4–10 sessions, and treatment of 8–20 sessions, with booster sessions for all but one of the patients. The framework of treatment was psychodynamic, with the use of hypnosis to foster abreaction. The follow-up, conducted between 4 and 24 months, comprised a clinical evaluation to determine whether symptoms had returned. The authors claimed that 12 of the 15 patients had a successful treatment. More importantly, the authors measured hypnotizability at the beginning of treatment, using the HIP (Spiegel & Spiegel, 1987). Although they did not calculate inferential statistics themselves, a binomial test for $p = .5$ that we conducted reveals a significant relationship between low hypnotizability and treatment failure ($p < .05$, two-tailed). This reanalysis provided support for the hypothesis that hypnotizability may be positively correlated with good treatment outcome in posttraumatic patients; nonetheless, the results must be qualified because the three treatment failures had "chronic" conditions, whereas the successful treatments included both "chronic" and "acute" conditions. Successful case reports with Vietnam veterans have also been provided by Brende and Benedict (1980), and Spiegel (1981). Van der Hart and Spiegel (1993) also described hypnosis-based treatment of psychotic conditions associated with trauma.

Recent Studies

Brom, Kleber, and Defares (1989) compared hypnosis to systematic desensitization and psychodynamic psychotherapy in the treatment of 112 individuals "who were diagnosed as suffering from posttraumatic stress disorders according to DSM-III" (p. 608). The majority of these patients had experienced the loss of a loved one, whereas the remaining patients had been traumatized directly; thus, some participants would not have met the current DSM-IV criteria for PTSD. The design included random assignment to an expert and testing at baseline, end of treatment, and 3 months after finishing treatment. Also a wait-list control group tested from Time 1 to Time 2 did not show change across these assessment periods. Before treatment started, patients had elevated scores on many symptoms subscales, including the Impact of Events Scale (IES). The authors found no significant difference in outcome among the three therapies evaluated (desensitization, hypnosis embedded in a behavioral framework, and psychodynamic therapy). The groups receiving hypnosis and desensitization had fewer sessions on average than the psychodynamic group ($M = 14.4$ and 15.0 sessions compared with 18.8 sessions for psychodynamic therapy). The "hypnotherapy" group had significantly lower IES scores at the end of therapy ($M = 33.7$, $SD = 22.9$) and at follow-up ($M = 31.7$, $SD = 22.0$) compared with its pretreatment testing ($M = 50.8$, $SD = 11.7$; $p < .05$; unbiased g's of 0.94 and 1.06, respectively). The group treated with hypnosis also had significantly lower IES scores at posttest and follow-up than the control group's baseline ($M = 51.1$, $SD = 14.1$, $p < .05$; Hedges's unbiased g's of 0.89 and 1.02, respectively). The wait-list group showed no change across assessment periods. The authors of the study concluded that hypnosis and desensitization are especially valuable for intrusion symptoms, and that psychodynamic therapy is particularly useful for avoidance symptoms. A meta-analysis of controlled clinical trials (Sherman, 1998) provided a comparison between the effects of the study by Brom and colleagues (1989) and those of other controlled studies. That comparison suggests that the major advantage of hypnosis may come at follow-up rather than at the end of the treatment (Sherman, 1998, pp. 422–423), a consistent result with meta-analyses of hypnosis for conditions other than PTSD (see Kirsch et al., 1999). Consistent with the proposed efficacy of hypnotic techniques for reexperiencing, a recent study with burn patients showed that adding hypnotic suggestions had a significant effect on pain ratings and trauma reexperiencing as compared with a standard care condition (Shakibaei, Harandi, Ghlomrezaei, Samoei, & Salehi, 2008).

The advice by Shalev, Bonne, and Eth (1996) to combine various forms of treatment for PTSD is worth heeding. A large group study by Bryant, Moulds, Guthrie, and Nixon (2005; Bryant et al., 2006) tested the effect of hypnosis as an adjunct to cognitive-behavioral therapy (CBT) in the treatment of ASD with patients ($N = 87$, of which 69 completed treatment) randomly assigned to six sessions of three different conditions: CBT, CBT + hypnosis (adding an induction and suggestions to engage fully in exposure), or supportive counseling (SC). Evaluators were masked to conditions and the treatment was manualized. Participants were assessed for PTSD at the end of treatment, at 6 months and at 3 years. At the end of treatment and at 6 months, participants were assessed with the Clinician-Administered PTSD Scale–2 (CAPS-2), the IES, and the Beck Depression (BDI) and the Beck Anxiety (BAI) Inventories. At posttreatment, participants in CBT + hypnosis and CBT alone had lower scores than SC participants in CAPS-2 Intensity, CAPS-2 Frequency, IES-Intrusion, IES-Avoidance, and BAI, with a similar pattern (except for the BAI), at the 6-month follow-up. Nonetheless, the effect sizes (Bryant et al., 2005, p. 338) showed that CBT + hypnosis produced greater therapeutic effects for intrusion than CBT at the end of the treatment, even though the authors opined that they barely used hypnotic strategies in that conditions. At the end of the 3-year follow-up, fewer CBT and CBT + hypnosis participants met criteria for PTSD, as compared with SC participants ($\chi^2 = 11.95$, $p < .005$; Bryant et al., 2006). There was no relationship between hypnotizability and treatment outcome.

Using a single-case, multiple-baseline design, Hossack and Bentall (1996) found that two sessions each of relaxation and visual–kinesthetic dissociation (somewhat similar to the split-screen technique described earlier) produced substantial improvement in intrusive and general symptomatology in three patients, partial recovery in one, and no improvement in another. Although the authors did not call their intervention "hypnosis," they used two common hypnotic techniques. Walters and Oakley (2002) employed hypnosis and self-hypnosis with a woman who had postabortion distress and PTSD. This was a multiple baseline design, with 39 specific target symptoms and administration of the Posttraumatic Stress Diagnostic Scale (PSDS) before and after treatment. There were great reductions in target symptoms measured after the end of the treatment, at the 3- and 12-month follow-ups. However, the study was limited, in that by conducting a multiple-baseline study across behaviors, identified behaviors or symptoms are supposed to be the target of treatment at different times, and the identified symptoms should be independent from each other (Barlow & Hersen, 1984). Nonetheless, this and other systematic, single-case designs on the effect of hypnosis on PTSD (Walters, 2005) support the use of hypnosis in the treatment of PTSD.

Ffrench (1995) described the use of hypnosis within a cognitive-behavioral framework. She treated a moderately hypnotizable victim of armed robbery whose symptoms initially were consistent with ASD, but whose diagnosis was changed to PTSD after 4 weeks. After eight sessions, the patient's scores decreased on the BDI (from 31 to 4) and the State–Trait Anxiety Inventory (STAI; from 99th to 58th percentile in the State scale, and from 99th to 64th percentile in the Trait scale). A follow-up 1 month after treatment showed that therapeutic gains had been maintained.

With respect to specific traumas, recent case studies of hypnosis for PTSD have included victims of robbery (Moore, 2001), sexual abuse, assault or rape (Benningfield, 1992; Ebert, 1988; Manning, 1996; Pantesco, 2005; Phillips, 1993; Roth & Batson, 1993; Smith, 1991, 2004; Spiegel, 1989), car and industrial accidents (Carter, 2005; Kingsbury, 1988; Leung, 1994), Holocaust survivors (Somer, 1994), and incarcerated women with PTSD (Salerno, 2005). Peebles (1989) described the treatment of a patient whose PTSD was brought on by failure of anesthesia during surgery, and Degun-Mather (2001, 2006) provided accounts of the successful treatment of a war veteran with 40 years of chronic PTSD and dissociative fugues, a victim of multiple childhood trauma, and a patient with a 12-year-long period of dissociative amnesia in her life, among others.

Hypnotic techniques have proven effective with individuals from other cultural groups exposed to traumatic events, as exemplified by case reports of Native American Vietnam War veterans with PTSD (Krippner & Colodzin, 1989), Asian survivors of mass violence (Lee & Lu, 1989), Hispanic burn patients (Dobkin de Ríos & Friedmann, 1987), a Chinese-born Indonesian woman (Kwan, 2006), and rural Guatemalan boys (Iglesias & Iglesias, 2005/2006).

There are also a few case reports describing the use of hypnotic techniques on children with posttraumatic symptomatology (Kluft, 1991). Rhue and Lynn's (1991) described the joint use of storytelling and hypnosis. Friedrich (1991) described four case studies, two of which included pre- and posttreatment data on the Child Behavior Checklist (CBCL), which includes various symptom subscales. A test on the subscale scores of these two children indicated that they were significantly better after treatment than before (means = 62.2 and 75.5, respectively; Wilcoxon's $z = 3.62$, $p < .0005$; Hedges's unbiased $g = 1.18$).

Hypnosis has been integrated with other strategies, including eye movement desensitization and reprocessing (EMDR; Beere, Simon, & Welch, 2001; Hollander & Bender, 2001), strategic therapy (Kingsbury, 1992), ego state therapy (Phillips, 1993; Watkins & Watkins, 1997), and systematic desensitization (Wilshire, 1996). Various other specific hypnotic techniques for the treatment of PTSD have also been described by MacHovec (1984), Torem (1992), and Gafner and Benson (2001).

Our review of the literature shows that hypnotic techniques have been used for more than 150 years in the treatment of posttraumatic conditions.

Although many case reports by clinicians from different eras and countries have consistently endorsed hypnosis for posttraumatic disorders, there were few randomized control studies with ASD or PTSD patients using DSM criteria. More randomized controlled and single-case designs are clearly needed (Cardeña, 2000), but the consistency of promising studies is revealing.

Summary and Recommendations

There are compelling theoretical reasons and clinical observations to recommend the use of hypnosis as an adjunct treatment for PTSD. Hypnosis is a procedure that may accelerate the therapeutic relationship and positive treatment outcome, which may be especially useful in the age of managed care. Hypnotic techniques may also facilitate the important task of working through traumatic memories, increase coping skills, and promote a sense of competency. They may also be valuable for patients who exhibit symptoms such as anxiety, dissociation, pain, and sleep and other problems for which hypnosis has been effective.

Although systematic outcome research has been limited, there is consistent clinical evidence that hypnosis can facilitate, intensify, and shorten treatment (Level B). The consistency of clinical reports and observations going back for almost two centuries, coupled with some controlled studies, suggest that hypnosis is an effective and safe adjunctive procedure in the treatment of PTSD and other posttraumatic conditions (Level A).

We should mention also that before attempting hypnosis, it may be useful to dispel false beliefs about the nature of hypnosis; administering a set of questions to evaluate patients' beliefs and attitudes about hypnosis may be valuable (Keller, 1996). The following is a list of *contraindications*:

1. In the rare cases of individuals who are refractory or minimally responsive to suggestions, hypnosis may not be the best choice because there is evidence that hypnotizability is related to treatment efficacy (Flammer & Bongartz, 2003). There are brief but effective measures to evaluate hypnotizability in the clinical setting (e.g., HIP: Spiegel & Spiegel, 1987; the Stanford Hypnotic Clinical Scale: Morgan & Hilgard, 1978–1979).

2. Some patients with PTSD may be very resistant to participation in hypnosis, perhaps due to religious or cultural beliefs. If the resistance is not dispelled by clarification of mistaken assumptions, other suggestive techniques may be tried, including emotional self-regulation therapy, done with open eyes and with sensory recall exercises rather than a hypnotic induction (Bayot, Capafons, & Cardeña, 1997; Kirsch et al., 1999).

3. For patients who have low blood pressure or are prone to falling asleep, hypnotic procedures such as "alert hand," which emphasizes alertness and activity rather than relaxation, may be substituted (Cardeña et al., 1998).

References

Alpern, H. S., Carbone, H. A., & Brooks, J. T. (1946). Hypnosis as a therapeutic technique in the war neuroses. *Bulletin of the U.S. Army Medical Department, 5*, 315–324.

Balson, P. M., & Dempster, C. R. (1980). Treatment of war neuroses from Vietnam. *Comprehensive Psychiatry, 211*, 167–175.

Barlow, D. H., & Hersen, M. (1984). *Single case experimental designs: Strategies for studying behavior change* (2nd ed.). New York: Pergamon.

Bayot, A., Capafons, A., & Cardeña, E. (1997). Emotional self-regulation therapy: A new and efficacious treatment for smoking. *American Journal of Clinical Hypnosis, 40*, 146–156.

Beere, D. B., Simon, M. J., & Welch, K. (2001). Recommendations and illustrations for combining hypnosis and EMDR in the treatment of psychological trauma. *American Journal of Clinical Hypnosis, 43*, 217–231.

Benningfield, M. F. (1992). The use of hypnosis in the treatment of dissociative patients. *Journal of Child Sexual Abuse, 1*, 17–31.

Bleckwenn, W. J. (1930). Narcosis as therapy in neuropsychiatric conditions. *Journal of the American Medical Association, 95*, 1168–1171.

Bremner, J. D., Scott, T. M., Delaney, R. C., Southwick, S. M., Mason, J. W., Johnson, D. R., et al. (1993). Deficits in short-term memory in posttraumatic stress disorder. *American Journal of Psychiatry, 150*, 1015–1019.

Bremner, J. D., Southwick, S., Brett, E., Fontana, A., Rosenheck, R., & Charney, D. S. (1992). Dissociation and posttraumatic stress disorder in Vietnam combat veterans. *American Journal of Psychiatry, 149*, 328–332.

Brende, J. (1985). The use of hypnosis in posttraumatic conditions. In W. E. Kelly (Ed.), *Post-traumatic stress disorder and the war patient* (pp. 193–210). New York: Brunner/Mazel.

Brende, J., & Benedict, B. (1980). The Vietnam combat delayed stress response syndrome: Hypnotherapy of "dissociative symptoms." *American Journal of Clinical Hypnosis, 23*, 38–40.

Brenman, M., & Gill, M. M. (1947). *Hypnotherapy.* New York: International Universities Press.

Breuer, J., & Freud, S. (1982). *Studies on hysteria.* New York: Basic Books. (Original work published 1895)

Brom, D., Kleber, R. J., & Defares, P. B. (1989). Brief psychotherapy for post-traumatic stress disorder. *Journal of Consulting and Clinical Psychology, 57*, 607–612.

Brown, D., Scheflin, A., & Hammond, C. (1998). *Memory, trauma treatment, and the law.* New York: Norton.

Brown, D. P., & Fromm, E. (1986). *Hypnotherapy and hypnoanalysis.* Hillsdale, NJ: Erlbaum.

Brown, W. (1919, June 14). Hypnosis, suggestion, and dissociation. *British Medical Journal,* pp. 734–736.

Bryant, R. A., Guthrie, R. M., & Moulds, M. L. (2001). Hypnotizability in acute stress disorder. *American Journal of Psychiatry, 158*, 600–604.

Bryant, R. A., Guthrie, R. M., Moulds, M. L., Nixon, R. D. V., & Felmingham, K. (2003). Hypnotizability and posttraumatic stress disorder: A prospective study. *International Journal of Clinical and Experimental Hypnosis, 51*, 382–389.

Bryant, R. A., Moulds, M. L., Guthrie, R. M., & Nixon, R. D. V. (2005). The additive benefit of hypnosis and cognitive-behavioral therapy in treating acute stress disorder. *Journal of Consulting and Clinical Psychology, 73*(2), 334–340.

Bryant, R. A., Moulds, M. L., Nixon, R. D. V., Mastrodomenico, J., Felmingham, K., & Hopwood, S. (2006). Hypnotherapy and cognitive behaviour therapy of acute stress disorder: A 3-year follow-up. *Behaviour Research and Therapy, 44*, 1331–1335.

Butler, L. D., Duran, R. E. F., Jasiukaitis, P., Koopman, C., & Spiegel, D. (1996). Hypnotizability and traumatic experience: A diathesis–stress model of dissociative symptomatology. *American Journal of Psychiatry, 153*, 41–63.

Camino Galicia, J. (1928). *Hipnotismo e hipnoterapia sus aplicaciones a la medicina* [Hypnotism and hypnotherapy: Their applications to medicine]. Madrid: A. Marzo.

Cardeña, E. (1994). The domain of dissociation. In S. J. Lynn & J. Rhue (Eds.), *Dissociation: Clinical, theoretical, and research perspectives* (pp. 15–31). New York: Guilford Press.

Cardeña, E. (1995, August). *Alterations of consciousness in hypnosis and trauma.* Early Career Award Address at the 103rd Annual Meeting of the American Psychological Association, New York.

Cardeña, E. (1997). The etiologies of dissociation. In S. Powers & S. Krippner (Eds.), *Broken images, broken selves* (pp. 61–87). New York: Brunner/Mazel.

Cardeña, E. (2000). Hypnosis in the treatment of trauma: A promising, but not fully supported, efficacious intervention. *International Journal of Clinical and Experimental Hypnosis, 48*, 221–234.

Cardeña, E. (2005). The phenomenology of deep hypnosis: Quiescent and physically active. *International Journal of Clinical and Experimental Hypnosis, 53*, 37–59.

Cardeña, E., Alarcón, A., Capafons, A., & Bayot, A. (1998). Effects on suggestibility of a new method of active-alert hypnosis. *International Journal of Clinical and Experimental Hypnosis, 3*, 280–294.

Cardeña, E., Butler, L. D., & Spiegel, D. (2003). Stress disorders. In G. Stricker & T. Widiger (Eds.), *Handbook of psychology* (Vol. 8, pp. 229–249). New York: Wiley.

Cardeña, E., Grieger, T., Staab, J., Fullerton, C., & Ursano, R. (1997). Memory disturbances in the acute aftermath of disasters. In J. D. Read & D. S. Lindsay (Eds.), *Recollection of trauma* (p. 568). New York: Plenum Press.

Cardeña, E., Lynn, S. J., & Krippner, S. (Eds.). (2000). *Varieties of anomalous experience: Examining the scientific evidence.* Washington, DC: American Psychological Association.

Cardeña, E., Maldonado, J., van der Hart, O., & Spiegel, D. (2000). Hypnosis. In E. B. Foa, T. M. Keane, & M. J. Friedman (Eds.), *Effective treatments for PTSD: Practice guidelines from the International Society for Traumatic Stress Studies* (pp. 350–354). New York: Guilford Press.

Cardeña, E., & Spiegel, D. (1991). Suggestibility, absorption and dissociation: An integrative model of hypnosis. In J. F. Schumaker (Ed.), *Human suggestibility: Advances in theory, research and application* (pp. 93–107). New York: Routledge.

Cardeña, E., & Spiegel, D. (1993). Dissociative reactions to the San Francisco Bay Area earthquake of 1989. *American Journal of Psychiatry, 150*, 474–478.

Carter, C. (2005). The use of hypnosis in the treatment of PTSD. *Australian Journal of Clinical and Experimental Hypnosis, 33*, 82–92.

Christianson, S., & Loftus, E. (1987). Memory for traumatic events. *Applied Cognitive Psychology, 1*, 225–239.

Classen, C., Koopman, C., Hales, R., & Spiegel, D. (1998). Acute stress disorder as a predictor of posttraumatic stress symptoms. *American Journal of Psychiatry, 155,* 620–624.

Crabtree, A. (1993). *From Mesmer to Freud: Magnetic sleep and the roots of psychological healing.* New Haven, CT: Yale University Press.

Crocq, L., & De Verbizier, J. (1989). Le traumatisme psychologique dans l'oeuvre de Pierre Janet [Psychological trauma in the work of Pierre Janet]. *Annales Médico-Psychologiques, 147,* 983–987.

Daly, E., & Wulff, J. (1987). Treatment of a post-traumatic headache. *British Journal of Medical Psychology, 60,* 85–88.

Degun-Mather, M. (2001). The value of hypnosis in the treatment of chronic PTSD with dissociative fugues in a war veteran. *Contemporary Hypnosis, 18,* 4–13.

Degun-Mather, M. (2006). *Hypnosis, dissociation and survivors of child abuse.* Chichester, UK: Wiley.

Dobkin de Ríos, M., & Friedmann, J. K. (1987). Hypnotherapy with Hispanic burn patients. *International Journal of Clinical and Experimental Psychology, 35,* 87–94.

Donatone, B. (2006). Hypnotic imagery rehearsal in the treatment of nightmares: A case report. *American Journal of Clinical Hypnosis, 49,* 123–127.

Dracu, C. V., Riggs, D. S., Hearst-Ikeda, D., Shoyer, B. G., & Foa, E. B. (1996). Dissociative experiences and posttraumatic stress disorder among female victims of criminal assault and rape. *Journal of Traumatic Stress, 9,* 253–267.

Dywan, J., & Bowers, K. (1983). The use of hypnosis to enhance recall. *Science, 222,* 184–185.

Ebert, B. W. (1988). Hypnosis and rape victims. *American Journal of Clinical Hypnosis, 31,* 50–56.

Edgette, J. H., & Edgette, J. S. (1995). *The handbook of hypnotic phenomena in psychotherapy.* New York: Brunner/Mazel.

Eich, E. (1995). Searching for mood dependent memory. *Psychological Science, 6,* 67–75.

Eichelman, B. (1985). Hypnotic change in combat dreams of two veterans with post-traumatic stress disorder. *American Journal of Psychiatry, 142,* 112–114.

Eisen, M. L., Anderson, A., Cooper, T., Horton, M., & Stenzel, C. (1994, August). *Repeated child abuse, parental addictions, interpersonal trust and hypnotizability.* Paper presented at the 102nd Annual Convention of the American Psychological Association, Los Angeles.

Ellenberger, H. F. (1970). *The discovery of the unconscious.* New York: Basic Books.

Erdelyi, M. H. (1994). Hypnotic hypermnesia: The empty set of hypermnesia. *International Journal of Clinical and Experimental Hypnosis, 42,* 379–390.

Ffrench, C. (1995). The meaning of trauma: Hypnosis and PTSD. *Australian Journal of Clinical and Experimental Hypnosis, 23,* 113–123.

Fischer, C. (1943). Hypnosis in treatment of neuroses due to war and to other causes. *War Medicine, 4,* 565–576.

Flammer, E., & Bongartz, W. (2003). On the efficacy of hypnosis: A meta-analytic study. *Contemporary Hypnosis, 20,* 179–197.

Foa, E. B., & Hearst-Ikeda, D. (1996). Emotional dissociation in response to trauma. In L. K. Michelson, & W. J. Ray (Eds.), *Handbook of dissociation* (pp. 207–226). New York: Plenum Press.

Foa, E. B., Hearst-Ikeda, D., & Perry, K. (1995). Evaluation of a brief cognitive behavioral program for the prevention of chronic PTSD in recent assault victims. *Journal of Consulting and Clinical Psychology, 63*, 948–955.

Foa, E. B., & Meadows, E. A. (1997). Psychosocial treatments for posttraumatic stress disorder: A critical review. *Annual Review of Psychology, 48*, 449–480.

Frederick, C., & McNeal, S. (1993). From strength to strength: "Inner strength" with immature ego states. *American Journal of Clinical Hypnosis, 35*, 250–256.

Friedrich, W. N. (1991). Hypnotherapy with traumatized children. *International Journal of Clinical and Experimental Hypnosis, 39*, 67–81.

Fromm, E., & Nash, M. R. (1997). *Psychoanalysis and hypnosis.* Madison, CT: International Universities Press.

Gafner, G., & Benson, S. (2001). Indirect ego-strengthening in treating PTSD in immigrants from Central America. *Contemporary Hypnosis, 18*, 135–144.

Gill, M. M., & Brenman, M. (1961). *Hypnosis and related states.* New York: International Universities Press.

Gillespie, R. D. (1943). *Psychological effects of war on citizen and soldier.* London: Chapman & Hall.

Gold, S. (2000). *Not trauma alone.* Philadelphia: Brunner/Routledge.

Grinker, R. R., & Spiegel, J. P. (1945). *Men under stress.* Philadelphia: Blakiston.

Hadfield, J. A. (1944). Treatment by suggestion and hypno-analysis. In E. Miller (Ed.), *The neuroses in war* (pp. 128–149). New York: Macmillan.

Hammond, D. C., Garver, R. B., Mutter, C. B., Crasilneck, H. B., Frischholz, E., Gravitz, M. A., et al. (1995). *Clinical hypnosis and memory: Guidelines for clinicians and for forensic hypnosis.* Des Plaines, IL: American Society of Clinical Hypnosis.

Hartland, J. (1965). The value of "ego-strengthening" procedures prior to direct symptom removal under hypnosis. *American Journal of Clinical Hypnosis, 8*, 89–93.

Hilgard, E. (1965). *The experience of hypnosis.* New York: Harcourt.

Hollander, H. E., & Bender, S. S. (2001). ECEM (eye closure eye movements): Integrating aspects of EMDR with hypnosis for treatment of trauma. *American Journal of Clinical Hypnosis, 43*(3–4), 187–202.

Hossack, A., & Bentall, R. P. (1996). Elimination of posttraumatic symptomatology by relaxation and visual-kinesthetic dissociation. *Journal of Traumatic Stress, 9*, 99–110.

Hyer, L. A., Albrecht, W., Poudewyns, P. A., Woods, M. G., & Brandsma, J. (1993). Dissociative experiences of Vietnam veterans with chronic posttraumatic stress disorder. *Psychological Reports, 73*, 519–530.

Iglesias, A., & Iglesias, A. (2005/2006). Hypnotic treatment of PTSD in children who have complicated bereavement. *American Journal of Clinical Hypnosis, 48*, 183–189.

International Society for the Study of Dissociation. (1994). *Guidelines for treating dissociative identity disorder.* Chicago: Author.

Janet, P. (1973). *L'automatisme psychologique* [The psychological automatism]. Paris: Société Pierre Janet. (Original work published 1889)

Janet, P. (1990). *Névroses et idées fixes* [Neuroses and fixed ideas] (Vol. 1). Paris: Société Pierre Janet. (Original work published 1898)

Jaycox, L. H., Foa, E. B., & Morral, A. R. (1998). Influence of emotional engagement and habituation on exposure therapy for PTSD. *Journal of Consulting and Clinical Psychology, 66*, 185–192.

Jiranek, D. (1993). Use of hypnosis in pain management in post-traumatic stress disorder. *Australian Journal of Clinical and Experimental Hypnosis, 21*, 75–84.

Jung, C. G. (1921–1922). The question of the therapeutic value of "abreaction." *British Journal of Medical Psychology, 2*, 13–22.

Kardiner, A., & Spiegel, H. (1947). *War stress and neurotic illness.* New York: Hoeber.

Kartchner, F. D., & Korner, I. N. (1947). The use of hypnosis in the treatment of acute combat reactions. *American Journal of Psychiatry, 103*, 630–636.

Keller, R. F. (1996). Assessment of client beliefs and expectations of hypnosis and treatment. *Psychological Hypnosis, 5*, 808–812.

Kingsbury, S. J. (1988). Hypnosis in the treatment of posttraumatic stress disorder: An isomorphic intervention. *American Journal of Clinical Hypnosis, 31*, 81–90.

Kingsbury, S. J. (1992). Strategic psychotherapy for trauma: Hypnosis and trauma in context. *Journal of Traumatic Stress, 5*, 85–96.

Kingsbury, S. J. (1993). Brief hypnotic treatment of repetitive nightmares. *American Journal of Clinical Hypnosis, 35*, 161–169.

Kirsch, I. (1994). Defining hypnosis for the public. *Contemporary Hypnosis, 11*, 142–143.

Kirsch, I. (1996). Hypnotic enhancement of cognitive-behavioral weight loss treatments: Another meta-reanalysis. *Journal of Consulting and Clinical Psychology, 64*, 517–519.

Kirsch, I., Capafons, A., Cardeña, E., & Amigó, S. (1999). Clinical hypnosis and self-regulation: An introduction. In *Clinical hypnosis and self-regulation therapy: A cognitive-behavioral perspective* (pp. 3–18). Washington, DC: American Psychological Association.

Kirsch, I., Montgomery, G., & Sapirstein, G. (1995). Hypnosis as an adjunct to cognitive behavioral psychotherapy: A meta-analysis. *Journal of Consulting and Clinical Psychology, 63*, 214–220.

Kluft, R. P. (1985). Dissociation as a response to extreme trauma. In R. P. Kluft (Ed.), *Childhood antecedents of multiple personality* (pp. 66–97). Washington, DC: American Psychiatric Press.

Kluft, R. P. (1991). Hypnosis in childhood trauma. In W. Wester & D. J. O'Grady (Eds.), *Clinical hypnosis with children* (pp. 53–68). New York: Brunner/Mazel.

Kluft, R. P. (1994). Applications of hypnotic phenomena. *Hypnos, 21*, 205–233.

Koopman, C., Classen, C., & Spiegel, D. (1996). Dissociative responses in the immediate aftermath of the Oakland/Berkeley firestorm. *Journal of Traumatic Stress, 9*, 521–540.

Krippner, S., & Colodzin, B. (1989). Multicultural methods of treating Vietnam veterans with post-traumatic stress disorder. *International Journal of Psychosomatics, 36*, 79–85.

Kritchevsky, M., Chang, J., & Squire, L. R. (2004). Functional amnesia: Clinical description and neuropsychological profile of 10 cases. *Learning and Memory, 11*, 213–226.

Kwan, P. S. (2006). The application of hypnosis in the treatment of a woman with complex trauma. *Australian Journal of Clinical and Experimental Hypnosis, 34*, 204–215.

Lee, E., & Lu, F. (1989). Assessment and treatment of Asian–American survivors of mass violence. *Journal of Traumatic Stress, 2*, 93–120.

Leung, J. (1994). Treatment of post-traumatic stress disorder with hypnosis. *Australian Journal of Clinical and Experimental Hypnosis, 22*, 87–96.

Lindemann, E. (1932). Psychological changes in normal and abnormal individuals under the influence of sodium amytal. *American Journal of Psychiatry, 88*, 1083–1091.

Lynn, S. J., & Cardeña, E. (2007). Hypnosis and the treatment of posttraumatic conditions: An evidence-based approach. *International Journal of Clinical and Experimental Hypnosis, 55*, 167–188.

MacHovec, F. (1984). The use of brief hypnosis for posttraumatic stress disorders. *Emotional First Aid, 1*, 14–22.

Maldonado, J. R., Butler, L., & Spiegel, D. (2000). Treatment of dissociative disorders. In P. E. Nathan & J. M. Gorman (Eds.), *A guide to treatments that work* (2nd ed., pp. 463–496). New York: Oxford University Press.

Maldonado, J. R., & Spiegel, D. (1994). Treatment of post traumatic stress disorder. In S. J. Lynn & J. Rhue (Eds.), *Dissociation: Clinical, theoretical and research perspectives* (pp. 215–241). New York: Guilford Press.

Maldonado, J. R., & Spiegel, D. (1998). Trauma, dissociation and hypnotizability. In R. Marmar & D. Bremmer (Eds.), *Trauma, memory and dissociation* (pp. 57–106). Washington, DC: American Psychiatric Press.

Manning, C. (1996). Treatment of trauma associated with childhood sexual assault. *Australian Journal of Clinical and Experimental Hypnosis, 24*, 36–45.

Marmar, C. R., Weiss, D. S., Schlenger, W. E., Fairbank, J. A., Jordan, B. K., Kulka, R. A., et al. (1994). Peritraumatic dissociation and posttraumatic stress in male Vietnam theater veterans. *American Journal of Psychiatry, 15*, 902–907.

Matthews, W. J., Bennett, H., Bean, W., & Gallagher, M. (1985). Indirect versus direct hypnotic suggestions—an initial investigation: A brief communication. *International Journal of Clinical and Experimental Hypnosis, 33*, 219–223.

McDougall, W. (1920–1921). The revival of emotional memories and its therapeutic value (III). *British Journal of Medical Psychology, 1*, 23–29.

McDougall, W. (1926). *An outline of abnormal psychology*. London: Methuen.

Mira, E. (1943). *Psychiatry in war*. New York: Norton.

Moore, M. (2001). Hypnosis and post-traumatic stress disorder. *Australian Journal of Clinical and Experimental Hypnosis, 29*(2), 93–106.

Morgan, A. H., & Hilgard, E. R. (1978–1979). The Stanford Hypnotic Clinical Scale for Adults. *American Journal of Clinical Hypnosis, 21*, 134–147.

Muraoka, M., Komiyama, H., Hosoi, M., Mine, K., & Kubo, C. (1996). Psychosomatic treatment of phantom limb pain with posttraumatic stress disorder: A case report. *Pain, 66*, 385–388.

Myers, C. S. (1916, March 18). Contributions to the study of shell-shock III. *Lancet*, pp. 608–613.

Myers, C. S. (1920–1921). The revival of emotional memories and its therapeutic value (II). *British Journal of Medical Psychology, 1*, 20–22.

Myers, C. S. (1940). *Shell shock in France 1914–18*. Cambridge, UK: Cambridge University Press.

Naples, M., & Hackett, T. P. (1978). The amytal interview: History and current uses. *Psychosomatics, 19*, 98–105.

Nash, M. R. (1992). Hypnosis, psychopathology, and psychological regression. In E. Fromm & M. R. Nash (Eds.), *Contemporary hypnosis research* (pp. 149–169). New York: Guilford Press.

Nijenhuis, E. R. S., Spinhoven, P., Van Dyck, R., van der Hart, O., & Vanderlinden, J.

(1996). The development and psychometric characteristics of the Somatoform Dissociation Questionnaire (SDQ-20). *Journal of Nervous and Mental Disease, 184,* 688–694.

Nijenhuis, E. R. S., & van der Hart, O. (1999). Forgetting and reexperiencing trauma: From anesthesia to pain. In J. M. Goodwin & R. Attias (Eds.), *Splintered reflections: Images of the body in trauma* (pp. 39–65). New York: Basic Books.

Nonne, M. (1915). Zur therapeutischen Verwendung der Hypnose bei Fällen von Kriegshysterie [The therapeutic use of hypnosis for cases of war hysteria]. *Medizinische Klinik, 11,* 1391–1396.

Overton, D. A. (1978). Major theories of state dependent learning. In B. T. Ho, D. W. Richards, & D. L. Chute (Eds.), *Drug discrimination and state dependent learning* (pp. 283–318). New York: Academic Press.

Ozer, E., Best, S., & Lipsey, T. (2003). Predictors of posttraumatic stress disorder symptoms in adults: A meta-analysis. *Psychological Bulletin, 129,* 52–73.

Pantesco, V. F. (2005). The body's story: A case report of hypnosis and physiological narration of trauma. *American Journal of Clinical Hypnosis, 47,* 149–159.

Peebles, M. J. (1989). Through a glass darkly: The psychoanalytic use of hypnosis with posttraumatic stress disorder. *International Journal of Clinical and Experimental Hypnosis, 37,* 192–206.

Pekala, R. J., Kumar, V. K., & Marcano, G. (1995). Anomalous/paranormal experiences, hypnotic susceptibility, and dissociation. *Journal of the American Society for Psychical Research, 89,* 313–332.

Phillips, M. (1993). Turning symptoms into allies: Utilization approaches with posttraumatic symptoms. *American Journal of Clinical Hypnosis, 35,* 179–180.

Piccione, C., Hilgard, E. R., & Zimbardo, P. G. (1989). On the degree of stability of measured hypnotizability over a 25 year period. *Journal of Personality and Social Psychology, 56,* 289–295.

Pitman, R. K., Altman, B., Greenwald, E., Longpre, R. E., Macklin, M. L., Poire, R. E., et al. (1991). Psychiatric complications during flooding therapy for posttraumatic stress disorder. *Journal of Clinical Psychology, 52,* 17–20.

Putnam, F. W. (1992). Using hypnosis for therapeutic abreactions. *Psychiatric Medicine, 10,* 51–65.

Putnam, F. W., & Carlson, E. B. (1998). Hypnosis, dissociation, and trauma: Myths, metaphors, and mechanisms. In J. D. Bremner & C. R. Marmar (Eds.), *Trauma, memory, and dissociation* (pp. 27–55). Washington, DC: American Psychiatric Press.

Rhue, J., & Lynn, S. J. (1991). Storytelling, hypnosis and the treatment of sexually abused children. *International Journal of Clinical and Experimental Hypnosis, 39,* 198–214.

Richmond, K., Berman, B. M., Docherty, J. P., Holdstein, L. B., Kaplan, G., Keil, J. E., et al. (1996). Integration of behavioral and relaxation approaches into the treatment of chronic pain and insomnia. *Journal of the American Medical Association, 276,* 313–318.

Rivers, W. H. (1918, February 2). The repression of war experience. *Lancet,* pp. 173–177.

Ross, T. A. (1941). *Lectures on war neuroses.* London: Edward Arnold.

Roth, S. H., & Batson, R. (1993). The creative balance: The therapeutic relationship and thematic issues in trauma resolution. *Journal of Traumatic Stress, 6,* 159–177.

Salerno, N. (2005). The use of hypnosis in the treatment of post-traumatic stress disorder in a female correctional setting. *Australian Journal of Clinical and Experimental Hypnosis, 33*(1), 74–81.

Sargant, W. (1942). Physical treatment of acute war neuroses. *British Medical Journal, 2*, 574–576.

Sargant, W., & Slater, E. (1940). Acute war neuroses. *Lancet, 2*, 1–5.

Scheff, T. J. (1980). *Catharsis in healing, ritual, and drama.* Berkeley: University of California Press.

Schoenberger, N., Kirsch, I., Gearan, P., Montgomery, G., & Pastyrnak, S. (1997). Hypnotic enhancement of a cognitive behavioral treatment for public speaking anxiety. *Behavior Therapy, 28*, 127–140.

Scoboria, A., Mazzoni, G., & Kirsch, I. (2006). Effects of misleading questions and hypnotic memory suggestion on memory reports: A signal detection analysis. *International Journal of Clinical and Experimental Hypnosis, 54*, 340–359.

Shakibaei, F., Harandi, A. A., Ghlomrezaei, A., Samoei, R., & Salehi, P. (2008). Hypnotherapy in management of pain and reexperiencing of trauma in burn patients. *International Journal of Clinical and Experimental Hypnosis, 56*, 185–197.

Shalev, A. Y., Bonne, O., & Eth, S. (1996). Treatment of posttraumatic stress disorder: A review. *Psychosomatic Medicine, 58*, 165–182.

Shalev, A. Y., Peri, T., Canetti, L., & Schreiber, S. (1996). Predictors of PTSD in injured trauma survivors: A prospective study. *American Journal of Psychiatry, 153*, 219–225.

Sherman, J. J. (1998). Effects of psychotherapeutic treatment for PTSD: A meta-analysis of controlled clinical trials. *Journal of Traumatic Stress, 11*, 413–436.

Shor, R. E., & Orne, E. C. (1962). *Harvard Group Scale of Hypnotic Susceptibility manual.* Mountain View, CA: Consulting Psychologists Press.

Simmel, E. (1919). *Kriegs-neurosen und psychisches trauma* [War neurosis and psychological trauma]. München/Leipzig: Otto Nemnich.

Smith, G. E., & Pear, T. H. (1917). *Shell shock and its lessons.* London: University Press.

Smith, M. L., Glass, G. V., & Miller, T. I. (1980). *The benefits of psychotherapy.* Baltimore: Johns Hopkins University Press.

Smith, W. H. (1991). Antecedent of posttraumatic stress disorder: Wasn't being raped enough? *International Journal of Clinical and Experimental Hypnosis, 39*, 129–133.

Smith, W. H. (2004). Brief hypnotherapy of severe depression linked to sexual trauma: A case study. *International Journal of Clinical and Experimental Hypnosis, 52*, 203–217.

Smucker, M. R., Dancu, C., Foa, E. B., & Niederee, J. L. (1995). Imagery rescripting: A new treatment for survivors of childhood sexual abuse suffering from posttraumatic stress. *Journal of Cognitive Psychotherapy, 9*, 3–17.

Somer, E. (1994). Hypnotherapy and regulated uncovering in the treatment of older survivors of Nazi persecution. *Clinical Gerontologist, 14*, 47–65.

Southard, E. E., & Fenton, N. (1919). *Shell-shock and other neuropsychiatric problems.* Boston: Leonard.

Spiegel, D. (1981). Vietnam grief work using hypnosis. *American Journal of Clinical Hypnosis, 24*, 33–40.

Spiegel, D. (1989). Hypnosis in the treatment of victims of sexual abuse. *Psychiatric Clinics of North America, 12*, 295–305.

Spiegel, D. (1992). The use of hypnosis in the treatment of PTSD. *Psychiatric Medicine, 10*, 21–30.

Spiegel, D. (1994). Hypnosis. In R. E. Hales, S. C. Yudofsky, & J. A. Talbott (Eds.), *The*

American Psychiatric Press textbook of psychiatry (pp. 1115–1142). Washington, DC: American Psychiatric Press.

Spiegel, D., & Cardeña, E. (1990). New uses of hypnosis in the treatment of posttraumatic stress disorder. *Journal of Clinical Psychiatry, 51,* 39–43.

Spiegel, D., & Cardeña, E. (1991). Disintegrated experience: The dissociative disorders revisited. *Journal of Abnormal Psychology, 100,* 366–378.

Spiegel, D., Detrick, D., & Frischholz, E. (1982). Hypnotizability and psychopathology. *American Journal of Psychiatry, 139,* 431–437.

Spiegel, D., Hunt, T., & Dondershine, H. E. (1988). Dissociation and hypnotizability in posttraumatic stress disorder. *American Journal of Psychiatry, 145,* 301–305.

Spiegel, H., & Spiegel, D. (1987). *Trance and treatment: Clinical uses of hypnosis.* Washington, DC: American Psychiatric Press.

Stutman, R. K., & Bliss, E. L. (1985). Posttraumatic stress disorder, hypnotizability, and imagery. *American Journal of Psychiatry, 142,* 741–743.

Tellegen, A., & Atkinson, G. (1974). Openness to absorbing and self-altering experiences ("absorption"), a trait related to hypnotic susceptibility. *Journal of Abnormal Psychology, 83,* 268–277.

Terr, L. (1991). Childhood traumas: An outline and overview. *American Journal of Psychiatry, 148,* 10–20.

Torem, M. S. (1992). "Back from the future": A powerful age progression technique. *American Journal of Clinical Hypnosis, 35,* 81–88.

Valdiserri, E. V., & Byrne, J. P. (1982). Hypnosis as emergency treatment for a teenage rape victim. *Hospital and Community Psychiatry, 33,* 767–769.

van der Hart, O., Boon, S., & van Everdingen, G. B. (1990). Writing assignments and hypnosis in the treatment of traumatic memories. In M. L. Fass & D. Brown (Eds.), *Creative mastery in hypnosis and hypnoanalysis* (pp. 231–253). Hillsdale, NJ: Erlbaum.

van der Hart, O., & Brown, P. (1992). Abreaction re-evaluated. *Dissociation, 5,* 127–140.

van der Hart, O., Brown, P., & van der Kolk, B. A. (1989). Pierre Janet's treatment of post-traumatic stress. *Journal of Traumatic Stress, 2,* 379–396.

van der Hart, O., & Horst, R. (1989). The dissociation theory of Pierre Janet. *Journal of Traumatic Stress, 2,* 397–412.

van der Hart, O., Nijenhuis, E. R. S., & Steele, K. (2006). *The haunted self: Structural dissociation and the treatment of chronic traumatization.* New York/London: Norton.

van der Hart, O., & Spiegel, D. (1993). Hypnotic assessment and treatment of trauma-induced psychoses. *International Journal of Clinical and Experimental Hypnosis, 41,* 191–209.

van der Kolk, B. A., McFarlane, A. C., & van der Hart, O. (1996). A general approach to treatment of posttraumatic stress disorder. In B. A. van der Kolk, A. C. McFarlane, & L. Weisaeth (Eds.), *Traumatic stress: The effects of overwhelming experience on mind, body, and society* (pp. 417–440). New York: Guilford Press.

van der Kolk, B. A., & van der Hart, O. (1989). Pierre Janet and the breakdown of adaptation in psychological trauma. *American Journal of Psychiatry, 146,* 1530–1540.

Vermetten, E., & Bremner, J. D. (2004). Functional brain imaging and the induction of traumatic recall: A cross-correlational review between neuroimaging and hypnosis. *International Journal of Clinical and Experimental Hypnosis, 52,* 280–312.

Vijselaar, J., & van der Hart, O. (1992). The first report of hypnotic treatment of traumatic grief: A brief communication. *International Journal of Clinical and Experimental Hypnosis, 40*, 1–6.

Walters, V. J. (2005). *Hypnotic imagery as an adjunct to the treatment of PTSD and extreme distress.* Unpublished doctoral dissertation, City University, London.

Walters, V. J., & Oakley, D. A. (2002). Hypnosis in post-abortion distress: An experimental case study. *Contemporary Hypnosis, 19*(2), 85–99.

Watkins, E. (2008, June). *Depressive rumination: Investigating mechanisms to improve treatment.* Paper presented at the conference on What makes therapy work?: Towards a science of cognitive, emotional, and behavioral change, Lund, Sweden.

Watkins, J. (1949). *Hypnotherapy of war neuroses.* New York: Ronald Press.

Watkins, J. (1987). *Hypnotherapeutic techniques: Clinical hypnosis* (Vol. 1). New York: Irvington.

Watkins, J. G., & Watkins, H. H. (1997). *Ego states: Theory and therapy.* New York: Norton.

Wegner, D. M., & Pennebaker, J. W. (1993). *Handbook of mental control.* Englewood Cliffs, NJ: Prentice-Hall.

Wilshire, D. (1996). Trauma and treatment with hypnosis. *Australian Journal of Clinical and Experimental Hypnosis, 24*, 125–136.

CHAPTER 18

Couple and Family Therapy for Adults

David S. Riggs, Candice M. Monson,
Shirley M. Glynn, and John Canterino

Clinicians have long recognized that the support provided by intimate and family relationships serves an important role in recovery from traumatic events (Barrett & Mizes, 1988; Beiser, Turner, & Ganesan, 1989; Davidson, Hughes, Blazer, & George, 1991; Solomon, Waysman, & Mikulincer, 1990). Likewise, they have noted that the aftereffects of trauma can significantly impact partners and families of those directly exposed to the event (e.g., Dirkzwager, Bramsen, Ader, & van der Ploeg, 2005; Riggs, Byrne, Weathers, & Litz, 1998; Waysman, Mikulincer, Solomon, & Weisenberg, 1993). As a result, authors have suggested including conjoint and family therapy when developing comprehensive treatment plans for posttraumatic stress disorder (PTSD) and other psychological sequelae of trauma (e.g., Figley, 1988, 1989; Glynn et al., 1995; Monson, Stevens, & Schnurr, 2005).

Since the first edition of this volume, several well-designed programs incorporating couple or family interventions targeting PTSD have been added to the literature. However, the empirical literature on couple and family interventions targeting the needs of patients with PTSD remains scant. Importantly, in this area the empirical literature is largely devoid of the well-controlled randomized trials that are necessary to identify efficacious treatments for PTSD.

With some exceptions, the existing interventions tend to focus on dyadic or conjoint interventions rather than on including the larger family. Regardless of whether the suggestion is to incorporate partners or families, authors have relied on many of the same reasons for including family members in treatment. We note whether an author clearly references one modality or the other, but the reader should be aware that many of the arguments for including family members in treatment would apply equally well for partners or for the larger family.

Theoretical Context

In the first edition of this volume, programs were divided, based on the rationale offered for including partners or family members. Some programs include couple/family therapy to address the impact and the effects of trauma on families and relationships of exposed individuals (Carroll, Rueger, Foy, & Donohoe, 1985; Jordan et al., 1992; Riggs et al., 1998; Solomon, Mikulincer, Fried, & Wosner, 1987; Waysman et al., 1993). These approaches aim to reduce the systemic disruption resulting from the trauma and the posttraumatic symptoms of one or more family members. These therapies focus more on relieving family distress than on reducing a particular individual's PTSD symptoms.

Other programs focus on the role of the partner and family members in helping the trauma survivor to recover from the symptoms arising from the trauma (Barrett & Mizes, 1988; Beiser et al., 1989; Davidson et al., 1991; Solomon et al., 1990). In this formulation, the partner or family members represent an important source of support for the identified patient. Couple/family interventions focus on improving the efficacy with which this support is provided. This model of couple/family treatment relies heavily on educational and skills training approaches to treatment, and draws less from the traditions and theories of couple and family therapy.

The distinction in focus between these approaches to therapy also leads to differences in evaluation of treatment efficacy. The efficacy of systemic treatments is typically evaluated with measures of family or relationship functioning, with a focus on communication. Interventions promoting family support to the identified individual with PTSD tend to treat trauma-related symptoms in that individual as the primary outcome.

These approaches are not mutually exclusive, and the programs that have been reported since the first edition of this volume (e.g., Glynn et al., 1999; Monson et al., 2005) have tended to blur the distinction. Indeed, even in the earlier programs there is some overlap in techniques and evaluation. Authors who suggest targeting the relationship or family system recognize the role of the family in providing support and promoting recovery. Similarly, those focused on educating and training the family acknowledge that trauma can impact family members who were not directly exposed (or multiple family members exposed to the same trauma). This distinction has lessened with recent efforts; consequently, this review is not organized by these distinctions. However, it should be noted that the different philosophies lead to somewhat different treatment approaches, units of analysis (system vs. individual), and measures of outcome.

Rationale for Systemic Treatment Approaches

In some cases (e.g., natural disasters, motor vehicle accidents [MVAs]), entire families experience the same trauma. In these cases, the family system is likely to be disrupted, and the logic behind offering treatment to the family is straightforward. However, even when only one family member is directly exposed to a trauma, the effects can extend to the rest of the family. For example, combat veterans with PTSD are at risk for significant relationship problems (Card, 1987; Carroll et al., 1985; Jordan et al., 1992; Riggs et al., 1998; Waysman et al., 1993). Veterans' PTSD also may negatively impact the mental health of partners and family members (Beckham, Lytle, & Feldman, 1996; Calhoun, Beckham, & Bosworth, 2002; Dirkzwager et al., 2005; Waysman et al., 1993). The presence of significant family and dyadic disruption provides an impetus for the application of many of the couple/family therapy approaches to posttraumatic symptoms reviewed here.

Systemic treatments aim to reduce the negative effects of trauma on the family or relationship rather than directly targeting the symptoms of one family member. Success is evaluated via improvement in family functioning, primarily improved communication and reduced conflict. Within this framework, two intervention strategies have been suggested: (1) family therapy—focused on alleviating conflict and promoting communication with the entire family system, and (2) couple therapy—focused on aiding dyadic communication and reducing conflict between spouses.

Rationale for Supportive Treatment Approaches

The awareness that intimate partners and family members are a key source of support (Beach, Martin, Blum, & Roman, 1993; McLeod, Kessler, & Landis, 1992; Syrotuik & D'Arcy, 1984) underlies programs that aim to educate family members and encourage support of traumatized individuals. Also, families high in expressed emotion (EE; criticism, hostility, emotional overinvolvement) can negatively impact individual PTSD treatment (Tarrier, Sommerfield, & Pilgrim, 1999). Promoting support and decreasing potential negative influences on PTSD treatment are particularly important given the aggravating or mitigating role of social relationships in recovery from trauma (Barrett & Mizes, 1988; Beiser et al., 1989; Brewin, Andrews, & Valentine, 2000; Davidson et al., 1991; Solomon et al., 1990).

Description of Techniques

The most detailed description of systemic family therapy with trauma survivors has been put forward by Figley (1983, 1985, 1986, 1988, 1995). This program aims to "*empower* the family to overcome and learn from their ordeal and, in so doing, be more prepared to handle future adversities" (Figley, 1995, p. 351; original emphasis). Therapists work to foster skills that help the family effectively exchange information, solve problems, and resolve conflicts. Figley (1986, 1995) describes five phases of therapy with traumatized families: (1) commitment to therapeutic objectives, (2) framing the problem, (3) reframing the problem, (4) developing a healing theory, and (5) closure and preparedness. The therapy is brief, and the therapist serves primarily as a facilitator, encouraging family members to develop and refine their own skills for dealing with extreme stressors. Success is measured by improvement in current family functioning and in the family's ability to cope with future difficulties better (Figley, 1995).

Initial sessions are used to establish rapport and trust among the therapist and family members, and to define the therapist's role as a consultant to the family. The therapy then examines the family's reaction to the trauma, previous attempts to cope, and obstacles to successful coping. Once difficulties are identified, the therapist works to promote supportive interactions and communication skills to enhance the exchange of ideas and self-disclosure. The family then reviews troubling memories related to the trauma. As family members share their reactions, the process fosters the development of a new consensus view of the trauma and the family's reaction. Finally, individual perspectives are brought together to form a "family healing theory"—or a single story about the trauma and its aftermath—that allows the family to agree on what has happened and how its members will cope with a similar event in the future (Figley, 1985).

Erickson (1989) adapted Williamson's (1982a, 1982b) consultation process to address the needs of a traumatized family. Like Figley (1995), Erickson's (1989) therapy aims to strengthen family cohesion through effective communication and support. Interventions are designed to help family members (1) recognize the trauma as a family crisis requiring a shared response, (2) recognize and respond to the needs of each member, (3) encourage appropriate self-disclosure, and (4) understand that the damage caused by the trauma is not irreparable. Initially, the survivor and family are seen separately and encouraged to talk about the trauma. Later, the survivor and the family are seen together and encouraged to explore the impact of the trauma on the family. Each family member, including the survivor, is asked to write an "autobiography" of his or her experience of the trauma. When the family is ready (therapist determined, criteria are not provided), the survivor briefly shares her story of the rape, for example, and (over several sessions) the family discusses in detail the events of the rape and its impact on the family.

Harris (1991) describes a five-step problem-solving intervention for families dealing with a recent trauma. The first stage is used to build rapport and trust between the therapist and family. The second stage involves (1) identifying problems, (2) improving communication, and (3) improving family support. In the third stage, the family examines possible solutions to the problems and decides on a course of action. With the survivor's permission, this stage includes a discussion of his or her psychological problems related to the trauma. In the fourth stage, the therapist encourages the family to take action to solve identified problems. The final stage of the intervention, follow-up, allows for further treatment of the family.

Other authors have presented general guidelines, but not specific techniques, for conducting family therapy with trauma survivors and their families. The suggestions include the following:

1. Removing the survivor from the role of identified patient (Williams & Williams, 1980).
2. Educating families about the impact of trauma (Mio & Foster, 1991; Williams & Williams, 1980).
3. Using both individual and family sessions (Mio & Foster, 1991; Rosenheck & Thompson, 1986).
4. Developing mutual support and communication skills (Williams & Williams, 1980).
5. Clarifying roles and values (Mio & Foster, 1991; Williams & Williams, 1980).
6. Identifying and breaking patterns of trauma repetition (Brende & Goldsmith, 1991).
7. Resolving specific emotional disruptions, such as rage, shame, or guilt (Brende & Goldsmith, 1991; Williams & Williams, 1980).

Behavioral family therapy (BFT), first introduced to help families manage symptoms of chronic mental illness, has been suggested for treatment of persons with PTSD (Mueser & Glynn, 1995). In BFT, the person with PTSD is seen with at least one relative for 16 sessions. The therapist uses the first three sessions to orient participants to the treatment and to conduct assessments of individual and couple strengths and weaknesses; two sessions that focus on education about PTSD and available services follow. The next three sessions focus on communication training, with an additional two sessions devoted to anger management. The final six to eight sessions are used to improve the couple's problem-solving skills.

Several interventions for couples—critical interaction therapy (D. R. Johnson, Feldman, & Lubin, 1995), emotionally focused marital/couple therapy (S. M. Johnson, 1989, 2002; S. M. Johnson & Williams-Keeler, 1998), and cognitive-behavioral couple treatment (CBCT; Monson, Schnurr, Stevens, & Guthrie, 2004)—in which one member has PTSD have been detailed in the literature. D. R. Johnson and colleagues' (1995) critical interaction therapy focuses on general patterns of dyadic interaction that commonly occur in Vietnam War veterans' families. The authors argue that trauma survivors' families engage in a behavior pattern, the "critical interaction," that reflects a "repetitive conflict that is covertly associated with the traumatic memory" (p. 404) and follows a set sequence of events. Critical interaction therapy uses a series of interventions to (1) teach the couple about the interactional process, (2) point out the connections to the veteran's trauma, (3) allow the veteran and partner to stop blaming one another and to offer support, and (4) promote better problem solving and communication. D. R. Johnson and colleagues detail a number of steps used to educate partners and to defuse these critical interactions, and promote positive discussion around the conflict.

Emotionally focused marital/couple therapy (EFT) is effective for treating marital distress; the techniques of EFT are detailed elsewhere (S. M. Johnson, 1996; S. M. Johnson & Greenberg, 1994), as is the application of EFT to cases in which one member of the couple has experienced trauma (S. M. Johnson, 2002). Briefly, the approach is short term (12–20 sessions) and experiential, with a focus on "reprocessing the emotional responses that organize attachment behaviors" (S. M. Johnson & Williams-Keeler, 1998, p. 29). EFT is divided into nine steps that according to Johnson and Williams-Keeler parallel the stages of therapy for trauma survivors described by McCann and Pearlman (1990). Steps 1–4 of EFT (assessment, identification of interaction patterns, identification of underlying feelings, and labeling negative interaction patterns as the problem) reflect the stabilization phase of trauma treatment. Steps 5–7 of EFT (owning relationship fears, acceptance by the partner, and asking that one's needs be met appropriately) reflect the building of capacities phase in trauma treatment. Steps 8 (developing new ways of coping) and 9 (integrating new interaction patterns) parallel the integration stage of McCann and Pearlman's treatment.

CBCT (Monson et al., 2004, 2005) for PTSD is a relatively new intervention program designed to address individual PTSD symptoms and relationship problems simultaneously. CBCT comprises 15 sessions, broken down into three phases. In the first two sessions, the clinician works to orient the couple to the treatment and to educate partners about PTSD and its impact on relationships. After this come six sessions that focus on communication skills training and overcoming experiential avoidance. The final phase of the treatment comprises six sessions that focus on delivering cognitive interventions aimed at changing the core beliefs and schemas related to safety, esteem, trust, power, and intimacy associated with the persistence of PTSD symptoms and problems within the relationship.

Another attempt to apply an existing couple-focused treatment to cases of PTSD was reported by Cahoon (1984). In this case, cognitive-behavioral techniques developed to improve relationships were offered to couples in which the man suffered from PTSD related to his Vietnam War combat experience. Treatment, focused primarily on teaching communication and problem-solving skills, was conducted in a group format in seven weekly sessions lasting 90–120 minutes.

Another variation on these programs, described by Devilly (2002), is an intensive group intervention, labeled a lifestyle management course, for veterans and their partners. Participants attended 5 days of courses led by experienced PTSD counselors. Topics included education about PTSD, managing stress, relaxation/meditation, self-care, diet and nutrition, communication, anger management, and problem solving. There were also open-topic groups (some were gender-specific, and others were combined) and discussions of self-esteem, alcohol, and depression.

Most suggestions to incorporate supportive treatments for spouses and/or family members occur in the context of larger treatment programs targeting PTSD. These programs typically include mechanisms for educating family members about PTSD and PTSD treatment, the provision of family support groups, and programs to help family members improve stress management skills.

The first supportive program described in the literature is incorporated into the Koach project, a monthlong, extensive, multifaceted treatment program developed in Israel for combat veterans (Solomon, Bleich, Shoham, Nardi, & Kotler, 1992). Of interest here is the inclusion of veterans' wives in treatment, as described by Rabin and Nardi (1991). Briefly, wives attended two sessions prior to the veterans' program, during which they were asked to discuss difficulties they were experiencing as a result of their husbands' symptoms, and were educated about posttraumatic symptoms and basic behavioral and cognitive principles as they relate to chronic PTSD. During the first week of the veterans' treatment, wives attended a daylong workshop to learn how to reinforce husbands' positive behavior, cognitive coping skills, and communication skills. In the second week, wives and family members participated in a "family day," with entertaining activities and informal talks between staff and wives. During the last 2 weeks of the program, veterans and wives participated in three couple groups to discuss common problems, to improve communication and problem-solving skills, and to encourage veterans to view their partners as sources of support.

A second example of a support-focused program, Support and Family Education (SAFE), was developed by Sherman (2003). This multisession educational program is flexible and has been used with families dealing with a range of mental illnesses (e.g., PTSD, major depression, bipolar disorder, and schizophrenia) and with various family members (e.g., spouse, parent, sibling). However, because the SAFE program was developed in the U.S. Veterans Health Administration (VHA), many cases involve PTSD. The SAFE program originally comprised 14 sessions covering a variety of topics of concern to family members of persons with mental illness. Most of the sessions involve topics that cut across illnesses (e.g., education about mental illness and services available), but several are specific to illnesses commonly seen in the VHA (i.e., depression, PTSD, schizophrenia). The developers recently added four new sessions that introduce information and skills not included in the original program (e.g., family problem-solving skills, minimizing stress). Unlike the other programs reviewed here, the SAFE program is clearly conceptualized as an educational rather than a therapeutic program, with 90-minute workshops presented once monthly on an ongoing basis. This allows family members to join or leave the program at any time, and to choose which specific workshops they will attend. Each session includes a didactic component, group discussion, and an opportunity for family members to ask questions of mental health experts.

Method of Collecting Data

We were unable to identify a comprehensive review of the use of couple/family therapy in the context of trauma other than that in the earlier edition of this volume. Therefore, this summary relies heavily on the earlier volume, and recently published original sources. We used the same procedures to identify resources for this chapter. Initially, we conducted searches of the Psyc-LIT and Published International Literature on Traumatic Stress (PILOTS) databases for articles and chapters that included at least one of the terms "marital therapy," "couples therapy," or "family therapy," and at least one of the terms "PTSD," "posttraumatic stress disorder," "trauma," "disaster," "combat," "rape," or "assault." To limit redundancy, we restricted this search to work published since 1998, when we conducted the original review. Once we identified potentially appropriate articles and chapters, we reviewed titles and abstracts to find those most likely to include empirical data and/or specific descriptions of therapeutic approaches. We used these articles and chapters for the bulk of this review. In addition, we identified relevant works cited in these articles and chapters; we obtained these works if they were not already included in the review.

Although many authors have discussed the potential value of incorporating couple/family therapy into programs to treat trauma survivors, few have outlined specific techniques or approaches that might be of value. Instead, couple/family therapy is often included with other, potential adjunct therapies that may be incorporated into a comprehensive treatment program. Often, the suggestion to include couple/family therapy constituted a single paragraph or brief section in a much larger discussion of treatment issues. In such cases, the authors seemed to rely on readers' existing knowledge of couple/family interventions, or referred readers to general descriptions of such approaches. Because a full review of couple and family therapies is beyond the scope of this chapter, we focus on specific couple or family techniques or interventions that have been suggested specifically for the treatment of trauma survivors.

Literature Review

Behavioral Family Therapy

In the only published randomized controlled trial of couple or family treatment for PTSD, Glynn and colleagues (1999) randomly assigned 42 Vietnam War veterans to one of three groups: (1) directed therapeutic exposure (DTE), (2) DTE followed by behavioral family therapy (BFT), or (3) a wait list (WL). BFT is designed to include a variety of family members, but most (89%) of the participants in this study were intimate partners of the veterans. Participants in the treatment conditions (DTE, DTE + BFT) completed 18 sessions of DTE over 9 weeks. Those in the combined condition then completed 16 sessions (12 weekly, 2 biweekly, 2 monthly) of BFT over 6 months. Participants in the WL condition were assessed 2 months after entering the study, then offered treatment with BFT.

The researchers examined the impact of treatment on veterans' PTSD symptoms, social adjustment, and problem-solving skills (see Table 18.1). Changes were assessed immediately after treatment and at a 6-month follow-up. The treatment groups improved more than the WL on positive PTSD symptoms (i.e., reexperiencing, arousal) but not negative PTSD symptoms (i.e., avoidance, numbing) or social adjustment. Comparisons between the two treatment groups were not statistically significant. At the 6-month assessment, there were no differences between the two treatment groups. When the authors examined veterans' problem-solving skills, they found that participants who completed BFT showed more improvement in problem solving than did participants who did not complete BFT.

About 33% of participants declined BFT sessions when they reached that point in the treatment. The refusal rate was the same in the DTE and WL conditions, suggesting that the inclusion of exposure did not lead to high dropout. One factor related to refusal of BFT was high levels of avoidance and numbing symptoms. The authors noted difficulties in adapting BFT for use with conjugal couples rather than the parent or sibling commonly seen when BFT is used with chronically mentally ill individuals, and particular difficulties when the relationship is fragile because of conflict that often accompanies PTSD. *Strength of evidence: A.*

Behavioral Marital Therapy

In a small dissertation study, Sweany (1988) randomly assigned 14 couples in which the male partner had combat-related PTSD to marital treatment based on behavioral marital therapy (Jacobson & Margolin, 1979) or to a WL condition. Treatment comprised eight weekly, 2-hour sessions focused on increasing positive interactions, improving communication, teaching problem-solving skills, and enhancing intimacy. Results indicated marginally significant group differences, with the treated group showing small improvements in relationship satisfaction, depression, and PTSD. Effect sizes were not calculable based on the data reported. Veterans' and partners' reports of relationship satisfaction improved significantly more in the treatment group than in the WL group. The treated veterans reported a significantly larger reduction in PTSD symptoms than did veterans in the control group. *Strength of evidence: A.*

Cognitive-Behavioral Couple Treatment

Monson and colleagues (2004, 2005) reported the results of a small, uncontrolled pilot study that included seven couples who received CBCT for PTSD (see Table 18.1). Couples were assessed prior to and immediately following treatment using standardized measures of PTSD, depression, anxiety, and relationship satisfaction. Results revealed improvements in veterans' PTSD, depression, and anxiety (Monson et al., 2004). Moreover, there were significant improvements in the wives' anxiety in general, and improvements in PTSD and depression among those wives with clinical levels of these problems prior to treatment (Monson et al., 2005). There was no improvement in the husbands' relationship satisfaction, but there was a trend toward improvement in the wives' satisfaction. There were improvements in social functioning more broadly (Monson et al., 2005). All the statistically significant improvements were associated with large within-group effect sizes (Cohen's $d > 1.0$). The absence of significant changes in relationship satisfaction may be due to the fact that the couples were generally satisfied at the time they entered treatment. *Strength of evidence: B.*

Lifestyle Management Courses

Devilly (2002) reported on the results of a lifestyle management course for male veterans with PTSD and many of their partners. A total of 111 male veterans (98 of whom were accompanied by a partner) attended the program held at a residential setting specializing in the care of veterans (see Table 18.1). Outcome was evaluated using standardized measures of PTSD, depression, anxiety, relationship satisfaction, stress, anger, alcohol use, and quality of life. Because the groups lasted only 1 week, Devilly argued that the post-treatment assessment likely reflected overall program satisfaction rather than meaningful symptom change, so the primary outcome evaluations were conducted on data collected 3- and 6-months after the program. Both veterans and their partners experienced significant reductions in anxiety, depression, and stress, and veterans also experienced a reduction in PTSD. There were also small improvements in anger and quality of life, though, in the latter case, only the objective measure, not the subjective quality of life, improved. There was no significant improvement in relationship satisfaction.

The author noted that many of the statistically significant findings were associated with relatively small effect sizes. Thus, even though the lifestyle

TABLE 18.1. Results of a Lifestyle Management Course for Male Veterans with PTSD

Study	Treatment tested	Population	Comparison groups	N	Duration of trial	Main outcome measures	Within-group effect size	Comparison	Between-N group effect size ITT	Between-N group effect size Completer	Results
Level A studies											
Glynn et al. (1999)	Direct therapeutic exposure (DTE)	Male Vietnam War combat veterans + family member	DTE	12 (1)	18 sessions over 9 weeks	PTSD positive symptom	(0.29)	DTE vs. WL		0.85	DTE > WL
	Behavioral family therapy (BFT)		DTE + BFT	17 (1)	18 sessions over 9 weeks + 16 sessions over 6 months		(0.71)	DTE + BFT vs. WL		0.65	DTE + BFT > WL
			Wait list (WL)	13 (1)	9 weeks		(−0.08)	DTE vs. DTE + BFT		0.07	DTE > DTE + BFT, ns
			DTE	12 (1)		PTSD negative symptom	(0.68)	DTE vs. WL		0.76	DET > WL, ns
			DTE + BFT	17 (1)			(0.38)	DTE + BFT vs. WL		0.45	DET + BFT > WL, ns
			WL	13 (1)			(0.21)	DTE vs. DTE + BFT		0.2	DTE > DTE + BFT, ns
			DTE	12 (1)		Social Adjustment Scale	(0.71)	DTE vs. WL		0.42	DTE > WL, ns
			DTE + BFT	17 (1)			(0.44)	DTE + BFT vs. WL		0.49	DTE + BFT > WL, ns
			WL	13 (1)			(0.17)	DTE vs. DTE + BFT		0.15	DTE > DTE + BFT, ns

Level B studies

Study	Treatment	Population	Intervention	N	Duration	Measure	Effect size
Devilly (2002)	Lifestyle management course	Male Vietnam War combat veterans + partners	Lifestyle management course	111	Approximately 35 hours during 1 week	Impact of Event Scale	(0.04)[a]
						Abbreviated Dyadic Adjustment Scale (Men)	(0.11)[a]
						Abbreviated Dyadic Adjustment Scale (Women)	(0.26)[a]
Monson et al. (2004)	Cognitive-behavioral couple therapy	Male Vietnam War combat veterans + partners	Cognitive-behavioral couple therapy	7	15 sessions over 15 weeks	CAPS	1.6[a]
						PCL—Self-report	0.64[a]
						PCL—Partner Report	1.18[a]
						Dyadic Adjustment Scale (Me)	0.05[a]
						Dyadic Adjustment Scale (Wome)	0.92[a]

Notes. ITT, intention to treat; ns, not significant; CAPS, Clinician-Administered PTSD Scale; PCL, PTSD Checklist.
[a]Effect size provided in original article.

469

management course improved symptoms, gains were considered to be of limited clinical importance. However, 10 to 25% of participants showed clinically meaningful improvement on the measures administered. It is also noteworthy that, as a group, couples who participated in the program were satisfied with their relationships prior to the intervention, limiting both opportunities for relationship improvements and generalizability of the findings. *Strength of evidence: B.*

One study (Cahoon, 1984) examined the effects of behavioral marital therapy with Vietnam War veterans and their partners. Participants were recommended for treatment by Vet Center therapists and were not randomly assigned. A minority of veterans asked to participate agreed to enter the program, and only nine couples completed the seven sessions. Veterans improved on affective and problem-solving communication, but these changes were not statistically significant. Pre- and posttreatment effect sizes were $d = 0.18$ and 0.41, respectively, for affective and problem-solving communication. Partners reported statistically significant improvements in dyadic distress and problem-solving communication. Pre- and posttreatment effect sizes for partners were $d = 0.34$ and 0.56, respectively, for general distress and problem-solving communication. There were also significant improvements in rap group leaders' ratings of the veterans' coping ability (pre- and posttreatment $d = 0.72$) and PTSD (pre- and posttreatment $d = 0.47$). *Strength of evidence: C.*

Emotionally Focused Couple Therapy

There are no published controlled studies of EFT with trauma survivors. However, data support the efficacy of EFT with distressed couples generally (Dunn & Schwebel, 1995; S. M. Johnson & Greenberg, 1985) and in cases in which the woman is depressed (Dessaulles, 1991). S. M. Johnson (2002) suggests that EFT has been effective with couples in which one or both partners have experienced trauma and presents several cases to illustrate of the application of EFT to trauma survivors. No outcome data are presented. Johnson (1989) describes the successful treatment of a couple in which the woman survived incest; however, no standardized assessments were included. The techniques of EFT, as they pertain to work with trauma survivors, are also illustrated with case examples by S. M. Johnson and Williams-Keeler (1998). *Strength of evidence: D.*

Spousal Education and Support Programs

Sherman (2006) reported on data collected from participants over the first 5 years of the SAFE program. One-hundred seventy family members had participated in at least one workshop, with about two-thirds returning for more than one session (average of 6.5 sessions). Though no outcome data are available, family members anecdotally reported high satisfaction with the program and that it improved their family relations. In addition, the number of sessions attended was significantly correlated with measures of self-care, caregiver distress, knowledge of mental illness, and awareness of VHA resources. The efficacy of the Koach program on veterans' PTSD symptoms is unclear (see Solomon et al., 1992). However, 68% of the men and their wives reported that their relationships improved (Rabin & Nardi, 1991). *Strength of evidence: D.*

Family Systems–Based Therapy

To date, no published controlled studies have examined the efficacy of family systems therapy for PTSD. Case descriptions were provided to illustrate the treatment techniques; however, none of the articles describing Figley's (1983, 1985, 1986, 1988, 1995) treatment included data from validated measures to support the efficacy of this treatment in alleviating PTSD or the systemic disruption associated with the disorder. Similarly, no data were presented in the article describing Erickson's (1989) treatment to support its efficacy in treating posttraumatic symptoms at the systemic or individual level. Notably, Erickson suggested that this treatment is most appropriate for "families who were functioning adequately before the [trauma] and whose dynamics and interaction can incorporate the kind of self-disclosure and supportiveness demanded" (p. 273). A clinical case is presented to illustrate treatment techniques recommended by Harris (1991), but no validated measures were used. At 3-month posttreatment, the survivor indicated that the rape was "no longer a major issue to be overtly confronted" and the family "reported a general feeling of happiness and comfort with one another" (p. 206). *Strength of evidence: D.*

Critical Interaction Therapy

To date, there are no published controlled studies that examine critical interaction therapy. The D. R. Johnson and colleagues (1995) article provided no data to support its efficacy in treating posttraumatic symptoms at the systemic or individual level. There were no clinical case studies presented to support the efficacy of this treatment, but the techniques were illustrated with case examples. *Strength of evidence: F.*

Summary and Recommendations

The literature on couple and family therapies with trauma survivors is severely lacking despite the recent publication of several articles. Empirical examinations in the literature had small samples, and many did not include a control group. The studies are also limited in that they included mostly combat veterans and their partners. Until results are replicated with larger samples and survivors of other types of trauma, it is premature to recommend couple therapy for the treatment of PTSD or PTSD-related family distress. In the clinically focused literature, careful case studies with standard assessments are lacking. Authors provide strong theoretical arguments and rationales for using couple/family therapies, usually combined with other treatments for posttrauma symptoms. However, the lack of empirical data makes it difficult to know whether and when these therapies should be used, or how to combine them with other treatment approaches.

Because dyadic or family disruption is often a problem for individuals with PTSD, it is recommended that clinicians evaluate the need for couple or family therapy when treating trauma survivors. In general, treatments are skills-focused, with emphasis on improving communication, problem solving, coping, and mutual support. The available data suggest that in some cases these treatments may be helpful in addressing disruption in the family or increasing support available to the trauma survivor. Therefore, when couple or family therapy appears warranted, it is recommended that this treatment focus on improving communication and reducing conflict among family members. This may entail communication around current problems and/or issues related to the trauma and its aftermath.

The paucity of empirical studies of couple/family therapy for PTSD means that decision criteria for when to use these approaches, and the consequences of not including them when they are warranted, remain largely unknown. However, authors generally suggest that family therapy is most appropriate when the family system is largely intact and functioning well prior to the trauma. In these cases, treatment can focus on the impact of the trauma on the system. When the system is dysfunctional prior to the trauma, more traditional family therapy may be necessary prior to addressing trauma-related problems. Interestingly, relationships that have had a relatively satisfactory adaptation to the presence of trauma-related symptoms appear overrepresented in samples participating in couple treatment (Devilly, 2002; Monson et al., 2004). Thus, although it might be more appropriate to include couple/family therapy in a treatment plan for an individual when significant disruption exists, we know little about the effects of such treatment in these cases.

Rarely, and almost only in the case of traumatized children, is family therapy suggested to be the sole or even primary treatment for posttraumatic symptoms. The available data do not support the use of couple or family therapy alone to treat PTSD, although the preliminary data on CBCT for PTSD are promising. Instead, couple/family therapy is an important adjunct to other forms of treatment aimed more directly at alleviating posttraumatic symptoms. Even in cases in which family therapy is recommended as the primary form of therapy (see Erickson, 1989; Figley, 1995), individual treatment with the trauma survivor is recommended to address PTSD symptoms. Therefore, at the present time, it is recommended that when couple and family therapy are used with people who have PTSD, they should be concurrent with, or follow, evidence-based treatments focused on alleviating PTSD symptoms.

Further Considerations

Family Violence

Families in which one or more members have PTSD appear at increased risk for family violence (Jordan et al., 1992; Riggs et al., 1998). There is considerable debate within the family violence field as to whether couple or family therapy is appropriate when violence is ongoing. The determination of what treatment is most effective and safest for family violence remains unclear, and this complex decision likely depends on many factors, including the severity and frequency of violence, as well as its objective and subjective consequences. Generally, we recommend that clinicians proceed cautiously in applying couple and family therapy in trauma-related cases in which violence is occurring within the family. Consultation with professionals familiar with the treatment of family violence is highly recommended.

Separation/Lack of Commitment

Though it is not discussed explicitly except in the cases of EFT and CBCT for PTSD, the lack of commitment to the current relationship on the part of the survivor and/or spouse is probably a contraindication for the use of couple therapy for PTSD.

Type of Trauma and Chronicity

Most studies that examined couple and family therapy for PTSD focused on the treatment of male combat veterans with PTSD. Furthermore, most of these investigations were conducted many years after the veterans were in combat. The potential utility of couple/family therapy with other types of trauma survivors, or the possibility that such interventions would have to be modified to address problems that are more likely in other traumatized populations (e.g., sexual dysfunction among rape survivors), has not been examined. The reliance on samples of veterans with very chronic PTSD also limits our knowledge about the potential utility of couple/family interventions provided soon after the trauma.

Comorbid Conditions

No discussion of comorbid disorders as they relate to the use of couple/family therapies was found in the literature reviewed here. However, couple therapy has been found to be helpful in treating depression (e.g., Jacobson, Dobson, Fruzetti, Schmaling, & Salusky, 1991) and alcohol abuse (e.g., O'Farrell, 1994), either alone or in conjunction with other interventions. As these disorders represent much of the comorbid psychopathology associated with PTSD, it is possible that such interventions will prove helpful in the case of PTSD with comorbid depression and/or substance use. However, clear recommendations regarding the use of couple or family therapy in cases of PTSD with comorbid psychological disorders are not possible at this time.

Dual-Trauma Couples

As we mentioned earlier, there are times when couples or entire families experience a particular trauma simultaneously (or one member is directly traumatized, while the others are traumatized indirectly by the same event). It is also possible that members of a family experienced distinct traumas (e.g., the wife of a combat veteran has been raped). Little is known about the added complexity of couple/family therapy when multiple family members have experienced different traumas (see Balcom [1996] and Nelson, Wangsgaard, Yorgason, Kessler, & Carter-Vassol [2002] for descriptions of some issues that might arise in these cases). It would seem likely that cases in which multiple family members have experienced traumas would be more amenable to the systemic interventions described earlier. However, it may be important to incorporate additional supportive techniques into the intervention. Alternatively, it might be possible to conceptualize treatment of multiply traumatized families as constituting a "group treatment" for traumatized individuals. However, it is important to remember that even when a couple or family has experienced the same event, individual reactions may be quite different. One should consider the potential need to hold individual sessions in conjunction with the couple or family work. Regardless of the specific approach taken with these cases, it is likely that the couple or family intervention will prove significantly more complicated than in cases in which a single family member is the direct victim of trauma. As is the case with regard to comorbidity, specific recommendations about how best to treat multiply traumatized families awaits further study.

Future Directions

Clinical descriptions and empirical data indicate that trauma and posttraumatic symptoms create substantial disruption in the relationships and families of survivors (e.g., Jordan et al., 1992; Riggs et al., 1998). It is also apparent that social support is important in recovery from trauma. Thus, it seems likely that interventions aimed at reducing family distress, improving support, and educating family members about effects of trauma could be useful in alleviating problems of trauma survivors. Although a number of authors have suggested programs for addressing the needs of families in the aftermath of trauma, only a few have empirically examined specific interventions.

The shortage of systematic research into couple and family therapy for treating posttraumatic difficulties means that many questions regarding how, when, and to whom such treatments should be delivered are also unanswered.

There is little or no guidance offered regarding decisions as to when couple/family therapy should be incorporated during the process of therapy for PTSD. In the absence of clear guidelines, it seems important that clinicians evaluate the presence of couple/family disruption and the functional link between the family problems and the individual's PTSD symptoms. A few contraindications for this approach have been suggested (e.g., family violence, lack of commitment, prior family dysfunction), but these are taken from general issues related to couple and family therapy. There are no empirical data to support these contentions in the specific case of PTSD.

Numerous other questions remain regarding specific aspects of the application of couple and family therapies to the problems of trauma survivors. First, it is not clear whether certain forms of couple/family therapy would be more successful than others for survivors of specific types of trauma. Similarly, it is not clear whether some treatments would be better than others when treating a family in which all members were exposed to a trauma, and others would be more effective for a family coping with a trauma directly experienced by a single member. Additional unanswered questions include whether the treatment of a family that was intact prior to the trauma (e.g., a family trying to cope with the daughter's rape) is different or similar to the treatment of a family that formed subsequent to a trauma (e.g., partners who married after a veteran returned from combat). The impact of the chronicity of PTSD symptoms (i.e., whether the treatment is begun in the immediate aftermath of the trauma or years later) has also not been examined with regard to couple/family treatments.

References

Balcom, D. (1996). The interpersonal dynamics and treatment of dual trauma couples. *Journal of Marital and Family Therapy, 22*(4), 431–442.

Barrett, T. W., & Mizes, J. S. (1988). Combat level and social support in the development of posttraumatic stress disorder in Vietnam veterans. *Behavior Modification, 12*, 100–115.

Beach, S. R., Martin, J. K., Blum, T. C., & Roman, P. M. (1993). Effects of marital and co-worker relationships on negative affect: Testing the central role of marriage. *American Journal of Family Therapy, 21*, 313–323.

Beckham, J. C., Lytle, B. L., & Feldman, M. E. (1996). Caregiver burden in partners of Vietnam War veterans with posttraumatic stress disorder. *Journal of Consulting and Clinical Psychology, 64*, 1068–1072.

Beiser, M., Turner, R. J., & Ganesan, S. (1989). Catastrophic stress and factors affecting its consequences among Southeast Asian refugees. *Social Science and Medicine, 28*, 183–195.

Brende, J. O., & Goldsmith, R. (1991). Post-traumatic stress disorder in families. *Journal of Contemporary Psychotherapy, 21*(2), 115–124.

Brewin, C. R., Andrews, B., & Valentine, J. D. (2000). Meta-analysis of risk factors for posttraumatic stress disorder in trauma-exposed adults. *Journal of Consulting and Clinical Psychology, 68*, 748–766.

Cahoon, E. P. (1984). *An examination of relationships between post-traumatic stress disorder, marital distress, and response to therapy by Vietnam veterans.* Unpublished doctoral dissertation, University of Connecticut, Storrs.

Calhoun, P. S., Beckham, J. C., & Bosworth, H. B. (2002). Caregiver burden and psychological distress in partners of veterans with chronic posttraumatic stress disorder. *Journal of Traumatic Stress, 15,* 205–212.

Card, J. J. (1987). Epidemiology of PTSD in a national cohort of Vietnam veterans. *Journal of Clinical Psychology, 43*(1), 6–17.

Carroll, E. M., Rueger, D. B., Foy, D. W., & Donohoe, C. P. (1985). Vietnam combat veterans with PTSD: Analysis of marital and cohabitating adjustment. *Journal of Abnormal Psychology, 94,* 329–337.

Davidson, J. R., Hughes, D., Blazer, D. G., & George, L. K. (1991). Post-traumatic stress disorder in the community: An epidemiological study. *Psychological Medicine, 21,* 713–721.

Dessaulles, A. (1991). *The treatment of clinical depression in the context of marital distress.* Unpublished doctoral dissertation, University of Ottawa, Canada.

Devilly, G. J. (2002). The psychological effects of a lifestyle management course on war veterans and their spouses. *Journal of Clinical Psychology, 58,* 1119–1134.

Dirkzwager, A. J. E., Bramsen, I., Ader, H., & van der Ploeg, H. M. (2005). Secondary traumatization in partners and parents of Dutch peacekeeping soldiers. *Journal of Family Psychology, 19,* 217–226.

Dunn, R. L., & Schwebel, A. I. (1995). Meta-analytic review of marital therapy outcome research. *Journal of Family Psychology, 9*(1), 58–68.

Erickson, C. A. (1989). Rape and the family. In C. R. Figley (Ed.), *Treating stress in families* (pp. 257–289). New York: Brunner/Mazel.

Figley, C. R. (1983). Catastrophes: An overview of family reactions. In C. R. Figley & H. I. McCubbin (Eds.), *Stress and the family: Vol. II. Coping with catastrophe* (pp. 3–20). New York: Brunner/Mazel.

Figley, C. R. (1985). From victim to survivor: Social responsibility in the wake of catastrophe. *Trauma and Its Wake,* pp. 398–415.

Figley, C. R. (1986). Traumatic stress: The role of the family and social support system. *Trauma and Its Wake, 2,* 39–54.

Figley, C. R. (1988). A five-phase treatment of post-traumatic stress disorder in families. *Journal of Traumatic Stress, 1*(1), 127–141.

Figley, C. R. (1989). *Helping traumatized families.* San Francisco: Jossey-Bass.

Figley, C. R. (Ed.). (1995). *Compassion fatigue: Coping with secondary traumatic stress disorder in those who treat the traumatized.* New York: Brunner/Mazel.

Foa, E. B., & Rothbaum, B. O. (1998). *Treating the trauma of rape: Cognitive-behavioral therapy for PTSD.* New York: Guilford Press.

Glynn, S. M., Eth, S., Randolph, E. T., Foy, D. W., Leong, G. B., Paz, G. G., et al. (1995). Behavioral family therapy for Vietnam combat veterans with posttraumatic stress disorder. *Journal of Psychotherapy Practice and Research, 4,* 214–223.

Glynn, S. M., Eth, S., Randolph, E. T., Foy, D. W., Urbatis, M., Boxer, L., et al. (1999). A test of behavioral family therapy to augment exposure for combat-related posttraumatic stress disorder. *Journal of Consulting and Clinical Psychology, 67,* 243–251.

Harris, C. J. (1991). A family crisis-intervention model for the treatment of post-traumatic stress reaction. *Journal of Traumatic Stress, 4,* 195–207.

Jacobson, N. S., Dobson, K., Fruzetti, A. E., Schmaling, K. B., & Salusky, S. (1991). Marital therapy as a treatment for depression. *Journal of Consulting and Clinical Psychology, 59,* 547–557.

Jacobson, N. S., & Margolin, G. (1979). *Marital therapy: Strategies based on social learning and behavior exchange principles.* New York: Brunner/Mazel.

Johnson, D. R., Feldman, S. C., & Lubin, H. (1995). Critical interaction therapy: Couples therapy in combat-related posttraumatic stress disorder. *Family Process, 34,* 401–412.

Johnson, S. M. (1989). Integrating marital and individual therapy for incest survivors: A case study. *Psychotherapy, 21*(6), 96–103.

Johnson, S. M. (1996). *The practice of emotionally focused marital therapy: Creating connection.* New York: Brunner/Mazel.

Johnson, S. M. (2002). *Emotionally focused couple therapy with trauma survivors: Strengthening attachment bonds.* New York: Guilford Press.

Johnson, S. M., & Greenberg, L. S. (1985). Emotionally focused couples therapy: An outcome study. *Journal of Marital and Family Therapy, 11,* 313–317.

Johnson, S. M., & Greenberg, L. S. (Eds.). (1994). *The heart of the matter: Perspectives on emotion in marital therapy.* New York: Brunner/Mazel.

Johnson, S. M., & Williams-Keeler, L. (1998). Creating healing relationships for couples dealing with trauma: The use of emotionally focused marital therapy. *Journal of Marital and Family Therapy, 24,* 25–40.

Jordan, B. K., Marmar, C. R., Fairbank, J. A., Schlenger, W. E., Kulka, R. A., Hough, R. L., et al. (1992). Problems in families of male Vietnam veterans with posttraumatic stress disorder. *Journal of Consulting and Clinical Psychology, 60*(6), 916–926.

McCann, I. L., & Pearlman, L. A. (1990). *Psychological trauma and the adult survivor: Theory, therapy, and transformation.* New York: Brunner/Mazel.

McLeod, J. D., Kessler, R. C., & Landis, K. R. (1992). Speed of recovery from major depressive episodes in a community sample of married men and women. *Journal of Abnormal Psychology, 101,* 277–286.

Mio, J. S., & Foster, J. D. (1991). The effects of rape upon victims and families: Implications for a comprehensive family therapy. *American Journal of Family Therapy, 19*(2), 147–159.

Monson, C. M., Schnurr, P. P., Stevens, S. P., & Guthrie, K. A. (2004). Cognitive-behavioral couple's treatment for posttraumatic stress disorder: Initial findings. *Journal of Traumatic Stress, 17,* 341–344.

Monson, C. M., Stevens, S. P., & Schnurr, P. P. (2005). Cognitive-behavioral couple's treatment for posttraumatic stress disorder. In T. A. Corales (Ed.), *Focus on posttraumatic stress disorder* (pp. 245–274). Hauppauge, NY: Nova Science.

Mueser, K. T., & Glynn, S. M. (1995). *Behavioral family therapy for psychiatric disorders.* Needham Heights, MA: Allyn & Bacon.

Nelson, B. S., Wangsgaard, S., Yorgason, J., Kessler, M. H., & Carter-Vassol, E. (2002). Single- and dual-trauma couples: Clinical observations of relational characteristics and dynamics. *American Journal of Orthopsychiatry, 72,* 58–69.

O'Farrell, T. J. (1994). Marital therapy and spouse-involved treatment with alcoholic patients. *Behavior Therapy, 25,* 391–406.

Rabin, C., & Nardi, C. (1991). Treating post traumatic stress disorder couples: A psychoeducational program. *Community Mental Health Journal, 27*(3), 209–224.

Riggs, D. S., Byrne, C. A., Weathers, F. W., & Litz, B. T. (1998). The quality of intimate relationships of male Vietnam veterans: Problems associated with posttraumatic stress disorder. *Journal of Traumatic Stress, 11,* 87–102.

Rosenheck, R., & Thompson, J. (1986). "Detoxification" of Vietnam War trauma: A combined family–individual approach. *Family Process, 25,* 559–570.

Sherman, M. D. (2003). The SAFE Program: A family psychoeducational curriculum developed in a Veterans Affairs medical center. *Professional Psychology: Research and Practice, 34,* 42–48.

Sherman, M. D. (2006). Updates and five-year evaluation of the S.A.F.E. Program: A family psychoeducational program for serious mental illness. *Community Mental Health Journal, 42,* 213–219.

Solomon, Z., Bleich, A., Shoham, S., Nardi, C., & Kotler, M. (1992). The "Koach" project for treatment of combat-related PTSD: Rationale, aims, and methodology. *Journal of Traumatic Stress, 5*(2), 175–193.

Solomon, Z., Mikulincer, M., Fried, B., & Wosner, Y. (1987). Family characteristics and posttraumatic stress disorder: A follow-up of Israeli combat stress reaction casualties. *Family Process, 26*(3), 383–394.

Solomon, Z., Waysman, M., & Mikulincer, M. (1990). Family functioning, perceived social support, and combat-related psychopathology: The moderating role of loneliness. *Journal of Social and Clinical Psychology, 9,* 456–472.

Sweany, S. L. (1988). *Marital and life adjustment of Vietnam combat veterans: A treatment outcome study.* Unpublished doctoral dissertation, University of Washington, Seattle.

Syrotuik, J., & D'Arcy, C. (1984). Social support and mental health: Direct, protective and compensatory effects. *Social Science and Medicine, 18,* 229–236.

Tarrier, N., Sommerfield, C., & Pilgrim, H. (1999). Relatives' expressed emotion (EE) and PTSD treatment outcome. *Psychological Medicine, 29,* 801–811.

Waysman, M., Mikulincer, M., Solomon, Z., & Weisenberg, M. (1993). Secondary traumatization among wives of posttraumatic combat veterans: A family typology. *Journal of Family Psychology, 7,* 104–118.

Williams, C. M., & Williams, T. (1980). Family therapy for Vietnam veterans. In T. Williams (Ed.), *Post-traumatic stress disorder of the Vietnam veteran* (pp. 221–231). Cincinnati, OH: Disabled American Veterans.

Williamson, D. S. (1982a). Personal authority via termination of the intergenerational hierarchical boundary: Part II. The consultation process and the therapeutic methods. *Journal of Marital and Family Therapy, 8,* 23–37.

Williamson, D. S. (1982b). Personal authority in family experiences via termination of the intergenerational hierarchical boundary: Part III. Personal authority defined, and the power of play in the change process. *Journal of Marital and Family Therapy, 8,* 309–323.

CHAPTER 19

Creative Therapies for Adults

David Read Johnson, Mooli Lahad, and Amber Gray

The creative arts therapies involve trained therapists' intentional use of art, music, dance/movement, drama, and poetry in psychotherapy, counseling, special education, or rehabilitation. Creative arts therapies, as professions, began during the 1940s, when a number of psychotherapists and artists began collaborating in the treatment of severely disturbed clients. Because many severely disturbed patients were unable to utilize the highly verbal modality of psychoanalysis, nonverbal forms of communication seemed to hold much promise. Creative arts therapies were nurtured in a few long-term psychiatric hospitals, such as St. Elizabeths in Washington, DC, the Menninger Clinic in Topeka, Kansas, and Chestnut Lodge in Rockville, Maryland, and by psychiatrists such as Jacob Moreno, who had introduced action-oriented techniques into psychotherapy in the 1930s. There are approximately 15,000 trained creative arts therapists in the United States, and several thousand in other parts of the world.[1] Creative arts therapists are trained in specialized university programs, usually a 2- to 3-year master's degree (music therapists may receive training at the bachelor's or master's degree level). Several PhD programs also exist. Scholarship from the faculties of over 100 universities is regularly reported in the eight professional journals in the field.

Theoretical Context

Initially, the creative arts therapies were justified by psychoanalytic concepts, such as projection, externalization, and abreaction, or, less convincingly, by assumptions of the value of artistic expression. More recently, however, it has become evident that the creative arts therapies owe their effectiveness to the same therapeutic elements contained in cognitive-behavioral treatments. Thus, although specific creative arts therapy treatments for trauma have not yet been sufficiently tested, many of the major components of creative arts therapy treatments have received a great deal of empirical support.

Imaginal exposure is perhaps the most important therapeutic element in trauma treatment. All forms of creative arts therapy treatment of trauma utilize imaginal exposure, in that the trauma scene is represented in the artwork, dramatic role play, movement, poetry, or music. Lahad (2006) has pointed out the similarities between the "as if" nature of creative imagination and imaginal exposure. Halfway between *in vivo* and *in vitro* exposure, the client not only imagines the trauma scene but also represents it in physical or constructional behavior. The concretization of the traumatic imagery may be especially helpful in overcoming the client's avoidant tendencies. In addition, the sensory stimulation provided by the arts media may also enhance the vividness of traumatic imagery. Moreno's psychodrama demonstrated the power of such imaginal exposure in the 1940s and 1950s, and stimulated renewed interest among psychologists in studying imagery (Singer, 2005; Weis, Smucker, & Dresser, 2003). Use of guided imagery became an important element in early flooding procedures for posttraumatic stress disorder (PTSD) (Keane, Fairbank, Caddell, & Zimmering, 1989) and continues in a variety of methods in cognitive-behavioral therapy (Krakow et al., 2001), as well as the creative arts therapies (Blake & Bishop, 1994; Orth, Doorschodt, Verburgt, & Drozdek, 2004).

Cognitive restructuring is another very important therapeutic factor in trauma treatment. Psychologists in the 1950s demonstrated the effectiveness of role playing in attitude change (Hovland, Janis, & Kelley, 1953), so much so that role playing has been integrated into most forms of education and many types of psychological intervention (McMullin, 1986). Role playing (and its relative, *covert modeling*), not surprisingly, have become standard elements in many forms of trauma treatment (e.g., Foa & Rothbaum, 1998). Playing out scenes, switching roles, and replaying more health-promoting options can be very effective means of changing or challenging a person's view of a situation. Placing clients in action elicits new behaviors that expand their repertoires of responses to challenging situations. "Role playing is a way to learn new behaviors and words for old ways of doing things. . . . The repeated practice of a behavior reduces anxiety and makes it more likely that a new behavior will be used" (Foa & Rothbaum, 1998, p. 217).

Cognitive interventions, including identification of distorted cognitions, cognitive reprocessing, and reframing, are essential components of the creative arts therapies. The aim is to impact clients' narratives of their traumatic experience, often termed "restorying." The use of journaling, writing, and storytelling are common narrative techniques in the creative arts therapies, especially following nonverbal interventions such as art, movement, or music (Lahad, 1992; Rose, 1999). Producing the trauma narrative is a component of many cognitive-behavioral forms of intervention (Cohen, Mannarino, & Deblinger, 2006; Rynearson, 2001). An increasing number of clinical studies that utilize storytelling and narrative with trauma survivors has been published (Fry & Barker, 2002; Meyer-Weitz & Sliep, 2005; Reisner, 2002).

Stress/anxiety management skills are also important elements of effective trauma treatment, especially relaxation techniques. These techniques were integrated into behavioral treatment for anxiety disorders in the 1960s, and have been utilized in trauma treatments, particularly as stress inoculation training (Meichenbaum, 1974). Techniques such as progressive muscle relaxation (Bernstein & Borkovec, 1973) and deep breathing are standard elements in most forms of creative arts therapy for trauma (Dayton, 1997; Gray, 2002; Levy, 1995). Attention to basic physiological functions, such as breathing, muscular tonality, and heart rate, may improve their regulation.

Resilience enhancement techniques have more recently received greater attention (Bonanno, 2005). Here the creative arts therapies can presumably make a useful contribution because most studies of resilience emphasize the importance of creativity, humor, spontaneity, flexibility, and activity, all of which are incorporated into creative arts therapy methods (Johnson, 1987; Lahad, 1999, 2000; Raynor, 2002). Creative activity increasingly is being recommended for traumatized clients (Bloom, 1997). Creative arts therapies may improve the self-esteem, hope, and prosocial behavior of clients with PTSD, and reduce feelings of shame and guilt, through the association of traumatic material to adaptive and aesthetic modes of expression. These modalities are also being utilized increasingly in community-based resilience programs (Gray, 2002; Losi, Reisner, & Salvatici, 2002; Mapp & Koch, 2004; Reisner, 2002).

Effective therapeutic interventions at the social level include testimony, public education, and destigmatization, which may be enhanced through creative forms. For example, theater and dance performances by trauma victims, exhibitions of victims' artworks, and public readings of victims' poetry serve to educate the public about trauma, destigmatize the condition of PTSD, and offer the victims themselves an avenue for reintegration into society (Jones, 1997; Losi et al., 2002; Mapp & Koch, 2004; Meyer-Weitz & Sliep, 2005; Sithamparanathan, 2003).

In summary, studies of the creative arts therapies will most likely indicate that their effectiveness is due to their use of empirically supported therapeutic factors of imaginal exposure, cognitive/narrative restructuring, stress management skills, resilience enhancement, and testimonial methods.

The Unique Contribution of the Creative Arts Therapies

The potential advantage of utilizing creative arts therapy procedures is most likely based on the nonverbal (behavioral) aspects of the artistic modalities. First, the symbolic media of the arts may provide more complete access to implicit (as opposed to explicit) memory systems, as well as visual–kinesthetic schemas (Johnson, 1987; van der Kolk, 1994). It seems possible that certain aspects of traumatic experience and associated distorted schemas are stored in these nonlexical forms. By providing a wider range of stimuli (visual, sonic, tactile, and kinesthetic), the creative arts therapies may increase the vividness of imaginal exposure. By providing concretized forms of representation (visual, written, and enacted), the creative arts therapies may help to decrease avoidance. Both of these effects should lead to greater habituation of the client's fear response. The behavioral nature of the creative arts therapies may also support or enhance cognitive restructuring strategies. All of these potential effects appear to be especially helpful with clients with dissociative tendencies (Kellerman & Hudgins, 2000; Kluft, 1992; Mills, 1995).

> Like other victims of childhood trauma, DID [dissociative identity disorder] patients are often uniquely responsive to nonverbal approaches. Art therapy, occupational therapy, sand tray therapy, movement therapy, other play therapy derivatives, and recreational therapy are reported as helpful toward achieving treatment goals, including integration. (International Society for the Study of Dissociation, 1997, p. 6)

Second, the claim that creative arts therapies are especially helpful to traumatized, inexpressive persons has been supported by the concept of "alexithymia," about which much has been written in the trauma field (Krystal, 1988). The inability to put feelings into words appears to be relatively common in patients with PTSD. Presumably, clients who are unable to find words to express their experience may find the nonverbal/behavioral forms of the creative arts a more welcoming means of expression (Lev-Wiesel, 1998; Levy, 1995). Creative arts therapies may facilitate the restoration of the developmental progression from sensory–motor to symbolic to lexical modes of representation, therefore aiding language skills acquisition (Greenberg & van der Kolk, 1989). This may be the reason why creative arts therapies have been especially useful with children (see Goodman, Chapman, & Gantt, Chapter 20, this volume).

Description of Techniques

Given the numerous formats and models in the creative arts therapies, it is a difficult task to describe them in a comprehensive manner. Nevertheless, we can outline some general principles. Generally, a typical session, whether with an individual, family, or group, begins with discussion about how clients are doing and what problems or concerns they have been facing. Then, instead of exploring these issues in continued verbal discussion, the therapist guides the client(s) into the use of a particular art medium, such as painting, movement, role playing, or listening to or creating poetry or music, as a means of working on the presenting problem. Often, the therapist leads the client in warm-up or relaxation exercises to help prepare for the work and/or focus on the issue (i.e., "stress management"). These activities typically open up and relax the client, and indicate to the therapist the client's mood or level of anxiety about the presenting issue.

The creative arts therapist attempts to understand the client's behavior in terms of the particular art medium: For example, the art therapist attends to the expressive qualities of different colors, lines, forms, patterns, and arrangements; the dance/movement therapist assesses the meaning of different movement patterns and qualities, efforts, rhythms, energy flow, articulation of body parts, and use of space; the drama therapist notes the patterns and types of gestures, roles, and flow of dramatic action; the poetry therapist attends to word choice, images, or metaphors selected; and the music therapist attends to the rhythm, harmony, pitch, timbre, and meter of the client's musical expressions. Cultural and social contexts are always taken into account in these observations.

The main part of the session is spent participating in the arts medium. In treatment models specifically designed for psychological trauma, the traumatic memories are worked on directly (i.e., "imaginal exposure"); for example, when a man is having trouble with memories of physical abuse by his father, the drama therapist may take on the role of his father as they role-play the scene. At other times, the client draws, sings, or improvises, and issues linked to the trauma are addressed by the therapist as they emerge. For example, the art therapist may ask the client to draw a picture of her home before the abuse began, or a picture of her feelings of anger, or her perception of her own body. The music therapist may help the client to produce an improvised song concerning the impact of the rape on her life. A dance movement therapist may assist the client to identify and demonstrate movement gestures that depict the feeling associated with a traumatic experience, as well as a contrasting, more positive feeling. The client in poetry therapy may write and then read a poem written as a letter to a buddy who died in Vietnam. In each of these activities, in addition to the client's manifest thoughts that arise about the subject, it is believed that the presence of the rhythms, melodies, colors, gestures, and actions of the arts media enhances the possibility that new aspects of the situation will be discovered. These sensory prompts may allow for a more vivid recollection of the trauma scene. Usually the therapist attempts to direct the client toward more healthy views of his or her traumatic experience (i.e., "cognitive restructuring"), by encouraging him or her to represent in the art medium a more hopeful or accurate perspective, or to articulate a more integrated narrative (i.e., "restorying"). The concretization of the client's issues in the art form tends to serve as a distancing tool, allowing the client to reflect on his or her own behavior in real-life situations.

The creative arts therapies have been used both to target specific PTSD symptoms and to address other, associated conditions and functional problems (Carey, 2006; Thomas, 2005). Exposure-based components address reexperiencing and avoidance symptoms, and relaxation and distraction-based components target hyperarousal symptoms. Group interaction components aim to improve interpersonal relationships, communication skills, and work functioning. Creativity/performance-based components aim to increase resilience and reduce shame caused by victimization. The multifaceted aspects of creative arts therapy treatment lend themselves to broadly defined treatment goals. Thus, Cruz and Essen (1994) note that many adult survivors of childhood trauma can benefit from the inclusion of arts therapies into their overall psychotherapy treatment program.

Literature Review

The creative arts therapies have been utilized with all types of trauma, though there are no data to indicate whether their efficacy varies according to type of traumatic event, single versus repeated traumatization, or age of traumatization (Cohen, Barnes, & Rankin, 1995; Dayton, 1997; Kellerman & Hudgins, 2000; Kluft, 1992; Spring, 1993; Winn, 1994). Clinical experience suggests that the creative arts therapies have been helpful for clients with acute trauma in accessing memories of their trauma or abuse (Steele, 2003). These therapies have been increasingly applied in cross-cultural interventions with survivors of war, torture, and disasters (Baker, 2006; Callaghan, 1993; Gray, 2001, 2002; Hardi & Erdos, 1998; Lahad, 1999, 2000; van der Velden & Koops, 2005). The creative arts therapies have also aided clients with chronic PTSD address conditions of demoralization and hopelessness (Dintino & Johnson, 1996; Feldman, Johnson, & Ollayos, 1994).

The dearth of experimental research on the creative arts therapies is due largely to the lack of training of practitioners in research methodology and the relatively few available doctoral-level programs in the creative arts therapies. Evidence from clinical case studies indicates that two areas of improvement have most often been noted: (1) primary symptoms of PTSD and (2) global clinical improvement. Noted less often are improvements in functional behaviors or clinical service utilization. The mean effect size of dance/movement therapy for core psychiatric symptoms, based on meta-analyses, has been estimated as 0.37 (range = 0.15–0.54; Cruz & Sabers, 1998). However, no estimates are available with specifically PTSD populations, nor, to our knowledge, have any meta-analyses been completed on the other creative arts therapy modalities. Most empirical work has focused on assessment, particularly in the discipline of art therapy. In a review of the empirical literature on graphic indicators of sexual abuse, Trowbridge (1995) found 12 studies that met inclusion criteria. In summarizing the results of this meta-analysis, she wrote, "Presence of the following indicators in children's drawings warrants further investigation: genitalia, hands omitted, fingers omitted, and head only drawn" (p. 492).

We found few empirical studies of the creative arts therapies in the treatment of trauma. Morgan and Johnson (1995) used a single-case experimental (A-B-A) design that demonstrated significant reductions in PTSD symptoms and frequency of nightmares after an art therapy intervention with Vietnam War veterans. Johnson, Lubin, Hale, and James (1997) found that the creative arts therapies produced higher rates of short-term symptom reduction among

Vietnam War veterans in an inpatient PTSD program, though, as a whole, the program showed modest therapeutic effects. The art therapy group was found to be most beneficial for the more symptomatic veterans. Similar results were found from another Department of Veterans Affairs (VA) inpatient PTSD program (Ragsdale, Cox, Finn, & Eisler, 1996).

Most of the evidence of efficacy is derived from clinical reports and case studies. The creative arts therapies have been cited as helpful in reduction of alexithymia (Duey, 1991; James & Johnson, 1996), increase in emotional control (Cohen et al., 1995; Slotoroff, 1994), improvement in interpersonal relationships (Carey, 2006; Dintino & Johnson, 1996), decrease in dissociation and anxiety (Duey, 1991; Greenberg & van der Kolk, 1989; Jacobson, 1994), decrease in nightmares and sleep problems (Daniels & McGuire, 1998; Hernandez-Ruiz, 2005; Morgan & Johnson, 1995), improved body image (Simonds, 1992), and reduction of depression (Clendenon-Wallen, 1991). In the nomenclature used in this volume, all of these reports would be coded as Level D or E in terms of support.

Specialized Methods Targeting PTSD

A number of creative arts therapy methods have been designed specifically to target PTSD symptoms and trauma-related pathology. Though none of these approaches has been empirically tested in randomized, controlled studies, each has shown promise as an effective technique for trauma symptomatology. Barry Cohen and his colleagues (1995; Cohen & Mills, 1999; Cox & Cohen, 2005) have developed a method of art therapy that carefully guides the client through increasing levels of exposure to traumatic imagery. Helen Bonny and her colleagues have developed a method called guided imagery and music that has been used successfully with traumatized populations (Blake & Bishop, 1994; Schulberg, 1997). In this approach, clients recall their traumatic experience while specifically selected music is playing. Kay Adams (1997) developed a form of journal therapy, in which the client's trauma narrative is developed, then restructured through a creative writing process. Mooli Lahad (1992) designed the six-part story method, a creative narrative technique that helps clients achieve successful coping responses. This method has been applied widely in community stress prevention settings, disaster relief, as well as psychotherapy (Lahad, 1999, 2000). More recently, Lahad (2006) has integrated this method with cognitive-behavioral therapy, using a set of cards that the client selects that serve as anchors to the traumatic recall. Kate Hudgins (2002) has designed the therapeutic spiral method of psychodrama that applies various methods of affect containment, cognitive restructuring, and testimony. The approach has been applied with refugees and disaster victims, as well as psychotherapy clients. Amber Gray (2002) has developed a dance/movement therapy intervention called the center post model, specifically for refugees and survivors of torture, war, and disasters. David Johnson and his colleagues (Dintino & Johnson, 1996; James & Johnson, 1996; Landers, 2002) have applied a drama therapy technique called developmental transformations to numerous trauma populations. Using improvisational role playing, the clients are gradually guided through recalling their traumatic experiences, then encouraged to transform them playfully into more health-promoting forms.

Known Risks and Side Effects

There are no known risks or side effects specific to the creative arts therapies when used by appropriately educated and trained therapists. Occasionally, as in most forms of trauma treatment, clients may become overwhelmed when accessing traumatic material too quickly or too intensively, though these reactions can often be prevented through specific structuring techniques within the session (Carey, 2006; Cohen et al., 2006).

Summary and Recommendations

Despite relatively wide use and application, the efficacy of the creative arts therapies has not yet been established through empirical research. Implementation of rigorous empirical research studies in this area is a primary priority for the field. Creative arts therapy professionals claim that these treatment modalities may be useful as either primary or adjunctive interventions (Johnson, 1987). There is clinical consensus that use of the creative arts may be helpful as an adjunct to the treatment of PTSD under the following conditions: (1) The arts therapy is conducted by a practitioner educated and trained in that approach; (2) the therapy is conducted with the permission of the client; and (3) the therapy is conducted in conjunction with other, ongoing treatments and therapists. The exact source of therapeutic benefits of the creative arts therapies in the treatment of PTSD has not been identified, but it is likely to be a combination of generic psychological processes (e.g., imaginal exposure, cognitive restructuring, stress management, resilience enhancement, and testimony), physiological processes, and specific contributions of nonverbal and creative elements. There is currently insufficient evidence to differentiate the impact of the creative arts therapies on PTSD, comorbid disorders, or associated symptoms.

In conclusion, we offer the following three recommendations regarding the creative arts therapies in the treatment of trauma.

1. The recognition, justification, and further development of the creative arts therapies in the treatment of psychological trauma will be most fully encouraged by more sophisticated empirical inquiries using control groups and randomized assignment.
2. Creative arts therapy treatments designed as specific treatments for PTSD will presumably have heightened therapeutic effects over nonspecific creative arts therapy approaches. We recommend the further design, development, and testing of such treatments.

3. The unique contribution of the creative arts therapies cross-culturally, particularly in underdeveloped countries, in translation of effective intervention models across linguistic barriers and diverse cultural traditions should be investigated further.

Note

1. American Art Therapy Association (*www.arttherapy.org*), American Dance Therapy Association (*www.adta.org*), American Music Therapy Association (*www.musictherapy.org*), American Society for Group Psychotherapy and Psychodrama (*www.asgpp.org*), National Association for Drama Therapy (*www.nadt.org*), National Association for Poetry Therapy (*www.poetrytherapy.org*), Israel Association of Arts Therapists (*www.yahat.org*), European Consortium for Arts Therapy Education (*www.ecarte.info*).

References

Adams, K. (1997). *The way of the journal.* Denver, CO: Sidran Press.

Baker, B. (2006). Art speaks in healing survivors of war: The use of art therapy in treating trauma survivors. *Journal of Aggression, Maltreatment and Trauma, 12,* 183–198.

Bernstein, D., & Borkovec, T. (1973). *Progressive muscle relaxation training.* New York: Research Press.

Blake, R., & Bishop, S. (1994). The Bonny method of guided imagery and music in the treatment of posttraumatic stress disorder with adults in the psychiatric setting. *Music Therapy Perspectives, 12,* 125–129.

Bloom, S. (1997). *Creating sanctuary.* New York: Routledge.

Bonanno, G. (2005). Resilience in the face of potential trauma. *Current Directions in Psychological Science, 14,* 135–138.

Callaghan, K. (1993). Movement psychotherapy with adult survivors of political torture and organized violence. *Arts in Psychotherapy, 20,* 411–421.

Carey, L. (2006). *Expressive and creative arts methods for trauma survivors.* London: Jessica Kingsley.

Clendenon-Wallen, J. (1991). The use of music therapy to influence the self-confidence of adolescents who are sexually abused. *Music Therapy Perspectives, 9,* 17–31.

Cohen, B., Barnes, M., & Rankin, A. (1995). *Managing traumatic stress through art.* Lutherville, MD: Sidran Press.

Cohen, B., & Mills, A. (1999). Skin/paper/bark: Body image, trauma, and the Diagnostic Drawing Series. In J. Goodwin & R. Attias (Eds.), *Splintered reflections: Images of the body in trauma* (pp. 203–221). New York: Basic Books.

Cohen, J. A., Mannarino, A., & Deblinger, E. (2006). *Treating trauma and traumatic grief in children and adolescents.* New York: Guilford Press.

Cox, C., & Cohen, B. (2005). The unique role of art making in the treatment of dissociative identity disorder. *Psychiatric Annals, 35,* 685–694.

Cruz, F., & Essen, L. (1994). *Adult survivors of childhood emotional, physical, and sexual abuse.* Northvale, NJ: Aronson.

Cruz, R., & Sabers, D. (1998). Dance/movement therapy is more effective than previously reported. *Arts in Psychotherapy, 25,* 101–104.

Daniels, L., & McGuire, T. (1998). Dreamcatchers: Healing traumatic nightmares using group dreamwork, sandplay, and other techniques of intervention. *Group, 22,* 205–227.

Dayton, T. (1997). *Heartwounds: The impact of unresolved trauma and grief on relationships.* Deerfield Beach, FL: Health Communication.

Dintino, C., & Johnson, D. (1996). Playing with the perpetrator: Gender dynamics in developmental drama therapy. In S. Jennings (Ed.), *Drama therapy: Theory and practice* (Vol. 3, pp. 205–220). London: Routledge.

Duey, C. J. (1991). Group music therapy for women with multiple personalities. In K. E. Bruscia (Ed.), *Case studies in music therapy* (pp. 513–528). Phoenixville, PA: Barcelona.

Feldman, S., Johnson, D., & Ollayos, M. (1994). The use of writing in the treatment of PTSD. In J. Sommer & M. Williams (Eds.), *The handbook of post-traumatic therapy* (pp. 366–385). Westport, CT: Greenwood Press.

Foa, E. B., & Rothbaum, B. O. (1998). *Treating the trauma of rape: Cognitive-behavioral therapy for PTSD.* New York: Guilford Press.

Fry, P., & Barker, L. (2002). Female survivors of abuse and violence: The influence of storytelling reminiscence on perceptions of self-efficacy, ego strength, and self-esteem. In J. Webster & B. Haight (Eds.), *Critical advances in reminiscence work* (pp. 197–217). New York: Springer.

Gray, A. (2001). The body remembers: Dance/movement therapy with an adult survivor. *American Journal of Dance Therapy, 23,* 29–43.

Gray, A. (2002). The body as voice: Somatic psychology and dance/movement therapy with survivors of war and torture. *Connections, 3,* 2–4.

Greenberg, M., & van der Kolk, B. (1989). Retrieval and integration with the "painting cure." In B. van der Kolk (Ed.), *Psychological trauma* (pp. 191–216). Washington, DC: American Psychiatric Press.

Hardi, L., & Erdos, E. (1998). Nonverbal therapy of traumatized war victims. *Torture, 8,* 82–85.

Hernandez-Ruiz, E. (2005). Effect of music therapy on anxiety levels and sleep patterns of abused women in shelters. *Journal of Music Therapy, 42,* 140–158.

Hovland, C., Janis, I., & Kelley, H. (1953). *Communication and persuasion.* New York: Basic Books.

Hudgins, K. (2002). *Experiential treatment for PTSD: The therapeutic spiral model.* New York: Springer.

International Society for the Study of Dissociation. (1997). *Treatment guidelines.* Washington, DC: Author.

Jacobson, M. (1994). Abreacting and assimilating traumatic, dissociated memories of MPD patients through art therapy. *Art Therapy, 11,* 4–52.

James, M., & Johnson, D. (1996). Drama therapy for the treatment of affective expression in post-traumatic stress disorder. In D. Nathanson (Ed.), *Knowing feeling: Affect, script, and psychotherapy* (pp. 303–326). New York: Norton.

Johnson, D. (1987). The role of the creative arts therapies in the diagnosis and treatment of psychological trauma. *Arts in Psychotherapy, 14,* 7–14.

Johnson, D., Lubin, H., Hale, K., & James, M. (1997). Single session effects of treatment components within a specialized inpatient posttraumatic stress disorder program. *Journal of Traumatic Stress, 10,* 377–390.

Jones, J. (1997). Art therapy with a community of survivors. *Art Therapy, 14,* 89–94.

Keane, T., Fairbank, J., Caddell, J., & Zimmering, R. (1989). Implosive (flooding) therapy reduces symptoms of PTSD in Vietnam combat veterans. *Behavior Therapy, 20,* 245–260.

Kellerman, P., & Hudgins, K. (2000). *Psychodrama with trauma survivors: Acting out your pain.* London: Jessica Kingsley.

Kluft, E. (Ed.). (1992). *Expressive and functional therapies in the treatment of multiple personality disorder.* Springfield, IL: Thomas.

Krakow, B., Hollifield, M., Schrader, R., Koss, M., Tandberg, D., Lauriello, J., et al. (2001). A randomized controlled study of imagery rehearsal therapy for chronic nightmares in sexual assault survivors with posttraumatic stress disorder. *Journal of the American Medical Association, 286,* 537–545.

Krystal, H. (1988). *Integration and self-healing: Affect, trauma, alexithymia.* Hillsdale, NJ: Analytic Press.

Lahad, M. (1992). Storymaking in assessment methods for coping with stress. In S. Jennings (Ed.), *Dramatherapy: Theory and practice II* (pp. 150–163). London: Routledge.

Lahad, M. (1999). The use of drama therapy with crisis intervention groups, following mass evacuation. *Arts in Psychotherapy, 26,* 27–33.

Lahad, M. (2000). Darkness over the abyss: Supervising crisis intervention teams following disaster. *Traumatology, 6,* 273–293.

Lahad, M. (2006). *Fantastic reality.* Haifa: Nord. (in Hebrew)

Landers, F. (2002). Dismantling violent forms of masculinity through developmental transformations. *Arts in Psychotherapy, 29,* 19–30.

Lev-Wiesel, R. (1998). Use of a drawing technique to encourage verbalization in adult survivors of sexual abuse. *Arts in Psychotherapy, 25,* 257–262.

Levy, F. (Ed.). (1995). *Dance and other expressive art therapies: When words are not enough.* New York/London: Routledge.

Losi, N., Reisner, S., & Salvatici, S. (2002). *Psychosocial and trauma response in war-torn societies: Supporting traumatized communities through arts and theatre.* Geneva: International Organization for Migration.

Mapp, I., & Koch, D. (2004). Creation of a group mural to promote healing following a mass trauma. In N. B. Webb (Ed.), *Mass trauma and violence: Helping families and children cope* (pp. 100–119). New York: Guilford Press.

McMullin, R. (1986). *Handbook of cognitive therapy techniques.* New York: Norton.

Meichenbaum, D. (1974). *Cognitive behavior modification.* Morristown, NJ: General Learning Press.

Meyer-Weitz, A., & Sliep, Y. (2005). The evaluation of Narrative Theatre training: Experiences of psychological workers in Burundi. *Intervention, 3,* 97–111.

Mills, A. (1995). Outpatient art therapy with multiple personality disorder: A survey of current practice. *Art Therapy, 12,* 253–256.

Morgan, C., & Johnson, D. (1995). Use of a drawing task in the treatment of nightmares in combat-related PTSD. *Art Therapy, 12,* 244–247.

Orth, J., Doorschodt, L., Verburgt, J., & Drozdek, B. (2004). Sounds of trauma: An introduction to methodology in music therapy with traumatized refugees in clinical and outpatient settings. In J. Wilson & B. Drozdek (Eds.), *Broken spirits: The treatment of traumatized asylum seekers, refugees, war and torture victims* (pp. 443–480). New York: Brunner/Routledge.

Ragsdale, K., Cox, R., Finn, P., & Eisler, R. (1996). Effectiveness of short-term specialized inpatient treatment for war-related posttraumatic stress disorder: A role for adventure-based counseling and psychodrama. *Journal of Traumatic Stress, 9,* 269–283.

Raynor, C. (2002). The role of play in the recovery process. In W. Zubenko & J. Capoz-zoli (Eds.), *Children and disasters: A practical guide to healing and recovery* (pp. 124–134). New York: Oxford University Press.

Reisner, S. (2002). Staging the unspeakable. In N. Losi, S. Reisner, & S. Salvatici (Eds.), *Psychosocial and trauma response in war-torn societies: Supporting traumatized communities through arts and theatre* (pp. 9–30). Geneva: International Organization for Migration.

Rose, S. (1999). Naming and claiming: The integration of traumatic experience and the reconstruction of self in survivors' stories of sexual abuse. In K. Rogers, S. Leydesdorff, & G. Dawson (Eds.), *Trauma and life stories: International perspectives* (pp. 160–179). London: Routledge.

Rynearson, E. (2001). *Retelling violent death.* Philadelphia: Brunner/Routledge.

Schulberg, C. (1997). An unwanted inheritance: Healing transgenerational trauma of the Nazi Holocaust through the Bonny method of guided imagery and music. *Arts in Psychotherapy, 24,* 323–345.

Simonds, S. (1992). Sexual abuse and body image: Approaches and implications for treatment. *Arts in Psychotherapy, 19,* 289–294.

Singer, J. (2005). *Imagery in psychotherapy.* Washington, DC: American Psychological Association.

Sithamparanathan, K. (2003). Interventions and methods of the Theatre Action Group. *International Journal of Mental Health, Psychosocial Work, and Counseling in Areas of Armed Conflict, 1,* 44–47.

Slotoroff, C. (1994). Drumming technique for assertiveness and anger management in the short term psychiatric setting for adult and adolescent survivors of trauma. *Music Therapy Perspectives, 12,* 111–116.

Spring, D. (1993). *Shattered images: Phenomenological language of sexual trauma.* Chicago: Magnolia Street.

Steele, W. (2003). Using drawing in short-term trauma resolution. In C. A. Malchiodi (Ed.), *Handbook of art therapy* (pp. 139–151). New York: Guilford Press.

Thomas, P. (2005). Dissociation and internal models of protection: Psychotherapy with child abuse survivors. *Psychotherapy: Theory, Research, Practice and Training, 42,* 20–36.

Trowbridge, M. M. (1995). Graphic indicators of sexual abuse in children's drawings: A review of the literature. *Arts in Psychotherapy, 22,* 485–494.

van der Kolk, B. (1994). The body keeps the score. *Harvard Review of Psychiatry, 1,* 253–265.

van der Velden, I., & Koops, M. (2005). Structure in word and image: Combining narrative therapy and art therapy in groups of survivors of war. *Intervention, 3,* 57–64.

Weis, J., Smucker, M., & Dresser, J. (2003). Imagery: Its history and use in the treatment of posttraumatic stress disorder. In A. Sheikh (Ed.), *Healing images: The role of imagination in health* (pp. 381–395). Amityville, NY: Baywood.

Winn, L. (1994). *Posttraumatic stress disorder and dramatherapy: Treatment and risk reduction.* London: Jessica Kingsley.

CHAPTER 20

Creative Arts Therapies for Children

Robin F. Goodman, Linda M. Chapman,
and Linda Gantt

Theoretical Context

Children experience traumas on many levels. Trauma overwhelms physiological structures and psychic functioning, impacting how the event is integrated and assimilated. The images and experiences are stored in incoherent, disorganized, and fragmented ways, often indescribable in words. According to van der Kolk, "Trauma interferes with declarative memory, or conscious recall of the event, but that implicit memory, emotional responses, skills, habits, and sensorimotor sensations related to the experience remain intact" (cited in Klorer, 2000, p. 14). Using the creative arts therapies (CATs) with children who have posttraumatic stress disorder (PTSD) provides a familiar mode of communication when direct verbal access to trauma-related experiences is not possible or advisable.

Rationale for the CATs

According to the most inclusive definition,

> the creative arts therapies include art therapy, dance/movement therapy, drama therapy, music therapy, poetry therapy, and psychodrama. These therapies use arts modalities and creative processes during intentional intervention . . . to foster health, communication, and expression; promote the integration of physical,

491

emotional, cognitive, and social functioning; enhance self-awareness; and facilitate change. . . . Participation in all the creative arts therapies provides people . . . ways to express themselves that may not be possible through more traditional therapies. (National Coalition of Creative Arts Therapies, 2006 [online source])

The CATs are based in diverse theoretical orientations; yet each modality has a rich history either in professional artists' work with individuals having a range of mental health needs, or in mental health professionals' keen interest or background in a particular art form. The different creative arts modalities have qualities especially conducive to trauma-related work. For example, art provides an avenue for exploring associations to color; auditory memories may find expression in music; remembered physical sensations may be revealed in dance/movement therapy; drama and psychodrama facilitate reenactment of interpersonal interaction; and poetry therapy provides a written exposure technique. Vivid words such as "trapped," "frozen," "dirty," or "haunted" lend themselves to being translated into images, movement, music, and drama (Naitove, 1982; Winn, 1994). Although reenactment at a symbolic level may occur with both play and CATs, we distinguish the CATs from play therapy (Gil, 2003), most broadly by the media and art-making processes. In the CATs, meaning is attached to what has been created or performed by the client; in contrast, the client attributes meaning to a ready-made object in play therapy.

According to Nader and Pynoos (1991), relief from PTSD is related to "the degree of perceived control over outcome, to the degree a satisfactory ending is achieved, to the degree that there is freedom to express the prohibited affect or to the degree a cognitive reworking is facilitated" (p. 376). Involvement in the creative arts can offer such relief. "Unique aspects of nonverbal media are applicable at each stage of post traumatic stress disorder treatment, initially gaining access to traumatic memories, working-through and integrating the split-off parts of the self, and finally in re-joining the world of others" (Johnson, 1987, p. 12). Although talking certainly occurs, the mechanism of change is thought to be specific to the nature of the CATs.

A CAT Perspective on Trauma

The presumed value of the CATs for trauma lies in several spheres:

- The creative arts are a part of every culture. They are available and familiar to children in various forms (Bergmann, 2002; Sutton, 2002); hence, they are not necessarily associated with therapy but with other normalizing aspects of life.
- CAT sessions are structured to allow for a safe, containing, and nonthreatening creative transitional space (Johnson, 1987; Kowski, 2007; Kozlowska & Hanney, 2001; Sutton, 2002) in which to explore and master elements of trauma.

- The creative arts provide grounding for threatening material and externalization of metaphors that can be viewed and shared (Loewy & Stewart, 2004; Winn, 1994).
- Materials and nonverbal modes of expression can be paired with psychological tasks in accordance with what a child can tolerate (Clements, Benasutti, & Henry, 2001; Klorer, 2003).
- The CATs allow for individualized intervention to fit a child's level of comfort and readiness to confront traumatic elements.
- The CATs symbolically address the trauma until direct expression can be achieved and tolerated. Metaphors can titrate exposure and provide safety from direct confrontation (Bowers, 1992).
- Engagement in creative activities is enjoyable, resulting in a sense of competence even without attaching verbal meaning (Bergmann, 2002; Kozlowska & Hanney, 2001).
- The creative arts can evoke specific imagery or be relaxing (Atwood & Donheiser, 1997; Cassity & Theobold, 1990; Monti et al., 2006; Winn, 1994).
- The CATs are especially valuable for young children, who have less linguistic sophistication and organization (Klorer, 2000; Lieberman, Van Horn, & Ippen, 2005).

The CATs from a Neuroscience Perspective

Progress in the neurosciences has contributed to an understanding of the complex effects of trauma and abuse, and the mechanism of change in therapy. A scientific understanding of the neural interaction that occurs during engagement in the CATs is rapidly growing, and a more detailed explanation of how imagery and the creative arts facilitate change is emerging (Belkofer & Konopka, 2003; Berrol, 2006; Kruk, 2004).

The somatic nervous system, in cooperation with proprioceptive functions, encodes traumatic experiences in the brain (Rothschild, 2000). During traumatic stress response, neurochemical dysregulation shuts down 80–90% of the brain's potential, mainly in the higher structures, in the service of survival (Pearce, 1992). When this happens, the body and brain record the experience primarily in somatic memory (Ogden & Minton, 2000; Steele, 2003; van der Kolk, 1996). Traumatic material is most commonly recalled consciously, in visual form (Cohn, 1993; Terr, 1991; Tower, 1983), followed by other sensory modes of information processing.

Recent neuroimaging studies suggest that traumatic material is stored in the right hemisphere of the brain, which is associated with visual–motor functioning and emotions (Schiffer, Teicher, & Papanicolaou, 1995; Schore, cited in Hontz, 2006; Siegel, 1999; van der Kolk, 1996). Rauch and colleagues (1996) used positron emission tomographic (PET) scans to determine that individuals with PTSD who were read transcripts of their own accounts of trauma demonstrated heightened activity in the right amygdalar areas of the temporal and frontal cortex and the right visual cortex. The left hemisphere, associated with language and cognitive problem solving, was "turned off." If the left prefrontal cortex is not "on," it will not store verbal information (Perry, Pollard, Blakely, Baker, & Vigilante, 1995). This is evidenced in the typical inability to recall traumatic experiences with linguistic narratives. Van der Kolk (1996) refers to this as "speechless in terror" (p. 234), presumably due to the loss of hippocampal volume. The hippocampus is necessary for encoding and retrieving items from long-term memory (Siegel, 1999). Additionally, Broca's area, the source of language and sequencing, is deactivated.

A lack of cortical consolidation or bilateral cooperation between hemispheres results in impairment of cortical consolidation of memory and integration. Gazzaniga (cited in McNamee, 2004) proposes that "the left brain will weave a story in order to convince itself and you that it is in full control"; furthermore, the "creative output of the right brain is a more reliable expression of experience or emotion" (p. 137).

Effective therapy has to access the right hemisphere of the brain, and art making increases this connectivity (Schore, cited in Hontz, 2006). The CATs operate at the sensorimotor level of information processing, activating the right hemisphere. They provide access to kinesthetic, somatic (Ben-Asher, Koren, Tropea, & Fraenkel, 2002), and nonverbal chaotic remnants of the trauma. The creative product or process serves as a container for the affect, aiding in emotional regulation.

Following activation of the subcortical structures, the limbic structures, the centers for emotional and perceptual processes, are activated. This can occur without processing by higher cortical functions (Bergmann, 2002). Coherent narratives, a core element of resolution, require hemispheric integration (Siegel, 1999). The act of creating offers the opportunity to externalize the imagery associated with the traumatic event. Words and meaning can be attached to these remnants (or fragments) now in tangible form; they can be organized and managed to create coherent narratives. "By activating both right and left hemisphere activity along with both visual and verbal neural pathways, therapeutic potential is maximized as the brain creates a visual, non-verbal narrative that is translated to a coherent linguistic narrative" (Chapman, Morabito, Ladakakos, Schreier, & Knudson, 2001, p. 102).

Description of Techniques

Treatment Variables

When planning CAT interventions a number of variables are considered.

- *Participants.* CAT is conducted with individuals (Ben-Asher et al., 2002; Finan & McCutcheon, 1995; Robb, 1996), families (Hanney & Kozlowska, 2002; Zimmerman, Wolbert, Burgess, & Hartman, 1987), client groups (Atwood & Donheiser, 1997; Powell & Faherty, 1990; Zaidi & Gutierrez-Kovner, 1995), staff groups (Byers, 1996), and community groups (Baráth, 2003; Kalmanowitz & Lloyd, 1999).

- *Format.* Treatments are time-limited, often for acute trauma (Chapman et al., 2001; Robb, 2002; Rousseau, Singh, Lacroix, Bagilshya, & Measham, 2004; Steele & Raider, 2001), or open-ended, often following chronic trauma (Kalmanowitz & Lloyd, 1999; Klorer, 2003). The treatment approach can be directive or nondirective.
- *Interactivity.* The level of interactivity varies among the different CATs and among individual therapists. Certain art forms are more interactive than others. For example, a music therapist may respond to a child via an interwoven melody (Bergmann, 2002; Kowski, 2007). Psychodrama and drama therapy often involve enactment of dynamic relationships (Winn, 1994), whereas, in art therapy, a therapist drawing on a child's work would be considered by many to be an intrusion.
- *Process versus product.* The creative arts allow for the potential to have a "finished product" (a piece of art, a composed song, a monologue, or a choreographed dance). or to focus on the creative process. Using paint spontaneously or improvising with a chosen instrument to reflect a feeling is quite different from painting a landscape or singing along to a favorite recording. The amount and ratio of teaching to exploring or free expression, as well as the degree of emphasis on a product, vary according to the therapist's orientation and the client's needs.
- *Single versus multiple CAT interventions.* Some programs are based on a particular CAT (Coulter, 2000; Steele & Raider, 2001); others use a combination of arts modalities (Akhundov, 1999; Baráth, 2003; Clendenon-Wallen, 1991). The choice of modality is due to therapist variables (e.g., preference) or to the situation (e.g., practicality).

Therapists employ an assorted combination of formats and work in diverse settings, such as short-term psychiatric units (Slotoroff, 1994) and outpatient clinics (Rabenstein & Lehmann, 2000). There are structured, time-limited, multimodality therapy groups (Powell & Faherty, 1990), as well as single-modality, ongoing, nondirective individual art therapy (Clements, 1996). The value of one format and orientation over another has not yet been identified, let alone confirmed.

Overlap of CATs with Other Treatment Modalities

Use of art with children diagnosed with PTSD dates back to some of the earliest trauma-related work. According to Nader and Pynoos (1991), reenactment play and art can be used in psychological first aid and interviewing "to identify traumatic imagery and avoidance, to introduce discussion of the child's individual traumatic experience, . . . to assess the embedded perceptual aspects of the trauma, [and] to transform those aspects" (p. 379), and for brief and long-term therapy "to identify the child's ongoing processing of traumatic aspects of the event and its aftermath, to address ongoing issues of helplessness, self-blame and passivity, to enhance mastery of traumatic intrusive phenomena, [and] to assess the child's progress" (p. 384).

Little has been added to the scientific literature on the use of drawing since Pynoos and Eth's (1986) description of their art-based interviewing technique. Yedidia and Itzhaky (2004) assessed trauma response via a Bridge Drawing and paired characteristics of the drawing to PTSD symptoms and conducted treatment accordingly. Gross and Hayne (1998), in a small study with young public school children without a known trauma history, concluded that drawing and talking about emotional experiences resulted in more information than talking alone, and that it was as accurate as talking alone. This has important implications for the use of the creative arts in trauma treatment and suggests that there is value in combining a directive, art-based approach with exposure techniques.

Currently, there seem to be two streams of clinical work and research using the CATs. In one, treatment is conceptualized around the creative modality and uses creative arts activities. In the other, art, dance/movement, music, and/or drama/psychodrama-based activities support intervention with a non-CAT theoretical premise, usually conducted by non-creative-arts therapists.[1] For example, many trauma-focused cognitive-behavioral therapy (CBT) interventions include drawing, songwriting or playacting to address affect identification or to create a trauma narrative (Goodman, 2004; TF-CBT Web, 2006). Art therapists Sobol and Schneider (1996) make a slightly different distinction, describing the therapy they conduct as a blend of art- and trauma-based models using a phase-specific sequence and more supportive, studio-based treatment.

In using a CAT as the primary intervention, the creative activity is viewed as therapeutic in and of itself. Attaching words about the creative output to the actual trauma happens over time, if at all. "Staying in the metaphor is necessary because often what is expressed in art is not ready to be acknowledged or verbalized consciously. . . . Therapy should focus on exploring the feeling component of what happened, and gaining mastery over feelings that are overwhelming for the child" (Klorer, 2000, pp. 17–18).

Current evidence-based, CBT-oriented practice considers exposure (either direct or indirect via the trauma narrative) to be a primary and necessary component of child trauma interventions (Cohen, Berliner, & March, 2000). Using CAT interventions that do not focus on awareness and recognition of the trauma diverges from such thinking. Unfortunately, research is needed to know whether expression and mastery alone via the CATs, with presumed subsequent changes in the brain, are enough to ameliorate symptoms, or whether linking what is expressed creatively to the actual trauma is necessary. Individual practice rather than science thus far has guided creative arts therapists.

Creative arts therapists do not generally assign their interventions to a specific trauma model, nor refer to common, trauma-related interventions, such as exposure. However, even though they may not use CBT terminology, exposure and cognitive processing are often elements of the work. Zimmerman and colleagues (1987) had children draw and talk about their trauma-related court experiences. Following a Los Angeles earthquake, Roje (1995) had schoolchildren draw a picture of the earthquake the way they "remember it," draw how they felt, and to discuss how to manage feelings and behaviors (p. 243). Baráth (2003) asked, "What is the smell, touch, and color of war?" and "What am I afraid of? How do I cope with it?" (p. 158). Hanney and Kozlowska's (2002) illustrated storybook technique, done with the entire family, is exquisitely similar to making illustrated trauma narratives. Loewy and Stewart (2004) used "story song" for working sequentially with a specific trauma-driven theme. Slotoroff (1994), an obvious exception to other creative arts therapists, reported specifically on his use of improvisational drumming and CBT to address anger and issues of power with adolescent survivors of trauma.

The use and benefit of exposure-related CAT techniques are difficult to determine because they are not regularly practiced or reported as such. Hagood (2000) referred to a finding from a British study that 60% of the art therapists working with sexually abused children used a nondirective approach. This usually equates to a process-oriented, non-CBT approach. Yet, in practice, therapists may do both (Winn, 1994). Hagood argues for using what the case requires, including CBT-oriented intervention.

Method of Collecting Data

We collected literature on the use of CATs for children with PTSD by searching the PsycINFO and the Published International Literature on Traumatic Stress (PILOTS) databases, inputting the terms "art," "dance," "drama," and "music therapy," as well as "children, adolescents, and trauma." Additional literature was obtained based on bibliographical references within selected abstracts, articles, and chapters. The overwhelming majority of literature (including chapters, articles, and research) was related to art therapy. (A PILOTS search yielded 189 art, 11 dance, 35 drama, and 26 music therapy citations.) The preponderance of art-related work is reflected in the following discussion of interventions.

Literature Review

Within the very limited scientific literature on the use of creative arts with any group, there is scant research addressing children with PTSD (see Table 20.1). In the literature that exists, child survivors of sexual and physical abuse (Atwood & Donheiser, 1997; Bowers, 1992; Glaister & McGuinness, 1992; Goodill, 1987; Harvey, 1995; Zaidi & Gutierrez-Kovner, 1995; Weltman, 1986) and war-related trauma (Baráth 2003; Bergmann, 2002; Berman et al., 2001; Kalmanowitz & Lloyd, 1999; Rousseau et al., 2004) were most frequently discussed.

TABLE 20.1. Studies with Randomized Control, Control, and No-Control Groups on Creative Arts Therapies for Children

Study	Target population[a]	Number/ length of sessions	Treatment(s)/control[b]	Major findings	Between- group effect sizes	Within- group effect sizes
Randomized studies						
Chapman et al. (2001)	*N* = 85 (7- to 17-yr-olds with traumatic injury)	1 session	*N* = 31 (1-session art therapy intervention) *N* = 27 (treatment as usual [TAU]) *N* = 27 (did not present PTSD symptoms at baseline)	No significant difference between groups; art therapy participants had significant decrease in avoidance at 1 mo.	N/A	N/A
Nonrandomized studies with a control group						
Coulter (2000)	*N* = 9 (56 admissions; 17 after start; 5 refused, 3 discharged before start; 6 not abused; 16 discharged before end) (9- to 17-yr-olds with sexual or physical abuse)	6 days a wk/8 wk/30- to 45-min sessions	*N* = 9 (music therapy: songwriting) *N* = 9 (recreational music [within subject])	No significant differences.	N/A	N/A
Nonrandomized, without a control group						
Pifalo (2002)	*N* = 13 (8- to 17-yr-olds; sexual abuse)	10-wk group	*N* = 13 (art therapy)	Pre- and posttreatment significant differences on 3 of 10 subscales of the Trauma Symptom Checklist (Anxiety, Posttraumatic Stress, Dissociation-Overt).	N/A	N/A
Steele & Raider (2001)	*N* = 168 (6- to 18-yr-olds; various traumas occurring between 1 wk and 17 yr prior to treatment)	8 sessions	*N* = 168 (art therapy, Structured Sensory Intervention for Traumatized Children, Adolescents and Parents (SITCAP) *N* = 150 (at 3-mo follow-up)	Assessed at intake, at end of 8 sessions and at 3 mo with modified Child PTSD Reaction Index and own child and parent measures. After termination, reported mean differences as significant for reexperience, avoidance, and arousal.	N/A	N/A

[a]*N* = subjects starting study or treatment.
[b]*N* = subjects in data analyses.

498

Case Studies: Individual and Group

The overwhelming majority of literature is in the form of individual or group case studies and vignettes (Cattanach, 1996; Coulter, 2004; Hagood, 2000; Robb, 1996). Typically, the case studies describe nondirective treatment. Structured interventions that are presented in more detail are usually conducted in groups. Specific protocols and manuals are not routinely followed, but a directed sequence of themes and topics is suggested.

Atwood and Donheiser (1997) described their group format for sexually abused preadolescent girls as a "blending of psychological theory and brief solution-focused therapy skills" (p. 197) that employs arts activities such as "reparative visualization" (p. 198) imagery, clay work, mask making, and life-size body drawing.

Powell and Faherty (1990) facilitated structured groups for sexually abused latency-age girls. Group members drew or acted out their sexual abuse experience and initial disclosure. Baráth (2003) paired art activities with themes based on a 12-step approach.

Morgan and White (2003) also used art in conjunction with a specific sequence of critical-incident stress-debriefing sessions with groups. They analyzed the pictures and concluded that art making was beneficial in increasing comfort and promoting expression. However, they seemed to use an impressionistic rather than objective rating system. In an interesting study, Bosnian refugee youth living in Canada were instructed to photograph "people, objects, or events important in their lives" (Berman, Fold-Gilboe, Moutrey, & Cekic, 2001, p. 28) over a 2-week period. What emerged was discussion filled with specific kinesthetic and detailed references to trauma-related events.

Although objective measures were absent, the majority of authors of case studies conclude that progress was made. The studies provided psychosocial background information, a trauma history, and qualitative descriptions of symptoms and behaviors. Rarely were formal evaluations mentioned, nor was a specific DSM-IV psychiatric diagnosis (American Psychiatric Association, 1994) provided. Outcomes were determined by what was created or performed and/or behavioral observations. Roje (1995) accurately outlined PTSD symptoms and described the children she worked with following an earthquake as having nightmares, intrusive thoughts, and avoidance of earthquake-related activity, but she did not specifically assess PTSD. The lack of baseline standardized assessments and diagnostic information on clients in the CAT literature has been especially problematic.

Uncontrolled Studies

Baráth (2003) reported on work in the former Yugoslavia with 99,000 children, teachers, and school staff. Among other results, Baráth reported significant decreases in PTSD symptoms for a sample of 5,628 children, comparing those with high versus low PTSD scores before and after crisis intervention

in one program. A total of 3,710 pieces of art from 530 children were analyzed for trauma symbols according to "carefully prepared instructions"
for using semantic differential scales. A positive change was noted, in that
the artwork was "progressively loaded with more positive emotions, greater
self-empowerment, and an increase in active coping" (p. 165). The massive
undertaking was impressive and encouraging given the extremely difficult
conditions, yet there are no details about any use of scientific rigor for data
collection or analysis.

Following field testing, Steele and Raider (2001) developed the Structured Sensory Intervention for Traumatized Children, Adolescents and Parents (SITCAP) program. They reported a significant reduction in reexperiencing, avoidance, and arousal following participation in their eight-session
intervention, as measured by pre- and posttesting and at 3-month follow-up.
This worthy example for the field follows a rather traditional CBT-oriented
model that used art activities for exposure, telling of the story via a trauma
narrative, and cognitive reframing. However, the results were based on pilot
data; there was neither randomization nor control groups. The results have
not yet been published in a peer-reviewed journal.

Pifalo (2002) used the Trauma Symptom Checklist for Children (TSCC)
to assess change in sexually abused children and adolescents in group art
therapy. She reported a pre- to posttreatment reduction in symptoms. The
results from the small study (13 subjects) must be regarded with caution, but
this foray into research is encouraging.

Of note are two studies based in music therapy. Coulter (2000) looked at
the changes in PTSD symptoms in nine adolescent subjects in songwriting and
recreational music groups. Although no differences were found, the author
reported trends toward a decrease in avoidance and intrusive thoughts, and
possible age effects. However, there were a number of design limitations, such
as mixing participants and non participants in the music group). Rather than
measure symptom change, a 12-week music therapy group (which included
art activities) for 11 adolescents who had been sexually abused, focused on
increasing self-confidence and self-esteem (Clendenon-Wallen, 1991). A pre-
to posttreatment test of self-confidence showed a significant increase in the
small sample, yet no measure of PTSD was provided.

In the uncontrolled research, few (if any) quantifiable variables were
employed to assess individual changes by pre- and posttesting. Clearly, this
would be a first step prior to comparing a particular CAT treatment to a no-
treatment control group. Once data are generated from such preliminary
research, then comparisons between (1) different creative arts and (2) a specific CAT and a noncreative arts treatment could be pursued.

Randomized Controlled Trials

To date, only one study can be considered to meet criteria for a randomized
controlled trial (RCT) specific to the CATs. Chapman and colleagues (2001)

investigated an art therapy treatment intervention for traumatically injured, hospitalized children and adolescents. In a prospective, randomized cohort design, participants were children ages 7–17 years who were admitted to a hospital with an injury requiring a minimum 24-hour hospitalization. Children were tested before treatment and after treatment at 1 week, 1 month, and 6 months) with the Children's Post Traumatic Stress Disorder Index (PTSD-I, Parent, Child, and Adolescent versions; Rodriguez, Steinberg, & Pynoos, 1997), the Posttraumatic Stress Diagnostic Scale (Foa, 1995), and the Family Environment Scale (Moos & Moos, 1994). Eighty-five patients were enrolled: 31 received a specific art therapy intervention; 27 received standard hospital care; and 27 did not present PTSD symptoms at baseline. Although there was no statistically significant reduction in overall PTSD scores, the intervention produced a reduction in all DSM-IV (American Psychiatric Association, 1994) PTSD Criteria C (avoidance) symptoms at 1 week. That decrease was sustained at 1 month.

Summary and Recommendations

Avenues for Future Research

It is imperative for the CATs to develop evidence-based PTSD clinical practice guidelines. This requires attention on many fronts.

• Evidence for the therapeutic value of the arts should move beyond the clinical report. Further exploration into the neurological underpinnings of the CATs is crucial to develop a sound theoretical model and to guide interventions.

• Valid and reliable assessment tools must be used to measure the efficacy of CAT interventions. CAT assessment tools need to be developed and validated against existing, valid PTSD measures to determine CAT-related symptom change.

• Best practices must be established for number and type of participants, session format, level of interactivity, strategies focusing on process, and recommendations for art making and performance.

• Manualized treatment protocols for acute and chronic PTSD must be developed. Then pilot data must be collected and RCTs conducted, with outcomes clearly identified. Treatment outcome investigations can then be replicated in multiple settings.

• The influence of development, cognitive ability, language skills, and psychological state must underlie and inform any research. It is imperative to control for age-appropriate differences.

• There is a notable lack of longitudinal research on children's drawings and on the effects of trauma on developmental level. Changes in drawings over time should be studied, along with changes in development and life situations (Carpenter, Kennedy, Armstrong, & Moore, 1997).

• Unfortunately, there is sporadic mention of adjunctive caregiver work. Creative arts therapists often specialize in treating either children or adults, and the settings in which clients are seen are often likewise segmented. Evidence is clear that caregiver involvement is an essential component of successful trauma-focused treatment (Lieberman, Van Horn, & Ippen, 2005; Pfeffer, Jiang, Kakuma, Hwang, & Metsch, 2002, Sandler et al., 2003); it is crucial that protocols be developed with this in mind. Family-oriented work has been conducted (Ambridge, 2001; Hanney & Kozlowska, 2002; Rabenstein & Lehmann, 2000; Steele & Raider, 2001; Zimmerman et al., 1987). But, there are not nearly enough examples in which caregivers are integrated into the intervention. Alternative models, such as individual child and caregiver sessions, as well as joint sessions as needed, should be explored. Both models are more frequently represented in the child trauma literature (e.g., Cohen, Mannarino, & Deblinger, 2006; Kolko, 1996).

• Creative arts therapists should be inventive in maximizing the value of the arts rather than translating and replicating existing interventions. For example, body mapping is being converted to color in "virtual art therapy" (Tripathi, 2006), and new computer-generated art and music offer new avenues. With respect to innovation, the value of the CATs and their application to severe mental illness is still untapped.

Conclusions

Based on the existing body of clinical work in the CATs, there is a clear consensus that the arts allow for access to trauma-related content that may not be as readily accessible with language, and that they offer unique treatment. Neuroscience offers valuable information on why the CATs might have such value, but there is little research to support the conclusions of thousands of devoted creative arts therapists. Scientific progress will require both increased research on existing fronts and innovation. The similarity between the interventions described by non-CAT mental health professionals and creative arts therapists is striking: The former are seemingly unaware of the latter. Virtually all work with children and adolescents uses nonverbal techniques. Hence, the professional boundaries are fluid. Creative arts therapists' sensitivity to, and familiarity with, the power of the arts, and non-CAT-trained clinician's knowledge of evidence-based techniques should be used to augment each other's work. Collaboration between creative arts therapists and other mental health professionals would enhance the work of both, with the clients benefiting the most.

Acknowledgments

We gratefully acknowledge the careful review of the chapter and input from dance/movement therapist Lenore W. Hervey, PhD, ADTR, NCC, REAT, and music therapist Juliane Kowski, MA, MT-BC. We also thank Megan Doyle for her contribution in retrieving references.

Note

1. Art, dance, drama, music, psychodrama, and poetry therapy each has its own established professional training standards, including an approval and monitoring process, a code of ethics and standards of clinical practice, and a credentialing process.

References

Akhundov, N. (1999, December). Psychosocial rehabilitation of IDP children: Using theatre, art, music and sport. *Forced Migration Review, 6,* 20–21.

Ambridge, M. (2001). Using the reflective image within the mother–child relationships. In J. Murphy (Ed.), *Art therapy with young survivors of sexual abuse* (pp. 69–85). Philadelphia: Taylor & Francis.

American Psychiatric Association. (1994). *Diagnostic and statistical manual of mental disorders* (4th ed.). Washington, DC: Author.

Atwood, J. D., & Donheiser, G. (1997). Me and my shadow: Therapy with sexually abused pre-adolescents. *Contemporary Family Therapy, 19*(2), 195–208.

Baráth, A. (2003). Cultural art therapy in the treatment of war trauma in children and youth: Projects in the former Yugoslavia. In S. Krippner & T. McIntyre (Eds.), *The psychological impact of war trauma on civilians: An international perspective* (pp. 155–170). Westport, CT: Praeger/Greenwood Press.

Belkofer, C., & Konopka, L. (2003, November). *A new kind of wonder: EEG and art therapy research.* Paper presented at the annual conference of the American Art Therapy Association, Chicago.

Ben-Asher, S., Koren, B., Tropea, E. B., & Fraenkel, D. (2002). Case study of a five-year-old Israeli girl in movement therapy. *American Journal of Dance Therapy, 24*(1), 27–43.

Bergmann, K. (2002). The sound of trauma: Music therapy in a post-war environment. *Australian Journal of Music Therapy, 13,* 3–16.

Berman, H., Ford-Gilboe, M., Moutrey, B., & Cekic, S. (2001). Portraits of pain and promise: A photographic study of Bosnian youth. *Canadian Journal of Nursing Research, 32*(4), 21–41.

Berrol, C. F. (2006). Neuroscience meets dance/movement therapy: Mirror neurons, the therapeutic process and empathy. *Arts in Psychotherapy, 33*(4), 302–315.

Bowers, J. J. (1992). Therapy through art: Facilitating treatment of sexual abuse. *Journal of Psychosocial Nursing, 30*(6), 15–23.

Byers, J. G. (1996). Children of the stones: Art therapy interventions in the West Banks. *Art Therapy: Journal of the American Art Therapy Association, 13,* 238–243.

Carpenter, M., Kennedy, M., Armstrong, A., & Moore, E. (1997). Indicators of neglect in preschool children's drawings. *Journal of Psychosocial Nursing, 35*(4), 10–17.

Cassity, M. D., & Theobold, K. A. K. (1990). Domestic violence: Assessments and treatments employed by music therapists. *Journal of Music Therapy, 27*(4), 179–194.

Cattanach, A. (1996). The use of dramatherapy and play therapy to help de-brief children after the trauma of sexual abuse. In A. Cattanach & A. Gersie (Eds.), *Dramatic approaches to brief therapy* (pp. 177–187). Philadelphia: Jessica Kingsley.

Chapman, L., Morabito, D., Ladakakos, C., Schreier, H., & Knudson, M. (2001). The effectiveness of art therapy interventions in reducing post traumatic stress disorder (PTSD) symptoms in pediatric trauma patients. *Art Therapy: Journal of the American Art Therapy Association, 18*, 100–104.

Clements, K. (1996). The use of art therapy with abused children. *Clinical Child Psychology and Psychiatry, 1*, 181–198.

Clements, P. T., Jr., Benasutti, K. M., & Henry, G. C. (2001). Drawing from experience: Using drawings to facilitate communication and understanding with children exposed to sudden traumatic deaths. *Journal of Psychosocial Nursing and Mental Health Services, 39*(12), 13–20.

Clendenon-Wallen, J. (1991). The use of music therapy to influence the self-confidence and self-esteem of adolescents who are sexually abused. *Music Therapy Perspectives, 9*, 73–81.

Cohen, J., Berliner, L., & March, J. (2000). Treatment of children and adolescents. In E. B. Foa, T. M. Keane, & M. J. Friedman (Eds.), *Effective treatments for PTSD: Practice guidelines from the International Society for Traumatic Stress Studies* (pp. 106–138). New York: Guilford Press.

Cohen, J. A., Mannarino, A. P., & Deblinger, E. (2006). *Treating trauma and traumatic grief in children and adolescents.* New York: Guilford Press.

Cohn, L. (1993). Art psychotherapy and eye movement desensitization reprocessing (EMDR) technique: An integrated approach. In E. Virshup (Ed.), *California art therapy trends* (pp. 275–290). Chicago: Magnolia Street.

Coulter, S. (2004). Working with a child exposed to community and domestic violence in Northern Ireland: An illustrated case example. *Child Care in Practice, 10*(2), 193–203.

Coulter, S. J. (2000). Effect of song writing versus recreational music on posttraumatic stress disorder (PTSD) symptoms and abuse attributions in abused children. *Journal of Poetry Therapy, 13*(4), 189–208.

Finan, H. T., & McCutcheon, M. (1995). Art as a therapeutic technique: Addressing the clinical issues of children of Vietnam veterans. In D. K. Rhoades, M. R. Leaveck, & J. C. Hudson (Eds.), *The legacy of Vietnam veterans and their families: Survivors of war: Catalysts for change* (pp. 372–383). Washington, DC: Agent Orange Class Assistance Program.

Foa, E. (1995). *Post Traumatic Stress Diagnostic Scale manual.* Minneapolis, MN: National Computer Systems.

Gil, E. (2003). Art and play therapy with sexually abused children. In C. A. Malchiodi (Ed.), *Handbook of art therapy* (pp. 152–166). New York: Guilford Press.

Glaister, J. A., & McGuinness, T. (1992). The art of therapeutic drawing: Helping chronic trauma survivors. *Journal of Psychosocial Nursing, 30*(5), 9–17.

Goodill, S. (1987). Dance/movement therapy with abused children. *The Arts in Psychotherapy, 14*(1), 209–214.

Goodman, R. F. (2004). Treatment of childhood traumatic grief: Application of cognitive-behavioral and client-centered therapies. In N. B. Webb (Ed.), *Mass trauma and violence: Helping families and children cope* (pp. 77–99). New York: Guilford Press.

Gross, J., & Hayne, H. (1998). Drawing facilitates children's verbal reports of emotionally laden events. *Journal of Experimental Psychology: Applied, 4*(2), 163–179.

Hagood, M. M. (2000). *The use of art in counseling child and adult survivors of sexual abuse.* London/Philadelphia: Jessica Kingsley.

Hanney, L., & Kozlowska, K. (2002). Healing traumatized children: Creating illustrated storybooks in family therapy. *Family Process, 14*(1), 37–65.

Harvey, S. (1995). Sandra: The case of an adopted sexually abused child. In F. Levy (Ed.), *Dance and other expressive arts therapies* (pp. 167–180). New York: Routledge.

Hontz, J. (2006, March 20). The healing canvas. *Los Angeles Times,* pp. F1, F11.

Johnson, D. R. (1987). The role of the creative arts therapies in the diagnosis and treatment of psychological trauma. *The Arts in Psychotherapy, 14*(1), 7–13.

Kalmanowitz, D., & Lloyd, B. (1999). Fragments of art at work: Art therapy in the former Yugoslavia. *The Arts in Psychotherapy, 26*(1), 15–25.

Klorer, P. (2000). *Expressive therapy with troubled children.* Northvale, NJ: Aronson.

Klorer, P. (2003). Sexually abused children: Group approaches. In C. A. Malchiodi (Ed.), *Handbook of art therapy* (pp. 339–350). New York: Guilford Press.

Kolko, D. J. (1996). Individual cognitive behavioral treatment and family therapy for physically abused children and their offending parents: A comparison of clinical outcomes. *Child Maltreatment, 1,* 322–342.

Kowski, J. (2007). "Can you play with me?": Dealing with trauma, grief and loss in analytical music therapy and play therapy. In V. Camilleri (Ed.), *Healing the inner-city child: Creative arts therapies with at-risk youth.* London: Jessica Kingsley.

Kozlowska, K., & Hanney, L. (2001). An art therapy group for children traumatized by parental violence and separation. *Clinical Child Psychology and Psychiatry, 6*(1), 49–78.

Kruk, K. (2004). *EEG and art therapy: Brain activity during art-making.* Paper presented at the annual conference of the American Art Therapy Association, San Diego, CA.

Lieberman, A. F., Van Horn, P., & Ippen, C. G. (2005). Towards evidence based treatment: Child–parent psychotherapy for preschoolers exposed to marital violence. *Journal of the American Academy of Child and Adolescent Psychiatry, 44,* 1241–1248.

Loewy, J. V., & Stewart, K. (2004). Music therapy to help traumatized children and caregivers. In N. B. Webb (Ed.), *Mass trauma and violence: Helping families and children cope* (pp. 191–215). New York: Guilford Press.

McNamee, C. (2004). Using both sides of the brain: Experiences that integrate art and talk therapy through scribble drawings. *Art Therapy: Journal of the American Art Therapy Association, 21*(3), 136–142.

Monti, D. A., Peterson, C., Kunkel, E. J. S., Hauck, W. W., Pequignot, E., Rhodes, L., et al. (2006). A randomized, controlled trial of mindfulness-based art therapy (MBAT) for women with cancer. *Psycho-Oncology, 15,* 363–373.

Moos, R., & Moos, B. (1994). *Family Environment Scale manual.* Palo Alto, CA: Consulting Psychologists Press.

Morgan, K. E., & White, P. R. (2003). The functions of art-making in CISD with children and youth. *International Journal of Emergency Mental Health, 5*(2), 61–76.

Nader, K., & Pynoos, R. (1991). Play and drawing techniques as tools for interviewing traumatized children. In C. Schaefer, K. Gitlin, & A. Sandgrund (Eds.), *Play diagnosis and assessment* (pp. 375–389). New York: Wiley.

Naitove, C. E. (1982). Arts therapy with sexually abused children. In S. Sgroi (Ed.), *Handbook of clinical intervention in child sexual abuse* (pp. 269–308). Lexington, MA: Lexington Books.

National Coalition of Creative Arts Therapies. (2006). Retrieved July 28, 2006, from *www.nccata.org/index.htm*

Ogden, P., & Minton, K. (2000). Sensorimotor psychotherapy: One method for processing traumatic memory. *Traumatology, 6*(3), Article 3. Retrieved September 29, 2006, from *www.sensorimotorpsychotherapy.org/articles.html*

Pearce, J. (1992). *Evolution's end: Claiming the potential of our intelligence.* San Francisco: Harper.

Perry, B., Pollard, R., Blakely, T., Baker, W., & Vigilante, D. (1995). Childhood trauma, the neurobiology of adaptation, and "use-dependent" development of the brain: How "states" become "traits." *Infant Mental Health Journal, 16,* 271–291.

Pfeffer, C. R., Jiang, H., Kakuma, T., Hwang, J., & Metsch, M. (2002). Group intervention for children bereaved by the suicide of a relative. *Journal of the American Academy of Child and Adolescent Psychiatry, 41*(5), 505–513.

Pifalo, T. (2002). Pulling out the thorns: Art therapy with sexually abused children and adolescents. *Art Therapy: Journal of the American Art Therapy Association, 19*(1), 12–22.

Powell, L., & Faherty, S. L. (1990). Treating sexually abused latency age girls: A 20 session treatment plan utilizing group process and the creative arts therapies. *The Arts in Psychotherapy, 17*(1), 35–47.

Pynoos, R., & Eth, S. (1986). Witness to violence: The child interview. *Journal of the American Academy of Child Psychiatry, 25,* 306–319.

Rabenstein, S., & Lehmann, P. (2000). Mothers and children together: A family group treatment approach. *Journal of Aggression, Maltreatment and Trauma, 3*(1), 185–205.

Rauch, S., van der Kolk, B., Fisler, R., Alpert, N., Orr, S., Savage, C., et al. (1996). A symptom provocation study of posttraumatic stress disorder using positron emission tomography and script-driven imagery. *Archives of General Psychiatry, 53*(5), 389–387.

Robb, M. (2002). Beyond the orphanages: Art therapy with Russian children. *Art Therapy: Journal of the American Art Therapy Association, 19*(4), 146–150.

Robb, S. (1996). Techniques in song writing: Restoring emotional and physical well being in adolescents who have been traumatically injured. *Music Therapy Perspectives, 14,* 30–37.

Rodriguez, N., Steinberg, A., & Pynoos, R. (1997). *PTSD Index for DSM-IV Instrument Information: Child version, adolescent version, parent version.* Unpublished manuscript.

Roje, M. (1995). LA '94 earthquake in the eyes of children: Art therapy with elementary school children who were victims of disaster. *Art Therapy, 12*(4), 237–243.

Rothschild, B. (2000). *The body remembers: The psychophysiology of trauma and trauma treatment.* New York: Norton.

Rousseau, C., Singh, A., Lacroix, L., Bagilishya, D., & Measham, T. (2004). Creative expression workshops for immigrant and refugee children. *Journal of the American Academy of Child and Adolescent Psychiatry, 43*(2), 235–238.

Sandler, I. N., Ayers, T. S., Wolchik, S. A., Tein, J.-Y., Kwok, O.-M., Haine, R. A., et al. (2003). The Family Bereavement Program: Efficacy evaluation of a theory-based prevention program for parentally bereaved children and adolescents. *Journal of Consulting and Clinical Psychology, 71*(3), 587–600.

Schiffer, F., Teicher, M., & Papanicolaou, A. (1995). Evoked potential evidence for right brain activity during the recall of traumatic memories. *Journal of Neuropsychiatry and Clinical Neurosciences, 7,* 169–175.

Siegel, D. J. (1999). *The developing mind: How relationships and the brain interact to shape who we are.* New York: Guilford Press.

Slotoroff, C. (1994). Drumming technique for assertiveness and anger management in the short-term psychiatric setting for adult and adolescent survivors of trauma. *Music Therapy Perspectives, 12,* 111–116.

Sobol, B., & Schneider, K. (1996). Art as an adjunctive therapy in the treatment of children who dissociate. In J. L. Silberg (Ed.), *The dissociative child: Diagnosis, treatment, and management* (pp. 191–218). Lutherville, MD: Sidran Press.

Steele, W. (2003). Using drawing in short-term trauma resolution. In C. A. Malchiodi (Ed.), *Handbook of art therapy* (pp. 139–151). New York: Guilford Press.

Steele, W., & Raider, M. (2001). *Structured sensory intervention for traumatized children, adolescents and parents: Strategies to alleviate trauma.* Lewiston, NY: Edwin Mellen Press.

Sutton, J. P. (Ed.). (2002). *Music, music therapy and trauma.* Philadelphia: Jessica Kingsley.

Terr, L. (1991). Childhood traumas: An outline and overview. *American Journal of Psychiatry, 148*(1), 10–19.

TF-CBT Web. (2005). *A web-based learning course for trauma-focused cognitive-behavioral therapy.* Retrieved August 26, 2006, from *tfcbt.musc.edu*

Tower, R. (1983). Imagery: Its role in development. In A. A. Skeikh (Ed.), *Imagery: Current theory, research and application* (pp. 222–251). New York: Wiley.

Tripathi, A. (2006). *Virtual but real cure for abused victims.* Retrieved July 28, 2006, from *www.ibnlive.com/printpage.php?id=14751&section_id=17*

van der Kolk, B. A. (1996). The body keeps the score: Approaches to the psychobiology of posttraumatic stress disorder. In B. A. van der Kolk, A. C. McFarlane, & L. Weisath (Eds.), *Traumatic stress: The effects of overwhelming experience on mind, body, and society* (pp. 214–241). New York: Guilford Press.

Weltman, M. (1986). Movement therapy with children who have been sexually abused. *American Journal of Dance Therapy, 9,* 47–66.

Winn, L. (1994). *Post traumatic stress disorder and dramatherapy: Treatment and risk reduction.* Bristol, PA/London: Jessica Kingsley.

Yedidia, T., & Itzhaky, H. (2004). A drawing technique for diagnosis and therapy of adolescents suffering traumatic stress and loss related to terrorism. In N. B. Webb (Ed.), *Mass trauma and violence: Helping families and children cope* (pp. 283–303). New York: Guilford Press.

Zaidi, L. Y., & Gutierrez-Kovner, V. M. (1995). Group treatment of sexually abused latency-age girls. *Journal of Interpersonal Violence, 10*(2), 215–227.

Zimmerman, M. L., Wolbert, W. A., Burgess, A. W., & Hartman, C. R. (1987). Art and group work: Interventions for multiple victims of child molestation (Part II). *Archives of Psychiatric Nursing, 1*(1), 40–46.

CHAPTER 21

Treatment of PTSD and Comorbid Disorders

Lisa M. Najavits, Donna Ryngala, Sudie E. Back,
Elisa Bolton, Kim T. Mueser, and Kathleen T. Brady

Theoretical Context

There is a central paradox in the field of posttraumatic stress disorder (PTSD) comorbidity: Comorbidity with PTSD is the norm, yet treatment outcome studies routinely exclude patients with significant comorbid conditions and fail to assess for them. The past several years have seen some change in these patterns, and there is now a growing body of work on treatments designed either specifically for comorbid conditions or for a particular condition and studied in comorbid samples.

The good news is that many of these studies evidence promising models and positive outcomes. But there are also some surprises that reiterate a basic fact in the area of comorbidity: Not all comorbid conditions are alike; thus, specificity by disorder appears to be a helpful approach at this point. Also, treatments are not necessarily specific, so a treatment designed to treat just one disorder, such as PTSD, may also have positive outcomes for comorbid conditions. Thus, when considering comorbidity and its treatment, it is helpful to explore the myriad possible relationships among the comorbid conditions (e.g., their development over time, course during treatment, and impact on each other), and also how treatment may impact them (e.g., both together or differentially). There are many possible results and, given the newness of this area of work, much that remains to be discovered.

In actual rates, approximately 80% of people with PTSD have a co-occurring psychiatric or substance use disorder (SUD [lifetime rates]; Breslau, Davis, Andreski, & Peterson, 1991; Kessler, Sonnega, Bromet, Hughes, & Nelson, 1995). Moreover, this is not unique to PTSD. For example, about 45% of people with at least one diagnosis have one or more additional ones as well (current rates; Kessler, Chiu, Demler, Merikangas, & Walters, 2005). In terms of treatment, there are a variety of approaches to comorbidity:

- *Integrated* (treat comorbid disorders at the same time, by the same provider, focusing on linkages between them).
- *Sequential* (treat one disorder, then the other).
- *Parallel* (also known as concurrent; i.e., treat each disorder but in separate treatments, often by separate providers, and sometimes in separate systems, such as mental health vs. substance abuse).
- *Single diagnosis* (treat just one disorder).

In general, the current state of the art is believed to be integrated treatment, which allows fluid attention to all disorders and how they are linked. However, at this point there is almost no empirical research on this question. Thus far, most research has addressed the early stages of treatment development—creating new treatments and evaluating them in basic outcome trials.

Finally, it is also worth noting that there are a variety of causal explanations for comorbidity (see Meyer, 1986; Weiss et al., 1998). Examples of such relationships include the following:

- Disorder *x* causes disorder *y*.
- Disorder *y* causes disorder *x*.
- Both *x* and *y* are caused by some other factor.
- Each disorder arises independently, without any relation between them.
- Each disorder may impact the course of the other (improving or worsening), even if not caused by it.

Evidence

In this chapter, we provide a comprehensive summary of the literature on treatment models for PTSD and comorbid disorders. We conducted a literature search for the following disorders:

Axis I: *substance use disorders* (alcohol, amphetamine, cannabis, cocaine, hallucinogen, inhalant, opioid, phencyclidine, sedative, polysubstance); *anxiety disorders* (agoraphobia, panic, phobias, obsessive–compulsive, generalized anxiety); *somatoform disorders* (somatization, conversion, pain, hypochondriasis, body dysmorphic disorders); *fac-

ticious disorder; dissociative disorders (dissociative amnesia, fugue, and identity disorders and depersonalization disorder); *sexual and gender identity disorders; eating disorders* (anorexia, bulimia nervosa); *primary sleep disorders; impulse disorders* (intermittent explosive disorder, kleptomania, pyromania, pathological gambling, trichotillomania); *mood disorders,* and *schizophrenia and other psychotic disorders.*

Axis II: *personality disorders* (paranoid, schizoid, schizotypal, antisocial, borderline, histrionic, narcissistic, avoidant, dependent, and obsessive–compulsive personality disorders).

Studies were included if they (1) addressed PTSD (or trauma-related symptoms) plus one or more additional disorders; (2) used a specific model of treatment; (3) provided outcome data; and (4) were published or in press.

We have classified each study into Levels A–F based on methodology (per this book's Introduction). However, it should be noted that a study may be one level for PTSD, yet another for the comorbid condition because the level of rigor may not hold across both. For example, some studies are post hoc analyses from PTSD treatment trials, with comorbidity examined only in a subset of patients who had the comorbid disorder. Also, all studies address just one or sometimes a few comorbid conditions, but no studies thus far have comprehensively reported the full array of Axis I and II disorders that may be comorbid. Given the state of the literature in this area, we have departed slightly from the original Levels A–F formulation, as follows:

- Level A means the study meets criteria for that level, yet it may be missing a small element (e.g., not randomizing to therapists as well as treatment conditions; or not reporting interrater reliability on assessments).
- Level B means it is a good study, but it has enough major methodological weaknesses that we cannot classify it as Level A; also, we include here only studies that had some sort of control condition.
- Level C are studies that have a decent or better pilot study (but without a control condition), and/or service or naturalistic studies (per the definition in the Introduction to this book). However, we have not used the criterion that level C studies can be interpreted as "sufficiently compelling to warrant use of the treatment technique" (per page 30 in the Introduction, this volume). In our view, a treatment model for comorbidity can only be formally recommended if there are positive outcomes from Level A empirical work on it.
- Levels D–F: All single-case studies are included here.

For each study, the rationale for the assigned rating is provided. Given the early stage of research, it should be noted that although many models may be helpful to patients, the study methodology still attains a low rating. This is not a reflection on the models themselves; rather it is just the state of the science in studying them thus far. We hope that the upcoming years will see further evolution in the progression of research on the models. Also, the methodology of Levels A–F itself will likely be refined over time. For example, it does not address areas that are increasingly viewed as essential for strong outcome trials, such as the amount and type of external treatments, power analysis, intention-to-treat (ITT) versus completer analysis, description of therapist training, and therapist effects. See, for example, CONSORT (Consolidated Standards of Reporting Trials, 2004) and Moncrief (in Bisson & Andrew, 2005).

We focus solely on results from pre- to posttreatment because internal validity is strongest for that, especially given the early state of the literature and variable follow-up periods. We report only statistically significant results. Research below is presented in alphabetical order of the co-occurring diagnoses. The review is organized into three main sections: (1) all Axis I and II disorders except mood disorders and serious mental illness; (2) mood disorders and serious mental illness; and (3) pharmacotherapy.

See Table 21.1 for all Level A studies of psychotherapy; see Table 21.2 for all Level A studies of pharmacotherapy.

Literature Review

All Axis I and II Disorders (Except Mood and Psychotic Disorders)

PTSD and Generalized Anxiety Disorder/Major Depressive Disorder

EMPIRICAL EVIDENCE (LEVEL A)

Cognitive-Behavioral Therapy. Blanchard and colleagues (2003) developed an individual cognitive-behavioral therapy (CBT) for motor vehicle accident (MVA) survivors with PTSD. It includes psychoeducation, relaxation training, *in vivo* exposure, exposure-based homework, behavioral activation, and cognitive restructuring. They conducted a randomized controlled trial (RCT) comparing it with supportive psychotherapy for 78 MVA survivors with full or subsyndromal PTSD. The study is included because it examined generalized anxiety disorder (GAD) and major depressive disorder (MDD), in addition to PTSD. However, neither the study nor treatment targeted GAD or MDD. Only 49% of the sample had MDD and 35% had GAD, and it is unclear how many had both. They excluded current SUD, serious mental illness, and cognitive impairment.

Participants were randomly assigned to CBT, the supportive psychotherapy, or a wait-list control. The supportive psychotherapy included psychoeducation about PTSD and three sessions reviewing life history, trauma, and loss. The supportive therapists were instructed not to encourage driving or to use CBT techniques. Dose of treatment was not constant and ranged from 8 to 12 sessions. There was a therapist × treatment confound (the three study therapists delivered both treatments), and all therapists had a CBT orienta-

TABLE 21.1. Psychosocial Treatments (Level A Studies)

Treatment tested	Population	Comparison treatment	n	Duration of treatment	Main PTSD outcome measure	PTSD within-group effect size	PTSD between-group effect size	Results	Main comorbid outcome measure	Comorbid within-group effect size	Comorbid between-group effect size	Results
CBT for PTSD (comorbid GAD and MDD; Blanchard et al., 2003)	Motor vehicle accident survivors[a]	Support[d] or wait list	CBT 27; support 27; wait list 24	8–12 wk	Clinician-Administered PTSD Scale (CAPS)	1.82	Support: 0.63 Wait list: 1.16	p = .002 p = .001	Categorical results only reported	—	—	—
Seeking Safety (SS) for PTSD and substance abuse (Najavits, 2002)	Low-income women[b]	Relapse prevention (RP) or treatment as usual (TAU)	SS 41; RP 34; TAU 32	12 wk	Composite score[d]	0.2	RP: 0.10; TAU: 0.60	ns p = .01	Composite score[e]	0.11	RP: 0.19 TAU: 0.71	ns p = .001
	Adolescent girls[c]	TAU	SS 18; Tau 15	12 wk	TSCC PTSD[f]	Not reported	Not reported	ns	PEI loss of control[g]	1.15	3.15	p = .01

Notes = Within-group differences are only reported for the treatment of interest (see individual articles for within-group differences of comparison groups). All calculations are Cohen's *d*. ns, not significant.

[a]Blanchard et al. (2003).

[b]Hien et al. (2004).

[c]Najavits et al. (2006).

[d]Composite PTSD score included the CAPS, the Impact of Event Scale, and the Clinical Global Impression.

[e]Composite substance abuse score consisted of the Substance Use Index and Clinician Global Impression.

[f]Trauma Symptom Checklist for Children, PTSD Scale.

[g]Personal Experiences Inventory.

TABLE 21.2. Pharmacotherapy Studies (Level A Only)

Medication tested	Population	Comparison treatment	n	Duration of treat-ment	Main PTSD outcome measure	Within-group effect size	Between-group effect size	Results
Sertraline (Brady & Clary, 2003)	Civilians	Placebo	SER 194 PBO 201	12 weeks	CAPS		0.37	$p = .0003$
Sertraline (Brady et al., 2005)	Civilians	Placebo	SER 49 PBO 45	12 weeks	CAPS		0.29	$p = .08$
Risperidone (Hamner et al., 2003)	Veterans	Placebo	RIS 19 PBO 18	5 weeks	CAPS	0.38 0.81	0.10	ns

Note. SER, sertraline; PBO, placebo; RIS, risperidone; CAPS, Clinician-Administered PTSD Scale; ns, not significant. All within- and between-group effect sizes are Cohen's *d*. Positive between-group effective size means greater drop in measurement outcome for the experimental group versus the placebo group.

513

tion. Results indicated that CBT was superior to supportive psychotherapy, which was superior to the wait list, on numerous variables including PTSD. CBT patients also showed greater reduction in MDD and GAD than the other two conditions, which did not differ. This study is Level A for the comparison of CBT versus wait-list control only. The supportive psychotherapy does not qualify as Level A due to artificial restriction of content (unable to encourage driving) and therapist assignment (CBT clinicians conducted it). Moreover, Level A refers to PTSD only because comorbid conditions were not present in all patients. The treatment is *single-diagnosis* because it addressed PTSD only.

SUMMARY

One study addressed comorbid MDD and GAD as a post hoc analysis of a PTSD trial. Blanchard and colleagues (2003) compared CBT for PTSD, supportive psychotherapy, and wait-list control for MVA survivors. CBT appears to be a promising treatment for MVA PTSD, and possibly MDD and GAD. However, the CBT was not integrated, nor did it attempt to address the MDD or GAD. Given high comorbidity in this population, future work could target interventions for MDD and/or GAD. More research is needed on the supportive psychotherapy condition, especially testing a more valid version of it.

PTSD and Obsessive–Compulsive Disorder

CLINICAL EVIDENCE (LEVEL C)

Inpatient Treatment for Obsessive–Compulsive Disorder. Gershuny, Baer, Jenike, Minichiello, and Wilhelm (2002) and Gershuny, Baer, Radomesky, Wilson, and Jenike (2003) reported on a residential obsessive–compulsive disorder (OCD) program for patients with OCD and PTSD. The interventions were behavioral, including OCD exposure and response prevention, and therapy groups. There was no modification of the model to treat PTSD. A naturalistic study (Gershuny et al., 2002) addressed 15 patients with treatment-refractory OCD plus multiple comorbidities, eight of whom had PTSD. The authors compared patients with and without PTSD. Results indicated that average lengths of stay were not significantly different, but patients with PTSD had worse outcomes on OCD and depression. Indeed, they showed no improvement in these, whereas the group without PTSD improved on both. Some patients with PTSD demonstrated worsening of symptoms following treatment. This was similar to case studies by the same team (Gershuny et al., 2003). They conclude that "behavioral treatment of OCD . . . may be adversely affected by the presence of comorbid PTSD and indeed may be contra-indicated for some patients" (Gershuny et al., 2002, p. 853). Indeed, a decrease in OCD was related to an increase in PTSD, whereas an increase in OCD symptoms was related to a decrease in PTSD (Gershuny et al., 2003). These studies are Level

C because they are naturalistic. The treatment is *single-diagnosis* because it was designed for OCD only.

SUMMARY

The effectiveness of response prevention and exposure for OCD is already established. However, Gershuny and colleagues (2002, 2003) indicated that it appears to be contraindicated for patients with comorbid PTSD. A modification that includes a manualized PTSD model may have better outcomes. This area is virtually unexplored and highlights the importance of understanding comorbid disorder combinations, as well as potential worsening when comorbidity is not adequately addressed.

PTSD and Panic Disorder

EMPIRICAL EVIDENCE (LEVEL B)

Multiple-Channel Exposure Therapy. Multiple-channel exposure therapy (M-CET; Falsetti, Resnick, David, & Gallagher, 2001) is a treatment for PTSD and panic disorder adapted from existing treatments for each: cognitive processing therapy for PTSD (Resick & Schnicke, 1993) and panic control treatment (Barlow & Craske, 1988). Twelve group sessions address psychoeducation, breathing retraining, cognitive restructuring, and introceptive and *in vivo* exposure. M-CET was compared to a minimal-attention condition of bimonthly telephone consultation. Twenty-two women with PTSD and panic attacks were randomly assigned to treatment ($n = 7$), control ($n = 10$), or control then treatment ($n = 5$). Current substance dependence was excluded. In preliminary results on a completer sample, Falsetti and colleagues (2001) reported greater reduction in PTSD and panic attacks in M-CET compared to the control, and both conditions improved in self-reported depression symptoms. M-CET appears promising for the dual diagnosis of PTSD and panic disorder. Note that this study is Level B because it represents preliminary data, reports results only for a completer sample, and is not fully randomized (i.e., some participants served in both conditions). The treatment is *integrated* because it was designed for PTSD and panic disorder.

Sensation Reprocessing Therapy. Hinton and colleagues (2004, 2005) developed sensation reprocessing therapy (SRT), a 12-session Southeast Asian cultural adaptation of individual CBT for PTSD and panic attacks. Drawing from existing models for each disorder (e.g., Falsetti & Resnick, 2000; Foa & Rothbaum, 1998), the researchers added culturally appropriate psychoeducation, visualization, cognitive restructuring, and mindfulness techniques. A pilot study (Hinton et al., 2004) randomly assigned 12 Vietnamese refugees to immediate treatment or a wait-list control. All refugees had PTSD and panic attacks, and were considered treatment resistant. Medications were not controlled during the study. Results showed improvement on various measures, including PTSD and anxiety, but due to the study's use of just one clinician, it is impossible to separate treatment from therapist effects. A later study (Hinton et al., 2005) was conducted with survivors of the Cambodian genocide in 1970, who, like the patients in the earlier study, had PTSD and panic attacks, and were treatment resistant. In addition, all patients had GAD, and psychotic patients were excluded. They were randomly assigned to immediate or delayed treatment (20 per condition), conducted by one clinician. Medication and supportive psychotherapy biweekly could occur concurrently. Results indicated superior outcomes for the immediate treatment compared to delayed treatment on numerous variables, including PTSD, anxiety, severity of panic attacks, and GAD. SRT is promising and is noteworthy for its cultural sensitivity. This study is Level B because it was not fully randomized (some patients participated in both conditions), and due to a crossover design, the two conditions did not have identical timing of assessments. There was also no mention of adherence nor assessor training. The treatment is *integrated* because it was designed for PTSD and panic attacks.

CLINICAL EVIDENCE (LEVEL D)

CBT for Panic plus Implosive Therapy. Saper and Brasfield (1998) offered an 18-session individual model: nine sessions of CBT for panic disorder with agoraphobia (adapted from Craske & Barlow, 1990) followed by nine sessions of implosive therapy for PTSD (Levis, 1985). A case study indicated diagnosis-specific impact: reduction of panic but not PTSD after the initial nine sessions (the panic treatment phase), and reduction of both disorders after 18 sessions (the panic plus PTSD treatment phases). This study is Level D because it used long-standing treatments but was a single-case study. The treatment is *sequential* because it sequenced separate treatments for PTSD and panic attacks.

CBT/Exposure. Tsao, Lewin, and Craske (1998) examined two group CBTs for panic disorder (cognitive-behavioral exposure and cognitive *in vivo* exposure) in terms of their impact on comorbid syndromes, although current SUD, psychosis, and suicidality were exclusionary. In a post hoc analysis, they collapsed across the two treatments to evaluate outcomes for those with PTSD. Of 33 treatment completers, seven had full or subclinical PTSD. Outcomes indicated reduction in panic and, for those with PTSD, a reduction in PTSD symptoms. This study addressed comorbid disorders more than most, and the finding that the treatments helped improve disorders that they were not designed to treat is consistent with much of the literature on comorbidity. This study is Level D because it does not provide sufficient evaluation of PTSD effects (only a few patients had PTSD, and the two treatments were combined when evaluating PTSD). The treatments are *single-diagnosis* because they were designed for panic only.

SUMMARY

Several therapies that have been developed to treat co-occurring PTSD and panic disorder simultaneously show promising preliminary results. However, sample sizes were small and methodologies were limited.

PTSD and Substance Use Disorder

Early attempts to treat this population advocated a sequential approach in which SUD first had to be treated successfully, and only then could treatment for PTSD begin. In fact, this stance remains common. However, research on integrated treatment consistently indicates that it is helpful for this comorbid population. Indeed among comorbidities, there is more evidence for PTSD and SUD than for any other at this point, perhaps because of its prevalence, high-risk nature, and the use of substances to self-medicate PTSD (e.g., Jacobsen, Southwick, & Kosten, 2001).

EMPIRICAL EVIDENCE (LEVEL A)

Seeking Safety. Seeking Safety (SS; Najavits, 2002) is an integrated model for PTSD and SUD. It is the most researched model for any diagnosis co-occurring with PTSD, with 12 published studies that range in levels from A to C. It is a present-focused CBT that provides psychoeducation and coping skills to help patients attain greater safety in their lives. It was designed for group or individual format; men or women; diverse settings (e.g., outpatient, inpatient, residential); and all types of trauma and substances. It offers 25 treatment topics, each representing a safe coping skill relevant to both PTSD and SUD, such as Asking for Help and Healing from Anger. All topics are independent; thus, they can be done in any order, with as few or many sessions as time allows. SS is also used with patients who have just one disorder (PTSD or SUD), or are subthreshold.

Published studies are two multisite controlled trials (Desai, Harpaz-Rotem, Rosenheck, & Najavits, in press; Morrissey et al., 2005), two RCTs (Hien, Cohen, Miele, Litt, & Capstick, 2004; Najavits, Gallop, & Weiss, 2006), a controlled nonrandomized trial (Gatz et al., 2007), and seven uncontrolled pilots (Cook, Walser, Kane, Ruzek, & Woody, 2006; Holdcraft & Comtois, 2002; Mcnelis-Domingos, 2004; Najavits, Schmitz, Gotthardt, & Weiss, 2005; Najavits, Weiss, Shaw, & Muenz, 1998; Weller, 2005; Zlotnick, Najavits, & Rohsenow, 2003). Other completed studies are available (*www.seekingsafety. org*) but are not yet published (including a dissemination study by Rugs, Hills, & Peters, 2004). The published studies were conducted with various populations, including outpatient women in group modality (Najavits et al., 1998), women in prison in group modality (Zlotnick et al., 2003); women in a community mental health setting in group format (Holdcraft & Comtois, 2002); low-income urban women in individual format (Hien et al., 2004), adolescent girls in individual format (Najavits et al., 2006), men and women veterans in group format (Cook et al., 2006), homeless women veterans in group and/ or individual format (Desai et al., in press), women with co-occurring disorders in group format (Morrissey et al., 2005), outpatient men in individual format (Najavits, Schmitz, Gotthardt, & Weiss, 2005), and women veterans in group format (Weller, 2005). One study by Brown and colleagues (2007) is not reviewed here because it evaluated implementation rather than outcome. Two outcome studies are omitted from the summary below because they included SS as one model among several but did not report differences between them (Holdcraft & Comtois, 2002; Morrissey et al., 2005).

All outcome studies evidenced positive results. Eight of the nine studies that reported on substance use found improvements in that domain (Hien et al., 2004; Najavits et al., 1998, 2005, 2006; Weller, 2005; Zlotnick et al., 2003). The ninth study (Cook et al., 2006) did not have quantitative results for substance use but reported that patients maintained abstinence, verified by urinalysis. All nine studies assessed PTSD and/or or trauma-related symptoms and found improvements in one or both areas. Improvements were also found in other domains, such as social adjustment, suicidal thoughts, problem solving, sense of meaning, and quality of life. Treatment satisfaction and attendance were reported to be high in all studies.

In the four controlled trials, SS outperformed treatment as usual (TAU) (Desai et al., in press; Gatz et al., 2007; Hien et al., 2004; Najavits et al., 2006). All allowed patients in SS to obtain unlimited TAU, thus essentially evaluating the impact of SS plus TAU versus TAU alone. This is a challenging test because patients had so much treatment other than SS. Results for the controlled trials were as follows. In Hien and colleagues (2004), with a study sample of 107 women, both SS and relapse prevention (an additional arm of the study that represents a "gold standard" treatment for SUD) had reductions in PTSD, substance abuse, and psychiatric symptoms, whereas the TAU nonrandomized control worsened. In the Najavits and colleagues (2006) study of 33 adolescent girls, SS outperformed TAU on numerous variables, including substance use and trauma symptoms. In the Desai and colleagues (in press) multisite study of 450 homeless women veterans, SS outperformed a nonrandomized TAU comparison condition on several variables, including PTSD, psychiatric symptoms, employment, and social support. This study is notable for having used case managers without prior therapy training to conduct SS. In the Gatz and colleagues (2007) study of 313 women in community treatment, SS outperformed the control in PTSD, coping skills, and treatment retention. It was also the only study to evaluate possible mechanisms of action, with a finding that increased coping skills partially mediated outcomes. Finally, one of the pilot studies (Najavits et al., 2005) combined SS with an adapted version of prolonged exposure (PE; Foa & Rothbaum, 1998) with dosage based on choice. Patients chose an average of 21 SS sessions and nine PE sessions.

Implementation of the model is enhanced by various materials, including the published manual in English, and translations into Spanish, French,

German, Dutch, and Swedish, video-based training, a website (*www.seeking-safety.org*), and numerous national trainings. The empirical evidence is classified as Level A because, among the studies, two were RCTs with sufficient methodological rigor (Hien et al., 2004, Najavits et al., 2006). The treatment is *integrated* because it was designed for PTSD and SUD.

In summary, SS is the only co-occurring PTSD model that is established as effective at this point based on criteria for empirically supported treatments (e.g., Chambless & Hollon, 1998). It has shown consistent positive outcomes on various measures, superiority to TAU, comparability to a "gold standard" treatment (relapse prevention), positive results in populations considered challenging (e.g., the homeless, prisoners, adolescents, and veterans), and high acceptability.

EMPIRICAL EVIDENCE (LEVEL B)

Collaborative Care. Collaborative care (CC) is a treatment in medical settings for acutely injured trauma survivors who may be at risk for developing PTSD and alcohol use disorder (Zatzick et al., 2004). It is a stepped care program that includes continuous case management and some combination of psychopharmacological therapy, CBT, and/or motivational interviewing (MI), although it is unclear whether the latter two therapies were delivered in group or individual modality). It begins with case management by a trauma support specialist who coordinates medical treatment across settings, and is available either directly or through a covering staff person 24/7. Patients who screen positive for alcohol use on admission or who have evidence of alcohol abuse also receive MI. Three months posttrauma, patients who meet criteria for PTSD are given a choice of CBT, pharmacotherapy, or a combination of both. The CBT includes psychoeducation, relaxation, exposure, cognitive restructuring, relapse prevention, and community integration. Although manualized, the treatment is flexible, with intervention components provided as needed based on patient presentation and preference. An RCT compared CC (*n* = 59) and TAU (*n* = 61). TAU was simply providing patients with a list of community resources, with no coordination. The sample was surgical inpatients at a trauma center who were not cognitively impaired and not psychotic. Twenty-five patients met criteria for PTSD and 12 of these were comorbid for substance abuse. At 12-month follow-up, TAU participants had significant increases in both PTSD and alcohol use disorder, whereas CC participants did not. However, the CC participants evidenced a significant decline only in alcohol use disorder, not PTSD, during that 1-year time frame. This study targets an important population at risk for PTSD and SUD, and offers guidelines for implementing a flexible, multimodal treatment package. It shows clinical promise based on this initial study. The study is Level B because it had no adherence ratings, no blind evaluator, not all participants had PTSD, and treatments were neither fully randomized nor uniform within condition (CC patients chose the specific treatment that they received: CBT, pharmacotherapy, or a combination of the two). The treatment is *integrated* because it was designed for potential PTSD and alcohol use disorder ("potential" because it attempts to prevent the development of the disorders).

EMPIRICAL EVIDENCE (LEVEL C)

Concurrent Treatment of PTSD and Cocaine Dependence. Concurrent Treatment of PTSD and Cocaine Dependence (CTPCD; Back, Dansky, Carroll, Foa, & Brady, 2001; Brady, 2001) is a 16-session individual therapy that combines CBT interventions with efficacy for PTSD (Foa & Rothbaum, 1998) or SUD (Carroll, 1998; Monti, Kadden, Rohsenow, Cooney, & Abrams, 2002). Sessions are 90 minutes and include psychoeducation; SUD interventions, such as coping skills and relapse prevention; and PTSD interventions, such as *in vivo* and imaginal exposure. A pilot study was conducted on 39 patients with PTSD and cocaine dependence. Exclusion criteria were psychosis, dissociative identity disorder, dementia, illiteracy, suicidality, and homicidality. Patients were paid for attending therapy sessions. "Treatment completion" was defined as having attended 10 or more sessions; 24 of the 39 patients dropped out before meeting this criterion. Most dropout occurred prior to the introduction of the exposure component. Pre- to posttreatment outcome analyses, conducted on treatment completers only, showed significant decreases in PTSD, depression, and SUD. A baseline comparison of treatment completers and noncompleters indicated that the former had more years of education and were less avoidant. The study offers impressive pilot evidence that some patients with these disorders can tolerate imaginal and *in vivo* exposure treatment and, indeed, benefit from it. However, the study is preliminary and there are concerns about treatment retention. It is defined as Level C because it was a pilot study without a control condition; also, participants were paid for attending treatment sessions, which may have had an impact on outcome. The treatment is *integrated* because it was designed for PTSD and SUD.

Transcend. Transcend is a 12-week, intensive, partial hospitalization program for combat veterans with PTSD and SUD (Donovan, Padin-Rivera, & Kowaliw, 2001). It draws on psychodynamic, CBT, constructivist, and 12-step models, and is conducted in closed cohorts of eight patients. Patients attend 10 hours of group therapy per week and are required to participate in ancillary individual and/or group substance abuse treatment, relaxation training, community service, and physical exercise. Six weeks are devoted to skills development, followed by 6 weeks of trauma processing. An uncontrolled pilot study was conducted on 46 male Vietnam War veterans diagnosed with PTSD and SUD, all of whom had to achieve 30 days of substance abstinence prior to joining. Positive results were found from pre- to posttreatment on PTSD symptoms for the sample that completed all assessments. SUD was not assessed at posttreatment because patients were not allowed to use substances during the program. In summary, Transcend is the only model developed and tested as a partial hospital program. It addresses a population known to struggle with PTSD and SUD (veterans), and achieved some positive outcomes in a pilot study. Whether its intensity can be replicated in other settings remains an open question. The study is defined as Level C because it had no control; also, it did not evaluate effects for the comorbid condition (SUD) because all participants had to have 30 days of abstinence prior to joining, and there was no assessment of substance use at posttreatment. The treatment is *integrated* because it was designed for PTSD and SUD.

Trauma Empowerment Recovery Model. The trauma empowerment recovery model (TREM; Harris & the Community Connections Trauma Work Group, 1998) is a group model originally designed for women abuse survivors with severe mental disorders. It comprises 33 weekly, 75-minute sessions conducted over 9 months, including psychoeducation, cognitive restructuring, survivor empowerment, skills building, and peer support. A controlled study (Toussaint, VanDeMark, Bornemann, & Graeber, 2007) reports on the use of a modified version of TREM in combination with a psychoeducational trauma workbook (Copeland & Harris, 2000) compared to TAU. TREM was modified to a 24-session version and followed an initial orientation with the trauma workbook. The study evaluated 170 women in residential substance abuse treatment ($n = 64$ in TREM vs. $n = 106$ in TAU). Inclusion criteria included substance use disorder and at least one additional Axis I or II disorder (with one disorder current and the other in the past 5 years), plus a history of physical or sexual abuse and at least two prior treatment episodes. Results showed that those receiving the TREM-plus-workbook approach had better outcomes on trauma-related symptoms but not on substance use. Participants in both conditions improved in substance use symptoms, with no difference between them. The study is defined as Level C because it was naturalistic, not all participants had PTSD, and there was no report of the Axis I and/or Axis II disorders that participants had other than SUD. The treatment under study is *integrated* because it was intended for multiple disorders; however, it was not designed specifically for PTSD and/or SUD, but for abuse survivors with a broad range of mental disorders that might include PTSD and/or SUD.

Substance Dependence–PTSD Therapy. Substance Dependence–PTSD Therapy (SDPT; Triffleman, Carroll, & Kellogg, 1999) is a 40-session individual therapy with two phases: Phase I is trauma-informed, addiction-focused; Phase II is trauma-focused, addiction-informed. It adapts existing models for each disorder (PTSD, SUD), including both coping skills training and *in vivo* PTSD exposure (e.g., Carroll, 1998; Foa & Rothbaum, 1998). In one study, the model (Triffleman, 2000) was compared to 12-step facilitation therapy (TSF; Nowinski, Baker, & Carroll, 1995), which uses 12-step principles to facilitate substance abstinence but does not include a PTSD component. Both treatments were conducted individually twice a week with a sample of 19 participants, both men and women, all of whom met criteria for lifetime substance dependence, lifetime PTSD, and at least current partial PTSD. Exclusion criteria were acute psychosis, severe depression, untreated mania, dissociative identity disorder, acute suicidality or homicidality requiring hospitalization, or continuing involvement in ongoing psychotherapies. Patients were randomly assigned to treatment. Results indicated a higher number of sessions attended in SDPT than in TSF among those who attended at least three sessions. No other differences between the two treatment conditions were found; thus, the researchers combined data from both to report results from the merged data (not separately by treatment). The outcomes essentially represent SDPT *or* TSF, and the effects for either treatment alone cannot be determined. The analysis across SDPT and TSF showed an effect for time, with the combined sample improving on PTSD by the end of treatment. Self-reported substance use improved only at the 1-month follow-up and not on urine screens. In summary, SDPT is a treatment designed as a thoughtfully constructed blend of interventions that have shown efficacy with either PTSD or SUD. At face value, the model has potential. However, it is difficult to draw conclusions based on this one study as SDPT did not outperform the control (TSF) on either PTSD or SUD, nor were results reported separately for SDPT. The study is defined as Level C because of these limitations. The treatment is *integrated* because it was designed for PTSD and SUD.

CLINICAL EVIDENCE (LEVEL F)

Acceptance and Commitment Therapy. Batten and Hayes (2005) published a case study using acceptance and commitment therapy (ACT; Hayes, Strosahl, & Wilson, 1999) for 96 sessions of individual therapy over 17 months. The treatment focuses on "reduction of experiential avoidance, acceptance of private events, and commitment to behavior change" (Batten & Hayes, 2005, p. 253). The patient was stated to have PTSD and SUD, but there was no standardized assessment for these disorders. She was assessed every 3 months on various measures, with improvement occurring mostly at 9 months and thereafter. It is challenging to know what to make of this study given its methodology. Nonetheless, ACT is a well-known treatment, and it would be helpful to understand whether it has potential for PTSD and SUD. This study is Level F because it is a single-case study for a new model. The treatment is not classified because it was not designed for specific disorders.

SUMMARY

PTSD and SUD commonly co-occur, and the treatment literature for these disorders is more robust than for any other PTSD comorbidities. All of the studies in this section report promising results and one model, SS, is now established as effective. However, except for SS, the studies investigating these treatments are few and typically have small samples and a single, uncontrolled pilot study. Verification of self-reported substance use via urinalysis is the exception rather than the norm. Nonetheless, this area has seen major strides in the past decade, showing that patients with PTSD and SUD can be treated successfully for both disorders from the start of treatment. This finding is a striking departure from the earlier received wisdom, which was to delay treatment of PTSD until the SUD was under control.

PTSD and Borderline Personality Disorder

CLINICAL EVIDENCE (LEVEL C)

Prolonged Exposure/Stress Inoculation Training. Feeny, Zoellner, and Foa (2002) reanalyzed data from a prior PTSD trial (Foa et al., 1999) to compare patients with and without borderline personality disorder (BPD) symptoms. The study had four conditions: prolonged exposure (PE), stress inoculation training (SIT), PE plus SIT, and a wait-list control group (see Foa & Rothbaum [1998] and elsewhere in this book for a description of PE and SIT). Treatment comprised nine twice-weekly individual sessions, 90–120 minutes each. The sample was 72 female assault victims, all with current PTSD and 12 with either full ($n = 7$) or partial ($n = 5$) BPD (identified as "borderline personality characteristics," or BPC). Exclusionary criteria included active SUD, severe mental illness, organic mental disorder, high risk for suicide, and/or self-harm within the prior 3 months. Because the BPC sample was small and all treatment conditions were equally effective in the main study (Foa et al., 1999), the treatment data were collapsed. Results were provided only for the completer sample ($n = 58$; i.e., no ITT analysis). Patients with and without BPC improved by the end of treatment on various measures, including PTSD, but those with BPC had significantly lower end-state functioning. The study is Level C because most patients did not have the comorbid condition and treatment conditions were collapsed due to this. The treatments under study are *single diagnosis* because they were designed for PTSD only.

Psychodynamic Imaginative Trauma Therapy and Eye Movement Desensitization and Reprocessing. Sachsse, Vogel, and Leichsenring (2006) conducted a naturalistic study of women attending an inpatient trauma-focused program, most of whom had "complex PTSD" as well as co-occurring MDD, BPD, somatization disorder, and/or a dissociative disorder. Neither the sample nor the results, however, describe the average number of disorders per person, nor a breakdown of results by co-occurring disorder. The treatment was conducted in two phases: an initial generic, inpatient stabilization for 2 weeks, followed by readmittance about 8 months later, during which patients received the trauma-focused treatment program. The latter comprised an average of two eye movement desensitization and reprocessing (EMDR) sessions and three to four individual psychodynamic sessions for "working through and reorientation" per month (typically for 2–4 months). The treatment is manualized in German (Reddemann, 2004). A comparison was conducted between patients who received only Phase 1 (no trauma-focused treatment; $n = 66$) and those who also received Phase 2 (the trauma-focused treatment; $n = 87$). Results indicated that patients who completed the trauma-focused treatment had significantly better outcomes than those who did not, on a range of variables, including trauma-related symptoms and some general psychiatric symptoms. The study is Level C because it is naturalistic and has a time confound (the 8-month delay for the trauma-focused condition). The treatment is defined as *single diagnosis* because it was designed for PTSD only.

SUMMARY

The only comorbid Axis II disorder with any empirical literature at this point is BPD, and the evidence on that is very limited. Two studies were found, both of which used a manualized PTSD treatment (but not treatment for BPD). In both studies, positive effects were found on several variables, including either PTSD or trauma-related symptoms (Feeny et al., 2002; Sachsse et al., 2006). One study compared outcomes for patients with and without borderline symptoms and found positive results for both groups, but lower end-state functioning for those with borderline symptoms (Feeny et al., 2002). The studies are limited, however, in methodology (both are Level C), lack of an integrated model designed for the dual diagnosis, and sampling issues (a small sample with BPD in Feeny et al. and mixed comorbid diagnoses in Sachsse et al. [2006]). Nonetheless, the results of these studies suggest that patients with comorbid BPD symptoms can benefit from PTSD therapy.

Mood and Psychotic Disorders

Mood Disorders

Different study selection criteria are used for mood disorders than are used in the rest of this chapter (see Acknowledgments at the end of the chapter). There are several PTSD treatment studies that report changes in depression levels (e.g., Cloitre, Koenen, Cohen, & Han, 2002; Schnurr et al., 2003, 2007). However, given the high rate of comorbidity of PTSD and depression, all treatment studies for PTSD include people with comorbid depression. Studies that report pre- and posttreatment depression scores for all participants, whether they carry a diagnosis of depression or not, simply indicate the effect of the treatment on depression scores. Because these studies do not address whether individuals with a diagnosed mood disorder respond to the treatment in the same manner as individuals without a mood disorder, we did not include these studies. Furthermore, we decided to focus just on published studies that fit the category of either RCT or naturalistic, uncontrolled studies in which treatment response in a group or subgroup with and without concurrent mood disorders was studied, or that included an interaction of diagnostic group and treatment condition. We did not find any studies that met these criteria.

Psychotic Disorders

Trauma and PTSD are highly comorbid with psychosis and/or severe mental illness (SMI) (Mueser, Rosenberg, Goodman, & Trumbetta, 2002). Rates of trauma exposure in individuals with SMI range from 51 to 97% (Mueser et al., 1998), multiple traumatizations are common, and, for some SMI subgroups (e.g., dually diagnosed), rates of exposure are even higher. Although PTSD is estimated in 42% of individuals with SMI, only 2% carried the diagnosis in their charts (Mueser et al., 1998). Indeed, PTSD is often overlooked in treatment, although it is believed to worsen SMI (Mueser et al., 2002). Individuals with SMI sometimes have delusions with trauma themes. This has led to questions about the validity of trauma/PTSD assessment in the SMI population. Fortunately, research has established satisfactory validity of PTSD measures in the context of SMI (Goodman et al., 1999; Mueser et al., 2001).

Although there are few published data to guide the treatment of patients with SMI and PTSD, descriptions of treatment programs for this population agree on a number of points (Frueh, Cusack, Grubaugh, Sauvageot, & Wells, 2006; Harris & the Community Connections Trauma Work Group, 1998; Mueser, Rosenberg, Jankowski, Hamblen, & Descamps, 2004). One consideration is SMI patients' high sensitivity to stress and vulnerability to relapse. Another concern is their high rate of cognitive impairment, either due directly to the effects of mental illness, such as schizophrenia; traumatic brain injury associated with exposure to certain forms of traumatic events (e.g., physical abuse, car accident); or the poor health care of this population. Further issues include the impact of psychotic symptoms in disorders such as schizophrenia, risk of self-injury in disorders such as major mood disorders, and the high rate of comorbid SUD in the SMI population. Finally, it is important that treatment for PTSD be integrated into comprehensive mental health services, and that models be flexible enough to adapt to a wide range of severe psychopathology and impose minimal exclusion criteria.

Individuals with SMI have been ruled out of most controlled research on PTSD treatment. Hence, there is a need to develop or adapt interventions for PTSD in this population. To our knowledge, three groups work along these lines: Mueser, Rosenberg, and colleagues; Frueh and colleagues; and Harris and the Community Connections Trauma Work Group. The TREM model by the latter group is covered in the previous section because it is one empirical study thus far that was conducted with patients with SUD who did not necessarily have SMI (although it was originally designed as a group therapy for women with SMI). Also, we do not cover a new, three-session psychoeducational program on PTSD for persons with SMI, because it was not intended to treat PTSD per se. A pilot study with 70 inpatients indicated increased knowledge about PTSD and high satisfaction (Pratt et al., 2005).

TRAUMA RECOVERY GROUP (LEVEL C)

Mueser and colleagues (2007) developed a group CBT for patients with PTSD and SMI. It offers eight modules: overview, crisis planning, breathing retraining, psychoeducation on PTSD, cognitive restructuring, coping with symptoms, a personal recovery plan, and termination. An individual version is 12–16 sessions, whereas the group treatment is 21 sessions (Mueser et al., 2007; Rosenberg, Mueser, Jankowski, Salyers, & Acker, 2004). Both treatments were designed to be provided at local community mental health centers by doctoral- or master's-level therapists. Both are Level C pilot studies. The individual program (Rosenberg et al., 2004) evidenced high retention, and improved PTSD and general psychiatric symptoms. The group therapy ($N = 80$) had somewhat lower retention, but completers showed improvement in PTSD, depression, and posttraumatic cognitions. Thus, results are promising, but further research is needed.

LEVEL F

Frueh and colleagues (2004) propose a CBT to target PTSD in patients with SMI in public-sector mental health clinics. The program includes education, anxiety management skills training, exposure therapy, and long-term follow-up care.

Summary and Conclusions

Research on PTSD treatment for patients with SMI is limited. It is promising, however, because treatment models have been developed, with pilot data on one model. Future studies will benefit from more scientific rigor, expanded assessment, and exploration of the optimal number of sessions and treatment components.

Pharmacotherapy of Comorbidity in PTSD

Despite high comorbidity rates with PTSD, most PTSD pharmacological treatment trials have excluded individuals with comorbid conditions to improve internal validity. As such, applicability of findings to patients seen in the average clinicians' office is suspect. Studies that have addressed comorbid PTSD are of two general types: (1) efficacy studies of standard PTSD treatments in individuals with comorbidity; and (2) adjunctive pharmacotherapy studies to treat specific comorbid disorders or symptoms in individuals with PTSD. Both types can provide helpful information for clinical practice.

Empirical Evidence (Level A)

SERTRALINE

Brady and Clary (2003) examined the efficacy and tolerability of sertraline compared to placebo among 395 outpatients with (1) PTSD only; (2) PTSD and comorbid anxiety; (3) PTSD and comorbid depression; and (4) PTSD, comorbid anxiety, and comorbid depression. This study is a secondary analysis of data from the pivotal trials used to support the U.S. Food and Drug Administration (FDA) indication for sertraline; some individuals with co-occurring anxiety and depression were included in that trial (Brady et al., 2000; Davidson et al., 2001). This was a 12-week, multisite, double-blind, randomized, flexible dose (50–200 mg/day) trial. A Clinician-Administered PTSD Scale–2 (CAPS-2) total severity score ≥ 50 at baseline was required for inclusion. Sertraline treatment resulted in greater improvement in PTSD symptoms compared to placebo, particularly for individuals with PTSD and comorbid anxiety alone, or comorbid anxiety and depression. Patients in the sertraline group had a lower endpoint Clinical Global Impressions Scale score than those who received placebo, regardless of comorbidity status. No between-group differences in side effect burden were revealed.

In another double-blind, 12-week, controlled trial (also Level A), Brady and colleagues (2005) investigated sertraline in 94 (51 men, 43 women) individuals with PTSD and comorbid alcohol dependence. Patients were randomized to receive a fixed 150 mg/day dose of sertraline or placebo. A cluster analysis revealed medication group by symptom cluster interactions. Those with less severe alcohol dependence and early-onset PTSD demonstrated greater improvement in alcohol outcomes when treated with sertraline compared to placebo. In contrast, in those with more severe alcohol dependence and later-onset PTSD, the placebo group demonstrated greater improvement in alcohol outcomes compared to the sertraline-treated group. This suggests possible subtypes of patients with PTSD and alcohol dependence who respond differently to sertraline.

In a post hoc analysis of this trial, Labbate, Sonne, Randall, Anton, and Brady (2004) examined the impact of having additional comorbid anxiety or affective disorders on outcomes for patients with PTSD and alcohol dependence. Participants were divided into four groups: (1) no comorbid depression or anxiety; (2) comorbid depression; (3) comorbid anxiety; and (4) both comorbid depression and anxiety. Findings revealed few differences in outcome among the four groups. Patients showed improvement in alcohol use and PTSD regardless of anxiety–affect comorbidity status. However, the study may not have been sufficiently powered for the post hoc analysis.

RISPERIDONE

Hamner and colleagues (2003) conducted a 5-week, randomized, double-blind, placebo-controlled trial of adjunctive risperidone (1–6 mg/day, average dose of 2.5 mg/day) among 37 outpatient men with combat-related PTSD and comorbid psychotic features. Patients were also receiving antidepressant or other pharmacotherapy, but were required to have been on stable dosages for 1 month prior to the trial. Patients were required to have a Positive and Negative Syndrome Scale (PANSS) score ≥ 60 at baseline. Schizophrenia, schizoaffective disorder, or other primary psychotic disorders were excluded. Findings showed that risperidone, in comparison to placebo, led to greater reduction in global psychotic symptoms associated with chronic PTSD but not overall PTSD symptoms. Several limitations may have affected the findings (e.g., small sample size, possible inadequate dosing, short duration), and further investigation of risperidone for the treatment of psychotic symptoms in PTSD patients is warranted.

Empirical Evidence (Level B)

DISULFIRAM, NALTREXONE, AND THEIR COMBINATION

Among 254 outpatients with alcohol dependence and various comorbid disorders, Petrakis and colleagues (2005) investigated the efficacy of disulfiram and naltrexone, or their combination. The 12-week, controlled, randomized trial with partial blinding (open-label disulfiram) was conducted at three Veterans Administration clinics. Almost half of the sample met criteria for PTSD. Patients were also treated with various psychotropic medications but had to be on stable dosages 2 weeks prior to the trial. Patients treated with naltrexone or disulfiram, compared to placebo, had better alcohol outcomes. Disulfiram patients reported less craving from pre- to posttreatment than did naltrexone patients. No clear advantage of combining disulfiram and naltrexone was observed; in fact, participants who received the combination of medications evidenced higher depression and distress over time.

In a secondary analysis of the same data, Petrakis and colleagues (2006) examined these two medications (naltrexone vs. disulfiram) in patients with (37%) and without (63%) comorbid PTSD. Those with PTSD receiving either active medication compared to placebo demonstrated better alcohol outcomes. Those with PTSD who received disulfiram showed improvement in alcohol craving, and in total PTSD and hyperarousal symptoms. PTSD reexperiencing symptoms improved among patients taking either active medication compared to their combination. The combination was also associated with more side effects among patients with PTSD.

ANTIDEPRESSANT (PAROXETINE OR BUPROPION) VERSUS CBT
VERSUS COMMUNITY MENTAL HEALTH REFERRAL

Green and colleagues (2006) examined the effect of PTSD comorbidity on treatment outcome in an uncontrolled trial of 267 low-income women with MDD. Patients were randomized to (1) CBT; (2) antidepressant medication (paroxetine or bupropion); or (3) a community mental health referral. One-third of the women had PTSD. Depression improved at similar rates in both groups (i.e., paroxetine vs. bupropion) over time. Over a 1-year follow-up, however, women with PTSD evidenced poorer physical functioning and more depression than those without PTSD.

Summary

Despite the high comorbidity of PTSD with SUD and other psychiatric disorders, there have been few pharmacotherapy studies in this complicated patient population. The studies that exist are promising, with most indicating that patients with PTSD and comorbidity respond as well to standard pharmacotherapies as those without comorbidity. Several studies provide useful data concerning adjunctive pharmacotherapies in specific comorbid conditions. More research is needed.

Summary and Recommendations

Virtually all of the literature on treatment for PTSD and comorbid conditions has arisen in the past few years. This speaks both to the emerging awareness of comorbidity and to the larger zeitgeist, in which there is strong interest in the development and evaluation of new psychotherapy models (both in the PTSD field and more broadly). Given the high rates of PTSD comorbidity and the often vulnerable nature of such populations, it is encouraging to see such a burst of energy in this area of work. Nonetheless, study methodology is generally quite limited, as might be expected at this early stage. The next decade will likely see scientific advances in types of studies (more RCTs), more empirical work on dissemination and training, and greater understanding of the comorbidities themselves (e.g., rates, causal relationships, and prognosis).

Treatment models for PTSD comorbidity offer a wide range of features, including the types of trauma for which they are designed, the use of group versus individual modality, and the variety of techniques offered. Some models are designed from the start for comorbidity, whereas others are a combination of existing approaches that have already been found effective for each separate disorder.

At this point, summary points are as follows:

- It is important to assess for comorbidity of both DSM-IV Axis I and Axis II disorders.
- Single-diagnosis treatments (currently the majority of PTSD treatments) may have impact on comorbid conditions, even if not originally designed for them.
- Nonetheless, treatments that directly address comorbidities are gener-

ally suggested as an important area of work that is likely to be beneficial.

- Only one psychosocial model thus far has been established as effective for PTSD and a comorbid disorder (Seeking Safety for PTSD/substance use disorder), using established criteria for empirically supported treatments (e.g., Chambless & Hollon, 1998).
- Two medications have had Level A RCTs with comorbid PTSD populations (sertraline, risperidone).
- Patients with PTSD and comorbid conditions can benefit from manualized interventions and also from pharmacotherapy.
- More research is needed.

Acknowledgments

Sections of this chapter were written by different authors: Theoretical Context, Evidence, and Summary and Recommendations (Najavits); Axis I and Axis II Disorders (Najavits & Ryngala); Mood and Psychotic Disorders (Bolton & Mueser); Pharmacotherapy of Comorbidity (Back & Brady); tables (Ryngala & Back). They are responsible for the accuracy of their sections. Our thanks to Erin Rowe for her secretarial assistance on this project.

References

Back, S., Dansky, B., Carroll, K., Foa, E., & Brady, K. (2001). Exposure therapy in the treatment of PTSD among cocaine-dependent individuals: Description of procedures. *Journal of Substance Abuse Treatment, 21*, 35–45.

Barlow, D. H., & Craske, M. G. (1988). *Mastery of your anxiety and panic.* Albany, NY: Graywind.

Batten, S. V., & Hayes, S. C. (2005). Acceptance and commitment therapy in the treatment of comorbid substance abuse and posttraumatic stress disorder: A case study. *Clinical Case Studies, 4*(3), 246–262.

Bisson, J., & Andrew, M. (2005). Psychological treatment of post-traumatic stress disorder (PTSD). *Cochrane Database of Systematic Review, 2*, 1–60.

Blanchard, E. B., Hickling, E. J., Devineni, T., Veazey, C. H., Galovski, T. E., Mundy, E. A., et al. (2003). A controlled evaluation of cognitive behavioral therapy for posttraumatic stress in motor vehicle accident survivors. *Behaviour Research and Therapy, 41*(1), 79–96.

Brady, K. T. (2001). Comorbid posttraumatic stress disorder and substance use disorders. *Psychiatric Annals, 31*, 313–319.

Brady, K. T., & Clary, C. M. (2003). Affective and anxiety comorbidity in posttraumatic stress disorder treatment trials of sertraline. *Comprehensive Psychiatry, 44*(5), 360–369.

Brady, K. T., Pearlstein, T., Asnis, G., Baker, D., Rothbaum, B., Sikes, C. R., et al. (2000). Efficacy and safety of sertraline treatment of posttraumatic stress disorder: A randomized controlled trial. *Journal of the American Medical Association, 283*(14), 1837–1844.

Brady, K. T., Sonne, S., Anton, R. F., Randall, C. L., Back, S. E., & Simpson, K. (2005). Sertraline in the treatment of co-occurring alcohol dependence and posttraumatic stress disorder. *Alcoholism: Clinical and Experimental Research, 29*(3), 395–401.

Breslau, N., Davis, G. C., Andreski, P., & Peterson, E. (1991). Traumatic events and posttraumatic stress disorder in an urban population of young adults. *Archives of General Psychiatry, 48*, 216–222.

Brown, V. B., Najavits, L. M., Cadiz, S., Finkelstein, N., Heckman, J. P., & Rechberger, E. (2007). Implementing an evidence-based practice: Seeking Safety group. *Journal of Psychoactive Drugs, 39*, 231–240.

Carroll, K. (1998). *A cognitive-behavioral approach: Treating cocaine addiction* (NIH Publication No. 98-4308). Rockville, MD: National Institute on Drug Abuse.

Chambless, D., & Hollon, S. (1998). Defining empirically supported therapies. *Jounal of Consulting and Clinical Psychology, 66*, 7–18.

Cloitre, M., Koenen, K. C., Cohen, L. R., & Han, H. (2002). Skills training in affective and interpersonal regulation followed by exposure: A phase-based treatment for PTSD related to childhood abuse. *Journal of Consulting and Clinical Psychology, 70*, 1067–1074.

Consolidated Standards of Reporting Trials (CONSORT). (2004). Consort statement. Retrieved February 18, 2004, from *www.consort-statement.org/statement/ revisedstatement.htm*

Cook, J. M., Walser, R. D., Kane, V., Ruzek, J. I., & Woody, G. (2006). Dissemination and feasibility of a cognitive-behavioral treatment for substance use disorders and posttraumatic stress disorder in the Veterans Administration. *Journal of Psychoactive Drugs, 38*, 89–92.

Copeland, M. E., & Harris, M. (2000). *Healing the trauma of abuse: A woman's workbook.* Oakland, CA: New Harbinger.

Craske, M. G., & Barlow, D. H. (1990). *Therapist's guide for the Mastery of Your Anxiety and Panic (MAP) program.* Albany, NY: Graywind.

Davidson, J., Pearlstein, T., Londborg, P., Brady, K. T., Rothbaum, B., Bell, J., et al. (2001). Efficacy of sertraline in preventing relapse of posttraumatic stress disorder: Results of a 28-week double-blind, placebo-controlled study. *American Journal of Psychiatry, 158*(12), 1974–1981.

Desai, R., Harpaz-Rotem, I., Rosenheck, R., & Najavits, L. (in press). Treatment of homeless female veterans with psychiatric and substance abuse disorders: Impact of "Seeking Safety" on one-year clinical outcomes. *Psychiatric Services.*

Donovan, B., Padin-Rivera, E., & Kowaliw, S. (2001). Transcend: Initial outcomes from a posttraumatic stress disorder/substance abuse treatment study. *Journal of Traumatic Stress, 14*, 757–772.

Falsetti, S. A., & Resnick, H. S. (2000). Cognitive-behavioral treatment for PTSD with panic attacks. *Journal of Contemporary Psychotherapy, 30*, 163–179.

Falsetti, S. A., Resnick, H. S., David, J., & Gallagher, N. G. (2001). Treatment of posttraumatic stress disorder with comorbid panic attacks: Combining cognitive processing therapy with panic control treatment techniques. *Group Dynamics: Theory, Research, and Practice, 5*(4), 252–260.

Feeny, N. C., Zoellner, L. A., & Foa, E. B. (2002). Treatment outcome for chronic PTSD among female assault victims with borderline personality characteristics: A preliminary examination. *Journal of Personality Disorders, 16*(1), 30–40.

Foa, E. B., Dancu, C. V., Hembree, E. A., Jaycox, L. H., Meadows, E. A., & Street, G. P. (1999). A comparison of exposure therapy, stress inoculation training, and their combination for reducing posttraumatic stress disorder in female assault victims. *Journal of Consulting and Clinical Psychology, 67*(2), 194–200.

Foa, E. B., & Rothbaum, B. O. (1998). *Treating the trauma of rape: Cognitive-behavioral therapy for PTSD.* New York: Guilford Press.

Frueh, B. C., Buckley, T. C., Cusack, K. J., Kimble, M. O., Grubaugh, A. L., Turner, S. M., et al. (2004). Cognitive-behavioral treatment for PTSD among people with severe mental illness: A proposed treatment model. *Journal of Psychiatric Practice, 10,* 26–38.

Frueh, B. C., Cusack, K. J., Grubaugh, A. L., Sauvageot, J. A., & Wells, C. (2006). Clinician's perspectives on cognitive-behavioral treatment for PTSD among persons with severe mental illness. *Psychiatric Services, 57,* 1027–1031.

Gatz, M., Brown, V., Hennigan, K., Rechberger, E., O'Keefe, M., Rose, T., et al. (2007). Effectiveness of an integrated, trauma-informed approach to treating women with co-occurring disorders and histories of trauma: The Los Angeles site experience. *Journal of Community Psychology, 35,* 863–878.

Gershuny, B. S., Baer, L., Jenike, M. A., Minichiello, W. E., & Wilhelm, S. (2002). Comorbid posttraumatic stress disorder: Impact on treatment outcome for obsessive–compulsive disorder. *American Journal of Psychiatry, 159*(5), 852–854.

Gershuny, B. S., Baer, L., Radomsky, A. S., Wilson, K. A., & Jenike, M. A. (2003). Connections among symptoms of obsessive–compulsive disorder and posttraumatic stress disorder: A case series. *Behaviour Research and Therapy, 41*(9), 1029–1041.

Goodman, L. A., Thompson, K. M., Weinfurt, K., Corl, S., Acker, P., Mueser, K. T., et al. (1999). Reliability of reports of violent victimization and PTSD among men and women with SMI. *Journal of Traumatic Stress, 12,* 587–599.

Green, B. L., Krupnick, J. L., Chung, J., Siddique, J., Krause, E. D., Revicki, D., et al. (2006). Impact of PTSD comorbidity on one-year outcomes in a depression trial. *Journal of Clinical Psychology, 62*(7), 815–835.

Hamner, M. B., Faldowski, R. A., Ulmer, H. G., Frueh, B. C., Huber, M. G., & Arana, G. W. (2003). Adjunctive risperidone treatment in post-traumatic stress disorder: A preliminary controlled trial of effects on comorbid psychotic symptoms. *International Clinical Psychopharmacology, 18*(1), 1–8.

Harris, M., & the Community Connections Trauma Work Group. (1998). *Trauma recovery and empowerment: A clinician's guide for working with women in groups.* Washington, DC: Community Connections, Inc./Free Press.

Hayes, S. C., Strosahl, K. D., & Wilson, K. G. (1999). *Acceptance and commitment therapy: An experiential approach to behavior change.* New York: Guilford Press.

Hien, D. A., Cohen, L. R., Miele, G. M., Litt, L. C., & Capstick, C. (2004). Promising treatments for women with comorbid PTSD and substance use disorders. *American Journal of Psychiatry, 161*(8), 1426–1432.

Hinton, D. E., Chhean, D., Pich, V., Safren, S. A., Hofmann, S. G., & Pollack, M. H. (2005). A randomized controlled trial of cognitive-behavior therapy for Cambodian refugees with treatment-resistant PTSD and panic attacks: A cross-over design. *Journal of Traumatic Stress, 18*(6), 617–629.

Hinton, D. E., Pham, T., Tran, M., Safren, S. A., Otto, M. W., & Pollack, M. H. (2004). CBT for Vietnamese refugees with treatment-resistant PTSD and panic attacks: A pilot study. *Journal of Traumatic Stress, 17*(5), 429–433.

Holdcraft, L. C., & Comtois, K. A. (2002). Description of and preliminary data from a women's dual diagnosis community mental health program. *Canadian Journal of Community Mental Health, 21,* 91–109.

Jacobsen, L. K., Southwick, S. M., & Kosten, T. R. (2001). Substance use disorders in patients with posttraumatic stress disorder: A review of the literature. *Amercican Journal of Psychiatry, 158,* 1184–1190.

Kessler, R. C., Chiu, W. T., Demler, O., Merikangas, K. R., & Walters, E. E. (2005). Prevalence, severity, and comorbidity of 12-month DSM-IV disorders in the National Comorbidity Survey Replication. *Archives of General Psychiatry, 62*(6), 617–627.

Kessler, R. C., Sonnega, A., Bromet, E., Hughes, M., & Nelson, C. B. (1995). Posttraumatic stress disorder in the National Comorbidity Survey. *Archives of General Psychiatry, 52,* 1048–1060.

Labbate, L. A., Sonne, S. C., Randall, C. L., Anton, R. F., & Brady, K. T. (2004). Does comorbid anxiety or depression affect clinical outcomes in patients with posttraumatic stress disorder and alcohol use disorders? *Comprehensive Psychiatry, 45*(4), 304–310.

Levis, D. J. (1985). Implosive theory: A comprehensive extension of conditioning theory of fear/anxiety to psychopathology. In S. Reiss & R. R. Bootzin (Eds.), *Theoretical issues in behavior therapy* (pp. 49–82). New York: Academic Press.

Mcnelis-Domingos, A. (2004, May). *Cognitve behavioral skills training for persons with co-occurring posttraumatic stress disorder and substance abuse.* Master's thesis, Southern Connecticut State University, New Haven.

Meyer, R. E. (1986). How to understand the relationship between psychopathology and addictive disorders: Another example of the chicken and the egg. In R. E. Meyer (Ed.), *Psychopathology and addictive disorders* (pp. 3–16). New York: Guilford Press.

Monnelly, E. P., Ciraulo, D. A., Knapp, C., & Keane, T. (2003). Low-dose risperidone as adjunctive therapy for irritable aggression in posttraumatic stress disorder. *Journal of Clinical Psychopharmacology, 23*(2), 193–196.

Monti, P. M., Kadden, R. M., Rohsenow, D. J., Cooney, N. L., & Abrams, D. B. (2002). *Treating alcohol dependence: A coping skills training guide* (2nd ed.). New York: Guilford Press.

Morrissey, J. P., Jackson, E. W., Ellis, A. R., Amaro, H., Brown, V. B., & Najavits, L. M. (2005). Twelve-month outcomes of trauma-informed interventions for women with co-occurring disorders. *Psychiatric Services, 56,* 1213–1222.

Mueser, K. T., Bolton, E. E., Carty, P. C., Bradley, M. J., Ahlgren, K. F., DiStaso, D. R., et al. (2007). The trauma recovery group: A cognitive-behavioral program for PTSD in persons with severe mental illness. *Community Mental Health Journal, 43,* 281–304.

Mueser, K. T., Goodman, L. A., Trumbetta, S. L., Rosenberg, S. D., Osher, F. C., Vidaver, R., et al. (1998). Trauma and posttraumatic stress disorder in severe mental illness. *Journal of Consulting and Clinical Psychology, 66,* 493–499.

Mueser, K. T., Rosenberg, S. D., Goodman, L. A., & Trumbetta, S. L. (2002). Trauma, PTSD, and the course of schizophrenia: An interactive model. *Schizophrenia Research, 53,* 123–143.

Mueser, K. T., Rosenberg, S. D., Jankowski, M. K., Hamblen, J., & Descamps, M. (2004). A cognitive-behavioral treatment program for posttraumatic stress disorder in severe mental illness. *American Journal of Psychiatric Rehabilitation, 7,* 107–146.

Mueser, K. T., Salyers, M. P., Rosenberg, S. D., Ford, J. D., Fox, L., & Cardy, P. (2001). A psychometric evaluation of trauma and PTSD assessments in persons with severe mental illness. *Psychological Assessment, 13,* 110–117.

Najavits, L. M. (2002). *Seeking safety: A treatment manual for PTSD and substance abuse.* New York: Guilford Press.

Najavits, L. M., Gallop, R. J., & Weiss, R. D. (2006). Seeking Safety therapy for adolescent girls with PTSD and substance use disorder: A randomized controlled trial. *Journal of Behavioral Health Services and Research, 33,* 453–463.

Najavits, L. M., Schmitz, M., Gotthardt, S., & Weiss, R. D. (2005). Seeking Safety plus Exposure Therapy: An outcome study on dual diagnosis men. *Journal of Psychoactive Drugs, 37,* 425–435.

Najavits, L. M., Weiss, R. D., Shaw, S. R., & Muenz, L. R. (1998). "Seeking safety": Outcome of a new cognitive-behavioral psychotherapy for women with posttraumatic stress disorder and substance dependence. *Journal of Traumatic Stress, 11,* 437–456.

Nowinski, J., Baker, S., & Carroll, K. (1995). *Twelve Step Facilitation Therapy manual: A clinical research guide for therapists treating individuals with alcohol abuse and dependence* (Vol. 1). Rockville, MD: National Institute on Alcohol Abuse and Alcoholism.

Petrakis, I. L., Poling, J., Levinson, C., Nich, C., Carroll, K., Ralevski, E., et al. (2005). Naltrexone and disulfiram in patients with alcohol dependence and comorbid psychiatric disorders. *Biological Psychiatry, 57,* 1128–1137.

Petrakis, I. L., Poling, J., Levinson, C., Nich, C., Carroll, K., Ralevski, E., et al. (2006). Naltrexone and disulfiram in patients with alcohol dependence and comorbid post-traumatic stress disorder. *Biological Psychiatry, 60,* 777–783.

Pratt, S. I., Rosenberg, S. D., Mueser, K. T., Brancato, J., Salyers, M. P., Jankowski, M. K., et al. (2005). Evaluation of a PTSD psychoeducational program for psychiatric inpatients. *Journal of Mental Health, 14,* 121–127.

Reddemann, L. (2004). *Psychodynamisch Imaginative Traumatherapie: PITT–das Manual.* Stuttgart: Pfeiffer bei Klett-Cotta.

Resick, P. A., & Schnicke, M. K. (1993). *Cognitive processing therapy for rape victims: A treatment manual.* Newbury Park, CA: Sage.

Rosenberg, S. D., Mueser, K. T., Jankowski, M. K., Salyers, M. P., & Acker, K. (2004). Cognitive-behavioral treatment of posttraumatic stress disorder in severe mental illness: Results of a pilot study. *American Journal of Psychiatric Rehabilitation, 7,* 171–186.

Rugs, D., Hills, H. A., & Peters, R. (2004). *Diffusion of research in practice in substance abuse treatment: A knowledge adoption study of gender-sensitive treatment.* Paper presented at the Complexities of Co-Occurring Conditions: Harnessing Services Research to Improve Care for Mental, Substance Use and Medical/Physical Disorders conference, Washington, DC.

Sachsse, U., Vogel, C., & Leichsenring, F. (2006). Results of psychodynamically oriented trauma-focused inpatient treatment for women with complex posttraumatic stress disorder (PTSD) and borderline personality disorder (BPD). *Bulletin of the Menninger Clinic, 70*(2), 125–144.

Saper, Z., & Brasfield, C. R. (1998). Two-phase treatment of panic disorder and post-traumatic stress disorder with associated personality features resulting from childhood abuse: Case study. *Journal of Behavior Therapy and Experimental Psychology, 29*(2), 171–178.

Schnurr, P. P., Friedman, M. J., Engel, C. C. J., Foa, E. B., Shea, M. T., Chow, B. K., et al. (2007). Cognitive behavioral therapy for posttraumatic stress disorder in women: A randomized controlled trial. *Journal of the American Medical Association, 297*, 820–830.

Schnurr, P. P., Friedman, M. J., Foy, D. W., Shea, M. T., Hsieh, F. Y., Lavori, P. W., et al. (2003). Randomized trial of trauma-focused group therapy for posttraumatic stress disorder: Results from a department of veterans affairs cooperative study. *Archives of General Psychiatry, 60*, 481–489.

Toussaint, D. W., VanDeMark, N. R., Bornemann, A., & Graeber, C. J. (2007). Modifications to the trauma recovery and empowerment model (TREM) for substance-abusing women with histories of violence: Outcomes and lessons learned at a Colorado Substance Abuse Treatment Center. *Journal of Community Psychology, 35*(7), 879–894.

Triffleman, E. (2000). Gender differences in a controlled pilot study of psychosocial treatments in substance dependent patients with post-traumatic stress disorder: Design considerations and outcomes. *Alcoholism Treatment Quarterly, 18*(3), 113–126.

Triffleman, E., Carroll, K., & Kellogg, S. (1999). Substance dependence posttraumatic stress disorder therapy. An integrated cognitive-behavioral approach. *Journal of Substance Abuse Treatment, 17*(1–2), 3–14.

Tsao, J. C. I., Lewin, M. R., & Craske, M. G. (1998). The effects of cognitive-behavior therapy for panic disorder on comorbid conditions. *Journal of Anxiety Disorders, 12*(4), 357–371.

Weiss, R. D., Najavits, L. M., Greenfield, S. F., Soto, J. A., Shaw, S. R., & Wyner, D. (1998). Reliability of substance use self-reports in dually diagnosed outpatients. *American Journal of Psychiatry, 155*, 127–128.

Weller, L. A. (2005). Group therapy to treat substance use and traumatic symptoms in female veterans. *Federal Practitioner, 22*, 27–38.

Zatzick, D., Roy-Byrne, P., Russo, J., Rivara, F., Droesch, R., Wagner, A., et al. (2004). A randomized effectiveness trial of stepped collaborative care for acutely injured trauma survivors. *Archives of General Psychiatry, 61*(5), 498–506.

Zlotnick, C., Najavits, L. M., & Rohsenow, D. J. (2003). A cognitive-behavioral treatment for incarcerated women with substance use disorder and posttraumatic stress disorder: Findings from a pilot study. *Journal of Substance Abuse Treatment, 25*, 99–105.

PART IV

TREATMENT GUIDELINES

Psychological Debriefing
for Adults

Description

Psychological debriefing (PD) was widely advocated for routine use following major traumatic events during the 1980s and 1990s. Several methods of PD have been described, including critical incident stress debriefing and multiple stressor debriefing. Most researchers have considered a PD to be a single-session, semistructured crisis intervention designed to reduce and prevent unwanted psychological sequelae following traumatic events by promoting emotional processing through the ventilation and normalization of reactions and preparation for possible future experiences. PD was initially described as a group intervention, one part of a comprehensive, systematic, multicomponent approach to the management of traumatic stress, but it has also been used with individuals and as a stand-alone intervention. Its purpose is to review the impressions and reactions of clients shortly after a traumatic incident. The focus of a PD is on the present reaction of those involved. Psychiatric labeling is avoided, and emphasis is placed on normalization. Participants are assured that they are normal people who have experienced an abnormal event.

General Strength of the Evidence

Identified studies vary greatly in their quality. Overall the quality of studies, including the randomized controlled trials, is poor. Studies included since the first edition's guidelines support and strengthen the original conclusion that there is no evidence to suggest that single-session individual PD is effective in the prevention of posttraumatic stress disorder (PTSD) symptoms shortly after a traumatic event or in the prevention of longer-term psychological sequelae (Level A). There remains an absence of evidence with regard to group PD. The single identified study of group PD was neutral, suggesting that there is unlikely to be a significant beneficial effect of group PD. Some negative outcomes following individual PD were found, but, overall, the impact of early individual PD was neutral when all the identified studies were considered collectively (Level A).

Course of Treatment

PD has generally been described as a group intervention lasting up to a few hours shortly after (often within a few days of) a traumatic event, and as one component of a critical incident stress management program. It has also been described as a single-session intervention for individuals, and as one component of a treatment package for chronic PTSD.

Recommendations

The current evidence suggests that individual PD should not be used following traumatic events (Level A), and that there is unlikely to be a significant beneficial effect of group PD; therefore, its use is not advocated (Level A). The effectiveness of group PD as a support process for homogeneous groups to enhance unit cohesion and unit performance, and as one component of a package of care such as critical incident stress management have yet to be determined. Given the current state of knowledge, the following steps are advocated.

1. Shortly after a traumatic event, it is important that those affected should be provided, in an empathic manner, practical, pragmatic psychological support and information about possible reactions, and about how to help themselves, how to access support from those around them, and where and when to access further help if necessary (Level C).

2. Any early intervention approach should be based on an accurate and current assessment of need prior to intervention. No formal intervention should be mandated for all exposed to trauma. Use of trauma support should be voluntary, except in cases in which event-related impairment is a threat to an individual's own safety or to the safety of others (Level C).

3. Interventions should be culturally sensitive, developmentally appropriate, and related to the local formulation of problems and ways of coping (Level C).

Summary

The evidence for a neutral overall effect of PD has strengthened since the publication of the first edition of the International Society for Traumatic Stress Studies (ISTSS) guidelines. There appears to be little advantage to investing limited resources into further evaluation of individual or group PD as a single-session intervention. It is not a psychological treatment or a substitute for psychological treatment when indicated. However, it is probable that certain components of PD are helpful. Future research should be on the development of new approaches rather than on PD as a stand-alone intervention. PD should be regarded as an intervention that had good face validity and was appropriate to subject to randomized controlled trials, but that was not shown to be effective in either significantly reducing distress or preventing long-term psychopathology. The PD era should not only inform the development of new interventions, but it should also serve as a stark reminder that psychological interventions can be extremely powerful and cause negative, as well as positive, effects. Therefore future research efforts should focus on evaluating tailored, multilevel systems of care for high-risk populations, such as emergency service workers, as well as on innovative applications of interventions proven to be effective in other posttrauma settings, such as cognitive-behavioral interventions.

Suggested Readings

Everly, G. S., Jr., & Mitchell, J. T. (1999). *Critical incident stress management (CISM): A new era and standard of care in crisis intervention.* Ellicott City, MD: Chevron.

National Collaborating Centre for Mental Health. (2005). *Post-traumatic stress disorder: The management of PTSD in adults and children in primary and secondary care.* London: Gaskell/BPS.

Watson, P. J., Friedman, M. J., Ruzek, J. I., & Norris, F. H. (2002). Managing acute stress response to major trauma. *Current Psychiatry Reports, 4,* 247–253.

Wessely, S., Rose, S., & Bisson, J. (2005). *A systematic review of brief psychological interventions ("debriefing") for the treatment of immediate trauma related symptoms and the prevention of posttraumatic stress disorder* [CD-ROM]. Oxford, UK: Update Software.

Acute Interventions
for Children and Adolescents

Description

Over the past several decades, there have been a variety of acute interventions for children and adolescents after traumatic experiences. Acute interventions comprise those provided in the first 6 weeks after exposure. Such strategies have included psychoeducation; bereavement support; various forms of psychological debriefing; eye movement desensitization and reprocessing (EMDR), clarification of cognitive distortions; discussion of thoughts and feelings; reinforcement of adaptive coping and safety behaviors, and use of support systems; structured and unstructured art and play activities; and massage. Interventions have been delivered in a variety of modalities, including individual, group, and classroom sessions; community-based programs; crisis intervention groups; psychoeducational materials; and crisis hotlines.

General Strength of the Evidence

There is a paucity of evidence regarding the effectiveness of acute posttrauma interventions for children and adolescents. Much of the material describing these efforts has not been published in mainstream psychological and psychiatric journals, but in journals devoted to other disciplines that have less stringent standards for methodological rigor. In addition, the majority of these reports provide only anecdotal findings; relatively few have used randomized designs with adequate control groups. Most studies to date have suffered from small sample size, lack of adequate control/comparison groups, and absence of long-term follow-up. Whereas some studies have geared evaluation metrics to specific intervention objectives, others have used available child or adolescent measures. Such standardized instruments may not be adequately sensitive in detecting the benefits of the intervention, especially if these domains are not intervention targets. Another problem is the time variability posttrauma in which the intervention is delivered, making cross-study comparisons difficult.

Systemic Approaches

Systemic approaches have included psychoeducation; consultation with school personnel, media, and parents; crisis hotlines; and community-based programs. The overall evidence regarding the benefits of these types of interventions falls within the Agency for Health Care Policy and Research (AHCPR) Level C category. The most comprehensive study documented the benefits of community-based services in four areas, including program responsiveness, visibility of staff, responsiveness to ethnic differences, and overall quality of the program. This type of community approach holds great promise, but more rigorous quantitative studies with appropriate controls are needed.

Art and Massage Therapies

One art therapy study (AHCPR Level A) showed no statistically significant differences between experimental and control groups. Due to lack of dose of exposure methodology, it is difficult to determine whether there were potential benefits of the intervention associated with different levels of trauma. Future studies need to use exposure groups in analyzing findings. In regard to massage therapy, one study meeting AHCPR Level A criteria demonstrated potential benefits in a number of outcome domains but did not evaluate PTSD postintervention. Future studies in this area need to examine the benefits of this type of therapy in regard to amelioration of PTSD.

Eye Movement Desensitization and Reprocessing

A variety of EMDR protocols or adaptations have been studied in the acute aftermath of trauma. EMDR treatment includes eight phases: history taking, preparation, assessment of a traumatic memory, desensitization, strengthening positive responses to traumatic memories and reminders, body scan for somatic symptoms, closure, and reassessment. Variability in the duration of EMDR interventions studied posttrauma has included interventions that have been provided during the acute phase and those that have been continued up to 1 year posttrauma (AHCPR Level B). As components of EMDR overlap with those that have been incorporated in many other approaches, future studies need to identify the active ingredients specific to this promising approach.

Debriefing

Three studies have examined the effectiveness of various forms of debriefing in children and adolescents after different types of trauma (AHCPR Levels A and B). Current evidence suggests that debriefing cannot effectively prevent the subsequent development of PTSD or other anxiety disorders in traumatized children and adolescents. Although these studies have combined debriefing with other acute interventions, and have differed in timing, debriefing is not recommended at this time.

Cognitive-Behavioral Approaches

Many clinicians are familiar with and have utilized cognitive-behavioral approaches in acute settings. Although these approaches have been found to be effective in longer-term treatment outcome studies of traumatized children and adolescents, no studies in the acute aftermath have formally evaluated outcome (AHCPR Level C). This approach holds great promise; however, more studies are needed in order to determine the effectiveness and optimal timing of cognitive-behavioral approaches.

Psychological First Aid

Psychological first aid (PFA) approaches include many of the intervention strategies that comprise other acute intervention protocols for children and adolescents. PFA allows tailoring of these interventions to meet the specific needs of children and families. In addition, many of the PFA recommendations are supported by a vast literature on the utility of enhancing coping, social support, and problem solving, and have been informed by clinicians with extensive experience. Although PFA has not yet been systematically studied, one PFA field operations guide has been based on years of experience in providing acute assistance to traumatized children and families, and has been found to be acceptable to and well received by consumers (AHCPR Level C). Establishing the evidence base for PFA approaches will require standardized protocols and trainings, documentation of fidelity, rigorous outcome evaluation, and longitudinal studies that document course of recovery.

Course of Treatment

There are currently no definitive data regarding the optimal length or timing of acute interventions for traumatized children and adolescents. The optimal length of intervention will likely vary broadly depending on the degree of exposure and loss, and severity of posttrauma adversity and distress. These factors make it difficult to identify a potentially optimal length of intervention that would fit across differentially affected individuals. In response to these considerations, more recent efforts have focused on tailoring flexible acute interventions to meet the specific needs of affected children and adolescents.

Recommendations

Given the current state of knowledge, a good deal more research on the effectiveness of acute interventions for children and adolescents impacted by a traumatic event is needed, thus precluding any definitive recommendations regarding intervention selection or timing. Five major categories of acute interventions have been used.

Summary

There are many gaps in our knowledge about providing optimal assistance to children and adolescents in the acute aftermath of trauma. There is a great need for both program evaluation and randomized controlled trials to examine the effectiveness of acute interventions across trauma types, age ranges, cultural groups, and different settings. In reviewing the literature, it is apparent that many studies have not utilized strict protocols or adhered to intervention guidelines. Future research needs to examine the optimal timing of acute interventions and the possible differential effectiveness of intervention strategies for differentially affected subpopulations.

Suggested Readings

Bisson, J. I., & Cohen, J. A. (2006). Disseminating early interventions following trauma. *Journal of Traumatic Stress, 19,* 583–595.

Brymer, M., Jacobs, A., Layne, C., Pynoos, R., Ruzek J., Steinberg, S., et al. (2006). *Psychological first aid: Field operations guide, second edition.* Washington, DC: National Child Traumatic Stress Network and National Center for PTSD. Available at *www.nctsn.org* and *www.ncptsd.va.gov*

McNally, R. J., Bryant, R. A., & Ehlers, A. (2003). Does early psychological intervention promote recovery from posttraumatic stress? *Psychological Science in the Public Interest, 4,* 45–79.

Stallard, P., Velleman, R., Salter, E., Howse, I., Yule, W., & Taylor, G. (2006). A randomised controlled trial to determine the effectiveness of an early psychological intervention with children involved in road traffic accidents. *Journal of Child Psychology and Psychiatry, and Applied Disciplines, 47,* 127–134.

Early Cognitive-Behavioral Interventions for Adults

Description

In the past decade, a number of randomized controlled trials (RCTs) have examined the efficacy of cognitive-behavioral therapy (CBT) to prevent the development of PTSD in the weeks and months following a traumatic event. Use of CBT to target PTSD in the early intervention context mirrors the techniques found to have efficacy with chronic PTSD in tertiary care. The published trials employed a family of CBT strategies, including psychoeducation, stress management skills training, cognitive therapy, and exposure therapy. The interventions were collaborative and experiential, and utilized homework and *in vivo* application of strategies learned in face-to-face therapy.

General Strength of the Evidence

Capitalizing on natural recovery trajectories, open and uncontrolled trials are considerably less revealing than RCTs; accordingly, only evidence from Level A RCTs was considered. With the exception of indices of effect size, the trials are not easily compared because they differ in terms of gender of the subjects, nature of the index trauma targeted, procedural variations (e.g., number of sessions, differing assessments), and specific CBT techniques employed. Nevertheless, as trauma types and contexts vary, practitioners need to know whether CBT is effective as an early intervention for the challenges their patients face. Accordingly, the reviewed CBT trials were categorized according to the types of trauma survivors (and subject gender) studied.

Mixed-Gender Motor Vehicle and Industrial Accidents

Four Level A RCTs targeting motor vehicle and industrial accident survivors were evaluated. CBT was robustly more effective in reducing PTSD symptom burden and in preventing chronic PTSD relative to supportive counseling, repeated assessments, and self-help booklets.

Mixed-Gender Accidents and Nonsexual Assaults

Treatment outcome was strong in the five Level A RCTs of men and women who experienced an accident or nonsexual assault. In some of the studies, CBT was found to be superior to supportive counseling in reducing PTSD symptoms and in preventing PTSD, although attrition rate was greater for the CBT arms. In some studies, CBT robustly reduced avoidance behaviors, yet there was little impact on other PTSD symptoms. In a trial of individuals with physical injury, CBT conferred little advantage compared to standard hospital care.

Female-Only Sexual and Nonsexual Assault Trials

CBT appears to hasten recovery in female assault survivors compared to supportive care, but supportive care also leads to marked improvement over time. In one of the best-designed studies to date, CBT did not provide any lasting advantage relative to an assessment-only condition. Trials that include assault survivors may have less positive results because adaptation to interpersonal violence, especially sexual violence, appears to be more complicated and multifaceted.

Course of Treatment

Early-intervention CBT ranges from five to 12 weekly sessions, 60–90 minutes in length.

Recommendations

CBT is recommended as an early intervention for survivors of relatively discrete accidents who endorse significant, enduring posttraumatic difficulties in the aftermath of trauma. It is more difficult to draw definitive recommendations from studies that include both physical and sexual assault survivors because the efficacy data from these are less compelling at this time. In the early aftermath of trauma (days and weeks), treatment with CBT should only be provided to sexual assault and nonsexual assault survivors following a period of sustained monitoring and support. For some assault and accident survivors, such a policy could readily be part of a treatment plan. One added benefit of routine monitoring within the first weeks is that it can also trigger self-referral to formal CBT, if symptoms or impairment are sufficiently severe. During a monitoring phase, assault survivors might be prepared for CBT treatments to enhance readiness and motivation for care.

Summary

Evidence for the efficacy of CBT in preventing chronic PTSD is unequivocally strong (Level A) among discrete trauma survivors (motor vehicle and industrial accidents), and is less clear-cut for traumatic events that involve interpersonal violence, such as sexual and nonsexual assault. The field needs more studies of the efficacy of a standardized CBT as an early intervention following trauma exposure, employing a standardized number of sessions, as well as comparable process and outcome measures. Clinical trials that target groups at high risk for trauma exposure, namely, emergency services personnel, first responders, and military combatants, would also be especially welcome.

Suggested Readings

Bryant, R. A., & Harvey, A. G. (2000). *Acute stress disorder: A handbook of theory, assessment, and treatment.* Washington, DC: American Psychological Association.

Litz, B. T. (Ed.). (2004). *Early intervention for trauma and traumatic loss.* New York: Guilford Press.

Cognitive-Behavioral Therapy for Adults

Description

Several forms of cognitive-behavioral therapy (CBT) have been studied as treatments for chronic adult posttraumatic stress disorder (PTSD) resulting from a range of traumatic events. However, the amount and quality of supporting evidence varies substantially for different CBT programs. *Exposure therapy* refers to a series of procedures designed to help individuals confront thoughts and safe or low-risk stimuli that are feared or avoided. Applied to the treatment of PTSD, most exposure therapy programs include imaginal exposure to the trauma memory and *in vivo* exposure to reminders of the trauma or triggers for trauma-related fear and avoidance, although some CBT programs have been limited to one type of exposure. *Systematic desensitization* is procedurally distinct from other forms of exposure therapy in that it involves the explicit pairing of the trauma-related memories and reminders with muscle relaxation to inhibit the fear, whereas other exposure therapy programs do not routinely seek actively to inhibit fear during exposure exercises.

Stress inoculation training (SIT) is a multicomponent anxiety management treatment program that includes education, muscle relaxation training, breathing retraining, role playing, covert modeling, guided self-dialogue, and thought stopping. SIT programs may also include *assertion training* and exposure therapy components, although studies of SIT for chronic PTSD have typically left out one or both of these components because they were included in the comparison condition under investigation. Training in progressive *muscle relaxation* is both a part of SIT and a stand-alone comparison treatment. *Biofeedback* training, another approach to promote relaxation, uses electrophysiological instruments to provide feedback about physiological states, thereby promoting deeper levels of relaxation. *Cognitive therapy* (CT), predicated on the idea that it is one's interpretation of an event rather than the event itself that determines emotional reactions, involves identifying erroneous or unhelpful cognitions, evaluating the evidence for and against these cognitions, and considering whether the cognitions are the result of cognitive biases or errors, in the service of developing more realistic or useful cognitions. In the treatment of PTSD, much of the focus of CT is on cognitions related to safety/danger, trust, and views of oneself.

Several CBT programs combine elements of one or more of the preceding treatments, most commonly combining some form of exposure therapy with components of SIT, CT, or both. For example, *cognitive processing therapy* (CPT) implements exposure to the trauma memory via writing a trauma narrative and repeatedly reading it, and is combined with CT focused on themes of safety, trust, power/control, esteem, and intimacy. Several other combination programs have varied the specific components that have been combined, and the manner in which they have been implemented. *Dialectical behavior therapy* (DBT) is a comprehensive treatment developed for the treatment of individuals with borderline personality disorder. An important aspect of DBT is skills training in affect regulation and interpersonal regulation. Some trauma survivors may have deficits in these skill areas that make it difficult for them to tolerate or benefit from trauma-focused interventions such as exposure therapy. Accordingly, such skills training has been proposed not as a treatment for PTSD per se, but as a preliminary intervention that may enhance at least some patients' (e.g., survivors of childhood abuse) ability to benefit from subsequent trauma-focused treatments such as exposure therapy. Most conventional CBT programs for PTSD are described in terms of techniques explicitly intended to reduce distress. *Acceptance and commitment therapy* (ACT), by contrast, assumes that much of human suffering is the result of attempts to control internal experiences, called "experiential avoidance." The solution, from this approach, is the *acceptance* of one's personal experiences and a *commitment* to live one's life in accordance with personal values, rather than the pursuit of experiential avoidance.

Recent innovations in treatments that have been the focus of empirical research include combined CBT programs that specifically target nightmares and use technology to assist in the delivery of treatment. Innovations in the use of technology to deliver treatment include the use of virtual reality technology and the administration of treatment via the Internet.

General Strength of the Evidence

Because the amount and quality of evidence varies for different CBT programs, strength of the evidence is summarized separately for each of the

CBT programs described earlier. The treatments are summarized in order of decreasing strength of supporting evidence.

Exposure Therapy

There is strong support for the efficacy of individual exposure therapy administered to a range of trauma populations (men and women; survivors of military trauma, physical and sexual assault, childhood sexual abuse, motor vehicle accidents, political violence) from 22 randomized Agency for Health Care Policy and Research (AHCPR) Level A studies and eight nonrandomized Level B studies. The evidence is particularly strong for the combination of imaginal plus *in vivo* exposure (11 Level A studies, four Level B studies). These studies consistently yielded positive results; patients treated with exposure therapy demonstrated significant improvement, and in randomized trials, exposure therapy was superior to various control conditions (wait list, relaxation, and supportive counseling).

Other variations of exposure therapy include imaginal exposure alone (nine Level A studies, two Level B studies) and *in vivo* exposure alone (two Level A studies, one Level B study). One Level A study that utilized a crossover design found that imaginal and *in vivo* exposure produced similar outcomes, although *in vivo* exposure was superior to imaginal exposure in reducing behavior avoidance. With one exception, an older randomized study of imaginal exposure with male Vietnam veterans, that did not directly assess PTSD symptoms, these studies all yielded significant improvement from pre- to posttreatment. In addition, the randomized studies yielded superior improvement compared to wait-list and supportive counseling comparison groups. Three of the Level A studies of imaginal exposure utilized a program called narrative exposure therapy (reconstruction of traumatic experiences in relation to the biography of the survivor), which has been implemented successfully with survivors of political violence. For example, one study was conducted with Sudanese refugees living in an Ugandan refugee settlement. Two additional studies, both with male veterans (one Level A, the other Level B), administered exposure therapy in group settings. The Level A study found similar, small but statistically significant, reductions in PTSD severity for both exposure and present-centered group therapies. The Level B study did not find any significant change in PTSD severity for either exposure therapy or skills building treatment utilizing SIT methods that targeted anxiety, stress, and anger.

In summary, the evidence from many well-controlled studies across and a wide range of trauma survivors is very compelling. Individually administered exposure therapy is effective. In fact, no other specific CBT program has such strong evidence for its efficacy. The evidence is strongest for the combination of imaginal plus *in vivo* exposure, although imaginal exposure alone was also found to be efficacious in a number of studies. Thus, individually administered exposure therapy receives an AHCPR Level A rating.

By contrast, there is very little support for efficacy of group-administered exposure therapy.

Cognitive Processing Therapy

There is consistent support for CPT from five studies (three Level A studies, one Level B study, and one Level C study). Two studies found CPT to be more effective than wait list among female rape survivors; one of the studies received a Level A rating. The two remaining Level A studies found CPT to be more effective than wait list among female survivors of sexual abuse in childhood and among (predominantly) male veterans in which the index trauma was related to combat in 78% of the cases, with noncombat physical and sexual assaults comprising the rest. The study that received a Level C rating utilized archival data from a service-based organization to test the applicability of CPT to a U.S. population of refugees from Afghanistan and Bosnia–Hertzgovina. Although based on significantly fewer studies than results for exposure therapy, CPT receives an AHCPR Level A rating.

Stress Inoculation Training

Support for the efficacy of SIT is mixed but generally supportive, particularly among female sexual assault victims. Four studies of individually administered SIT that targeted PTSD symptoms (two Level A studies, two Level B studies) of female sexual assault victims found significant reductions from pre- to posttreatment, and the two randomized studies found it to be more effective than wait list and supportive counseling. Among veterans, researchers in one Level A study reported in a footnote that in addition to the exposure therapy and wait-list control conditions, the original design of the study included stress inoculation group training, but the data were not reported because only five subjects completed the treatment. A second (Level B) study that provided SIT to veterans in a group format did not find any significant improvement on PTSD severity. A third study with veterans, utilizing SIT that targeted anger, found a greater reduction on anger and reexperiencing than that which was found with use of routine clinical care. The strength of the two controlled studies of PTSD among female sexual assault victims earned SIT a Level A rating with this population. Evidence for the efficacy of SIT among veterans is limited and mixed.

Cognitive Therapy

CT was found to be effective in reducing posttrauma symptoms and received support from two controlled studies of civilian traumas, both of which were rated Level A.

Systematic Desensitization

The efficacy of systematic desensitization for PTSD has been evaluated in six studies (two Level A studies, three Level B studies, and one Level C study). All but one of these studies suffered from serious methodological problems. The one well-conducted, Level A study of systematic desensitization was superior to wait list but did not differ from hypnotherapy or psychodynamic treatment, neither of which has strong independent support from other RCTs. Thus, systematic desensitization has not received strong support from well-controlled studies and receives a Level B– or C+ rating.

Assertion Training

The only Level B study that evaluated the efficacy of assertion training found that assertion training did not differ from comparison conditions. Thus, assertion training has not received strong support in the treatment of PTSD.

Relaxation and Biofeedback

No studies have directly examined the efficacy of relaxation by comparing it with a wait list. However, relaxation has served as a comparison group against which other treatments have been compared. With regard to CBT, three Level A studies have found relaxation to be less efficacious than exposure therapy, CT, and their combination. There is only one Level A study of biofeedback for PTSD in which either biofeedback or eye movement desensitization and reprocessing (EMDR) was added to treatment as usual (TAU). Biofeedback was not supported because the addition of EMDR was superior to TAU (see Chapter 11, this volume, for review and guidelines regarding EMDR), but the addition of biofeedback was not. Thus, neither relaxation training nor biofeedback has received support as treatments for PTSD.

Dialectical Behavior Therapy and Acceptance and Commitment Therapy

Three studies (two Level A studies, one Level B study) evaluated the sequential application of skills training followed by trauma-focused treatment (imaginal exposure in two studies, trauma-focused writing in one study). Significant improvement from pre- to posttreatment was observed in all three studies, and treatment in the Level A studies was superior to wait list. The only study that evaluated the effects of the skills training component on PTSD found minimal change that did not differ from wait list. Furthermore, the design of the study did not permit the determination of whether skills training facilitated subsequent treatment with imaginal exposure because the study did not compare the combined treatment with imaginal exposure alone. In support of the underlying model that preliminary skills training may enhance subsequent trauma-focused treatment, one study found that therapeutic alliance and negative mood regulation skills during the skills training portion of treatment predicted PTSD improvement during the imaginal exposure portion of treatment. To date, no published studies have evaluated ACT as a treatment for PTSD. Thus, neither DBT nor ACT has received support as an effective treatment for PTSD.

Combination Treatment and Comparisons among Treatments

Numerous individually administered CBT programs targeting PTSD, that have combined elements of exposure therapy, SIT, and CT, have been studied in 25 Level A and 13 Level B studies across a range of trauma populations. All of these studies have found significant improvement from pre- to posttreatment, and the randomized studies have consistently found CBT to be superior to comparison conditions (wait list, supportive counseling, TAU). Imagery rehearsal therapy is a somewhat unique treatment, in that it uses a combination of imaginal exposure and CT plus instruction in sleep hygiene specifically to target nightmares and sleep problems. Unlike more conventional exposure therapy, imaginal exposure is to the content of the nightmare rather than the trauma memory, and rescripting involves intentionally altering the nightmare content in some fashion. Three studies (two Level A studies, one Level B study) have found significant reductions in PTSD severity from pre- to posttreatment, and the two randomized studies found greater improvement than that in the wait list. Unlike more conventional exposure therapy, imagery rehearsal therapy has been successfully administered in groups.

Nine Level A studies have directly compared one CBT program with a different program (e.g., exposure therapy vs. SIT) or have compared a combined treatment program with one or more of the constituent treatments (e.g., exposure therapy alone vs. exposure therapy combined with CT). Six additional Level A studies have compared some form of exposure therapy (alone or in combination with SIT or CT) with EMDR. All of these studies have found significant improvement for the CBT programs (including EMDR), with little evidence of superiority for one program over another, and they have found that the combined treatments are generally not more efficacious than the component treatments.

Collectively, these studies indicate that CBT programs including one or more components of exposure therapy, SIT, and CT are broadly effective. However, with the exception of intense exposure therapy (imaginal plus *in vivo* exposure), few specific treatment programs have been evaluated in more than three Level A studies, and most have been studied with a limited range of trauma populations (e.g., CT has not been studied in veterans).

Medication and CBT

One small, Level A pilot study directly compared exposure therapy plus SIT with paroxetine, one of two medications with U.S. Food and Drug Administration (FDA) indications for PTSD. Although the study did not include a placebo condition, significant improvement was obtained from pre- to posttreatment for both treatments, with no difference between them. Four Level A studies have found that adding CBT to ongoing medication management for medication partial responders results in greater improvement than medication continuation alone.

Use of Technology in Administering CBT

One Level A study and one Level B study have investigated the use of virtual reality technology to administer exposure therapy. Both studies found reductions in PTSD severity from pre- to posttreatment, and the randomized study found that virtual reality exposure therapy was superior to wait list. No study has compared virtual reality exposure therapy with more traditionally delivered CBT. Five studies (four Level A studies, one Level B study) have evaluated combined CBT programs administered via the Internet, although one of these studies included some in-person contact with a study therapist. All studies found significant improvement from pre- to posttreatment, and the Level A studies found CBT to be superior to wait list (three studies) or supportive counseling similarly administered via the Internet (one study). No studies have evaluated the efficacy of CBT administered via the Internet with the same treatment delivered in person.

Course of Treatment

CBT programs for PTSD are generally short-term, averaging approximately 8–12 individual therapy sessions. A small number of studies have demonstrated significant improvement with as few as one to four sessions of CBT. Sessions typically last between 60 and 90 minutes, are administered once or twice weekly, and involve patients' completion of homework between sessions. One difference between research studies and standard clinical practice is that studies need to specify ahead of time the number of sessions to be offered, independent of patients' individual needs. However, some patients may require longer treatment than others to obtain optimal benefits, such as patients with significant comorbidities or those whose clinical picture is complicated by chronic pain problems. In such cases, common clinical practice is to extend treatment as long as there are signs of progress. Consistent with the clinical practice of extending treatment based on the patient's response to treatment, one study of exposure therapy (alone and in combination with

CT) found that patients who did not achieve an excellent outcome by Session 8 substantially benefited from just a few additional sessions.

Recommendations

Based on the evidence summarized here, we recommend the following:

1. CBT that comprises exposure therapy (imaginal and *in vivo* exposure), CT, SIT, or one of the many combination programs that incorporate some form of exposure with formal CT (e.g., CPT) or SIT is recommended as a first-line treatment for chronic PTSD.

2. RLX, biofeedback, and assertiveness training cannot be recommended as primary treatments for PTSD, although they may be useful as ancillary interventions for specific problems in certain patients with PTSD.

3. Skills training in affect and interpersonal regulation, based on DBT, prior to implementing trauma-focused interventions, such as imaginal exposure, may be useful for individuals who have difficulty tolerating trauma-focused interventions. However, due to insufficient evidence, *routine* application of skills training prior to trauma-focused treatment is not recommended *at this time*.

4. Due to the current lack of evidence on the efficacy of ACT, we cannot recommend it as a first-line treatment for PTSD, although acceptance-based strategies, some of which are incorporated into DBT, may be useful ancillary interventions for some individuals.

5. With the exception of imagery rehearsal targeting nightmares, CBT for PTSD should be administered in one-on-one therapy sessions. However, given the limited evidence for this treatment relative to other CBT programs to date, imagery rehearsal therapy is not recommended as a first-line treatment for PTSD. It may be most useful as an ancillary treatment, if residual sleep problems remain after a course of other CBT.

6. CBT is intended to be a short-term treatment, and 8–12 sessions lasting 60–120 minutes, administered once or twice weekly, may be used as a general guideline for planning the duration of treatment. However, some patients may be responsive to fewer sessions, while others with more complex cases may require a somewhat longer course of treatment. Accordingly, it is recommended that treatment not be arbitrarily terminated based on the number of sessions. Rather, treatment duration should be determined by a combination of the patient's progress and current symptom status: If the patient has shown improvement but continues to experience significant PTSD, continued treatment is likely to result in further benefit.

7. Recent technological advances show promise in making treatment easier to implement and more readily available. For example, virtual reality technology may make it easier to implement certain kinds of exposure exercises that would otherwise be difficult to implement *in vivo* (e.g., riding in a

military helicopter for Vietnam veterans), and use of the Internet can make access to CBT available in underserved communities. However, practical considerations limit the utility of these treatments at this time. Virtual reality technology is currently still relatively expensive, few therapists have access to it, and treatment programs are available for only a limited number of traumas. In addition, use of the Internet to deliver treatment allows a therapist to treat someone he or she has never seen in person and who may very well be receiving that treatment in a different state or even country. This raises ethical and legal issues that need to be worked out prior to making strong recommendations for the routine use of this service delivery mechanism.

Summary

The evidence in support of the effectiveness of individually administered CBT for the treatment of PTSD in adults is now quite compelling: Numerous CBT programs have been shown to work in well-controlled studies meeting high methodological standards. Considering both the quantity and quality of evidence supporting each treatment, the evidence in favor of exposure therapy is the most convincing, as it has 22 RCTs to support its use across a wide range of traumatized populations. Across studies, exposure therapy has been implemented in numerous ways, including imaginal exposure, *in vivo* exposure, and writing about the trauma. The most frequent—and therefore, the most supported—method of implementing exposure is the combination of imaginal exposure to the trauma memory plus *in vivo* exposure to feared and avoided but low-risk people, places, situations and activities. In fact, no other CBT modality has received as much support as exposure therapy.

The next-best-supported CBT program is CPT, which has received support in three RCTs of survivors of sexual assault, including childhood sexual abuse, and military-related traumas. SIT and CT have both received support from two RCTs each. Numerous, additional well-controlled, randomized studies support the use of combination CBT programs, most of which have utilized some form of exposure therapy plus elements of other CBT programs, such as SIT, CT, or skills training in affect and interpersonal regulation based on principles of DBT. Direct comparisons between different CBT programs (e.g., exposure therapy vs. CT) have generally found comparable outcomes across different treatments. Similarly, studies that have compared combined treatment programs with the constituent programs (e.g., exposure therapy plus SIT vs. exposure therapy alone) have found comparable outcomes for the individual treatments and the combination treatments.

Treatments that did not receive support as stand-alone therapies for PTSD were RLX, biofeedback, assertiveness training, DBT, and ACT. The limited research on RLX and biofeedback indicates that they are less efficacious than other CBT programs, and the single study of assertiveness training found that it is no more efficacious than supportive counseling. There are insufficient data at this time to evaluate the efficacy of ACT for PTSD or related symptoms.

It has been proposed that skills training in affect and interpersonal regulation, based on DBT, prior to implementing trauma-focused interventions, such as imaginal exposure, may be useful for individuals who have difficulty tolerating trauma-focused interventions and who have associated features of PTSD, such as impaired affect regulation, dissociative symptoms, interpersonal problems, and personality changes that may arise from chronic trauma (e.g., survivors of childhood abuse or domestic violence, and prisoners of war or refugees). The studies that have evaluated the administration of skills training followed by trauma-focused CBT have found this combination to be efficacious for PTSD symptoms, as well as for problems such as emotion regulation, dissociative experiencing, and interpersonal dysfunction. Given the evidence to date, it is unknown to what extent the first-line treatments, DBT-based interventions, or their combinations may be successful in reducing associated features of PTSD often seen in chronically traumatized populations.

In general, CBT for PTSD has been administered as a one-on-one therapy, and group exposure therapy has not been found to be particularly effective. A notable exception to this is the use of imagery rehearsal therapy to target nightmares, which has been implemented successfully in a group therapy setting. Two recent technological innovations that received empirical support are the use of virtual reality technology to implement exposure therapy and the delivery of CBT via the Internet. In particular, use of the Internet to deliver treatment has the potential to provide CBT to people in locations where it would not otherwise be available.

Suggested Readings

Cloitre, M., Cohen, L. R., & Koenen, K. C. (2006). *Treating survivors of childhood abuse: Psychotherapy for the interrupted life.* New York: Guilford Press.

Foa, E. B., Hembree, E. A., & Rothbaum, B. O. (2007). *Prolonged exposure therapy for PTSD: Emotional processing of traumatic experiences: Therapist guide.* Oxford, UK: Oxford University Press.

Follette, V. M., & Ruzek, J. I. (2006). *Cognitive-behavioral therapies for trauma* (2nd ed.). New York: Guilford Press.

Resick, P. A., & Schnicke, M. K. (1993). *Cognitive processing therapy for rape victims: A treatment manual.* Newbury Park, CA: Sage.

Schauer, M., Neuner, F., & Elbert, T. (2005). *Narrative exposure therapy: A short-term intervention for traumatic stress disorder after war, terror or torture.* Göttingen, Germany: Hogrefe & Huber.

Taylor, S. (2006). *Clinician's guide to PTSD: A cognitive-behavioral approach.* New York: Guilford Press.

Cognitive-Behavioral Therapy for Children and Adolescents

Description

A number of effective trauma-specific cognitive-behavioral therapy (CBT) models are currently available. These models share common components, summarized by the acronym PRACTICE, whose components are as follows: *Parental* treatment, including parenting skills; *Psychoeducation* about common child and parent reactions to trauma; *Relaxation* and stress management skills; *Affective* expression and modulation skills; *Cognitive* coping skills; *Trauma narrative* and cognitive processing of the child's traumatic experiences; *In vivo desensitization* to trauma reminders; *Conjoint* child–parent sessions; and *Enhancing safety* and future development. Some CBT models for traumatized children only include some of these components; others add additional components and/or include ancillary services, such as case management. Additional tenets of these treatments include the following: (1) skills development (e.g., affective regulation and addressing safety needs) is provided prior to exposure components; (2) parental inclusion in therapy is optimal when possible; (3) recognition that trauma impacts multiple facets of children's lives; therefore, interfacing with schools, medical providers, justice system, child protection, child welfare, and other systems of care is often necessary to provide optimal interventions for traumatized children.

General Strength of the Evidence

Several individual posttraumatic stress disorder (PTSD)–targeted CBT models for children or adolescents have evidence of efficacy in Level A or B studies.

Trauma-focused CBT (TF-CBT) is the most thoroughly tested of these models, with six Level A studies completed for children between 3 and 17 years of age by three independent research teams in the United States and Australia. These studies demonstrated that TF-CBT is superior to comparison conditions for improving a variety of child symptoms, including PTSD, depression, internalizing symptoms, general behavioral symptoms, and shame. All of these studies were conducted with sexually abused children. The largest study included over 200 children, most of whom had experienced multiple-trauma histories in addition to sexual abuse. TF-CBT was also used in three Level B studies for children who had experienced terrorism and traumatic grief; these studies also demonstrated significant improvement in PTSD symptoms. TF-CBT has been culturally adapted and evaluated for Latino children and is currently being used and evaluated with Dutch, German, Norwegian, African, Pakistani, and other international populations of children.

Cognitive-based CBT has been compared to a wait-list control in a pilot Level A study for U.K. children exposed to single-incident traumatic events and has shown positive findings for PTSD, anxiety, and depression.

Seeking Safety (SS) is an integrated treatment model for comorbid PTSD and substance use disorder (SUD). Direct exposure techniques are not typically included (but can be done adjunctively). A Level A study of U.S. adolescents showed significantly better outcomes for SS than for treatment as usual (TAU) in various domains at posttreatment, including substance use and associated problems, trauma-related symptoms, cognitions related to PTSD and SUD, psychiatric functioning, and several additional areas of pathology not targeted in the treatment (e.g., anorexia, somatization, generalized anxiety). Some gains were sustained at 3-month follow-up.

KIDNET, a child-friendly form of narrative exposure therapy (NET), was developed in Germany specifically to treat survivors of multiple and severe trauma. NET includes psychoeducation, narration, and cognitive processing, with a focus on children's and human rights to help regain dignity. One KID-NET study described as Level A was published in German in a book chapter and presented at a peer-reviewed conference shortly before publication of these guidelines.

Trauma systems therapy (TST) combines individual therapy, such as TF-CBT with a systematic approach for children who have experienced complex trauma or challenging family situations, or who need medication management, residential or inpatient placement, and/or other complex clinical needs. TST was found to be superior to usual care in a Level B study of U.S. children and adolescents.

Promising practices for complex trauma are currently being tested. Two such models, Structured Psychotherapy for Adolescents Recovering from Chronic Stress (SPARCS) and Life Skills/Life Story are being tested in residential, as well as outpatient, settings for U.S. teens with complex trauma histories.

Course of Treatment

The CBT models for childhood PTSD described earlier are provided over the course of 8–24 sessions, but they are intended to be implemented with flexibility, so that each component can be adjusted to the needs of the individual child.

Recommendations

Several trauma-focused cognitive-behavioral child and adolescent interventions effectively decrease PTSD symptoms. Additionally, these interventions provide traumatized children and teens with skills that generalize beyond PTSD symptoms to include a variety of other domains, such as depression, anxiety, behavioral problems, shame, grief, and adaptive functioning. Therapists working in community or nonclinic settings often see multiply traumatized children: those with comorbid psychiatric conditions; those with challenging family situations, including children living in foster care, residential settings, and domestic violence shelters or refugee camps, or other unsafe settings; those who are taking a variety of psychotropic medications; and/or those with significant behavioral problems. TF-CBT, SS, TST, and KIDNET have been used and tested with some of these populations; SPARCS, Life Skills/Life Stories, and KIDNET were developed specifically for these youth. Some of the interventions described earlier have been used internationally and have been culturally adapted for diverse child populations.

Growing numbers of community therapists are using these interventions, particularly TF-CBT, through the Substance Abuse and Mental Health Services Administration (SAMHSA)–funded National Child Traumatic Stress Network (*www.nctsn.org*) and other state or nationally funded efforts. These include a free Web-based training (*www.musc.edu/tfcbt*), the use of learning collaboratives (*www.ihi.org*), and the adaptation of these treatments for children of different cultural groups.

Summary

Several models of non-school-based CBT have efficacy for treating child or adolescent PTSD in Level A or B studies. All of these models share basic principles and components described by the PRACTICE acronym. SS adds interventions for SUD prevention, and TST adds components for complex trauma management. Additional promising practices are being testing for complex trauma. Some of these models have been adapted and are being evaluated for children in diverse cultures. Thus, several effective forms of CBT are available for clinicians' use with traumatized children and teens, and preliminary information suggests that these interventions are acceptable and appropriate for children of diverse cultures.

Suggested Readings

Cohen, J. A., Mannarino, A. P., & Deblinger, E. (2006). *Treating trauma and traumatic grief in children and adolescents.* New York: Guilford Press.

Najavits, L. M. (2002). *Seeking safety: A treatment manual for PTSD and substance abuse.* New York: Guilford Press.

Saxe, G. N., Ellis, B. H., & Kaplow, J. B. (2006). *Collaborative treatment of traumatized children and teens: The trauma systems therapy approach.* New York: Guilford Press.

Schauer, E., Neuner, F., Elbert, T., Ertl, V., Onyut, P. L., Odnenwald, M., et al. (2004). Narrative exposure therapy in children: A case study in a Somali refugee. *Intervention, 2,* 18–32.

Psychopharmacotherapy for Adults

Description

There is a strong rationale for pharmacotherapy as an important treatment in posttraumatic stress disorder (PTSD). Alterations in a number of key neurobiological mechanisms appear to be associated with this disorder. These include dysregulation of adrenergic, hypothalamic–pituitary–adrenocortical (HPA), serotonergic, glutamatergic, gamma-aminobutyric acid (GABA)-ergic, and dopaminergic systems. Furthermore, there is considerable overlap between symptoms of PTSD, depression, and other anxiety disorders. Finally, PTSD is frequently comorbid with psychiatric disorders that are responsive to pharmacological treatment (e.g., major depression and panic disorder). Medication treatment is one of the most feasible treatments for PTSD. It is generally accepted by most patients, although the occurrence of side effects, lack of patient compliance with prescribed medication regimens, patient and family concerns about pharmacotherapy, and the high commercial cost of new therapeutic agents lessen their full impact.

Despite these scientific findings, pharmacotherapy for PTSD has primarily been guided by empirical evidence that a specific drug has efficacy against a specific symptom. Indeed, at present there are very few data in all psychiatric disorders, including PTSD, linking psychobiological abnormalities to specific medication effects. In research (and in clinical practice) almost every class of psychotropic agent has been prescribed for patients with PTSD. Most studies involve antidepressants: selective serotonin reuptake inhibitors (SSRIs), serotonin–norepinephrine reuptake inhibitors (SNRIs), monoamine oxidase inhibitors (MAOIs), tricyclic antidepressants (TCAs), and other serotonergic agents (trazodone and nefazodone). Antiadrenergic drugs tested include the alpha-1 receptor (prazosin), the alpha-2 receptor agonists (clonidine and guanfacine) and the beta receptor antagonist (propranolol). Recent developments include tests of mood-stabilizing anticonvulsants and augmentation strategies with atypical antipsychotics for SSRI partial responders.

General Strength of the Evidence

The strength of the evidence is best for the different classes of antidepressant agents tested in most of the randomized clinical trials (RCTs) on pharmacotherapy. There is also good evidence from augmentation trials with atypical antipsychotic agents. Finally, there are encouraging results with the antiadrenergic agent, prazosin, the antidepressant, mirtazapine, and older antidepressants, such as MAOIs and TCAs.

SSRIs (Sertraline/Paroxetine/Fluoxetine—Level A)

SSRIs can be recommended as a first-line treatment for PTSD. They not only reduce PTSD symptoms and produce global improvement but are also effective against comorbid disorders and associated symptoms. They have fewer side effects and greater safety than other antidepressants, but they may produce insomnia, agitation, gastrointestinal symptoms, and sexual dysfunction. Results with veterans are difficult to interpret because of the severity and chronicity of PTSD in veteran cohorts tested thus far.

SNRI (Venlafaxine—Level A)

Large, multisite trials indicate that venlafaxine can be recommended as a first-line treatment for PTSD. It is as effective as SSRIs and useful for comorbid depression. Its most significant contraindication is that it may exacerbate hypertension.

Other Second-Generation Antidepressants

- *Mirtazapine—Level A.* Mirtazapine has been shown to be effective in small, randomized trials. It may produce somnolence, increased appetite, and weight gain.
- *Bupropion—Level C.* Bupropion has been effective in small, open-label trials.
- *Nefazodone—Level A.* In the United States, Serzone, but not generic nefazodone, has been withdrawn from the market because of liver toxicity, although it appears to be as effective as SSRIs. Different regulatory decisions may apply in other countries.

- *Trazodone—Level C.* Trazodone has only modest efficacy, although it is a useful adjunct to SSRIs to promote sleep. It may be too sedating during the day and may also produce priapism.

MAOIs (Phenelzine—Level A)

MAOIs have been shown to be effective for DSM-IV Criterion B symptoms and global improvement, with some efficacy against Criterion D symptoms; however, they have not been tested extensively. They are also effective antidepressants and antipanic agents. Compliance with MAOI dietary restrictions is an important limitation of MAOI treatment. Furthermore, they are contraindicated in patients likely to use alcohol, illicit drugs, or certain drugs prescribed for other clinical conditions. Cardiovascular, hepatotoxic, and other side effects also must be monitored with MAOIs.

TCAs (Imipramine/Amitriptyline/Desipramine—Level A)

Imipramine and amitriptyline have been shown to be moderately effective treatments, whereas desipramine has been without effect in RCTs. Taken as a whole, TCAs generally are moderately effective in reducing DSM-IV Criterion B symptoms and promoting global improvement. They appear to be less effective than MAOIs in this regard, but they have fewer serious side effects. Side effects from TCAs include hypotension, cardiac arrhythmias, anticholinergic side effects, sedation, and behavioral activation.

Antiadrenergic Agents

Antiadrenergic agents appear to reduce arousal, reexperiencing, and possibly dissociative symptoms. They have been tested inconsistently in clinical trials. They are generally safe, although blood pressure and pulse rate must be monitored routinely. Special caution must be observed when prescribing these agents for patients with low blood pressure or those who are receiving antihypertensive medications.

- *Prazosin—Level A* effectively reduces traumatic nightmares. In one study, it also reduced overall PTSD symptom severity.
- *Propranolol—Level B* has shown promise as both a treatment for children and as a prophylactic agent to prevent the later development of PTSD. It may exacerbate asthmatic and depressive symptoms.
- *Clonidine—Level C* has shown promise in open trials for PTSD and dissociative symptoms.
- *Guanfacine—Levels A and C* was ineffective in a randomized trial despite promising open-label results.

Anticonvulsants (Lamotrigine—Levels A and B; Tiagabine—Level A; Carbamazepine/Valproate/Topiramate—Level B; Gabapentin/Vigabatrin—Level F)

Many open-label trials with anticonvulsants have had promising but inconclusive results; these medications have many side effects (see Table 9.3). A large, randomized trial with tiagabine had negative results, whereas a small trial with lamotrigine was modestly favorable. Anticonvulsants cannot be recommended for PTSD treatment at this time.

Benzodiazepines (Alprazolam—Level A; Clonazepam—Level B)

Although these drugs are both effective anxiolytics and antipanic agents, they are contraindicated for PTSD treatment. They produce their typical antiarousal effects without reducing either reexperiencing or avoidant/numbing symptoms. In addition, they should not be prescribed for patients with past or present alcohol/drug abuse dependency. Finally, they also may produce psychomotor slowing and exacerbate depressive symptoms. Benzodiazepines do not have any advantage over other classes of medications; therefore, they cannot be recommended for use as monotherapy in PTSD at this time.

Other Serotonergic Agents (Cyproheptadine—Level A; Buspirone—Level F)

A randomized trial with cyproheptadine was negative, and reports on the beneficial effects of buspirone have been anecdotal. There is no basis for recommending either drug at this time.

Atypical Antipsychotics (Risperidone/Olanzapine—Level A; Quetiapine—Level B)

Several small, randomized trials have shown the effectiveness of augmentation with atypical antipsychotics for partial responders to SSRIs or other treatment-refractory patients. These agents may also be useful for patients with PTSD who exhibit extreme hypervigilance/paranoia, physical aggression, social isolation, or trauma-related psychotic symptoms. They may produce weight gain, and olanzapine treatment has been associated with type 2 diabetes. Conventional antipsychotic agents are contraindicated in PTSD.

Course of Treatment

Current research findings suggest that controlled drug trials in PTSD should last at least 8–12 weeks because shorter trials have generally been ineffective.

More recent and much larger-scale studies (with SSRIs) suggest that maximum benefit, for some, may not be achieved until the 36th week of treatment.

Recommendations

Although some medications qualify as Level A treatments, their overall efficacy is not as great as that achieved with some cognitive-behavioral treatments. Furthermore, discontinuation of medication following a successful response is often followed by relapse. Finally, most medications have side effects that, if significant, may make it impossible for certain patients to remain in treatment despite reduction of symptoms. Regardless of these considerations, many patients prefer medication to psychotherapy; medication may be the only available option, if there are no qualified CBT therapists in the area; many patients tolerate side effects without problems; and many achieve complete remission and are willing to remain on medication as long as necessary.

Summary

The best evidence supports the use of SSRIs and SNRIs as first-line drugs for PTSD. There is also good evidence that augmentation with atypical antipsychotic agents is effective. Recent results with prazosin and mirtazapine are also promising. MAOIs are moderately effective and TCAs are mildly effective agents, although both may produce adverse side effects. Evidence supporting the use of anticonvulsants is weak, not because of negative findings, but because there have been so few randomized trials with either class of drugs. There is good evidence to suggest that benzodiazepines are not useful in treating PTSD. Finally, there is reason to believe that new, as yet untested, pharmacological agents that work through different mechanisms of action may prove to be more effective than medications that are currently available.

Suggested Readings

Davidson, J., Bernik, M., Connor, K. M., Friedman, M. J., Jobson, K. O., Kim, Y., et al. (2005). A new treatment algorithm for posttraumatic stress disorder. *Psychiatric Annals, 35,* 887–900.

Friedman, M. J., & Davidson, J. R. T. (2007). Pharmacotherapy for PTSD. In M. J. Friedman, T. M. Keane, & P. A. Resick (Eds.), *Handbook of PTSD: Science and practice* (pp. 376–405). New York: Guilford Press.

Psychopharmacotherapy for Children and Adolescents

Description

There are few controlled trials to guide practitioners and a sparse literature supporting medication use in childhood PTSD. Medication may play a role in targeting specific posttraumatic stress disorder (PTSD) symptoms and associated disorders and in helping to improve functioning in day-to-day life. A reasonable first approach in highly symptomatic children is to begin with a broad-spectrum agent, such as a selective serotonin reuptake inhibitor (SSRI), which should target anxiety, mood, and reexperiencing symptoms. Adrenergic agents, attention-deficit/hyperactivity disorder (ADHD) medications, mood stabilizers, or atypical neuroleptics, used either alone or in combination with a SSRI, may be useful interventions to target severe symptoms and/or comorbid conditions. Reduction in even one disabling symptom through pharmacotherapy may have a positive ripple effect on a child's overall functioning.

General Strength of the Evidence

There are few well-conducted, controlled trials of medication treatments of PTSD in childhood. The scant literature is not of sufficient rigor to calculate comparison effect sizes. The following is the strength of evidence for specific medications.

Adrenergic Agents (Clonidine, Guanfacine, Propranolol— Levels B, C, E)

The alpha-2 agonists clonidine and guanfacine and the beta-antagonist propranolol reduce sympathetic tone and may be effective in treating symptoms of hyperarousal, impulsivity, activation, sleep problems, and nightmares seen in PTSD. Clonidine, in relatively low doses, has been shown in open-label trials to reduce anxiety and arousal, and to improve concentration, mood, and behavioral impulsivity. Guanfacine has been helpful in reducing PTSD-associated nightmares. Propranolol may reduce arousal symptoms in survivors of childhood sexual abuse.

Because they reduce central nervous system (CNS) adrenergic tone target reexperiencing and hyperarousal symptoms, adrenergic agents are a rational treatment strategy in PTSD. Additionally, the alpha-2 adrenergic agents may be more effective than the psychostimulants for ADHD symptoms in maltreated or sexually abused children with PTSD.

Dopaminergic Agents (Risperidone, Quetiapine—Levels E, F)

Uncontrolled trials of children with PTSD and high rates of psychiatric comorbididty (e.g., bipolar disorder) have indicated remission of PTSD symptoms with risperidone treatment. Case series juvenile justice reports involving children with PTSD indicated that quetiapine (50–200 mg/day) provided significant improvements in dissociation, anxiety, depression, and anger symptoms over the 6-week treatment period. With scant evidence as to their utility in PTSD symptoms per se, the atypical neuroleptics are currently reserved for patients with refractory PTSD or for those who exhibit paranoid behavior, parahallucinatory phenomena or intense flashbacks, self destructive behavior, explosive or overwhelming anger, or psychotic symptoms.

Serotonergic Agents (Fluoxetine, Sertraline, Citalopram— Levels A, B)

Perhaps the best evidence is for SSRIs in pediatric PTSD. In children, SSRIs are approved for use in depression (fluoxetine) and in obsessive–compulsive disorder (OCD; fluoxetine, sertraline, and fluvoxamine). SSRIs may be useful in children with PTSD because of the variety of symptoms associated with serotonergic dysregulation, including anxiety, depressed mood, obsessional thinking, compulsive behaviors, affective impulsivity, rage, and alcohol or substance abuse.

The SSRIs have received the most clinical attention and are likely first-line choices for children, owing to their "broad-spectrum" activity. Citalopram reduces PTSD symptoms at a rate on par with reported rates in adult populations. Sertraline has also been shown to be helpful in reducing PTSD symptoms in one of the only randomized trials in the child literature.

The SSRIs are generally safe and well tolerated, although recent concerns have led to FDA black box warnings regarding increased suicidal ideation and behavior in depressed children treated with these medications.

Cyproheptadine, an antihistaminic serotonin (5-HT) antagonist, has shown limited utility in reducing traumatic nightmares in open trials. Because of its sedative action and generally safe side effect profile, it may be a useful agent in treating sleep-onset problems and nightmares in children with PTSD. Anecdotal evidence suggests that agents such as trazadone, a sedating 5-HT antagonist antidepressant, and cyproheptadine used alone or in conjunction with the SSRIs, may be particularly useful in sleep dysregulation and trauma-related nightmares that frequently occur in patients with PTSD.

Adrenergic and Serotonergic Agents (TCAs, Venlafaxine— Levels A, C)

Low-dose imipramine (1 mg/kg) to treat symptoms of acute stress disorder (ASD) and sleep disturbance was shown to be effective in one randomized study, resulting in full remission of ASD symptoms. TCAs, owing to cardiac and anticholinergic side effects, should be considered for sleep problems associated with trauma or when use of safer agents, such as the SSRIs, has failed.

Gamma-Aminobutyric Acid (GABA)-ergic/Benzodiazepine Agents (Lorazepam, Diazepam, Clonazepam—Level E)

Little, if any, data support benzodiazepine effectiveness in treating the core symptoms of PTSD. These agents (e.g., clonazepam, lorazepam) may have a minor role to play in reducing acute and intense symptoms of anxiety or agitation, or as a short-term, adjunctive treatment to facilitate exposure tasks in psychotherapy.

Opioid Antagonists (Nalaxone, Naltrexone—Level E)

Opioid antagonists have been utilized with mixed results in adults with PTSD. No clinical trials of these agents in treatment of children and adolescents with PTSD have been published.

Miscellaneous Agents/Agents Affecting Multiple Neurotransmitters

A number of successful open-label trials (Level C) have been conducted successfully with carbamazepine (300–1,200 mg/day, serum levels 10–11.5 µg/ml), with significant improvement in all PTSD symptoms except for continued abuse related nightmares.

Anecdotal experience suggests that traumatized children in fact have favorable responses in reduction of hyperactivity, impulse dyscontrol, and attention impairment with ADHD medications such as methylphenidate, dextroamphetamine, or atomoxetine. Similarly, bupropion is often considered a second-line agent for treating ADHD symptoms and may be a useful agent when affect dysregulation or depressed mood co-occurs with ADHD symptoms.

Course of Treatment

Certainly, the initial step in the treatment of PTSD is psychoeducation of the child, parents, and adult caregivers. Clinicians are advised to "start low and go slow" with medication dosages and titration schedules because children are not simply "small adults." Cognitive-behavioral therapy (CBT) in school-age and older children and adolescents is likely to be the treatment of first choice. Many experts use a blend of cognitive, behavioral, dynamic and family-based interventions for childhood PTSD.

Recommendations

Despite the lack of data, medication use in children with PTSD has become a standard of care. The acceptability of pharmacotherapy to the patient and parent is one criterion on which to base decisions to prescribe medication. Another is the presence of severe comorbid psychiatric conditions that respond to medications also used to treat PTSD. Medication may be favored as a first-line choice when the intensity of PTSD is interfering with a child's ability to engage in psychotherapy. Finally, medication treatment may also be indicated when there is no access to psychotherapy. No medication currently has an FDA label indication for the treatment of childhood PTSD.

Summary

The state of knowledge regarding medication treatments for children and adolescents lags substantially behind that for adults. Medication may play a role in reducing debilitating symptoms of PTSD in children's day-to-day lives and provide relief as they confront difficult material in therapy. Broad-spectrum agents, such as the SSRIs, are a good first choice. Comorbid conditions, such as ADHD or aggressive behavior, should, of course, be targeted with pharmacotherapy known to be effective for these disorders. Reduction in even one disabling symptom, such as insomnia or hyperarousal, may have a positive ripple effect on a child's overall functioning.

Suggested Readings

Friedman, M. J., & Davidson, J. R. T. (2007). Pharmacotherapy for PTSD. In M. J. Friedman, T. M. Keane, & P. A. Resick (Eds.), *Handbook of PTSD: Science and practice* (pp. 376–405). New York: Guilford Press.

Friedman, M. J., Donnelly, C. L., & Mellman, T. A. (2003). Pharmacotherapy for PTSD. *Psychiatric Annals, 33*, 57–62.

Eye Movement Desensitization and Reprocessing

Description

Eye movement desensitization and reprocessing (EMDR) is a multistage treatment for posttraumatic stress disorder (PTSD). It entails eight stages, including history gathering, treatment planning, patient preparation, systematic assessment of trauma-relevant target(s), desensitization and reprocessing, installation of alternative positive cognitions, body scan for continuing discomfort or trouble spots, and closure designed to address constructive coping needs for future use by treated patients. First introduced in 1989, the treatment has benefited from a dramatic improvement in research quality over the past 15 years.

General Strength of the Evidence

Evidence supporting the efficacy of EMDR has advanced from case reports to well-controlled randomized trials and multiple, systematic meta-analytic reviews. Consequently, this critical review of the evidence is based exclusively on a review of randomized controlled trials (RCTs) of EMDR for PTSD published in peer-reviewed journals since publication of the guidelines in the first edition of this volume. The treatment has been compared to other front-line treatments, most recently including medications that target PTSD. It has performed comparably in all such trials. Additionally, several investigations have examined elements of the conceptual framework offered to explain the treatment's effectiveness. Compared to other treatments targeting PTSD, the status of the evidence supporting EMDR is substantial and of high quality. The treatment warrants an Agency for Health Care Policy and Research (AHCPR) Level A rating for treatment of adults with a diagnosis of PTSD. EMDR applied to children warrants an AHCPR Level B rating.

Course of Treatment

Using EMDR requires extensive assessment to identify the range of traumatic event exposure across the patient's lifespan. Multiple aspects of each traumatic event also require assessment: affective and physiological response elements; negative self-representations; and alternative, desired positive self-representation. Treatment comprises eight stages. The length of treatment is based on the number of traumatic events identified and on the patient's response and potential. Sessions can vary in length depending on patient characteristics and response.

Recommendations

EMDR is widely applicable to civilian PTSD cases and also has some efficacy with combat-related PTSD. What is yet to be studied in the combat population is the degree to which "service-connected" disability status influences treatment outcome with EMDR, as acknowledged earlier by EMDR practitioners. Additionally, the literature is silent regarding the extent to which comorbid physical injury (a common occurrence in combat-related PTSD) complicates EMDR treatment. Finally the impact of chronicity of symptoms on EMDR treatment has not been specifically controlled in RCTs, although one 5-year follow-up investigation revealed a lack of long-term durability for chronic combat-related PTSD. These factors comprise important sources of "severity" among individuals with combat-related PTSD. Nonetheless, the success of EMDR in early trials with combat veterans warrants continued application and study with this population.

The treatment is relatively brief in terms of the functional duration, although the duration of treatment cannot be determined a priori and must be guided by the patient's needs. The treatment appears to be well tolerated by most patients, and possibly to a degree not characteristic of alternative psychological treatments, but this issue requires further systematic study. Children also seem to benefit to an adapted procedure. Existing data support the use of EMDR in children and adolescents; however, compared to adults, there have been considerably fewer RCTs evaluating EMDR in children and adolescents diagnosed with PTSD. Further research with this population is recommended. EMDR is robust in the face of some variations in procedure, while retaining its effectiveness (i.e., eye movements and other parallel stimulation).

Patient Characteristics

It is unknown what patient characteristics predict improvement, other than the observation that single-episode traumas appear to respond more favorably to treatment. Additionally, a recent pharmacological comparison revealed specifically that traumas originating during the developmental period are more resistant than those originating later in life when targeted for treatment during adulthood. As indicated in the previous edition of this volume, there remains little empirically based guidance for treating patients with comorbid disorders, other than that found in good clinical practice. In this connection, elevated depression scores do seem to respond favorably to EMDR, even when they are not targeted specifically for intervention.

Process Studies

Recent investigations suggest the possibility that the dosed exposure, combined with postexposure "mindful awareness" features contained in EMDR, might confer advantages over conventional exposure to trauma memories. In some ways, the treatment of panic disorder has similarly benefited from this approach entailing a specific focus on interoceptive sources of distress immediately following specific arousal induction procedures (Barlow, 2002).

Combination Treatment with Trauma-Focused Medication

Many patients seen in practice are either already taking FDA-approved medications for PTSD or may initiate a medication trial during treatment. As important as understanding individual efficacy is understanding the empirical basis for combined efficacy of medication and psychological interventions because their joint use is a likely reality in practice. More (drugs plus psychological therapy) is not always better in these matters, and practitioners should be informed by empirical findings concerning such combination treatments.

Tolerability and Acceptability

Finally, more information is needed on client acceptability of treatment in an effort to elucidate further the extent to which this treatment is suited to client preferences. The repeated finding of high dropout rates with PTSD treatment demands that we understand the role of patient and therapist tolerance and acceptability as they affect efficacious interventions.

Summary

EMDR is rated as a Level A treatment for its use with adults. Quality clinical trials support its use for patients with PTSD. More studies need to be completed with EMDR adapted for use with children and adolescents. It currently has a Level B rating for treatment with this population.

Suggested Readings

Barlow, D. (2002). *Anxiety and its disorders: The nature and treatment of anxiety and panic* (2nd ed.). New York: Guilford Press.

Shapiro, F. (2001). *Eye movement desensitization and reprocessing: Basic principles, protocols, and procedures* (2nd ed.). New York: Guilford Press.

Shapiro, F., & Maxfield, L. (2002). Eye movement desensitization and reprocessing (EMDR): Information processing in the treatment of trauma. *Journal of Clinical Psychology, 58,* 933–946.

Tinker, R. H., & Wilson, S. A. (1999). *Through the eyes of a child: EMDR with children.* New York: Norton.

Group Therapy

Description

Group therapy for posttraumatic stress disorder (PTSD) is widely practiced in clinical settings. Group approaches may vary across a number of dimensions, specifically, theoretical orientation (e.g., cognitive-behavioral, interpersonal), length (fixed-length vs. open-ended), trauma focus (whether trauma-related material is explicitly discussed), and group membership (e.g., sex, trauma type, open enrollment vs. cohort). There are several potential advantages of group therapy, including the opportunity to deliver effective treatment efficiently, the implicit inclusion of social support and social contact, and the availability of social learning through modeling. For persons with PTSD, in particular, group therapy may be especially useful for providing opportunities to develop trusting relationships and a sense of interpersonal safety, thus, ameliorating the isolation and alienation that often accompany PTSD.

General Strength of the Evidence

The research evidence for group therapy for PTSD shows positive change from pre- to posttreatment, with effect sizes ranging from small to large. There are relatively few well-designed randomized studies with sufficient sample size to provide definitive conclusions about the effects of specific forms of group therapy. Of the randomized studies, five are at an Agency for Health Care Policy and Research (AHCPR) Level A rating; three of these found significant effects for the group therapy being studied—two for cognitive-behavioral therapy (CBT) groups and one for interpersonal group therapy. Thus, most of the evidence comes from studies rated at AHCPR Level B or C. At present, there is no evidence for superiority of any specific type of group treatment compared to others, nor is there evidence for the relative superiority of the group modality over individual therapy.

In summary, the empirical support for group therapy as a modality for treating PTSD is largely based on pre- to posttreatment change. There are promising findings from a few AHCPR Level A studies and several Level B studies for superiority of specific groups relative to wait-list controls. At present, there is not sufficient evidence to warrant recommendation of a specific type of group therapy, to recommend group therapy in favor of individual therapy, or to predict for whom group therapy might be more or less effective.

Course of Treatment

The group therapy protocols investigated in articles reviewed in Chapter 12 ranged from 6 to 52 sessions, with a modal treatment length of 12 sessions, and with most protocols including 10–25 sessions. Reviewed group therapies tended to be closed (with members of a group comprising a single cohort, rather than fluid group membership) and to meet weekly for approximately 1.5–2 hours. In each study, group therapy was sufficient to result in significant reductions in PTSD symptoms.

Summary and Recommendations

At present, the available data suggest that group therapy for PTSD is associated with improvement in symptoms, and specific forms of cognitive-behavioral and interpersonal group treatments are superior to no treatment. Group therapy may be an acceptable alternative to individual therapy for many patients, but research is needed to establish the relative efficacy of group versus individual treatments. The majority of studies of group treatment have included participants whose PTSD symptoms are due to childhood sexual abuse or combat trauma.

1. Group therapy is recommended as a useful component of treatment for PTSD related to different types of traumatic experiences.
2. There is no evidence supporting superiority of any type of group therapy relative to others, although cognitive-behavioral group therapy remains the most frequently studied and has the largest amount of empirical support.
3. The effect of individual characteristics on group therapy outcome has received little study. Preliminary evidence suggests that the inclusion of participants with borderline personality disorder may negatively impact the outcome of process–interpersonal group therapy.

Suggested Readings

Baldwin, S. A., Murray, D. M., & Shadish, W. R. (2005). Empirically supported treatments or Type I errors?: Problems with the analysis of data from group-administered treatments. *Journal of Consulting and Clinical Psychology, 73,* 924–935.

Foy, D. W., Ruzek, J. I., Glynn, S. M., Riney, S. A., & Gusman, F. D. (1997). Trauma focused group therapy for combat-related PTSD. *Journal of Clinical Psychology, 3,* 59–73.

Krakow, B., Hollifield, M., Johnston, L., Koss, M., Schrader, R., Warner, T. D., et al. (2001). Imagery rehearsal therapy for chronic nightmares in sexual assault survivors with posttraumatic stress disorder. *Journal of the American Medical Association, 286,* 537–545.

Schnurr, P. P., Friedman, M. J., Foy, D. W., Shea, M. T., Hsieh, F. Y., Lavori, P. W., et al. (2003). Randomized trial of trauma-focused group therapy for posttraumatic stress disorder. *Archives of General Psychiatry, 60,* 481–488.

School-Based Treatment for Children and Adolescents

Description

Socioeconomically disadvantaged children have the greatest difficulty accessing mental health services, and traumatized individuals are also less likely than their nontraumatized counterparts to seek health services. Thus, our most vulnerable youth are those least likely ever to receive traditional, clinic-based mental health care. Schools can serve an important role in addressing unmet mental health needs following trauma, if children receive high-quality mental health services for trauma in schools.

The variety of school interventions for trauma can be categorized as (1) schoolwide, curricular interventions; (2) interventions designed for "at-risk" students; or (3) school-based treatment for children with trauma-related symptoms (traumatic stress). Most school programs developed to date are intended for "at-risk" students and include a screening or identification process to determine which students might benefit from the intervention. School intervention programs for traumatic stress (including posttraumatic stress disorder [PTSD] and related symptoms), are trauma-focused, developmentally oriented, and incorporate the core components common to many trauma-focused interventions. Common components include cognitive, behavioral, interpersonal, and emotion regulation and skills building approaches; these components are often characterized simply as cognitive-behavioral techniques (CBT). This guideline reviews programs developed specifically for use in schools (not clinical interventions delivered on the school campus) that focus on trauma and are designed for intervention rather than prevention of symptoms.

General Strength of the Evidence

In this newly developing field, there have been few rigorous evaluations to date. Of over 30 programs reviewed, only five have evidence of impact from randomized or quasi-experimental controlled trials (two with Level A randomized trials, and three with Level B studies with uncontrolled comparison groups). Three programs have been developed specifically for use in schools and focus on a broad array of traumas: the cognitive-behavioral intervention for trauma in schools (CBITS; supported by Level A and B studies), the multimodality trauma treatment (MMTT), and the UCLA Trauma/Grief Program (both supported by Level B studies). All three draw on evidence-based practices for trauma, largely cognitive-behavioral techniques, and all three have empirical support for the reduction of trauma-related symptoms. There also have been some notable international efforts in regions affected by disaster or ongoing terrorist threat. The classroom-based intervention program provides a psychoeducational curriculum for children that addresses critical needs of children and youth exposed to threat and terror (supported by a Level B study). The program, Overshadowing the Threat of Terrorism (OTT), has been used and evaluated in Israel for symptoms related to ongoing terrorism exposure (supported by an Level A study). Effect sizes in these studies show moderate to large effects. The Maile Project, a four-session psychosocial intervention used 2 years after Hurricane Iniki, also shows some promise. Evaluated in a Level A study, it showed no group differences in self-reported symptoms but a positive effect in clinician ratings on a small subsample. Many other promising programs that incorporate aspects of CBT or other techniques have not yet been evaluated with a control group.

Course of Treatment

School-based programs are commonly time-limited, but many include a mechanism for referral at the end of the intervention into more intensive or ongoing care.

Recommendations

More study of school-based programs is needed, but some appear to be effective in symptom reduction and show promise in reaching vulnerable youth. Several manual-based approaches are available, along with training and consultation from the developers.

Successful school-based intervention programs are tailored for the school setting and compatible with the school's educational mission. Hence, important adjustments to clinic-based CBT are required for successful school interventions. Specifically, school programs tend to be delivered in group format, to have more limited parental involvement, and to have less comprehensive facilitation of the trauma narrative and its processing. Although these limitations may necessitate a referral to treatment in a mental health specialty setting to allow more parental involvement, to continue individual work, or to allow further reduction of other mental health symptoms, the school-based setting provides opportunities that cannot be found in clinical settings. Beyond offering increased access to children who are unlikely to attend clinic-based treatment, school-based services offer access to teachers and can focus on improving children's functioning, such as academic performance, classroom behavior, and age-related peer interactions. Furthermore, interventions utilizing the school context allow the school environment to play a role in children's progress.

Summary

With growing interest in delivering trauma-focused interventions in schools, where the most vulnerable youth may be served, a number of programs have been developed. Most programs are time-limited and target students with elevated symptoms of PTSD, although there is a good deal of variety in format, focus, and length. To date, evaluations of these programs have been sparse, with only five programs evaluated in experimental or quasi-experimental controlled trials. These programs do show promise, however, that students can experience symptom reduction and improved behavior as a result of participating in the interventions.

Suggested Readings

Cole, S. F., O'Brien, J. G., Gadd, M. G., Ristuccia, J., Wallace, D., & Gregory, M. (2005). *Helping traumatized children learn: Supportive school environments for children traumatized by family violence.* Boston: Massachusetts Advocates for Children.

Jaycox, L. H., Morse, L., Tanielian, T., & Stein, B. D. (2006). *How schools can help students recover from traumatic experiences: A toolkit for supporting long-term recovery.* Santa Monica, CA: RAND Corporation.

Jaycox, L. H., Stein, B. D., Amaya-Jackson, L. M., & Morse, L. K. (in press). School-based interventions for traumatic stress. In S. W. Evans, M. Weist, & Z. Serpell (Eds.), *Advances in school-based mental health interventions* (Vol. 2). Kingston, NJ: Civic Research Institute.

U.S. Public Health Service. (2000). *Report of the Surgeon General's Conference on Children's Mental Health: A National Action Agenda.* Washington, DC: U.S. Department of Health and Human Services.

Psychodynamic Therapy for Adults

Description

Psychodynamic treatment seeks to reengage normal mechanisms of adaptation by addressing what is unconscious and, in tolerable doses, making it conscious. The psychological meaning of a traumatic event is progressively understood within the context of the survivor's unique history, constitution, and aspirations. This includes collaborative sifting and sorting through wishes, fantasies, fears, and defenses stirred up by the event. Transference and countertransference are universal phenomena that should be recognized by therapists but may or may not be addressed explicitly depending on the treatment modality and therapist judgment. Psychodynamic treatment requires insight and courage, and is best approached in a therapeutic relationship that emphasizes safety and honesty. The therapist–patient relationship is itself a crucial factor in the patient's response. The wide range and broad public health implications of posttraumatic responses are best understood and addressed within the adaptational, dimensional context of psychodynamic principles rather than in descriptive, categorical terms that typify the prevailing medical model of posttraumatic stress disorder (PTSD). Psychodynamic psychotherapy approaches PTSD by way of the mind. As such, it offers a unique and useful clinical tool.

General Strength of the Evidence

Only a few empirical investigations with randomized designs, controlled variables, and validated outcome measures have been reported. Case reports and tightly reasoned scholarly works comprise the bulk of the psychodynamic literature (Level D). These can neither provide ultimate tests for psychodynamic hypotheses nor define the limits of psychopathology, theory, or technique. They are, however, an essential part of the scientific effort to understand the human impact of psychological trauma. Randomized clinical trials and other efficacy study methods demonstrate that a treatment works within a controlled setting but are difficult to apply to the complex, interactive, and progressive processes involved in psychodynamic interventions. Effectiveness research (which examines outcomes in real-world settings rather than in the laboratory) may provide a powerful new lens for psychodynamic studies.

Course of Treatment

Formal psychoanalysis involves four to five 45- to 50-minute sessions each week over the course of 2–7 (or more) years. Psychodynamic psychotherapy most commonly involves one to two meetings per week and may be relatively short-term (a few months) or open-ended (lasting years). Brief psychodynamic psychotherapy involves once or twice weekly meetings for an average of 12–20 sessions. Supportive psychotherapy may be brief and focal or long-term and open-ended. Supportive psychotherapy typically involves one session per week, but sessions may be more or less frequent depending on the patient's needs and tolerance.

Recommendations

The decision to undertake psychodynamic psychotherapy and the choice of modality depend on the depth, complexity, and severity of the patient's problems, his or her attributes, the presence of maladaptive psychological defenses, and the patient's goals for treatment. Indications for more expressive treatment include strong motivation, significant suffering, ability to regress in the service of the ego, tolerance for strong affects and frustration, psychological mindedness, intact reality testing, ability to form meaningful and enduring relationships, reasonably good impulse control, and ability to sustain a job. Patients who are significantly lacking in one or more of these attributes are more likely to benefit from more supportive, less insight-oriented treatment. All psychodynamic psychotherapies combine expressive and supportive elements. Formal psychoanalysis is primarily an expressive psychotherapy that aims at decreasing symptoms, increasing self-understanding, improving ego strength, and bringing about fundamental change in the patient's intrapsychic balance (by focusing on long-standing conflicts, relationship problems, and developmental issues in the context of analysis of the transference). Psychodynamic psychotherapy is also a primarily expressive technique, but it differs from formal psychoanalysis in that it does not aim at fundamental changes in intrapsychic structure and does not necessarily center upon interpretation of the transference. Brief psychodynamic psychotherapy (either expressive or supportive) may be indicated when the situation is relatively acute and the patient's issues are focal. Contraindications to expressive therapies include long-standing ego weakness, acute life crisis, poor tolerance for anxiety and/or frustration, poor capacity for insight, poor reality testing, severely impaired object relations, limited impulse control, low intelligence or organic cognitive dysfunction (including significant traumatic brain injury), difficulty with self-observation, and tenuous ability to form a therapeutic alliance. These attributes do not preclude psychodynamic psychotherapy, but modifications of technique may be indicated to help the patient take part in treatment.

Summary

Psychodynamic psychotherapy has a long and rich tradition in the mental health field. Its roots stretch back more than 100 years. With the introduction of PTSD into the diagnostic nomenclature, authors contributed considerable scholarly work to adapt existing treatments to this psychiatric condition. Yet few empirical studies exist in the literature today. Given the large number of psychodynamically trained clinicians in the field, more systematic research in this area is warranted.

Suggested Readings

American Psychoanalytic Association. (2006). *Empirical studies of psychoanalytic treatments, process, and concepts.* Retrieved July 14, 2007, from *www.apsa.org/research/empiricalstudiesinpsychoanalysis/tabid/449/default.aspx*

Gabbard, G. O. (2005). *Psychodynamic psychiatry in clinical practice: Fourth edition.* Washington, DC: American Psychiatric Press.

Herman, J. (1992). *Trauma and recovery.* New York: Basic Books.

Horowitz, M. J. (2003). *Treatment of stress response syndromes.* Arlington, VA: American Psychiatric Publishing.

Kudler, H. (2007). The need for psychodynamic principles in outreach to new combat veterans and their families. *Journal of the American Academy of Psychoanalysis and Dynamic Psychiatry, 35*(1), 39–50.

Psychodynamic Therapy for Child Trauma

Description

In psychodynamic child trauma treatment, therapeutic interventions are shaped by the therapist's understanding of the child's inner life in the context of the child's immediate world/daily life and history. The psychodynamic psychotherapist focuses on the specific meanings the child gives to the traumatic event based on his or her constitutional, developmental, and environmental circumstances and history. Parents and/or other significant adults are engaged as allies in treatment to reestablish reassuring routines and the psychological safety that are essential to recovery. A core aspect of psychodynamic psychotherapies is that the ultimate goal is to promote personality coherence and healthy development rather than to alleviate symptom severity alone.

General Strength of the Evidence

Five randomized controlled trials (RCTs; Level A) support the efficacy of psychodynamic methods. Three RCTs, conducted by two independent research teams, have examined the efficacy of child–parent psychotherapy (CPP), a dyadic, relationship-based intervention. They involved the following populations: (1) preschoolers exposed to domestic violence, (2) maltreated preschoolers, and (3) maltreated infants. A fourth RCT focused on Attachment and Biobehavioral Catch-Up (ABC), a relationship-based intervention for maltreated children in foster care. The fifth RCT involved a psychoanalytically based individual treatment for sexually abused girls. Of note, in the first four trials, the majority of participants were members of ethnic minorities.

Together, the studies show that psychodynamic treatments have positive effects in terms of reducing child and caregiver symptomatology; changing children's attributions of parents, themselves, and relationships; altering attachment classifications; and reducing children's cortisol levels. One study shows promise of long-term effects. A 6-month follow-up of CPP showed that improvements in children's and parents' symptoms continue posttreatment.

In addition to the randomized trials, over 20 clinical case studies document the effectiveness of psychodynamic treatment following exposure to a range of traumas, including dog attacks; invasive medical procedures; domestic violence; sexual abuse; witnessing the murder of a parent; and complex, chronic trauma.

Course of Treatment

The course of treatment varies with the model. CPP is typically conducted over 50 weekly sessions that take place in the home or in a clinic. Sessions generally include the parent(s) and the child. Individual parent or child sessions may be added as needed. The goal of treatment is to support and strengthen the parent–child relationship as a vehicle to long-term healthy child development. Targets of intervention include mothers' and children's maladaptive representations of themselves and each other, and interactions and behaviors that interfere with the child's mental health. With trauma-exposed samples, treatment incorporates a focus on trauma experienced by the parent, the child, or both. Over the course of treatment, parent and child are guided in creating a joint narrative of the traumatic event, identifying and addressing traumatic triggers that generate dysregulated behaviors, reinforcing mutual traumatic expectations between parent and child, and placing the traumatic experience in perspective.

ABC involves 10 home-based sessions. Foster parents learn to reinterpret children's alienating behaviors, process their own issues that interfere with their ability to provide nurturing care, and create an environment that nurtures the child's regulatory capacities. Trowell and colleagues' (2002) intervention involved 30 sessions of brief, focused psychoanalytic treatment with three phases: (1) engagement; (2) focusing on issues relevant to the participant, and (3) separation, ending, and reworking key topics.

Recommendations

The research supporting the efficacy of relationship-based treatments is compelling and highlights the importance of involving caregivers when treating young children exposed to trauma. It recommends a focus on not only symptomatology but also the key developmental tasks of early childhood that are often disrupted by trauma. These tasks include developing a primary attachment relationship; forming internal working models of self, others, and the world; and learning to regulate affect. However, the research suggests that doing this work may take time; the majority of the trials involved a yearlong treatment period. Given clinic and funding demands that call for shorter protocols, two things are needed: (1) additional studies, including case studies, examining whether and under what conditions a brief version may be effective; and (2) changes in policy allowing for longer, more intensive treatments that reflect the importance of establishing meaningful change at this critical developmental period.

With respect to psychodynamically oriented interventions for older children, only one study was found that involved children over the age of 6. In light of evidence suggesting the effectiveness of psychodynamic treatment with adults, it would seem that additional research with older children is warranted. While these treatments are developed and studied, clinicians must weigh the option of using them as opposed to other methods for which an evidence base exists. Knowledge of the evidence and a sound clinical rationale should guide this decision.

Summary

Growing evidence supports the use of psychodynamic approaches in the treatment of traumatized children. Data are especially compelling for young children and are noteworthy because they show that psychodynamic methods have ecological validity for different cultural groups, and for children and mothers who have experienced multiple, chronic traumas. In addition, consistent with the goal of psychodynamic treatment, the research suggests that treatment results in not only symptom reduction but also changes in relationships and movement toward a more healthy developmental trajectory.

Reference

Trowell, J., Kolvin, I., Weeramanthri, T., Sadowski, H., Berelowitz, M., et al. (2002). Psychotherapy for sexually abused girls: Psychopathological outcome findings and patterns. *British Journal of Psychiatry, 180,* 234–247.

Suggested Readings

Lieberman, A. F., Compton, N. C., van Horn, P., & Ghosh Ippen, C. (2003). *Losing a parent to death in the early years: Guidelines for the treatment of traumatic bereavement in infancy and early childhood.* Washington, DC: Zero-to-Three Press.

Lieberman, A. F., & van Horn, P. (2005). *Don't hit my mommy: A manual for child–parent psychotherapy with young witnesses of family violence.* Washington, DC: Zero-to-Three Press.

Psychosocial Rehabilitation

Description

Traditional posttraumatic stress disorder (PTSD) treatments target the internal life of the individual; psychosocial rehabilitation operates at the nexus of the person and the larger community. Many persons with trauma histories show significant impairments in multiple life functioning domains—kin relationships, romantic relationships, employment, friendships, and so forth, and psychosocial rehabilitation techniques can address these difficulties. A class of eight psychosocial rehabilitation techniques has been reviewed here: (1) health education and psychoeducational techniques; (2) supported education; (3) self-care/independent living skills training; (4) supported housing; (5) family skills training; (6) social skills training; (7) vocational rehabilitation; and (8) case management. These interventions are grounded in learning theory and utilize techniques that emanate from this framework (model coaching, shaping, prompting, programmed generalization, etc.). Psychosocial rehabilitation techniques are recommended for the treatment of PTSD in traumatized adults with deficits in community functioning. These techniques may be especially relevant to persons who have been multiply traumatized or have had a more chronic course of PTSD.

General Strength of the Evidence

With rare exception, psychosocial rehabilitation techniques have been evaluated primarily in persons with serious psychiatric illnesses. Although it is fair to assume that many participants in existing studies have co-occurring (and often undiagnosed) PTSD, results from randomized trials targeting persons with PTSD are sorely lacking. Some controlled data suggest that educational interventions in PTSD may improve outcomes, whereas the one randomized trial of family intervention for PTSD found that family treatment did not confer statistically significant benefits over exposure treatment alone. In short, education about PTSD meets the Level A category of evidence of the Agency for Health Care Policy and Research (AHCPR)—several randomized trials. All the other psychosocial rehabilitation domains are still at Level C—case reports, naturalistic studies, clinical observations and recommendations, and the like. The major impediment here is a dearth of studies testing these interventions with well-diagnosed samples of persons for whom PTSD is a primary problem.

Course of Treatment

Consistent with the fundamentals of offering learning-based interventions, the provision of psychosocial rehabilitation interventions is grounded in a thorough assessment of the individual with PTSD. The needs of individuals with PTSD vary widely. A person who was recently assaulted on the job may decide to find another place to work; here, a supported employment program may be helpful, whereas a homeless combat veteran who has been struggling with chronic PTSD and co-occurring substance use problems may need housing assistance. It is also important to recognize that individuals differ greatly in the outcomes that are of value to them. A key tenet of the recovery model of serious mental illness is consumer-directed treatment, wherein the clinician serves as a consultant to the person with the disorder, helping him or her clarify treatment goals and select effective interventions' to meet those goals. Furthermore, the relative importance of treatment goals may vary over time. For example, a person with PTSD may initially want to go back to school, in which case participation in a supported education program may be in order; however, going to school may strain his or her marriage and exacerbate PTSD symptoms, in which case participation in a family program to strengthen relationships may be a subsequent important goal. Although the length of psychosocial interventions may vary, the skills development and practice, which are key components of these programs, tend to require months, and sometimes years, of treatment. For example, family psychoeducational programs for serious psychiatric illnesses generally must be provided for at least 9 months to achieve optimal benefits, and evidence-based supported employment programs are considered "time-unlimited").

Recommendations

Two sets of recommendations follow from the literature on psychosocial rehabilitation in PTSD. In the clinical domain, it is becoming increasingly apparent that PTSD may be associated with a wide array of disabilities that may not improve with treatments that focus exclusively on ameliorating core PTSD symptoms. More comprehensive interventions, in line with the psychosocial interventions outlined here, may be needed. It is imperative that a clinician working with a person with PTSD conduct a comprehensive assessment to identify deficiencies in role functioning, and to determine whether the person with the disorder wished to engage in interventions to remediate these problems. In considering whether to embark on a psychosocial rehabilitation program, the individual with the disorder should be encouraged to consider the appropriate staging and timing of intervention, so that he or she is not overwhelmed by the requirements of multiple, concurrent treatment activities. If the individual with the disorder deems that effort toward a particular goal is warranted and timely, the clinician should help that person access the treatment, either by providing it him- or herself (e.g., conduct social skills training or family psychoeducation) or by liaising with a facility that can provide the intervention (e.g., a Veterans Administration [VA]–supported employment program, a community college–supported education program).

It is clear that there is much work to be done in the research domain to evaluate the efficacy of extant psychosocial rehabilitation techniques with PTSD, and to modify and to test them systematically. Although controlled studies of these interventions are finally being conducted with samples whose primary problem is PTSD, the state of this research is in its infancy. With the increasing prevalence of PTSD diagnoses, and high rates of comorbidities and disabilities, more work is urgently needed

Summary

Many persons with PTSD have difficulties meeting their social roles as worker, student, partner, parent, friend, or family member. There has been increasing emphasis on improving community functioning in person with serious psychiatric illnesses, and many of the techniques developed as part of this effort may be effective for person with PTSD. Research is needed in this area; meanwhile, clients and clinicians should collaboratively adapt proven psychosocial rehabilitation services to address consumer-identified problems and undertake systematic comparisons of their relative effectiveness for PTSD.

Suggested Readings

Bond, G. R. (2004). Supported employment: Evidence for an evidence-based practice. *Psychiatric Rehabilitation Journal, 27,* 345–359.

Glynn, S. M., Cohen, A. N., Dixon, L. B., & Niv, N. (2006). The potential impact of the recovery movement on family interventions for schizophrenia: Opportunities and obstacles. *Schizophrenia Bulletin, 32*(3), 451–463.

Hypnosis

Description

Hypnosis is a procedure, generally established by an induction, during which
suggestions for alterations in behavior and mental processes, including sensations, perceptions, emotions, and thoughts, are provided. An induction procedure typically entails instructions to disregard extraneous concerns and
focus on the experiences and behaviors that the therapist suggests, or that
may arise spontaneously. Although many inductions use some type of relaxation instructions, others emphasize instead mental alertness and physical
activity. Hypnosis can bring about a narrow focus of attention, enhanced suggestibility, and alterations in consciousness (e.g., in time perception, in body
image). Individuals differ in their level of responsiveness to hypnotic suggestion, which is positively related to treatment efficacy. Hypnosis, which is not
a therapy per se but an adjunct to psychodynamic, cognitive-behavioral, or
other therapies, has been shown to significantly enhance therapeutic efficacy
in a variety of clinical conditions. The use of hypnosis in clinical practice
requires appropriate professional training and credentialing. Health care
professionals should only use its techniques within their areas of professional
expertise.

General Strength of the Evidence

The literature contains two randomized, controlled clinical trials of hypnosis
for various types of posttraumatic symptomatology. The older study showed
that hypnosis significantly decreased intrusion and avoidance symptoms, and
seemed to do it in fewer sessions than the comparison treatments. The newer
study found that hypnosis plus cognitive-behavioral therapy (CBT) had a

larger therapeutic effect for reexperiencing than did CBT alone at the end of treatment, although at a 3-year follow-up the effects of CBT and CBT plus hypnosis were equivalent. Thus, early treatment including hypnosis produced greater symptom reduction. There is also a series of systematic single-case designs that supports the use of hypnosis for posttraumatic conditions with adults and with children, in addition to an extensive literature that supports the efficacy of hypnosis for posttraumatic conditions, mostly based on service and case studies, going back to the 19th century (Levels C and D).

Course of Treatment

Hypnotic techniques can be easily integrated with diverse approaches to the treatment of traumatic stress syndromes, including exposure to trauma-related stimuli in a context that helps patients manage their reactions to them, cognitive restructuring of the meaning of the traumatic experience, and coping skills training—using hypnosis to help manage trauma-related hyperarousal. In a three-stage model of treatment, hypnotic techniques may be used in the following ways:

1. In the initial phase, hypnosis can be used to stabilize the patient by providing techniques to enhance relaxation and establish cues to induce a calm state outside of the therapeutic context. Specific suggestions may also be used to enhance ego strength and a sense of safety, to contain traumatic memories, and to reduce, or at least better control, symptoms such as anxiety or nightmares. Finally, hypnosis is widely believed to intensify the therapist–patient relationship, which can then enhance therapeutic purposes.

2. In the second stage of working through and resolving traumatic memories, various hypnotic techniques can help to pace and control the investigation, integration, and resolution of traumatic memories. In this context, the patient may learn to modulate his or her emotional and cognitive distance from the traumatic material, and better integrate traumatic memories. Projective and restructuring techniques, such as an imaginary split screen to represent different aspects of the traumatic experience, may be especially advantageous in this stage.

3. Finally, goals in the third stage include achieving a more adaptive integration of the traumatic experience into the patient's life, maintaining more adaptive coping responses, and furthering personal development. Hypnotic techniques may be helpful in providing strategies to focus intentionally and shift attention as necessary; they may also be helpful in self-integration, through, for instance, rehearsals in fantasy of a more adaptive self-image, of new activities, and so on.

Throughout these three basic stages, hypnosis may be used to facilitate eight important tasks for patients with posttraumatic stress disorder (PTSD): confronting the traumatic material, facilitating the conscious experience of aspects of the trauma that might have been dissociated, confessing embarrassing or painful deeds or emotions, providing appropriate consolation and sympathy for painful experiences, condensing various aspects of trauma into representative and more manageable images, enhancing concentration and mental control instead of falling prey to unbidden and distressing mental episodes, and facilitating an adaptive congruence in various areas of the patient's personal and social life. In the case of a recent traumatic event, without a history of chronic pathology, our observation has been that hypnotic techniques can facilitate recovery in a matter of a few sessions. Chronic and more complicated clinical pictures typically require lengthier treatment.

Summary

Indications

1. Hypnotic techniques may be especially useful for symptoms often associated with posttraumatic conditions, such as dissociation and nightmares, for which hypnotic techniques have been successfully used (Level C).

2. Patients with PTSD who manifest at least moderate hypnotizability may benefit from the addition of hypnotic techniques to their treatment (Level D).

3. Hypnotic techniques may be easily integrated into diverse approaches, including psychodynamic or cognitive-behavioral therapies, and pharmacotherapy. Although clinical observations suggest such integration for PTSD, we need more data that directly evaluate whether the addition of hypnosis enhances the efficacy of those treatments.

4. Because confronting traumatic memories may be very difficult for some patients with PTSD, hypnotic techniques may provide a means to modulate their emotional and cognitive distance from such memories as patients work through them therapeutically (Level D).

5. For patients with PTSD who may have experienced dissociative phenomena at the time of traumatic events, a similar state induced in hypnosis may potentially enhance a fuller recall of those events, especially if there are no other strong cues to the event (Level F).

Contraindications

1. In the rare cases of individuals who are refractory or minimally responsive to hypnotic suggestions, hypnotic techniques may not be beneficial because there is some evidence that hypnotizability is related to treatment outcome.

2. Some patients with PTSD may resist the use of hypnosis because of mistaken preconceptions or other reasons. If this resistance is not softened

after mistaken assumptions about hypnosis are dispelled, other suggestive techniques that do not involve the term "hypnosis" or an induction procedures, such as emotional self-regulation therapy, may be employed (Level F).

3. For patients with low blood pressure or proneness to fall asleep, a hypnotic procedure that emphasizes alertness rather than relaxation can be tried (Level F).

Potential complications of using hypnosis for PTSD include exaggerated confidence in the veracity of memories produced during hypnosis and the possible creation of pseudomemories, or "false memories," especially among highly suggestible individuals given misleading information. A number of studies have shown that hypnosis facilitates improved recall of both true and confabulated material, with no change in overall accuracy. Providing accurate information about the nature of hypnosis and memory, and warning patients about the potentially unwarranted confidence in memories obtained through hypnosis or other techniques, may minimize this concern. Clinicians should be especially careful with patients who may want to use hypnotic techniques to access "unremembered" episodes of previous abuse.

There may also be legal ramifications to the use of hypnosis for accessing memories of traumatic events, for instance, in the case of witnessing a crime, when the ability of victims to testify in court may be challenged if they were hypnotized. In these situations, it is wise to discuss such issues in advance with the attorneys and police officials involved in the case, and to record electronically all contacts with the patient.

Suggested Readings

Degun-Mather, M. (2006). *Hypnosis, dissociation and survivors of child abuse.* Chichester, UK: Wiley.

Kirsch, I., Capafons, A., Cardeña, E., & Amigó, S. (Eds.). (1998). *Clinical hypnosis and self-regulation therapy: A cognitive-behavioral perspective.* Washington, DC: American Psychological Association.

Lynn, S. J., & Cardeña, E. (2007). Hypnosis and the treatment of posttraumatic conditions: An evidence-based approach. *International Journal of Clinical and Experimental Hypnosis, 55,* 167–188.

Spiegel, H., & Spiegel, D. (2004). *Trance and treatment: Clinical uses of hypnosis* (2nd ed.). Washington, DC: American Psychiatric Press.

Couple and Family Therapy for Adults

Description

Experts suggested that it is important to consider including therapy for families or couples when addressing posttraumatic stress disorder (PTSD) and other psychological sequelae of trauma. Approaches to couple/family treatment have grown out of two theoretical traditions. Some programs include couple/family therapy to address the impact of trauma and its effects on families and the relationships of traumatized individuals. These programs tend to focus more on relieving family distress than on reducing a particular individual's PTSD symptoms. Other programs focus on the role of the partner and family members in helping the trauma survivor to recover from symptoms arising from the trauma. In this formulation, interventions focus on improving the efficacy with which this support is provided. The two approaches are not mutually exclusive, and there is clearly some overlap in techniques and evaluation. Programs that have been developed more recently tend to blur the distinction even more.

General Strength of the Evidence

The literature on couple and family therapies with trauma survivors is severely limited. The few empirical studies have significant limitations. Most utilized small samples and did not include a control or comparison group.

Indeed, only one published article and one unpublished doctoral dissertation have reported the results of randomized controlled trials of family or couple therapy. The existing studies are limited further by their focus on combat veterans and their partners. Until results are replicated with larger samples and survivors of other types of trauma, it is premature to recommend couple therapy for the treatment of PTSD or PTSD-related family distress. The clinically focused literature on the use of couple/family treatments with trauma survivors is similarly limited. Despite several descriptions of such treatments, careful case studies with standard assessments are absent.

The strength of the evidence for specific treatment programs is as follows:

- *Behavioral family therapy* includes education about PTSD and PTSD services, communication training, anger management, and improving couple problem-solving skills (Level A).
- *Behavioral marital therapy* focuses on increasing positive interactions, improving communication and problem-solving skills, and enhancing intimacy (Level A).
- *Cognitive-behavioral couple treatment for PTSD* comprises 15 sessions in which the clinician educates the couple about PTSD and its impact on relationships, introduces communication skills, helps the couple to overcome experiential avoidance, and applies cognitive interventions to change the core beliefs related to persistent PTSD symptoms (Level B).
- *Lifestyle management courses* include education about PTSD, managing stress, relaxation/meditation, self-care, diet and nutrition, communication, anger management, and problem solving, as well as discussions of self-esteem, alcohol, and depression (Level B).
- *Emotionally focused couple therapy* includes efforts to identify negative interaction patterns and label them as a problem, encourage acceptance by the partner, appropriately ask for one's needs to be met, develop new ways of coping, and integrate new interaction patterns (Level D).
- *Spousal education and support programs* typically include didactic, discussion, and question–answer components aimed at topics including education about mental illness and available services, training in problem-solving skills, stress management (Level D).
- *Family systems–based therapy* often includes developing a conceptualization of trauma as a family issue, educating families about trauma, developing support and communication skills, clarifying individual roles within the family, and resolving emotional disruption (Level D).
- *Critical interaction therapy* identifies patterns of dyadic processes that commonly occur in families of trauma survivors and uses a series of interventions to teach about the process, point out connections to the trauma, encourage partners to offer support, and promote better problem solving and communication (Level F).

Course of Treatment

The literature includes descriptions of a number of different couple/family treatment approaches that may be used following trauma but not generally agreed-upon programs or protocols for administering the treatment. The lack of strong empirical evidence for the use of couple/family treatments for trauma survivors further complicates attempts to delineate an expected course of treatment. With these limitations in mind, below is an outline of some of the common characteristics across the various treatments described in the literature.

Most programs incorporate the couple/family work into a larger treatment program that targets the psychological sequelae of trauma. Typically, this means that the individual(s) who experienced the trauma directly (and sometimes other family members) participate in individual therapy concurrently with or prior to the couple/family therapy. In general, the couple/family intervention is viewed as time-limited, though the number and frequency of sessions differ across programs. Early sessions are typically devoted to educating participants about the treatment program, trauma, and PTSD. The remaining sessions tend to focus on teaching specific skills, with an emphasis on improving communication, problem solving, coping, and mutual support. Often, interventions are designed to allow the families or couples to process the impact of the trauma on their lives. The specific skills taught, the manner and order in which they are taught, and the relative emphasis placed on skills training and processing varies across treatment programs.

Recommendations

Because dyadic and/or family disruption can be a problem for individuals with PTSD, it is recommended that clinicians evaluate the possible need for couple or family therapy when treating trauma survivors with PTSD. When couple or family therapy is warranted, it is recommended that this treatment focus on improving communication and reducing conflict among family members. This may entail communication about current problems and/or issues related to the trauma and its aftermath. Studies suggest that, in some cases, these treatments may help to address family disruption and increase support for the patient. However, there is little empirical support for including such treatments. Furthermore, decision criteria for when to use these treatments and the consequences of not including them are largely unknown.

When addressing the needs of traumatized children, rarely is family or couple therapy suggested to be the sole, or even primary, treatment for posttrauma symptoms. The preliminary data on cognitive-behavioral couple treatment for PTSD are promising and suggest that treatment incorporating skills training to improve communication and specific interventions targeting PTSD symptoms is possible. However, ability to make clear recommendations awaits further research.

Couple/family therapy is generally presented as an important adjunct to other forms of treatment aimed more directly at alleviating posttraumatic symptoms. Even in cases when family therapy is identified as the primary form of therapy, individual treatment with the trauma survivor is recommended to address PTSD symptoms. Therefore, it is recommended that couple and family therapy should be used concurrently with, or following, evidence-based treatments that focus on alleviating PTSD symptoms.

Experts suggest that couple/family therapy is most appropriate when the family system has functioned well prior to the trauma. When the system is dysfunctional prior to the trauma, alternative therapy approaches may be needed prior to treatment focused on the family's reactions to the trauma. Again, the empirical literature offers little to guide this decision. Recent studies of couple treatment have utilized samples whose participants report being generally satisfied with their relationships, so it is unclear how effective the treatments might be with dissatisfied couples. Thus, although it might be more appropriate to include couple/family therapy in a treatment plan for an individual when significant disruption exists, we know little about the effects of such treatment in these patients.

Summary

Experts provide strong theoretical arguments and rationales for using couple/family therapies, usually combined with other treatments for post-trauma symptoms. However, the lack of empirical data makes it difficult to know whether these programs are helpful in reducing family disruption or in promoting recovery from trauma. It is also unclear when couple/family interventions should be used, or how to combine them with other treatment approaches.

Suggested Readings

Figley, C. R. (1989). *Helping traumatized families*. San Francisco: Jossey-Bass.

Glynn, S. M., Eth, S., Randolph, E. T., Foy, D. W., Urbatis, M., Boxer, L., et al. (1999). A test of behavioral family therapy to augment exposure for combat-related post-traumatic stress disorder. *Journal of Consulting and Clinical Psychology, 67,* 243–251.

Monson, C. M., Stevens, S. P., & Schnurr, P. P. (2005). Cognitive-behavioral couple's treatment for posttraumatic stress disorder. In T. A. Corales (Ed.), *Focus on post-traumatic stress disorder* (pp. 245–274). Hauppauge, NY: Nova Science.

Creative Therapies for Adults

Description

The creative arts therapies are the intentional use by a trained therapist of art, music, dance/movement, drama, and poetry in psychotherapy, counseling, special education, or rehabilitation. All forms of creative arts therapy treatment of trauma utilize techniques that have elements in common with *imaginal exposure*, in that the trauma scene is represented in the artwork, dramatic role play, movement, poetry, or music. Similarly, many forms of creative art therapies utilize techniques that have some elements in common with *cognitive restructuring*, such as role playing (and its relative *covert modeling*). Playing out scenes, switching roles, and replaying more health-promoting options are means of changing or challenging a person's view of a situation. Identification of distorted cognitions, cognitive reprocessing, and reframing are implemented through the use of journaling, writing, storytelling, and other narrative techniques. *Stress/anxiety management skills*, such as progressive muscle relaxation and deep breathing, are standard elements in most forms of creative arts therapy for trauma. *Resilience enhancement techniques* in the creative arts therapies are implicit in their use of creativity, humor, spontaneity, flexibility, and activity. Finally, *testimony, public education, and destigmatization* are realized through theater and dance performances by trauma survivors, exhibitions of survivors' artwork, and public readings of their poetry.

The potential advantage of utilizing a creative arts therapy procedure is most likely based on the nonverbal (behavioral) aspects of the artistic modalities. First, the symbolic media of the arts may provide more complete access to implicit (as opposed to explicit) memory systems, as well as visual–kinesthetic schemas. By providing a wider range of stimuli (visual, sonic, tactile, and kinesthetic), the creative arts therapies may increase the vividness of imaginal exposure. By providing concretized forms of representation (visual, written, enacted), the creative arts therapies may help to decrease avoidance. The behavioral nature of the creative arts therapies may also support or enhance cognitive restructuring strategies. Second, the claim that creative arts therapies are especially helpful to traumatized, inexpressive persons has been supported by the concept of *alexithymia*, about which much has been written in the trauma field. The inability to put feelings into words appears to be relatively common in patients with posttraumatic stress disorder (PTSD). Presumably, clients who are unable to find words to express their experience may find the nonverbal/behavioral forms of the creative arts a more welcoming means of expression.

General Strength of the Evidence

Specific creative arts therapy treatments for trauma have not yet been empirically tested. Evidence for the effectiveness of the creative arts therapies is based on numerous clinical case studies by a wide range of practitioners over several decades Agency for Health Care Policy and Research (AHCPR; Level D). Progress has most often been noted in (1) the primary symptoms of PTSD and (2) global clinical improvement. Noted less often are improvements in functional behaviors or clinical service utilization. The creative arts therapies have been cited as being helpful in the reduction of alexithymia, increase in emotional control, improvement in interpersonal relationships, decrease in dissociation and anxiety, decrease in nightmares and sleep problems, improved body image, and reduction of depression.

Course of Treatment

The wide range of treatment formats used in the creative arts therapies vary in length, structure, and degree of integration with verbal therapies. More recently developed treatments are time-limited, structured interventions, similar in form to cognitive-behavioral treatment formats.

Recommendations

1. The recognition, justification, and further development of the creative arts therapies in the treatment of psychological trauma will be most fully encouraged by empirical inquiries using control groups and randomized assignment.
2. Creative arts therapy treatments designed as specific treatments for PTSD presumably will have heightened therapeutic effects over non-

specific creative arts therapy approaches. The further design, development, and testing of such treatments are recommended.

3. The unique contribution of the creative arts therapies cross-culturally, particularly in underdeveloped countries, in translation of effective intervention models across linguistic barriers and diverse cultural traditions should be further investigated.

Summary

Despite relatively widespread use and application over a substantial time period, the efficacy of the creative arts therapies has not yet been established through empirical research. The implementation of rigorous empirical research studies in this area is a primary priority for the field. Creative arts therapy professionals claim that these treatment modalities may be useful as either primary or adjunctive interventions. There is clinical consensus that the use of the creative arts therapies may be helpful as an adjunct to the treatment of PTSD under the following conditions: (1) The arts therapy is conducted by a practitioner educated and trained in that approach; (2) the therapy is conducted with the permission of the client; and (3) the therapy is conducted in conjunction with other, ongoing treatments and therapists. The exact source of therapeutic benefits of the creative arts therapies in the treatment of PTSD has not been identified, but is likely to be derived from imaginal exposure, cognitive restructuring, stress management, resilience enhancement, and testimony, as well as physiological processes and specific contributions of nonverbal and creative elements.

Suggested Readings

Adams, K. (1997). *The way of the journal.* Denver, CO: Sidran Press.

Cohen, B., Barnes, M., & Rankin, A. (1995). *Managing traumatic stress through art.* Lutherville, MD: Sidran Press.

Dayton, T. (1997). *Heartwounds: The impact of unresolved trauma and grief on relationships.* Deerfield Beach, FL: Health Communication.

Hudgins, K. (2002). *Experiential treatment for PTSD: The therapeutic spiral model.* New York: Springer.

Johnson, D. (1987). The role of the creative arts therapies in the diagnosis and treatment of psychological trauma. *Arts in Psychotherapy, 14,* 7–14.

Kluft, E. (Ed.). (1992). *Expressive and functional therapies in the treatment of multiple personality disorder.* Springfield, IL: Thomas.

van der Kolk, B. (1994). The body keeps the score. *Harvard Review of Psychiatry, 1,* 253–265.

Winn, L. (1994). *Posttraumatic stress disorder and dramatherapy: Treatment and risk reduction.* London: Jessica Kingsley.

Creative Arts Therapies
for Children

Description

The creative arts therapies (CATs) include art, dance/movement, drama, music, poetry, and psychodrama. They share a commitment to the value and use of creative arts processes to enhance, improve, and change physical, emotional, cognitive, and social functioning. The CATs have a tradition of use with children and teens (who often are accustomed to using the arts, or who have less sophisticated verbal skills) as a way to access nonverbal material or content that is unavailable to words. Hence, the CATs are especially well suited to work with children who have experienced trauma.

Significant advances in the past decade in the scientific basis and understanding of the relationship between brain functioning and processing of traumatic events has generated burgeoning interest in the role of the CATs in treating trauma and posttraumatic stress disorder (PTSD). The kinesthetic and sensory experiences inherent in the CATs activate the right hemisphere of the brain, allowing access to nonverbal memory. The art making and engagement in creative activities allows the externalization of internal images, thoughts, and feelings, in addition to enabling titration and containment of affect.

General Strength of the Evidence

Historically, CAT research has been based on assessments and clinical experience. Although there is no empirical evidence supporting the efficacy of the CATs, an abundance of CAT case studies describe treatment success, the majority published in academic CAT journals, and a preponderance using art therapy. To date, there is one small Level A randomized controlled art therapy study (Chapman et al., 2001) and other attempts at using objective measures to assess change.

Course of Treatment

Treatment has been conducted with individuals and groups in both inpatient and clinic settings. There are different schools of thought regarding theoretical orientation and practice. Interventions vary along a continuum from

- Therapist-directed activities and themes to more client-directed, unstructured sessions that are either time-limited or open-ended.
- An emphasis on the creative process as the agent of change to a focus on the product.
- Using verbal processing of creative output to foster hemispheric integration of past trauma to letting the process or product "speak for itself."
- Using a single CAT to incorporating multiple CATs.

CAT clinicians and researchers differ in their assimilation of non-CAT theoretical principles and practices. Most notably, a number of creative arts therapists use or adapt cognitive-behavioral therapy (CBT) interventions to their work (e.g., "draw what you saw"). Likewise, creative arts activities are often integrated into many CBT therapy sessions (e.g., "Let's role-play what you wish you had done").

Recommendations

Currently, treatment protocols and research paradigms are sporadically being developed to measure the efficacy of the CATs in medical, mental health, and educational settings, among others. Future work should focus on the following:

1. Exploring the relationship between neurological functioning and creative arts processes.

2. Using existing standardized measures of PTSD, in addition to developing appropriate creative arts–based assessment tools.

3. Including caregivers in treatment.

4. Developing manualized treatment protocols to better delineate the format and structure of interventions that can then be compared across settings and with other treatments.

5. Conducting controlled outcome studies of CATs PTSD treatments.

Additionally, it is recommended that those who use the arts with traumatized children have knowledge and experience in the area, and be properly trained in the specific creative arts modality, the creative process, nonverbal dialogue, and containment and stabilization via the arts. The CATs can promote powerful access to trauma-related experiences, and extreme care must be taken to avoid retraumatization and to foster coping.

Collaboration with other professionals is recommended to engage in dialogue and debate, and to learn how the CATs and other professions can build on the strengths and knowledge of one another to develop the best practices for PTSD treatment.

Summary

As the emerging effective paradigms of PTSD treatment are formally investigated, the CATs have great potential to contribute in-depth knowledge of nonverbal dialogue and the kinesthetic, sensory, auditory, and visual processes and their role in perception, cognition, and change in therapy. More CATs studies and collaboration with other mental health professions in the future are essential for the progress of effective, evidence-based treatment. The CATs are unique in their focus on gaining access to traumatic content and affect via nonverbal modalities and provide a ready avenue to explore the new frontier of brain and experience-based trauma therapies.

Reference

Chapman, L., Morabito, D., Ladakakos, C., Schreier, H., & Knudson, M. (2001). The effectiveness of art therapy interventions in reducing posttraumatic stress disorder (PTSD) symptoms in pediatric trauma patients. *Art Therapy: Journal of the American Art Therapy Association, 18*, 100–104.

Suggested Readings

Klorer, P. (2003). Sexually abused children: Group approaches. In C. A. Malchiodi (Ed.), *Handbook of art therapy* (pp. 339–350). New York: Guilford Press.

Webb, N. B. (Ed.). (2004). *Mass trauma and violence: Helping families and children cope.* New York: Guilford Press.

Treatment of PTSD and Comorbid Disorders

Description

Approximately 80% of people with posttraumatic stress disorder (PTSD) have a co-occurring psychiatric disorder (lifetime rates), yet treatments to address such comorbid conditions have only recently been developed and studied. There are several ways to approach the treatment of comorbid disorders: *integrated* (treatment of comorbid disorders at the same time, by the same provider); *sequential* (treatment of one disorder, then the other); *parallel* (treatment of each disorder, but in separate treatments); and *single diagnosis* (treatment of just one disorder).

When considering comorbidity and its treatment, it is also helpful to explore the many possible relationships between the comorbid conditions (e.g., their development over time, course during treatment, and impact on each other), as well as how treatment may impact them, both together or differentially.

General Strength of the Evidence

Treatment models for PTSD comorbidity offer a wide range of features, including the types of trauma for which they are designed, the use of group versus individual modality, and the variety of techniques offered. Some models are designed from the start for comorbidity, whereas others are a combination of existing approaches already found effective for each separate disorder. Some studies address models that, designed for only one diagnosis, also showed impact on comorbid conditions.

Overall, this research area is at an early stage in both the psychosocial and pharmacotherapy areas. There are only a few Level A studies, and only one model is established as effective. Most studies address Axis I comorbid conditions, with only a few studies of comorbid Axis II disorders. Study methodologies generally have a variety of limitations, and some are reanalyses of existing datasets in which comorbidity was addressed post hoc and on only a subset of patients. No studies thus far have reported the full array of comorbid Axis I and II disorders. In terms of the Agency for Health Care Policy and Research (AHCPR) standards that guide this volume, in the area of comorbidity, a study may be one level for PTSD, yet another for the comorbid condition.

Substance Use Disorder

Seeking Safety (Level A)

Seeking Safety (SS) is an integrated, present-focused coping skills model for PTSD and substance use disorder (SUD). It offers 25 topics, each representing a safe coping skill (e.g., *asking for help*). The model is designed for high flexibility (e.g., length and pacing of treatment; group or individual format; men or women; all types of trauma and substances). It is the most researched model for any diagnosis co-occurring with PTSD, with 12 published studies that range from Levels A to C. Studies have addressed diverse samples, including clients in community treatment, adolescents, homeless clients, veterans, prisoners, and others. SS is the only co-occurring PTSD model that is established as effective at this point using criteria for empirically supported treatments. It has shown consistent positive outcomes on various measures, consistent superiority to treatment as usual (TAU), comparability to a "gold standard" treatment (relapse prevention), and high acceptability.

Collaborative Care (Level B)

Collaborative care (CC) is a multidisciplinary, integrated prevention model for PTSD and SUD for medically injured trauma survivors at risk for developing PTSD and alcohol use disorder. The model combines motivational interviewing, cognitive-behavioral therapy (CBT), psychopharmacology, and case management, with dose and treatments varying by clients' presentation. The researchers compared CC and TAU; results after 1 year indicated that patients in CC were less likely to have PTSD and SUD than those in TAU. The study did not mention blind evaluators or adherence ratings, and it was not fully randomized, but this prevention model remains promising.

Concurrent Treatment of PTSD and Cocaine Dependence (Level C)

This model combines treatments that have efficacy for PTSD and SUD separately (relapse prevention, coping skills, *in vivo* and imaginal exposure). It is an integrated, 16-week individual treatment. A one-arm pilot study indicated that those who stayed in treatment had reductions in PTSD, depression, and SUD. The study offers impressive pilot evidence that some patients with PTSD and SUD can tolerate and benefit from PTSD exposure treatment; however, concerns center on treatment retention and paying patients to attend sessions.

Transcend (Level C)

Transcend is an integrated, 12-week partial hospitalization program of CBT, constructivist, psychodynamic, and 12-step models. An uncontrolled pilot study with 46 Vietnam veterans entering treatment evidenced significant reductions in PTSD symptoms; SUD was not assessed because all patients had to have 30 days of sobriety before starting. Transcend is currently the only model developed specifically for a partial hospitalization setting; it shows promise in treating veterans with PTSD and SUD.

Trauma Empowerment Recovery Model (Level C)

The trauma empowerment recovery model (TREM), a group model originally designed for women abuse survivors with severe mental disorders, has been adopted more broadly. The model includes psychoeducation, cognitive restructuring, survivor empowerment, skills building, and peer support. In a controlled study, TREM was modified to a 24-session version (from 33 sessions) and followed an initial orientation with a trauma workbook. The study evaluated women in residential substance abuse treatment, comparing TREM plus workbook to TAU. The former had better outcomes on trauma-related symptoms. Both improved in substance use symptoms, with no difference between them.

Substance Dependence–PTSD Therapy (Level C)

Substance dependence–PTSD therapy (SDPT) is an integrated, 40-session individual therapy that addresses PTSD and SUD in a phase-based approach using existing models for each disorder (e.g., coping skills training and *in vivo* exposure). A study compared SDPT to 12-step facilitation (TSF) in a sample with at least current partial PTSD and lifetime SUD. Results indicated that among participants who attended at least three sessions, more sessions were attended in SDPT than in TSF. No other differences were found between the treatment conditions; thus, the researchers combined the data. At face value, the model has potential. However, it is difficult to draw conclusions because SDPT did not outperform TSF relative to PTSD or SUD, nor are results reported separately for SDPT.

Acceptance and Commitment Therapy (Level F)

In a case study using acceptance and commitment therapy (ACT) for 96 sessions of individual therapy, the patient was stated to have PTSD and SUD, but without standardized assessment. She was assessed every 3 months on various measures, with improvement mostly at 9 months and thereafter. It is challenging to know what to make of this study given its methodology. Nonetheless, ACT is widely known, and it would be helpful to understand whether it has potential for PTSD and SUD.

Generalized Anxiety Disorder/Major Depressive Disorder

Cognitive-Behavioral Therapy for PTSD (Level A)

CBT has been evaluated among motor vehicle accident (MVA) survivors with full or subthreshold PTSD and comorbid disorders. A randomized controlled trial (RCT) compared CBT to supportive psychotherapy (SP) and wait list, and examined generalized anxiety disorder (GAD) and major depressive disorder (MDD) in addition to PTSD. However, the model was not designed for GAD or MDD. CBT was found superior to SP, which was superior to the wait list on numerous variables. CBT also showed greater reduction in MDD and GAD symptoms than the other conditions. This study is Level A for the comparison of CBT versus wait-list control only; SP does not qualify as Level A due to therapist assignment (CBT clinicians conducted it) and other concerns. Other issues include varying dose of treatment (8–12 sessions) and the fact that comorbid conditions were not present in all patients. Given the frequency of MVAs, this model addresses an important area.

Panic

Multiple-Channel Exposure Therapy (Level B)

Multiple-channel exposure therapy (M-CET) is a manualized, 12-week group model integrating cognitive processing therapy for PTSD (CPT) and exposure for panic. When M-CET was compared to a minimal attention control condition, the M-CET group had greater reductions in PTSD and panic symptoms, and both improved in depression. However, the study is only on a completer sample and is not fully randomized (i.e., some participants were in both conditions). More research is needed on this promising model.

Sensation Reprocessing Therapy (Level B)

Sensation reprocessing therapy (SRT), an integrated treatment for Southeast Asians, combines CPT for PTSD, exposure for panic, mindfulness, and cultural adaptation. The pilot studies compared SRT to a wait-list control in a Vietnamese population and in a Cambodian population and found that the SRT condition produced greater reductions in PTSD and other anxiety symptoms. However, only one clinician conducted all sessions; there was lack of full randomization (some patients were in both conditions), lack of identical timing of assessments, and no mention of adherence. SRT is especially noteworthy for its cultural sensitivity.

CBT for Panic Disorder plus Implosive Therapy (Level D)

A case study using a sequential approach examined nine sessions of CBT for panic disorder with agoraphobia followed by nine sessions of implosive therapy for PTSD. Results indicate diagnosis-specific impact: reduction of panic but not PTSD symptoms after the panic treatment phase, and reduction of symptoms of both disorders after the panic plus PTSD phases.

CBT/Exposure (Level D)

In a post hoc analysis on two group CBTs for panic disorder (both with an exposure component), the two treatments were combined to evaluate PTSD outcomes. Results indicated reduction in panic symptoms, and for those with PTSD, a reduction in PTSD symptoms. However, only a few patients had PTSD, and the two treatments were combined.

Obsessive–Compulsive Disorder

Obsessive–Compulsive Disorder Inpatient Treatment (Level C)

A naturalistic study and several case studies on a residential obsessive–compulsive disorder (OCD) treatment program examined a behavioral program (exposure and response prevention), with no modification for PTSD. Patients with PTSD showed worse outcomes on OCD and depression symptoms, and some had an increase in PTSD symptoms. Researchers concluded that this OCD treatment may be iatrogenic for comorbid PTSD.

Borderline Personality Disorder

Prolonged Exposure/Stress Inoculation Training (Level C)

In a reanalysis of data from a PTSD treatment trial to evaluate outcomes for borderline personality characteristics (BPC), three treatments developed for PTSD only, not BPC, were compared: prolonged exposure (PE), stress inoculation training (SIT), PE plus SIT, and wait list. Data from all conditions were collapsed due to the small BPC sample. All patients improved by end of treatment on various measures including PTSD. Although groups did not differ with regard to loss of diagnosis following treatment, those with BPC were less likely to achieve good end-state functioning.

Psychodynamic Imaginative Trauma Therapy and EMDR (Level C)

A naturalistic study of psychodynamic imaginative trauma therapy (PITT) and eye movement desensitization and reprocessing (EMDR) on patients with "complex PTSD" and multiple comorbidities was examined. The treatment was designed for PTSD only. All patients received 2 months of inpatient care, were discharged, then, 8 months later, a subset of patients reentered the hospital and received trauma treatment (PITT, a psychodynamic model, plus EMDR). Those who completed the trauma-focused component improved more than those who did not.

Psychotic Disorders

Trauma Recovery Group (Level C)

Trauma recovery group is a CBT program for PTSD and serious mental illness (SMI), with components that include crisis planning, breathing retraining, psychoeducation, coping with symptoms, and personal recovery. An individual version is 12–16 sessions, whereas the group treatment is 21 sessions. In uncontrolled pilot studies, the individual model evidenced high retention, and improved PTSD and general psychiatric symptoms. The group model had lower retention, but completers showed improvement in PTSD and other symptoms. SMI is an important comorbidity, and future research is warranted.

Psychopharmacology

Despite the high comorbidity of PTSD with other disorders, there have been few pharmacotherapy studies in this complicated patient population. Existing studies are promising, with most indicating that patients with PTSD and comorbidity respond as well to standard pharmacotherapies as those without comorbidity. Several studies provide useful data concerning adjunctive pharmacotherapies in specific comorbid conditions.

Level A studies have been conducted on sertraline and risperidone. Level B studies have been conducted on disulfiram, naltrexone, and their combination, and antidepressant (paroxetine or bupropion) versus CBT versus community mental health referral.

Overall results suggesting positive findings. There is also initial evidence for possible subtypes based on subjects with PTSD or comorbid conditions who respond differentially (e.g., to sertraline); possible subtypes based on chronicity of PTSD who respond differentially (e.g., to risperidone); a finding for better outcomes with medications provided separately than combined (for disulfiram and naltrexone); a finding of improved outcomes on alcohol use among those with PTSD (for disulfiram or naltrexone compared to placebo); and a finding of worse outcomes for patients with MDD and PTSD compared to MDD alone using antidepressant medication (paroxetine or bupropion).

Summary and Recommendations

Virtually all of the literature on treatment for PTSD and comorbid conditions has arisen in the past few years. Given the high rates of PTSD comorbidity and the often vulnerable nature of such populations, it is encouraging to see such a burst of energy. In addition to the disorders stated earlier, a number of other disorders frequently co-occur with PTSD. As yet, there are insufficient clinical trials addressing these disorders in the context of PTSD, for example, dissociative disorders and Axis II disorders, such as avoidant or antisocial personality disorders.

Overall, only four treatments have a Level A study: SS, CBT for PTSD in MVA survivors, and the medications sertraline and risperidone. Most treatments, both psychosocial and pharmacological, have a single study, with a few having two. SS is established as effective, with 12 published studies. Study methodologies generally have a variety of limitations, and some are reanalyses of existing datasets in which comorbidity was addressed post hoc and on only a subset of patients. Most studies address Axis I comorbid conditions, with only a few studies of comorbid Axis II disorders. Future studies will benefit from more scientific rigor, expanded assessment, and exploration of the optimal number of sessions and treatment components. It is hoped that the next decade will see more RCTs, more empirical work on dissemination and training, and greater understanding of the comorbidities themselves (e.g., rates, causal relationships, and prognosis). The study of PTSD comorbidity is a relatively new area of research in which there is room for a great deal of growth.

At this point, we present a few summary points:

1. Addressing comorbid conditions in treatment is recommended.
2. There are various ways to address comorbidity, but integrated treatment is generally the most highly recommended; research is needed to address whether it actually outperforms other approaches.
3. Single-diagnosis treatments (the majority of PTSD treatments thus far) may have impact on comorbid conditions even if not originally designed for them.
4. Patients with PTSD and comorbid conditions can benefit from psychosocial treatments, as well as from pharmacotherapy.

5. Most studies thus far are uncontrolled pilot studies; only four Level A studies were found (for SS, CBT for MVA survivors, sertraline, and risperidone); only SS meets criteria for efficacy.
6. Axis II comorbid conditions have been especially underaddressed.
7. Almost all studies address CBT-based models rather than other theoretical orientations.
8. Only one model was suggested to have negative outcomes (behavioral treatment of OCD).
9. More research is needed on these disorders and other, commonly occurring disorders not named, especially studies with strong methodology (Level A).

Suggested Readings

Mueser, K. T., Rosenberg, S. D., Goodman, L. A., & Trumbetta, S. L. (2002). Trauma, PTSD, and the course of schizophrenia: An interactive model. *Schizophrenia Research, 53*, 123–143.

Najavits, L. M. (2007). Psychosocial treatments for posttraumatic stress disorder. In P. E. Nathan & J. M. Gorman (Eds.), *A guide to treatments that work* (3rd ed., pp. 513–529). New York: Oxford University Press.

Weiss, R. D., Najavits, L. M., & Hennessy, G. (2004). Overview of treatment modalities for dual diagnosis patients: Pharmacotherapy, psychotherapy, and twelve-step programs. In H. R. Kranzler & B. J. Rounsaville (Eds.), *Dual diagnosis: Substance abuse and comorbid medical and psychiatric disorders* (2nd ed., pp. 103–128). New York: Marcel Dekker.

PART V

CONCLUSION

CHAPTER 22

Integration and Summary

Matthew J. Friedman, Judith A. Cohen, Edna B. Foa,
and Terence M. Keane

In this book, our goal was to provide critical reviews of the various treatment approaches to posttraumatic stress disorder (PTSD). Each chapter is dedicated to a specific approach, leaving unaddressed the important clinical questions of how patients' needs dictate choices among these treatments, the timing of the use of these treatments, or the methods to promote integration of these treatments.

Although there are some systematic comparisons of different treatment modalities (see, e.g., Brom, Kleber, & Defares, 1989; Foa et al., 1999; Foa, Rothbaum, Riggs, & Murdock, 1991; Marks, Lovell, Noshirvani, Livanou, & Thrasher, 1998; Resick, Nishith, Weaver, Astin, & Feurer, 2002; Rothbaum et al., 2006; Taylor et al., 2003), we have not reached the point where we can predict which treatments are most suitable for which patients under which conditions. To address these limitations we have provided information in each chapter on the efficacy of each treatment by the inclusion of effect sizes for all randomized clinical trials (RCTs). Hence, practitioners can examine the strength of the evidence that favors one treatment or another before deciding what to offer their patients.

Although the treatment guidelines for any given approach indicate the degree of empirical support available for that specific treatment, empirical data to guide the combination of psychosocial treatments and medications in PTSD are generally unavailable. Indeed, there is only one RCT with adults on augmentation of sertraline treatment with prolonged exposure therapy

(Rothbaum et al., 2006), and a small RCT for combined cognitive-behavioral therapy (CBT) and sertraline treatment in children (Cohen, Mannarino, Perel, & Staron, 2007). There are more studies in the literature that compare combinations of one CBT treatment with another (e.g., Foa et al., 1999; Foa, Hembree, et al., 2005; Marks et al., 1998); on the whole, these studies tend to show that combination treatments do not enhance the efficacy of any single treatment (e.g., Foa, Rothbaum, & Furr, 2003). On the other hand, in a handful of small studies, beneficial outcomes were observed when selective serotonin reuptake inhibitor (SSRI) pharmacotherapy was augmented with atypical antipsychotics (see Chapter 9 by Friedman, Davidson, & Stein, this volume). Despite the paucity of empirical studies on combined treatment, many patients with PTSD do receive more than one form of therapy concurrently (e.g., pharmacotherapy and some form of psychotherapy, or combinations of CBT procedures). As a result, different treatment combinations, sequences, and integration are important topics for future studies.

Although there are only a few PTSD studies on the outcome of medication and psychosocial treatments, such combinations were studied in other anxiety disorders, such as panic disorder (e.g., Barlow & Craske, 1994), obsessive–compulsive disorder (OCD; e.g., Foa, Liebowitz, et al., 2005), and social anxiety disorder (e.g., Davidson et al., 2004; Heimberg et al., 1998). This may be due to the fact that well-controlled studies of combined medication and CBT often yield disappointing results: Just like combinations of CBT procedures, combined treatments are typically not much more effective than single modalities (Foa, Franklin, & Moser, 2002). Notably, for future studies, there are several ways in which treatment modalities can be combined, some of which may show more promise than others. For example, the failure to find that the combination of CBT and pharmacotherapy was not much more effective than CBT alone or medication alone in treating anxiety disorders may be a function of the simultaneous introduction of treatments rather than the adoption of a sequential strategy. We hope that at least one chapter in the next edition of this book will have data from many RCTs on combined treatments for PTSD in adults and children.

Therefore, at present, the integration of treatment techniques remains the art of the clinician. As most clinicians know, the exercise of such "art" has many constraints. Not all clinicians are skilled in providing different techniques: Psychologists customarily do not prescribe medication, and few psychiatrists are adequately trained in CBT. Moreover, not all patients desire, or have the resources to engage in, more than one form of therapy. Importantly, as with other mental disorders, patients with PTSD who present to clinics pose unique and heterogeneous problems that require flexible decision making and solutions, including when to amend, modify, or alter the course of a treatment protocol. Epitomizing these clinical dilemmas is the dictum: *Science is mainly generic, whereas Reality is always specific.* By analogy, when implementing in one's clinical practice, the treatments discussed in the various chapters of this book, it is not a generic "PTSD" that one treats, but a particular patient, or group of patients, with PTSD who present with life situations and circumstances unique to a particular clinical setting.

Questions Addressed in This Chapter

- How should one choose among treatment modalities?
- What can one expect from treatment, and how does one define realistic goals?
- How can one combine various treatment techniques?
- How does one approach complex clinical pictures and comorbid conditions?
- How long should a treatment be followed? Booster sessions? Follow-up?
- Do some features of PTSD require a special approach that cuts across treatment modalities?
- How does one make sense of clinical difficulties and assess failure?
- What do we know about strategies for preventing PTSD among recently traumatized individuals?

In this concluding chapter, we provide an overview to assist the clinician in evaluating the information provided in each of the previous chapters. It is our intention to help the clinician know how to optimize the treatment of individual patients with PTSD. To this end, we address the preceding questions. We begin, however, by outlining what we have learned from each of the chapters, and what questions are left open.

General Issues

Although we have learned a great deal about the treatment of PTSD since the publication of the initial volume, one of the first general lessons we learned is that there is a need for more research. Today, the questions being asked by chapter authors are indeed more precise and perhaps even more sophisticated. For example, in CBT, for which there is considerable empirical evidence, there are still some unanswered questions. Most other chapters, however, conclude that the available empirical evidence does not permit strong conclusions about the efficacy of the treatment approach examined. Furthermore, in most other reviewed approaches to treatment, the ensuing recommendations are tentative, and based on clinical impression and expert opinion.

Lack of evidence, however, should not be confounded with negative evidence (i.e., evidence of lack of efficacy); moreover, some patients fail to benefit from treatments that possess the most empirical support. Nevertheless, with most patients, evidence-based treatments should be favored over treatments without such evidence when the mental health professional has the skills to provide them.

Another general point is that most of the treatment approaches described earlier are not specific to PTSD, but are based on principles, theories, or basic experiments that apply to other mental disorders as well. By analogy, when clinicians are called to choose between treatment options, they must first use their general skills and knowledge as diagnostician and therapist. *The treatment of PTSD, therefore, is to be provided by skilled clinicians only.* This is a very important issue because the most effective treatments, CBTs, are practiced by the smallest number of clinicians (Rosen et al., 2004). In response to this mismatch between need for evidence-based practice and availability of suitably skilled practitioners, there have been a few major initiatives to disseminate CBT, thereby increasing the pool of qualified therapists. To our knowledge, the most ambitious of such programs is within the U.S. Department of Veterans Affairs (VA), where hundreds of clinicians are being trained in prolonged exposure (PE) and/or cognitive processing therapy (CPT) for the treatment of PTSD. Other important initiatives to disseminate CBT are currently in progress in Australia and in the United Kingdom (where there is an incentive for practitioners to utilize evidence-based treatments by virtue of a higher rate of reimbursement for providing such treatments). Also, eye movement desensitization and reprocessing (EMDR) has been widely disseminated via workshops. Also proposed are efforts to train social work and clinical psychology students in evidence-based treatments, including those that are effective for PTSD, while the students are still in graduate school.

Finally, as noted in our Introduction, diagnosis and careful evaluation must precede treatment. In the case of PTSD, these should include the following:

1. Formal diagnoses of PTSD and comorbid disorders.

2. Determination of the most disturbing problem, which may or may not be the PTSD symptoms themselves (e.g., marriage breakup, violence, depression, severe behavior problems in children).

3. Evaluation of the patient's resources (e.g., stable family, work, and housing; supportive parents for children) and his or her deficiencies (e.g., substance misuse, poverty, ongoing traumatization).

4. Evaluation of the patient's (or the parent's, for children) motivation and ability to commit to the prescribed course of the selected therapy, and to its particular demands (e.g., completing homework assignments in CBT, adhering to the medication regimen). *Indeed, engaging patients with PTSD in the therapeutic process (or in complying with prescribed medication) is a first and critical stage of the treatment.*

Overview of the Chapters

In this section we do not review specific findings or recommendations about specific treatment approaches; these can be readily found in both the chapter and clinical guideline about that specific treatment. Instead, we make a few observations, ask a few questions, point to some promising current developments, and offer opinions about important developments for the future.

Acute Interventions and Debriefing

Various early interventions have been employed with individuals who have undergone recent traumatic experiences. The available, strong empirical evidence suggests that early provision of CBT can prevent chronic PTSD among trauma survivors. There is also strong evidence showing that single-session psychological debriefing (PD) is ineffective in preventing the development of chronic PTSD. An important difference between research on CBT and PD is that in the various populations that have usually been examined, most of the CBT work has focused on people (often with acute stress disorder [ASD] or with severe PTSD symptoms) with a high risk to develop PTSD, whereas PD has generally been provided to any trauma survivor, future PTSD risk notwithstanding. From a public health perspective, the optimal approach would be first to identify those survivors at highest risk to develop PTSD and to restrict the testing of a putative prophylactic treatment to them alone.

When discussing early interventions of any sort, it is important to consider the expected outcomes from such approaches. If the major concern is prevention of PTSD, which is the focus of this book, rather than to normalize posttraumatic distress among survivors by providing safety and shelter, attending to basic needs, improving communication, reuniting families, and so forth, then one might draw very different conclusions. Thus, although some early interventions may not prevent the later development of PTSD, they may serve other, important functions that have not been adequately documented in current research findings. Consequently, the question of whether preventive treatment should be provided to all trauma survivors or only to those with identifiable symptoms (or dysfunction) has not been explored systematically. Other questions left unanswered include the following:

1. Can any single, brief "immediate" intervention be expected to have enough power to reverse the complex interaction of variables that cause PTSD?
2. What is the optimal time for introducing preventive interventions?
3. Should such interventions be clinical in nature, or should they address situational and social stressors that occur shortly after the traumatic event(s) (e.g., relocation, uncertainty, pain, and rejecting attitudes of others)?

Given the paucity of controlled trials on PD and the many complex questions that have yet to be systematically addressed, it is the opinion of these editors that it is much too early to conclude that PD is an ineffective intervention for all acutely traumatized individuals. Even if subsequent studies confirm these early findings on the prevention of PTSD, we must be careful not to misinterpret the practical implications of such results. These same studies have also shown that the vast majority of people who receive PD report that this intervention facilitated their recovery from acute posttraumatic distress. Because most traumatized people do not develop PTSD, one possibility is that PD is very useful for many survivors posttrauma but not for those at greatest risk for developing PTSD. In short, there remain many open questions regarding PD. Is it effective in preventing PTSD and in modifying the trajectory of PTSD? What clinical outcomes should be expected? When should PD be administered to optimize its impact, and who should receive it? Can it prevent the ultimate development of PTSD or related psychological conditions? More work in these areas would be greatly welcomed by the clinical and research community.

Finally, we expect that the next edition of this book will include research on psychological first aid (PFA), an evidence-informed early intervention developed jointly by the National Center for PTSD and National Center for Child Traumatic Stress, which embodies practical assistance and general principles for postdisaster assistance. It shares with PD the expectation that it will be beneficial for almost any trauma survivor, but it differs from PD in that it does not include any emotional processing. Although there is great enthusiasm for this new, developmentally sensitive approach, there is no substitute for data. We await the results of such studies with great anticipation.

Cognitive-Behavioral Therapy

The various forms of behavioral, cognitive, and CBT techniques are the most studied interventions for PTSD in adults. Cahill, Rothbaum, Resick, and Follette (Chapter 7, this volume) concluded that CBT techniques are clearly effective. This conclusion is shared by all other clinical practice guidelines for PTSD. It should be noted that exposure therapy (including both PE and CPT) was judged as the only evidence-based approach for PTSD in the recent report of the U.S. Institute of Medicine (2008) report. Indeed, treatments that include exposure therapy emerged in our review as the consensual choice for the most powerful and reliable treatment for PTSD at this time.

However, not all patients who receive CBT benefit from treatment, and it is yet unclear what factors predict success. First, as with any other treatment, therapists must be trained in the various interventions that come under the heading of CBT, and some interventions (e.g., cognitive therapy) require more training than others (e.g., relaxation). Second, the treatment is demanding for both the therapist and the patient because it requires that the therapist be disciplined and focus on employing the particular intervention rather than on attending to issues that are extraneous to treatment goals. Third, the patient needs to be motivated and able to adhere to treatment requirements, including active engagement with treatment demands both during the session and at home. Although most of the studies have been conducted in specialty clinics, where therapists are highly trained and experienced in motivating their patients to comply with treatment demands, Foa and her colleagues (Foa, Hembree, et al., 2005) have demonstrated the transportability of PE therapy to community clinics that serve female survivors of rape. Similarly, Schnurr and colleagues (2007) have shown that new therapists can be efficiently trained to provide good-to-excellent PE, despite lack of previous experience delivering such treatment.

Importantly, the administration of CBT, like the administration of any therapy for PTSD, needs to adhere to general, responsible clinical practices, such as careful assessment of suicidality that may dictate preliminary therapy (e.g., the administration of medication or short-term hospitalization). Likewise, patients inundated with personal problems may require attention for those problems before they attend to their PTSD symptoms. This means that whereas some patients are ready to participate in a straight CBT protocol, others require a global treatment plan in which CBT is only one of several therapeutic components.

Although several CBT studies have compared the efficacy of specific interventions (e.g., cognitive therapy, exposure) and their combinations, only one study (mentioned earlier; Rothbaum et al., 2006) has examined the combination of CBT and other treatment approaches (e.g., SSRI pharmacotherapy). An extremely encouraging development is that some studies have monitored long-term follow-up and shown the stability of successful treatment for 9 months (Resick et al., 2002), 1 year (Foa, Hembree, et al., 2005), and even over a 5-year period (Tarrier & Summerfield, 2004). This is especially impressive considering the fact that successful pharmacotherapy responders must remain on medication, whereas a single 10- to 12-session successful course of CBT appears to maintain such improvement for years.

Also, because CBT programs routinely include several components, the relative contribution of each to program success is as yet unknown. In this respect, we know little about the extent to which it is crucial to focus the treatment on recollections of the traumatic event (reliving or imaginal exposure), or on erroneous cognitions or their current consequences (e.g., avoidance and negative self-perception). Indeed, based on the success of both PE and CPT, it is generally believed that remission can only be achieved through active processing of traumatic material. There is, however, some evidence to suggest that an approach focusing on symptom management rather than trauma processing may also be effective for some people. A few RCTs involving stress inoculation therapy (SIT) or present-centered therapies (PCT) may be effective for some people. Studies on SIT, reported by Cahill and colleagues (Chapter 7, this volume), although few in number, have had promising results. (It is important to note, however, that SIT includes cognitive and

exposure components.) Two studies with PCT (involving symptom management and problem-solving techniques) have shown positive results, although,
in both studies, treatment that focused on processing of the trauma was more
effective (McDonagh-Coyle et al., 2005; Schnurr et al., 2007). Clearly, more
research is needed on different approaches, not only to determine efficacy
but also to discover whether certain (e.g., trauma-focused) treatments are
better for some, whereas present-centered approaches are better for others.
Given the present state of knowledge, however, there is little evidence favoring these present-centered approaches. Therefore, we can only recommend
PE and CPT as first-line CBT treatments for PTSD at this time.

Some studies indicate that CBT has more modest effects among male
veterans with PTSD than among female assault victims. Is this differential
efficacy due to gender differences, trauma differences (e.g., combat vs. sexual
trauma), or does it suggest differences in PTSD chronicity, severity, or comorbidity? We do not have answers to these questions because information about
factors that predict treatment response is scarce. Such information, however,
is crucial for the clinical management of patients and decisions about treatment implementation. Recent findings that show positive results following PE
(Cahill, Hembree, & Foa, 2006) among combat veterans in Israel, CPT treatment among male Vietnam War veterans (Monson et al., 2006), and traffic
accident survivors (Blanchard et al., 2004) suggest that male gender per se
may not be a contraindication for CBT treatment.

It is important to note that CBT therapists routinely measure and monitor progress during therapy (e.g., by repeated evaluation of subjective distress
during exposure, inspecting homework diaries during cognitive therapy).
Our knowledge about all treatments would be greatly enhanced if this practice were adopted by therapists using other approaches.

Finally, exciting recent developments have provided CBT treatment utilizing virtual reality technology, Internet delivery systems, and telehealth
methodology. Such approaches are at a relatively preliminary stage with
regard to rigorous tests, although a few reports are noteworthy (e.g., Litz,
Engel, Bryant, & Papa, 2007; Welch & Rothbaum, 2007). We look forward to
further developments in this area that raise the possibility of providing effective PTSD treatments for people who currently cannot benefit from available
alternatives.

Pharmacotherapy

Research has identified a number of pharmacological agents, mainly among
the antidepressants, capable of significantly reducing PTSD symptoms. It is
important to recognize that no medication tested thus far was developed with
the unique pathophysiology of PTSD in mind. Indeed, all tested agents were
originally developed and approved for some other psychiatric, neurological,
or medical disorder. The list includes antidepressants, antiadrenergic agents,
anticonvulsants, the new generation of antipsychotics, and anxiolytics. Impor-

tantly, although the pharmacotherapy of PTSD, like that of most other anxiety disorders, seems capable of controlling symptoms, it does not yet have a clear effect on the course of the disorder. In that sense, hopes for recovery, as opposed to remission, are not supported by current research, especially because pharmacotherapy responders must either remain on medication indefinitely or be at significant risk for relapse. (In this regard, PTSD outcomes are no different than pharmacotherapy outcomes for depression and other anxiety disorders.) It is possible that new agents, with different pharmacological modes of action that are more potent in correcting biological abnormalities associated with PTSD, will someday find their way into general practice. Indeed, already some promising candidate medications are being developed and tested.

At present, remission rates from pharmacotherapy are considerably lower than those achieved with CBT. Partly for this reason there is no consensus on whether it is appropriate to consider SSRIs as evidence-based treatments for PTSD. Whereas some practice guideline, including this one (along with the American Psychiatric Association [2004] and the U.S. Veterans Affairs/ Department of Defense [VA/DoD] clinical practice guidelines [VA/DoD Clinical Practice Working Group, 2003]) have done so, others have not (Institute of Medicine, 2008; National Collaborating Centre for Mental Health, 2005). In addition, pharmacotherapy may effectively treat comorbid depression and anxiety disorders (e.g., panic disorder, social phobia, or OCD). An intriguing question, mentioned earlier, concerns combined treatments. A few studies have suggested that partial responders to medication may achieve full remission after CBT is added (Rothbaum et al., 2006). Several small studies indicate that partial responders to SSRIs do much better when the medication is augmented with atypical antipsychotic agents (see Friedman, Davidson, & Stein, Chapter 9, this volume). We expect this new and very important research area to draw a great deal of attention in future years. This suggests that augmentation techniques, such as the ones used in resistant depression, might also work in PTSD. A related issue is that patients with PTSD are often treated with several compounds. Although our research to date has generally focused on one medication at a time, systematic investigations of combination therapy, either concurrently or sequentially, are definitely needed.

Unlike many other disorders, PTSD has an identifiable starting point; hence, it may be amenable to preventive pharmacotherapy. A few small trials with promising results suggest that administration of propranolol or hydrocortisone or imipramine shortly after the traumatic event might prevent the later development of PTSD. This is obviously an exciting and important area for further research.

Treatment of Children and Adolescents

Some of the most impressive advances in research since the publication of the first edition of this book have occurred in the area of treatments for children and adolescents. To briefly summarize some of these, there is now evidence that an attachment/psychodynamic-based treatment, child–parent psychotherapy (CPP), reduces PTSD symptoms in preschoolers exposed to domestic violence; CPP was provided in homes and clinics in English and Spanish to multiply-traumatized mothers and their young children. Cognitive-behavioral intervention for trauma in schools (CBITS) has been shown to improve PTSD and depressive symptoms in children exposed to violence; CBITS has the clear advantage of being provided in school settings, where difficult-to-access children may be reached. Several trauma-focused, cognitive-based models for children now also possess evidence of efficacy. The most tested model, trauma-focused CBT (TF-CBT), has been evaluated in several additional studies, including a multisite study of more than 200 children, most of whom experienced multiple traumas, that combined TF-CBT + sertraline (noted earlier). Other CBT-based treatments include a child-friendly version of narrative exposure therapy (KIDNET) for refugee children and Seeking Safety (SS) for youth with comorbid PTSD and substance abuse. A child EMDR trial with sound methodology has also demonstrated positive results (see Cohen, Mannarino, Deblinger, & Berliner, Chapter 8, this volume).

Additional progress with regard to the development of psychological first aid and novel Web-based dissemination models offer examples of how rapidly the child PTSD field has progressed. However, challenges remain in providing effective treatments for children with PTSD. Pharmacological studies are few, and this is likely to continue to be the case for a variety of reasons, including legitimate concerns about possible medication side effects. Some therapists continue to use interventions that are known to be ineffective or even dangerous for children (e.g., rebirthing or other restrictive interventions). Despite these challenges, the child trauma field has much to be proud of and continues to make important strides forward.

Eye Movement Desensitization and Reprocessing

Among the advances highlighted in this edition are solid studies demonstrating the efficacy of EMDR. Most, but not all, clinical practice guidelines now consider EMDR an evidence-based treatment for PTSD. In the United Kingdom, the National Collaborating Centre for Mental Health (2005) guidelines concluded that the evidence is stronger for EMDR than for pharmacotherapy. On the other hand, in the United States, the Institute of Medicine (2008) report concluded that there is sufficient empirical evidence to support the efficacy of exposure therapies, but insufficient evidence for the efficacy of both EMDR and pharmacotherapy. Nevertheless, we are persuaded by the evidence and rank EMDR as an evidence-based, Level A treatment for PTSD in adults. Importantly, the quality of research on EMDR has improved greatly since the first edition of this book, and it is on this basis that we derive our decision.

As noted by Spates, Koch, Cusack, Pagoto, and Waller (Chapter 11, this volume), many dismantling studies continue to cast doubt on the proposed mechanism of action given that EMDR without eye movements (or some other repetitive motor activity) appears to be as effective as EMDR that includes such movements. In view of its success, it becomes very important to understand how EMDR works. Keane (1998) noted the need for a compelling theoretical model for understanding EMDR 10 years ago; the absence of a conceptual model that highlights the role of its treatment components will limit progress in understanding how, why, and for whom this treatment works. Is EMDR a variant of CBT, in which the exposure is achieved through a different protocol (Lohr, Lilienfeld, Tolin, & Herbert, 1999)? Does it achieve its results through the process proposed by Shapiro (Shapiro & Maxfield, 2002) or through a different mechanism of action? Or is its success due to a unique combination of proven, client-centered approaches (Hyer & Brandsma, 1997; Lohr et al., 1999)? In this regard, it is clear that several of the eight stages of EMDR include components that overlap with many other therapies, such as obtaining a patient's history, treatment planning, establishing a therapeutic relationship, education about PTSD, assessment, identifying maladaptive and adaptive cognitions, and imaging the traumatic memory. Which components are essential for the favorable outcomes observed to date?

Group Therapy

Group therapy is recommended as a useful component of treatment for PTSD related to a variety of traumatic experiences. Interestingly, studies of the efficacy of group psychotherapy seem to indicate that interventions addressing the trauma directly produce similar effects to those of interventions that do not address the trauma, such as assertive training and supportive interventions: All active group interventions yielded significant improvement relative to no-treatment or wait-list controls. In other words, a variety of approaches, including cognitive-behavioral, interpersonal, process–interpersonal, and insight-oriented, have all been associated with positive outcomes. However, there are relatively few RCTs with sufficient sample size to warrant definitive recommendations. This is unfortunate because group approaches are widely used and efficient in terms of clinical resources, and especially so with individuals exposed to a similar traumatic experience (e.g., sexual, military, disaster).

Although research on group therapy is even more challenging than clinical trials on individual treatments, we hope that investigators will take up this challenge to help answer questions that are very important to practitioners. Such questions include head-to-head comparisons of different group modalities to determine whether one is superior to the others, or questions of treatment matching to determine which people might benefit most from which group approach. Most important is the question of relative efficacy of group compared to individual therapy and, to be more specific, which group approaches might be better than which individual approaches.

It is possible that the mutual support, empowerment, collective problem solving, and shared perspectives provided within any group format are more powerful than the specific therapeutic approach that differentiates one group treatment from another. On the other hand, it is possible that the focus on the person's unique problems, and the absence of possible interruption of the therapeutic process by some group members, favors individual therapy. We need to find out which is more effective, for whom, and under what circumstances because the comparison between individual and group therapy will have a great impact on the field. To this end, future research should compare individual and group therapy, and evaluate specific processes in both treatment formats in well controlled studies with larger samples, in which patients are randomly assigned to different conditions.

Psychodynamic Therapy

Kudler, Krupnick, Blank, Herman, and Horowitz (Chapter 14, this volume) provide a thoughtful review of psychodynamic theory and treatment techniques, allowing the reader to reflect on the role of basic interpersonal processes and interactions between therapist and patient in the treatment of PTSD. Indeed, one of the strengths of the psychodynamic approach is its focus on generic elements of therapeutic encounters, including therapy for PTSD. On the other hand, there is very little empirical research on the efficacy of psychodynamic treatment for PTSD. This is partly due to the fact that a typical goal of psychodynamically oriented psychotherapy is to affect factors such as the capacity for human relatedness or one's incomplete view of one's past, rather than to reduce symptoms of specific disorders such as PTSD (which is the aim of therapies such as CBT and medication), for which we do not have satisfactory assessment methodology. Given the current emphasis of the practice guidelines on PTSD, Kudler and colleagues do not focus on those patients for whom psychodynamic therapies might provide the best approach: the repeatedly traumatized, deeply injured, and chronically impaired survivors of protracted interpersonal trauma, sometimes diagnosed with "complex PTSD." Such patients' most salient problems have less to do with DSM-IV PTSD symptoms, and more to do with interpersonal and intrapsychic deficiencies, mistrust of others, self-devaluation, dissociation, somatization, impulsivity, self-destructive behavior, and poor affective modulation. It should be clearly stated, therefore, that the effectiveness of psychodynamic psychotherapies for "complex PTSD" and related problems is simply not addressed in the empirical literature.

Psychosocial Rehabilitation

Psychosocial rehabilitation techniques have been proven to be valuable in the treatment of severe and persistently mentally ill (SMI) patients, especially with regard to work therapy and case management. Indeed, an emerging empirical literature demonstrates the efficacy of such approaches with patients with schizophrenia and affective disorders in a variety of public sector programs. Because PTSD is often a comorbid disorder for such patients (Mueser et al., 1998), and because patients with severe and chronic PTSD are often found among SMI cohorts and in homeless shelters (Friedman & Rosenheck, 1996), it makes sense to design and test psychosocial rehabilitation programs. Such treatments would have some distinctive therapeutic components given the unique social avoidance, hyperarousal, and related psychopathology of PTSD in comparison to other psychiatric disorders. Most importantly, patients referred for such treatment would be evaluated primarily in terms of self-care, independent living, family function, social skills, and maintenance of gainful employment rather than in terms of reduced PTSD symptoms. We hope that these specific areas will be evaluated systematically, and that reha-bilitation techniques specific to PTSD-related impairments will be developed and studied. Some encouraging preliminary studies exist, and there is a need for systematic replication of observational studies to ensure that the rehabili-tative approach to patients with PTSD is examined in earnest.

Hypnosis

As noted by Cardeña, Maldonado, and van der Hart in Chapter 17 (this volume), hypnosis is one of the oldest psychotherapy techniques applied to trauma-related disturbances. This rich history makes hypnosis a natural can-didate when the therapist considers therapeutic options. Yet, despite this fas-cinating history on which the authors rely in their clear description of how to integrate hypnosis into the general treatment of PTSD, we have very little empirical evidence for the efficacy of this technique. There are only two RCTs: an older study that showed similar outcomes from hypnotherapy and from other treatments (Brom et al., 1989), and a more recent study demonstrating a small therapeutic effect for hypnosis + CBT when compared to CBT alone on the reexperiencing symptoms only (Bryant, Moulds, Guthrie, & Nixon, 2005); both groups were equivalent 3 years later.

Marital and Family Therapy

Marital and family therapy for PTSD encompasses two approaches: support-ive and active (or "systemic") treatment. One problem with assessing family therapy for PTSD is that reduction in PTSD symptoms may not be the appro-priate outcome variable for therapy that has as its goal improvement of the marital unit. Although PTSD-related distress may be alleviated when family relationships improve, such an outcome is not specific to PTSD and may be seen in other disorders, such as schizophrenia. Clearly, the impact of PTSD on families is extensive. Treating the impact of PTSD on the family is valu-able given the profound changes across many domains of functioning. On the other hand, family therapy that focuses primarily on the person with PTSD, without fortifying the family, may not address other family members' needs for support. It would seem that a critical role for marital and family therapy is the attempt to achieve a clinically meaningful balance between addressing dysfunctional symptoms and behavior of the patient with PTSD and the distress of family members whose needs also require attention. This is an open and very important area for future research.

Unfortunately, there has been very little research in this area since publication of the first edition of this book. It is encouraging that two recent approaches (Devilly, 2002; Monson, Schnurr, Stevens, & Guthrie, 2004) have attempted to improve both the quality of the relationship and PTSD symptoms. We look forward to further research in this important area.

Creative Therapies

As with hypnosis, rehabilitation, and marital and family therapies, creative arts therapies address important dimensions of PTSD and may often be effective during impasses that other treatment techniques fail to address. Therefore, the reader is invited to consider the information provided about these techniques and their specific targets that may apply to his or her patients. Better efficacy in reduction of PTSD symptoms may be achieved once a breakthrough is attained via creative arts therapies. Interestingly, creative arts therapies do not escape the typical problems encountered in treating PTSD, that is, the balance between addressing current problems (e.g., alexithymia) and delving into past trauma, and between uncovering and reshaping traumatic material and finding new, "future-oriented" ways of expression. It is interesting to consider the possibility that creative arts therapies provide a unique (and usually nonverbal) format in which to provide imaginal exposure, cognitive restructuring, and anxiety management—approaches that overlap with CBT. This intriguing possibility requires rigorous scientific examination. Although creative arts therapies may capture the imagination of the therapist, it is important to keep in mind that, as with many other therapies discussed in this volume, empirical evidence for their efficacy with PTSD and other, related symptoms is not available.

Treatment of PTSD and Comorbid Conditions

Because 80% of people with PTSD are likely to have at least one additional psychiatric disorder (Kessler, Sonnega, Bromet, Hughes, & Nelson, 1995), comorbidity is the rule rather than the exception. Although research in this area is at an early stage, it is a mark of genuine progress that an entire chapter is dedicated to this topic; no such chapter appeared in the first edition of this book. The greatest advances have been made with regard to comorbid PTSD and substance use disorder (SUD) in which the Seeking Safety model has been rigorously tested and shown to be effective (Najavits, Gallop, & Weiss, 2006). This integrated, present-focused, coping skills model is notable because it was designed specifically for both comorbid disorders. Such proactive targeting of commonly co-occurring disorders is the exception rather than the rule because other evidence regarding effective comorbid treatment is generally from studies in which PTSD was the targeted disorder, but researchers found, retrospectively, that simultaneous improvement in other co-occurring disorders (e.g., depression or generalized anxiety disorder) contributed to the ultimate clinical outcome of a specific treatment. For PTSD and other psychiatric conditions, the treatment of concomitant psychiatric disorders is another key area that demands future research.

Summary

Now that we have briefly reviewed the chapters on each specific treatment and identified cross-cutting issues in the treatment outcome literature, we are ready to tackle our key questions enunciated at the beginning of this chapter. Here, very few experimental data guide our answers. But practicing clinicians cannot wait for slow-paced scientific research to come to the rescue. Patients with PTSD demand treatment immediately. Decisions must be made about choice of treatment, treatment combinations, reasonable expectations from treatment, length of treatment and follow-up, PTSD-specific treatment issues that cut across treatment modalities, how to approach complex clinical pictures and comorbid conditions, how to make sense of clinical difficulties and, most importantly, how to assess failure.

Choosing a Goal for Treatment

As noted earlier, the choice of treatment should be informed by the patient's needs, abilities, and preferences. The first step in making a decision about choice of treatment involves defining the treatment goals and considering whether they are achievable. With most individuals with PTSD, reduction of PTSD symptoms is among the main targets. But in some patients, whose comorbid symptoms and conduct symptoms are more distressing and disabling, these symptoms may need to be addressed first. For many patients, symptom reduction is the major focus of treatment. For some, however, stabilization and prevention of relapse may take precedence. In other cases, the initial goal of treatment is to help patients realize that they need to address their PTSD problems by seeking psychological or medical treatment (e.g., instead of drinking or acting out). Still others may have stressful life events or adverse life conditions that must be addressed first, to bring reactivation of PTSD or deterioration to a halt. Many children are brought to treatment for behavior problems unrelated to trauma issues, and their traumatic experiences and/or PTSD symptoms are discovered serendipitously. For some of these families, addressing the trauma issues will be irrelevant or undesired. In this situation, it will be critical for the clinician to address children's behavior problems concurrently, if not primarily, or the family may not return to therapy. Finally, whereas the patients themselves are the identified focus, treatment may need to involve other individuals, such as family members and others who are reciprocally involved in a significant relationship that has been adversely affected by the expression of PTSD symptoms.

• *How should one choose among treatment modalities?* Currently, there are no clear guidelines for choosing among treatment modalities. However, several criteria for making such choices are recommended. Among those, expected efficacy should be first because without such efficacy, the core concept of "treatment" is violated. This is why this practice guideline has placed such emphasis on efficacy throughout this volume. Following efficacy, one should evaluate the effectiveness of specific treatments on associated disorders and conditions. Potential difficulties, side effects, and negative effects (i.e., iatrogenic) of treatment must also be considered. Acceptability and consent should come next, followed by an evaluation of cost, length, and cultural appropriateness of the treatment. Accessibility is a key consideration for both children and adults. For children, acceptability is of particular importance because some treatments that may be available in school settings are much easier for children to access than those to which parents or other caregivers must bring their children every week. Even if efficacy or effectiveness of a school-based treatment were somewhat less than that of a clinic-based treatment, if a clinician knew that a particular family was unlikely to attend the clinic-based treatment, then it would be preferable to refer the child to the less effective, school-based treatment because the child would at least be likely to receive that treatment (i.e., receiving pretty good treatment is better than not receiving very good treatment). Finally, one should evaluate one's own resources and skills, as well as potential forensic implications of treatment. These general considerations have special implications for the treatment of traumatized survivors with PTSD.

Criteria for Choosing Treatment for PTSD

- Expected efficacy for amelioration of PTSD severity
- Associated disorders and problems
- Difficulties, side effects, and negative effects
- Acceptability and consent
- Cultural appropriateness
- Length, cost, and availability of resources
- Legal, administrative, and forensic implications
- Accessibility and acceptability to the family

Efficacy, as used here, relates specifically to prevention, amelioration, or eradication of PTSD symptoms. All things being equal, the selected treatment should be one that has proven successful in empirical studies.

Associated disorders and conditions relate to all or some dimensions and associated features of PTSD, such as depression, suicidality, violent behavior, or drinking habits. In some cases, treatment may have to stabilize an unstable condition (or patient) to prevent adverse events (loss of job) or conduct (drinking) before addressing PTSD per se. For example, suicidal behavior may require hospitalization; alcohol dependence, detoxification; and severe depression may require antidepressant medication. Whenever possible, it is desirable to select a treatment that might be expected to ameliorate the urgent problem and the PTSD simultaneously. For example, an SSRI would be a good choice for both severe depression and PTSD. Hospitalization would be indicated for suicidal symptoms, but it might also provide an opportunity to initiate PTSD treatment. And combined alcoholism–PTSD treatment may be the best choice when drinking behavior is the most urgent problem.

Side effects include effects that are pertinent to each treatment technique (e.g., loss of appetite with some drugs), as well as those pertinent to PTSD (e.g., temporary exacerbation of symptoms with trauma-focused treatment). Difficulties, side effects, and negative effects may also result from interactions between therapists and traumatized patients. One should remember that PTSD is associated with increased physiological and psychological reactivity, which may be specific (e.g., related to one's traumatic experiences) or nonspecific (e.g., generated by environmental demands).

In contrast to some views, *acceptability* and *consent* are neither categorical (yes or no) nor a priori statements given by the patient at the outset of therapy. Acceptability and consent are dynamic processes that are often fragile and brittle. Trust may have to be renewed, or regained, explicitly or implicitly, at each treatment encounter, particularly in survivors of dehumanizing, man-made traumas. Furthermore, patient preference must be weighed carefully in the choice of treatment. For example, some patients may be strongly opposed to medication, whereas others may be opposed to trauma-focused treatment that necessitates work on traumatic memories. In both cases, therapists' beliefs about what treatments are best must be subordinated to the likelihood that a patient will accept and comply with the treatment that has been prescribed.

Acceptability across *cultural boundaries* is particularly relevant in the case of refugees, who may or may not be prepared to accept the way their suffering is appraised and treated in another culture (e.g., as a mental disorder). Cross-gender problems may be seen in survivors of gender-related traumata. Indeed, many trauma survivors may wonder how much their therapist can "truly understand" and genuinely relate to their traumatic experiences, which they often perceive as ineffable. Treatments must also be developmentally, culturally, and contextually appropriate. Therapies developed for school-age children need to be adapted to make them more acceptable for younger children or teens. Implementation of child treatments has to be individualized for children of different cultures, genders, trauma experiences, and developmental levels. For example, different therapeutic activities, books, games, and educational materials would be needed for a 5-year-old Mexican American girl who experienced sexual abuse and for a 12-year-old refugee African boy who witnessed the murder of his parents; these children would need different materials than would a 16-year-old African American girl who experienced domestic violence.

Conceptually, issues of *cost* and *availability of resources* are extremely important in many societies, especially in poorer nations and in inner-city ghettos within wealthier nations. The cost of some SSRIs may be prohibitive in underdeveloped countries and poor provinces, and the likelihood of finding a skilled psychologist or psychiatrist is very low in disaster areas in Africa or in Central and South America. The likelihood of finding a qualified CBT therapist is not very great, even in the developed nations, although current dissemination efforts may change that significantly. Child psychiatrists are rare across the world. Indeed, in any mass disaster, the number of victims is likely to overwhelm the best efforts to provide skilled professional help. Whereas such shortages may exist in other conditions as well (e.g., AIDS), there are currently few simplified treatment protocols for PTSD like those emerging for the prevention of AIDS in poorer countries. One example of such a protocol is a culturally modified version of TF-CBT for HIV-affected, sexually abused children in Zambia, which has been developed and is being delivered by local paraprofessionals. The development of low-cost treatment for traumatized survivors with PTSD is a major task for the future of our field.

Finally, for many traumatized individuals, *legal, administrative,* or *forensic* elements are likely to be (or to become) associated with the treatment. Prevalent examples are litigation, financial coverage for the treatment, recognition of disability and entitlement for pension, reparations, and/or compensation. There are many ways that such elements can be linked with, or affect, the conduct of treatment and its expected outcome. Therapists should identify such issues and make their implications for therapy explicit in each individual case.

- *How can one combine various treatment techniques?* Combined treatments are common for PTSD despite the fact that limited empirical data support this practice. Indeed, in one of the few studies pertinent to this question, Foa and colleagues (1999) found that prolonged exposure alone and stress inoculation therapy (SIT) alone had better outcomes than a treatment that combined prolonged exposure and SIT. Several studies found that cognitive restructuring did not augment exposure therapy alone (Foa et al., 1999). In practice, most CBT approaches combine several different modalities, as do most pharmacotherapeutic approaches in which patients with PTSD frequently receive two or more different types of drugs. Another common clinical occurrence is that many patients with PTSD who receive some sort of individual psychotherapy also receive at least one medication. Such patients may receive group, marital, or family therapy, in addition to individual psychotherapy and drug treatment. Although clinicians often prescribe combined treatments with the belief that such combinations augment treatment outcome, such clinical practices need to be tested in rigorous experimental protocols. We have noted previously the one study in which partial responders to SSRI treatment showed significantly better outcomes after augmentation with CBT (Rothbaum et al., 2006). We also have cited several small studies in which SSRI partial responders exhibited significant improvement after augmentation pharmacotherapy with atypical antipsychotic agents (see Friedman et al., Chapter 9, this volume). Research of this type is a very high priority given the frequency of partial rather than complete remission following a particular course of therapy, and given how often patients with PTSD are concurrently prescribed more than one treatment.

The scant empirical evidence for combined approaches should not be interpreted as evidence against the efficacy of such treatments. Given the importance of this issue and the widespread prevalence of combined PTSD treatment in current clinical practice, we strongly recommend that treatments be introduced one at a time, in a sensible sequence that takes into account the patient's choices and the therapist's experience. After the therapist has chosen (and the patient has accepted) a specific initial treatment, there must be an adequate clinical trial of this approach to determine its effectiveness. If clinical goals are achieved, there is no need for additional treatments. If treatment is ineffective, or if it produces intolerable side effects, it must be discontinued and a different approach initiated. In the usual clinical scenario, however, patients achieve enough improvement to suggest that the initial treatment was effective, but that improvement was insufficient to cause them to be satisfied with the results. This is the time to introduce a second treatment, while maintaining the first treatment as initially prescribed. Again, treatment success (or failure) will be determined by whether predefined goals have been achieved. If so, efforts should be made to reduce or terminate the first treatment because it may have been superceded by the more potent, second treatment. A common problem is that once started, a treatment may be maintained indefinitely, even though its usefulness is questionable. We believe that combined treatments probably have a very important place in PTSD treatment and must be clarified by future research. We also believe that any treatment, combined or not, should be evaluated periodically to ensure that it is still needed to maintain desirable clinical outcomes.

- *How to approach complex clinical pictures and comorbid conditions?* We have already discussed complex clinical conditions in which psychiatric crises must be addressed before initiating treatment for PTSD. These include suicidal behavior, alcohol dependence, incapacitating depression, and, in children, severe behavior problems (see the section on choosing treatment for PTSD). We have also discussed combined treatments in which two or more clinical approaches have been prescribed for PTSD. These two issues must be reconsidered when PTSD is associated with at least one comorbid psychiatric disorder. As noted previously and discussed extensively by Najavitz and colleagues in Chapter 21 (this volume), comorbidity is a problem faced frequently by clinicians. Most commonly, PTSD is associated with comorbid affective (e.g., depression, dysthymia) or anxiety (panic, social phobia, obsessive–compulsive) disorders or alcohol–drug abuse/dependency. In addition, the high prevalence of PTSD among SMI patients with schizophrenia and chronic affective disorder is receiving increased recognition (Mueser et al., 1998). Finally, comorbid personality, and dissociative and somatoform disorders (often associated with prolonged childhood trauma) are another treatment challenge frequently seen in clinical practice.

As reviewed by Najavitz and colleagues (Chapter 21, this volume), a small body of research has begun to test interventions for PTSD and comorbid substance use disorder, major depression, generalized anxiety disorder, OCD, borderline personality disorder, and psychotic disorder. Because the quality of the research is mixed, the strength of evidence is mixed. Seeking Safety has emerged as a Level A treatment for comorbid PTSD and SUD, but evidence regarding other treatments is uneven in quality.

There are several ways to design a treatment plan when PTSD is associated with a comorbid disorder. Given the dictum "less is more," pharmacotherapists and CBT practitioners should start with a single treatment that might be expected to normalize both disorders simultaneously. For example, an SSRI would appear to be a logical first choice when PTSD is comorbid with depression, panic disorder, or OCD. However, it is all too common in children, as well as adults, to see patients on a "cocktail" of medications because, when one medication did not work, instead of discontinuing it, another was added to "augment" it. Before long, the patient is on 3, 4, 5, or 10 medications, without any possible way of determining which are (or are not) improving or (worsening) any of the patient's symptoms. Time then has to be spent weaning the patient off of all of these medications and starting over again (if the patient can be weaned off). This problem, which is not restricted to PTSD, is common to many situations in which patients have challenging comorbid problems that do not seem to respond to simple treatments. However the dictum of "more is more" rarely works well.

Similarly, a CBT protocol for PTSD could incorporate specific modules that address panic, social phobia, and OCD. CBT can also incorporate relapse prevention components (Foy, Glynn, Ruzek, Riney, & Gusman, 1997) to address alcohol–drug abuse/dependency. Finally, we recommend simultaneous treatment of PTSD and comorbid chemical abuse/dependency (Kofoed, Friedman, & Peck, 1993) rather than the all-too-frequent approach, in which they are treated sequentially, usually starting with detoxification and alcohol–drug rehabilitation before progressing to PTSD treatment (except in extreme cases in which the severity of addiction or chemical dependency makes PTSD treatment impossible). These guidelines would not apply when the therapist's choice of PTSD treatment is without proven efficacy with the comorbid disorder. Several CBT programs (e.g., prolonged exposure, cognitive processing therapy) have demonstrated that in addition to reduction in PTSD severity, depression and general anxiety also decrease. However, if the preferred approach is psychodynamic, group, or marital therapy, a separate treatment must be prescribed for the comorbid disorder. If the comorbid disorder is the first order of business because of urgency or severity, it must be addressed before PTSD treatment can begin. For example, if PTSD is comorbid with severe depression, antidepressant medication might be the best initial step. PTSD treatment should be delayed until depressive symptoms are under control. At that point, psychodynamic, group, or marital therapy can be initiated. As detailed previously (see the section on combined treatments), we recommend that all treatments (whether for the comorbid disorder or for PTSD) be introduced one at a time and be given an adequate clinical trial before discontinuation or addition of other treatments. We also reiterate our recommendation that all treatments (for PTSD, as well as for comorbid disorders) be evaluated periodically to ensure that they are still needed to maintain desirable clinical outcomes.

• *How long should a treatment be followed?* We know very little about long-term maintenance of favorable treatment outcomes for two major reasons: because we lack the relevant scientific data, and because of the nature of PTSD itself. First, with the notable exception of CBT, in which treatment effects have been maintained up to 5 years, most posttreatment outcome studies rarely monitor clinical status beyond 1 year. Clearly, long-term research is needed to help us develop reasonable expectations for longitudinal maintenance of therapeutic gains. With regard to pharmacotherapy, the classic research design is a discontinuation study, in which successfully medicated patients are randomized to placebo or continuation drug conditions to determine relapse rates with and without treatment over a long follow-up period. With regard to CBT, EMDR, and other time-limited psychotherapies, the operative questions are (1) how long the beneficial outcomes from treatment can be sustained; and (2) whether treatment benefits can (or should) be fortified by periodic booster sessions, and, if so, how often and for how long such booster sessions should be scheduled.

Second, people who have recovered naturally from an episode of PTSD are at greater risk for subsequent episodes if exposed to traumatic or trauma-related stimuli in the future. It is our hope that the coping skills acquired from psychotherapy will make individuals less vulnerable to future relapse than people with PTSD who have not received such treatment. An important focus for the future, therefore, must be to design interventions that foster resilience and prevent relapse. In the long run, such treatments will be much more valuable than approaches limited to amelioration of current symptoms.

• *Are there features of PTSD that require special attention beyond the active ingredient of treatment?* No matter what treatment or combination of treatments seem best, diagnosticians and therapists must keep in mind several unique features of PTSD. The initial assessment must be approached cautiously because patients are asked to retrieve and to relate traumatic memories that they usually try to avoid and suppress. Clinicians must respect such defenses, establish an atmosphere of trust and security, and show patience as reluctant patients' traumatic narratives unfold. The understandable ambivalence exhibited by patients with PTSD between desire for symptom relief and fear that therapy will increase their suffering by reexposing them to painful thoughts, memories, and feelings is the usual context in which the therapeutic contract must be negotiated. Realistic treatment goals must be carefully discussed. The staging and pace of treatment must be carefully considered. For severe and chronic PTSD, especially when associated with protracted trauma (as in childhood sexual abuse), it is often necessary to evaluate issues of safety and security in the home environment, as well as in the therapist's office. For example, trauma-focused psychotherapy may not be advisable for patients who continue to be exposed to traumatic events (e.g., because of ongoing domestic violence or physical/sexual abuse). In such cases, the initial phase of treatment is the establishment of safety and security. Only after this has been achieved can exposure or some other trauma-focused treatment be initiated. In this regard, it is important to remember that, for reasons addressed previously, trauma-focused treatment is not necessarily the treatment of choice for everyone.

The therapeutic alliance is paramount when implementing any of the recommended treatments presented in this review. For example, trust is an important concern for all patients with PTSD, so therapists must demonstrate both trustworthiness and professional competence. Negotiating a therapeutic contract that clearly specifies the process, time frame, and goals of treatment is one way to accomplish this. Another way is to avoid making promises that may be difficult to keep. For example, one should never promise a full recovery because it may not occur, and the risk of relapse is an ever-present possibility, even following complete remission of symptoms. This is another way to build trust, establish credibility, and generate appropriate expectations. Attention to these matters is a prerequisite for any effective therapeutic alliance with patients with PTSD.

• *How to understand treatment resistance and failure?* As with many mental disorders, PTSD, particularly in its chronic phase, is sometimes resistant to treatment. Despite repeated descriptions of difficulties and poor treatment outcomes in PTSD, *treatment resistance* for this disorder is poorly defined. Specifically, the following questions have not received convincing answers: Which treatments are being "resisted"? Which symptoms are particularly tenacious? When is it clear that a treatment is ineffective, and what should be done in such case (e.g., add more treatment, change dose, or start a new therapeutic approach)? These questions are especially difficult to answer because of the heterogeneity of treatment approaches to PTSD and traumatized populations (e.g., survivors of prolonged atrocities, survivors of torture, and survivors of discrete incidents).

At this time, the acknowledged reasons for treatment resistance in PTSD include those seen in other disorders (e.g., chronicity, comorbidity, poor compliance, adverse life circumstances), along with more specific, yet poorly explored, reasons (extreme or repeated traumatization, traumatization during critical developmental stages, etc.). No clear guidelines can be given to clinicians who encounter treatment resistance in their patients except to use their clinical wisdom to probe and eventually to improve their approach to the patient, to find out what might have gone wrong (too fast or too slow an exploration, incomplete mapping of current life stressors, lack of home practice, over- or underdosage of medication), and to use the variety of options offered in this book to refine and enrich their versatility as therapists.

Conclusion

This second edition of best practice guidelines of the International Society for Traumatic Stress Studies is still a work in progress. Although there has been considerably more research on CBT, pharmacotherapy, and EMDR than on other approaches, on balance, we still know relatively little about other treatments for PTSD monotherapies, and precious little about combined treatment approaches.

The good news is the rapid growth of rigorous clinical research in recent years. The number of new clinical trials since publication of the first edition of this volume is impressive, and the quality of the research is improving with each passing year. Many new questions are emerging, and more sophisticated research designs and analytic methods now permit us to answer previously unanswerable questions. Indeed, we fully expect that many questions posed throughout this book will have solid empirical answers within the foreseeable future. Until that time, however, we hope that the analyses of treatment research and recommendations by experts within this practice guideline will assist clinicians in the field and promote more effective treatment of PTSD internationally. In closing, we would like to thank all of those who contributed their valuable professional knowledge and skill to the creation of these best-practice guidelines.

Acknowledgments

This chapter updates the final chapter that appeared in the first edition of this book (Foa, Keane, & Friedman, 2000). Arieh Shalev was lead author of that chapter, at that time. We are indebted to him for providing the structure and many of the insights that we have retained from that original version.

References

American Psychiatric Association. (2004). Practice guidelines for the treatment of patients with acute stress disorder and posttraumatic stress disorder. *American Journal of Psychiatry, 161,* 1–31.

Barlow, D. H., & Craske, M. G. (1994). *Mastery of Your Anxiety and Panic II* (Treatment manual). Albany, NY: Graywind.

Blanchard, E. B., Hickling, E. J., Freidenberg, B. M., Malta, L. S., Kuhn, E., & Sykes, M. A (2004). Two studies of psychiatric morbidity among motor vehicle accident survivors 1 year after the crash. *Behaviour Research and Therapy, 42,* 569–593.

Brom, D., Kleber, R. J., & Defares, P. B. (1989). Brief psychotherapy for posttraumatic stress disorders. *Journal of Consulting and Clinical Psychology, 57*(5), 607–612.

Bryant, R. A., Moulds, M. L., Guthrie, R. M., & Nixon, R. D. V. (2005). The additive benefit of hypnosis and cognitive-behavioral therapy in treating acute stress disorder. *Journal of Consulting and Clinical Psychology, 73,* 334–340.

Cahill, S. P., Hembree, E. A., & Foa, E. B. (2006). Dissemination of prolonged exposure therapy for posttraumatic stress disorder: Successes and challenges. In Y. Neria, R. Gross, R. Marshall, & E. Susser (Eds.), *Mental health in the wake of terrorist attacks* (pp. 475–495). Cambridge, UK: Cambridge University Press.

Cohen, J. A., Mannarino, A. P., Perel, J. M., & Staron, V. (2007). A pilot randomized controlled trial of combined trauma-focused CBT and sertraline for childhood PTSD symptoms. *Journal of the American Academy of Child and Adolescent Psychiatry, 46,* 811–819.

Davidson, J. R.T., Foa, E. B., Huppert, J. D., Keefe, F. J., Franklin, M. E., Compton, J., et al. (2004). Fluoxetine, comprehensive cognitive behavioral therapy, and placebo in generalized social phobia. *Archives of General Psychiatry, 61,* 1005–1013.

Devilly, G. J. (2002). The psychological effects of a lifestyle management course on war veterans and their spouses. *Journal of Clinical Psychology, 58,* 1119–1134.

Foa, E. B., Dancu, C. V., Hembree, E. A., Jaycox, L. H., Meadows, E. A., & Street, G. P. (1999). A comparison of exposure therapy, stress inoculation training, and their combination for reducing posttraumatic stress disorder in female assault victims. *Journal of Consulting and Clinical Psychology, 6*(7), 194–200.

Foa, E. B., Franklin, M. E., & Moser, J. (2002). Context in the clinic: How well do cognitive-behavioral therapies and medications work in combination? *Biological Psychiatry, 52,* 989–997.

Foa, E. B., Hembree, E. A., Cahill, S. P., Rauch, S. A. M., Riggs, D. S., Feeny, N. C., et al. (2005). Randomized trial of prolonged exposure for posttraumatic stress disorder with and without cognitive restructuring: Outcome at academic and community clinics. *Journal of Consulting and Clinical Psychology, 73,* 953–964.

Foa, E. B., Keane, T. M., & Friedman, M. J. (Eds.). (2000). *Effective treatments for PTSD.* New York: Guilford Press.

Foa, E. B., Liebowitz, M. R., Kozak, M. J., Davies, S., Campeas, R., Franklin, M. E., et al. (2005). Randomized, placebo-controlled trial of exposure and ritual prevention, clomipramine, and their combination in the treatment of obsessive–compulsive disorder. *American Journal of Psychiatry, 162,* 151–161.

Foa, E. B., Rothbaum, B. O., Briggs, D. S., & Murdock, T. B. (1991). Treatment of posttraumatic stress disorder in rape victims: A comparison between cognitive-behavioral, procedures and counseling. *Journal of Consulting and Clinical Psychology, 59,* 715–723.

Foa, E. B., Rothbaum, B. O., & Furr, J. M. (2003). Augmenting exposure therapy with other CBT procedures. *Psychiatric Annals, 33,* 47–53.

Foy, D. W., Glynn, S. M., Ruzek, J. I., Riney, S. J., & Gusman, F. D. (1997). Trauma focus group therapy for combat-related PTSD. *In Session: Psychotherapy in Practice, 3,* 59–73.

Friedman, M. J., & Rosenheck, R. A. (1996). PTSD as a persistent mental illness. In S. Soreff (Ed.), *The seriously and persistently mentally ill: The state-of-the-art treatment handbook* (pp. 369–389). Seattle, WA: Hogrefe & Huber.

Heimberg, R. G., Liebowitz, M. R., Hope, D. A., Schneier, F. R., Holt, C. S., Welkowitz, L. A., et al. (1998). Cognitive behavioral group therapy vs. phenelzine therapy for social phobia: 12-week outcome. *Archives of General Psychiatry, 55,* 1133–1141.

Hyer, L. A., & Brandsma, J. M. (1997). EMDR minus eye movements equals good psychotherapy. *Journal of Traumatic Stress, 10,* 515–522.

Institute of Medicine. (2008). *Treatment of posttraumatic stress disorder: An assessment of the evidence.* Washington, DC: National Academies Press.

Keane, T. M. (1998). Psychological and behavioral treatments for posttraumatic stress disorder. In P. E. Nathan & J. Gorman (Eds.), *A guide to treatments that work* (pp. 398–407). New York: Oxford University Press

Kessler, R. C., Sonnega, A., Bromet, E., Hughes, M., & Nelson, C. B. (1995). Posttraumatic stress disorder in the National Comorbidity Survey. *Archives of General Psychiatry, 52,* 1048–1060.

Kofoed, L., Friedman, M. J., & Peck, R. (1993). Alcoholism and drug abuse in patients with PTSD. *Psychiatric Quarterly, 64,* 151–171.

Litz, B. T., Engel, C. C., Bryant, R. A., & Papa, A. (2007). A randomized, controlled proof-of-concept trial of an Internet-based, therapist-assisted self-management treatment for posttraumatic stress disorder. *American Journal of Psychiatry, 164,* 1676–1683.

Lohr, J. M., Lilienfeld, S. O., Tolin, D. F., & Herbert, J. D., (1999). Eye movement desensitization and reprocessing: An analysis of specific versus nonspecific treatment factors. *Journal of Anxiety Disorders, 13,* 185–207.

Marks, I. M., Lovell, K., Noshirvani, H., Livanou, M., & Thrasher, S. (1998). Treatment of posttraumatic stress disorder by exposure and/or cognitive restructuring: A controlled study. *Archives of General Psychiatry, 55,* 317–325.

McDonagh-Coyle, A., Friedman, M. J., McHugo, G. J., Ford, J. D., Sengupta, A., Mueser, K. T., et al. (2005). Randomized trial of cognitive-behavioral therapy for chronic posttraumatic stress disorder in adult female survivors of childhood sexual abuse. *Journal of Consulting and Clinical Psychology, 73,* 515–524.

Monson, C. M., Schnurr, P. P., Resick, P. A., Friedman, M. J., Young-Xu, Y., & Stevens, S. P. (2006). Cognitive processing therapy for veterans with military-related posttraumatic stress disorder. *Journal of Consulting and Clinical Psychology, 74,* 898–907.

Monson, C. M., Schnurr, P. P., Stevens, S. P., & Guthrie, K. A. (2004). Cognitive-behavioral couple's treatment for posttraumatic stress disorder: Initial findings. *Journal of Traumatic Stress, 17,* 341–344.

Mueser, K. T., Trumbetta, S. L., Rosenberg, S. L., Vidauer, R. M., Goodman, L. B., Osher, F. C., et al. (1998). Trauma and posttraumatic stress disorder in severe mental illness. *Journal of Consulting and Clinical Psychology, 66,* 493–499.

Najavits, L. M., Gallop, R. J., & Weiss, R. D. (2006). Seeking Safety therapy for adolescent girls with PTSD and substance use disorder: A randomized controlled trial. *Journal of Behavioral Health Services and Research, 33,* 453–463.

National Collaborating Centre for Mental Health. (2005). *Post-traumatic stress disorder: The management of PTSD in adults and children in primary and secondary care.* London: Gaskell.

Resick, P. A., Nishith, P., Weaver, T. L., Astin, M. C., & Feurer, C. A. (2002). A comparison of cognitive-processing therapy with prolonged exposure and a waiting condition for the treatment of chronic posttraumatic stress disorder in female rape victims. *Journal of Consulting and Clinical Psychology, 70,* 867–879.

Rosen, C. S., Chow, H. C., Finney, J. F., Greenbaum, M. A., Moos, R. H., Sheikh, J. I., et al. (2004). VA practice patterns and practice guidelines for treating posttraumatic stress disorder. *Journal of Traumatic Stress, 17,* 213–222.

Rothbaum, B. O., Cahill, S. P., Foa, E. B., Davidson, J. R. T., Compton, J. S., Connor, K. M., et al. (2006). Augmentation of sertraline with prolonged exposure in the treatment of posttraumatic stress disorder. *Journal of Traumatic Stress, 19,* 625–638.

Schnurr, P. P., Friedman, M. J., Engel, C. C., Foa, E. B., Shea, M. T., Chow, B. K., et al. (2007). Cognitive behavioral therapy for posttraumatic stress disorder in women: A randomized controlled trial. *Journal of the American Medical Association, 297,* 820–830.

Shapiro, F., & Maxfield, L. (2002). Eye movement desensitization and re-processing (EMDR): Information processing in the treatment of trauma. *Journal of Clinical Psychology, 58,* 933–946.

Tarrier, N., & Sommerfield, C. (2004). Treatment of chronic PTSD by cognitive therapy and exposure: 5-year follow-up. *Behavior Therapy, 35,* 231–246.

Taylor, S., Thordarson, D. S., Maxfield, L., Fedoroff, I. C., Lovell, K., & Ogrodniczuk, J. S. (2003). Comparative efficacy, speed, and adverse effects of three PTSD treatments: Exposure therapy, EMDR, and relaxation training. *Journal of Consulting and Clinical Psychology, 71,* 330–338.

VA/DoD Clinical Practice Guideline Working Group. (2003). *Management of posttraumatic stress* (Office of Quality and Performance Publication No. 10Q-CPG/PTSD-04). Washington, DC: Veterans Health Administration, Department of Veterans Affairs and Health Affairs, Department of Defense.

Welch, S. S., & Rothbaum, B. O. (2007). Emerging treatments for PTSD. In M. J. Friedman, T. M. Keane, & P. A. Resick (Eds.), *Handbook of PTSD: Science and practice* (pp. 469–496). New York: Guilford Press.

Index

Page numbers followed by *f* indicate figure, *t* indicate table.

643